ALL

HORSE

SYSTEMS

GO

ALL HORSE SYSTEMS GO

The Horse Owner's Full-Color Veterinary Care and Conditioning Resource for Modern Performance, Sport and Pleasure Horses

Nancy S. Loving, DVM

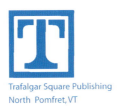

Trafalgar Square Publishing
North Pomfret, VT

First published in 2006 by
Trafalgar Square Publishing
North Pomfret, Vermont 05053

Printed in China

Copyright © 2006 Nancy S. Loving

All rights reserved. No part of this book may be reproduced, by any means, without written permission of the publisher, except by a reviewer quoting brief excerpts for a review in a magazine, newspaper, or Web site.

Disclaimer of Liability
This book is not to be used in place of veterinary care and expertise. The author and publisher shall have neither liability nor responsibility to any person or entity with respect to any loss or damage caused or alleged to be caused directly or indirectly by the information contained in this book. While the book is as accurate as the author can make it, there may be errors, omissions, and inaccuracies.

Library of Congress Cataloging-in-Publication Data
Loving, Nancy S.
  All horse systems go : the horse owner's full-color veterinary care and conditioning resource for modern performance, sport, and pleasure horses / Nancy Loving.
     p. cm.
  Includes bibliographical references and index.
  ISBN-13: 978-1-57076-326-7hc
  ISBN-10: 1-57076-326-7hc
  ISBN-13: 978-1-57076-332-8pb
  ISBN-10: 1-57076-332-1pb
  1. Horses—Diseases—Atlases. 2. Horses—Anatomy—Atlases. I. Title.
  SF951.L68 2005
  636.1'0896—dc22
                                         2005028711

Illustrations:
All the photographs in the book were taken by the author except where noted. The line drawings are by Laurie Prindle with the exception of those on pages 8, 10, 21,(*bottom left*), 28, 39, 55 (*top left*), 285, 291, and 374, which are by Patricia Peyman Naegeli. The chart on page 460 is reprinted with permission from *Feeding and Nutrition* by John Kohnke, B.V.Sc., RDA, Birubi Pacific, 1992.

Book design by Carrie Fradkin
Cover design by Heather Mansfield
Typeface: Fairfield, Myriad

10 9 8 7 6 5 4 3 2 1

This book is dedicated with love to

Barb, for her eternal inspiration to be more, in as many ways possible

Roger, for believing in me in every way, and for always being there

Bea and Mart, for such unwavering love and encouragement

Dwight, for getting the ball rolling and shooting it into the pocket

and

Flash the cat, for all his help on the keyboard.

ACKNOWLEDGMENTS

It would be hard to adequately express thanks to those who made the inner contents of this book possible:

The many devoted and diligent researchers, sports physiologists, and equine practitioners who continuously quest for answers to better the health and welfare of horses in all pursuits.

Those wonderful horse-owning clients who have entrusted the care of their horses to me for a couple of decades and have generously allowed so many of the photographs that appear in this book.

And, to all the gallant horses that have taught me so much along the way, and whose indomitable spirits are an inspiration to all of us.

Contents

CHAPTER 1
An Introduction — 1

A Horse's Body in Motion — 2
Custom-Tailored Training — 3
Strategies to Optimize Performance — 5

CHAPTER 2
Conformation for Performance — 7

Anatomy and Function — 7
Head — 11
Neck — 13
Withers — 18
Chest — 20
Shoulder — 20
Forelimb Alignment — 22
Upper Arm — 22
Forearm — 24
Knee — 24
Cannon Bone — 24
Pastern — 25
Back — 26
Hindquarters — 28
Stifle — 31
Hocks — 31
The Lower Portion of the Rear Limb — 34
Conformation Related to Specific Athletic Pursuits — 34

CHAPTER 3
The Hoof — 39

Hoof Structure and Growth — 39
  The Hoof Wall — 40
  The White Line — 44
  The Sole — 44
  The Bars — 44
  The Frog — 44
  Interactive Structures of the Foot — 45
  Foot Health, Genetics, and Performance — 46
Hoof Characteristics — 47
  Hoof Wall Integrity — 47
  Hoof Color — 47
  Hoof Size — 48
  Hoof Angle — 48
  Hoof Balance — 53
The Hoof as a Visual Record of Stress — 54
  Abnormal Hoof Contours — 54
  Hoof Wall Flares — 56
  Coronary Band Response to Uneven Stresses — 56
  Sheared Heels — 56
  Hoof Cracks — 57
Shoes and Pads — 58
  Shoeing: Injury versus Protection — 58
  Padding the Foot — 64
The Use of Hoof Dressings and Supplements — 66
  Reasons for Moisture Loss in the Hoof — 66
  Hoof Dressings — 67
  Feed Supplements for Hoof Nutrition — 67
  Maintaining Healthy Hooves — 68
The Many Faces of Hoof Lameness — 69
  Identifying a Beginning Problem — 69
  Sole Bruises, Abscesses, and Corns — 70
  Thrush, White Line Disease, and Canker — 73
  Laminitis — 74
    Characteristics of Laminitis, 74 • What is Laminitis? 75 • Metabolic Causes of Laminitis, 75 • Mechanical Causes of Laminitis, 80 • Consequences of Laminitis, 81 • Prevention of Laminitis Using Cryotherapy, 82 • Therapy for Laminitis, 82 • Recognizing Chronic Laminitis, 84
  Navicular Syndrome — 85
    What is Navicular Syndrome? 85 • Structure of the Navicular Apparatus, 86 • Etiology, 86 Understanding Diagnostic Tests for Heel Pain, 88 Palliative Treatment for Navicular Syndrome, 91

CHAPTER 4
Developing Strong Bones — 95

Bone as a System — 95
  The Remodeling Process — 96

Importance of Bone to Performance	98
Bone Size	98
Bone Density	99
Interaction of Bone with Tendons, Ligaments, and Muscle	99
Conditioning Bone to Reach Peak Strength	100
High-Speed Training	100
Skeletal Strength	101
Skeletal Maturity	102
Musculoskeletal Stress from Exercise	102
Effects of Overtraining	102
Inactivity and Layup	105
Extracorporeal Shock Wave Therapy	106
Different Machine Types	106
What Does ESWT Do?	106
Nutritional Disease of Bone	107
Nutritional Secondary Hyperparathyroidism	107

CHAPTER 5

Joints: Health, Problems and Therapies — 109

Parts of a Joint	109
Properties of Articular Cartilage	110
Joint Function	110
Signs and Symptoms of Joint Injury	112
Lameness and Pain	112
Heat and Swelling	113
Soft Tissue Injury Over Joints	114
Capped Hock, 114 • Capped Elbow, 114 Hygroma, 114	
Flexion Tests	115
Injurious Effects of Inflammation	115
Long-Term Expectations of Osteoarthritis	116
Gait Considerations of Specific Areas with Joint Pain	117
Signs of Stifle Pain, 117 • Signs of Hock Pain, 119 Ringbone, 121	
Prevention and Management of Osteoarthritis	122
Controlling Inflammation	122
Shoeing Strategies to Minimize Joint Pain	123
Medical Treatment of Degenerative Joint Disease	124
Surgical Options for Joints	128
Alternative Therapeutic Options for Joints	129
Management Strategies for Joint Problems	130
Ongoing Research into Joint Therapy	131
Joint Diseases	131
Developmental Orthopedic Disease	131
Epiphysitis, 132 • Osteochondrosis, 133 Wobbler Syndrome, 134 • Angular Limb Deformities, 134	
Lyme Disease	136

CHAPTER 6

Muscle Endurance — 137

The "Nuts and Bolts" of Muscle Tissue	137
Levers and Pulleys	137
Muscle Contraction	138
Food for Muscle Energy	139
Muscle Fuels	139
Energy Production	140
Muscles Produce Energy, 140 • Metabolism, 140 • Conserving Glycogen, 141 • Use of Energy, 142	
Muscle Fiber Types	143
Slow Twitch High Oxidative Muscle Fibers	143
Fast Twitch High Oxidative Muscle Fibers	143
Fast Twitch Low Oxidative Muscle Fibers	144
Measuring Fiber Types with a Muscle Biopsy	144
Response of Skeletal Muscle to Exercise	144
General Training Responses	144
Aerobic Skeletal Muscle Adaptations	145
Anaerobic Skeletal Muscle Adaptations	147
Muscle Conditioning	148
Long Slow Distance Training, 148 • Strength Training, 148 • Interval Training Techniques, 149	
Muscle Exercises	150
Resistance, 150 • Faster Gaits, 150 • Hill Work, 150 • Deep Footing, 150 • Benefits of Cross-Training, 150 • Sport-Specific Strengthening Exercises, 151 • Dressage, 151 • Jumping, 151 Reining, 151 • Cutting, 151	
"Detraining" the Muscles	151
Monitoring Muscular Efficiency	152
Thermistor	152
Blood Lactate	152
Warm-Up and Cool-Down Strategies	153
Warm-Up Exercises	153
Cool-Down Exercises	156
Cover-Ups, 159	
Dietary Manipulation of Muscle Performance	160
Ergogenic Acids	160
Electrolytes	162
Effects of Electrolyte Depletion, 163 • Neuromuscular Depression, 163 • Neuromuscular Hyperirritability, 163 • Thumps, 164	
Encouraging Water Intake	165
Muscle Injury or Disease	165
Muscle Fatigue: Losing the Peak	165
Tying-Up Syndrome aka Exertional Rhabdomyolysis aka Myositis	166
Clinical Signs, 166 • Recurrent Exertional Rhabdomyolysis, 166 • The Significance of Discolored Urine, 167 • The Significance of	

Myositis, 169 • *Measuring Muscle Damage by Enzyme Levels,* 170 • *What to Do with a Tied-Up Horse While Exercising,* 170 • *Preventive Thinking,* 171

Muscle Spasms Caused by Ear Ticks	171
Equine Polysaccharide Storage Myopathy	172
White Muscle Disease	173
Fibrotic Myopathy	173
Dryland Distemper aka Pigeon Fever	174
Hyperkalemic Periodic Paralysis	176
Therapy for Muscle Injury and Pain	**177**
Cold Therapy	177
Therapeutic Ultrasound	178
Acupuncture	178
Electrical Therapies	178

CHAPTER 7
Strong Tendons and Ligaments 181

The Difference between Tendons and Ligaments	**181**
Prevention of Soft Tissue Injury	**182**
Conditioning	182
Other Strategies	182
Predisposing Factors to Soft Tissue Injury	**183**
Conformation	183
Poorly Conditioned for the Task	184
Difficult Terrain	184
Quick Turns	184
Concussion Injury	184
Injury-Prone Areas	**184**
Cannon Bone Region	185
Fetlock Region	187
Signs of Injury: Diagnostic Aids	**189**
Pain, Heat, and Swelling	189
Diagnostic Ultrasound	190
Tendon and Ligament Repair	**190**
Fibrin and Granulation Tissue Repair Process	191
Exercises That Promote Healing	191
Healing Time	192
Successful Outcome versus Recurrence	192
Tendon and Ligament Therapy	**192**
Controlling Swelling and Inflammation	192

Thermal Treatment, 192 • *Cold Therapy,* 193 *Bandaging,* 194 • *Heat Therapy,* 194 • *Other Beneficial Therapies,* 195 • *Therapeutic Ultrasound,* 197 • *Extracorporeal Shock Wave Therapy,* 198

Tendon Disease: Flexural Contracture	**198**
Congenital Flexural Contracture	198
Acquired Flexural Contracture	199
Club Foot	200
Treatment of Flexural Contracture	200
Weak Flexor Tendons	201
Systemic Illness as Cause of Limb Swelling	**201**
Lymphangitis	202

CHAPTER 8
The Horse's Back 203

Horse Communication of Back Pain	**203**
Identification of Back Pain	205
Misleading Signs of Back Pain	207
Considering the Cause of Back Pain	**207**
Trauma	207
Lameness	211
Vertebral Problems	212
Therapy and Solutions for Managing Back Pain	**214**
Rest	214
Massage, Therapeutic Ultrasound, and Electrostimulation	214
Acupuncture	215
Anti-Inflammatory Medication	215
Manipulative Therapy	215
Joint Therapy	215
Exercise	215
Stretching	216
Long-Term Strategies to Manage Back Injury	216

CHAPTER 9
Cardiovascular Conditioning and Health 219

The Cardiovascular System	**219**
The Heart	219
Blood Vessels	219
The Spleen	219
Definitions of Exercise Efforts	**220**
Submaximal Exercise (Endurance)	220
Maximal Exercise (Sprint or Gallop)	220
Combination Exercise	220
Functional Cardiovascular Adaptations	**220**
Heart Rate	220
Cardiovascular Adaptations at Exercise	220
Invaluable Equipment	**222**
The Cardiotachometer	222
The Thermistor	224
Conditioning Techniques	**224**
Value of Repetition	225
Value of Walking	225
Value of Swimming	225
Long Slow Distance Training	226
Strength Training	227

Interval Training	227
Long Fast Distance Training	229
Evaluating Cardiovascular Conditioning	**229**
Fitness Indicators	229

Heart Rate Recovery, 229 • Cardiac Recovery Index, 230 • Other Metabolic Parameters to Assess Cardiovascular Fitness, 231

Standard Exercise Test	232
Maintaining Peak Form	233
Exercise Intolerance and Poor Performance	**233**
Overtraining	234
Dehydration	235
Stress Indicators	239
Heart Irregularities	240
Anemia	241

CHAPTER 10

Respiratory Conditioning and Health 245

The Respiratory System	**245**
The Upper Respiratory Tract	246
The Lower Respiratory Tract	249
Functional Adaptations of the Respiratory System	251
Situations That Overtax or Compromise the System	252
Respiratory Health and Illness	**254**
Defense against Foreign Particles	254
Factors Affecting Air Quality	256
Maintaining Air Quality	256
Stress Factors	258
Upper Respiratory Problems	258

Recurrent Laryngeal Neuropathy aka Roaring, 258

Lower Respiratory Problems	259

Inflammatory Airway Disease, 259 Recurrent Airway Obstruction aka Heaves, 260 • Managing IAD and Heaves, 261 Exercise Induced Pulmonary Hemorrhage, 262 • Respiratory Viruses, 264 • Bacterial Infection, 273

Preventing Respiratory Illness	279

CHAPTER 11

The Digestive System: Oral Cavity, Dental Care, and Intestinal Tract 281

Importance of Dental and Oral Cavity Health	**281**
Nutritional Demands	282
Problems Related to the Oral Cavity	282
Signs of Dental Problems	**284**
Eruption Patterns	285
Tooth and Mouth Issues	**286**
Wolf Teeth	286
Retained Caps	286
Abnormalities of Wear	286
Cribbing	288
Temporomandibular Joint	289
Equine Dentistry	**289**
Intestinal Anatomy: Structure and Function	**291**
The Stomach	291
The Small Intestines	292
The Large Intestines	292

The Large and Small Colon, 293

Intestinal Transit	293
Digestive Tract Disease	**293**
Diarrhea	293
Choke	295
Colic	297

Signs to Watch For, 297 • Interpreting a Horse's Pain, 298 • Vital Signs, 299 • Other Veterinary Diagnostic Tools, 301 • Types of Colic, 303 Spasmodic Colic, 303 • Impaction Colic, 303 Gaseous Colic, 308 • Intestinal Displacement or Torsion, 308 • Lipoma, 309 • Sand Colic, 310 Colic Caused by Diet or Management, 315 • Colic Related to Exercise, 316 • Gastric Ulcer Syndrome, 318 • Plants That Affect the Intestinal Tract, 320 The Best Colic Therapy is Prevention, 322

CHAPTER 12

The Digestive System: Nutritional Management 325

Basic Nutritional Requirements	**325**
Energy	325
Roughage	326

Hay, 326 • Pasture, 328 • Other Roughage Alternatives, 328 • Concentrates, 329 Fat for Energy, 330 • Probiotics, 331

Protein	332

Soy Products, 332

Water Requirements	332
Electrolyte Supplementation	333
Minerals and Trace Microminerals	337
Vitamins	338
Meeting Nutrient Requirements	**339**
The Idle and Lightly Worked Horse	339
The Hard-Working Athlete	339
Effects of Feeding on Gastrointestinal Function	340
Hot Climate Feeding	**341**
Heat Increment	341

Grains vs. Roughage, 341 • Fat for Energy, 342

Protein Requirements in Hot Weather	342

Protein's Role in Sweating, 343 • Excess Protein in Hot Climates, 343

Electrolyte Supplements	344
Improving Performance in Hot Weather	344
Cold Weather Feeding	**344**
Body Condition Scoring System	**345**
Nutritional Diseases	**350**
Obesity	350
Obesity-Related Diseases	352

CHAPTER 13
The Skin as an Organ — 355

The Role of the Skin as an Organ	**355**
Skin's Role in Thermoregulation	355
Dissipating the Heat, 356 • Natural Cooling Methods, 357 • External Cooling Methods, 358	
Heat Stress	359
Hot Weather, 359 • Level of Conditioning, 360 Transport Issues, 360 • Excess Sweating, 361 Anhidrosis, 361 • Determining Danger of Heat Stress, 361 • Preventing Heat Stress, 362	
Skin Diseases	**363**
Diagnosing Skin Diseases	363
Mechanical Skin Concerns	364
Saddle Sores and Girth Galls, 364	
Scratches	367
Causes of Scratches, 367 • Syndromes Confused with Scratches, 369 • Fungal Infection, 369 • Chorioptic Mange Mite, 369 • Rain Scald, 369 • White Pastern Disease, 369	
Managing Sunburn	371
Fungal Infection	372
Ringworm, 372	
Skin Problems Associated with Hair Loss	374
Skin Scald, 374 • Patchy Shedding, 374 Selenium Toxicity, 374 • Rain Scald or Dermatophilus Infection, 375	
External Parasites	376
Flies and Gnats, 376 • Fly and Insect Control Strategies, 381 • Mange Mites, 384 • Other External Parasites, 385 • Onchocerca Worm, 385 Pelodera Strongyloides, 386 • Lice, 386 • Ticks, 387 Summer Sores, 388 • Black Widow Spider, 389	
Allergic Skin Reactions	389
The Role of the Immune System, 389 • Hives, 389	
Hyperelastosis Cutis	392
Skin Growths	392
Warts, 392 • Equine Sarcoid, 392 • Melanoma, 397 • Squamous Cell Carcinoma, 399	
Sheath Cleaning	399

CHAPTER 14
Equine First Aid, Medication, and Restraint — 403

Wound Management	**403**
Initial Treatment	403
Assessing the Damage	403
Debridement	404
Shaving	404
Scrubbing	405
Lavage	405
Antiseptic Cleaning Compounds	405
Compounds That Slow Healing	406
Promoting Wound Healing	407
Contraction, 407 • Systemic Antibiotics, 410 Sutures, 411 • Spray-On Protectants, 412 Topical Ointments and Gels, 412 • Managing Proud Flesh, 416 • Bandaging Recommendations, 416 • Remodeling of a Wound, 419 Hyperbaric Oxygen Therapy, 420	
Puncture Wounds	421
Tendon or Joint Punctures, 421 • Anaerobic Bacteria, 422	
Blunt Trauma	423
Kick Wounds, 423 • Seroma or Hematoma, 423 • Sequestrum, 424	
Rope Burns	424
Characteristics of Rope Burns, 425 • Treating Rope Burns, 426	
Hemorrhage Control	426
First Aid Kit	**428**
Fever	**429**
Reasons for Fever	429
Dangers of Fever	429
Cooling Techniques	429
Snakebite	**430**
The Body's Response	430
Treatment	431
Injectable Medication	**432**
The Label	433
Safe Storage	434
Pre-Injection Procedure	435
Intramuscular Injection	436
Injection Target, 436 • Choice of Needle, 437 Adverse Reactions, 438	
Intravenous Injection	440
Administering IV Injections, 440 IV Catheter, 441	
Subcutaneous Injection	441
Intradermal Injection	442
Non-Steroidal Anti-Inflammatory Drugs	**442**
Method of Action	442
Cautionary Situations	443

Types of NSAIDs	444
NSAID Toxicity	445
Alternatives to NSAIDs	446
Safe and Effective Restraint	**446**
Understanding Horse Behavior	447
Creating Calmness	447
Handling Procedures	448
Methods of Restraint	449
Physical Restraint, 450 • Chemical Restraint, 453	

CHAPTER 15
Preventive and Mental Horse Health — 455

Herd Health	**455**
Health Inspection	455
Vaccination Status	456
Brand Inspection	457
The Value of Blood Tests	457
Coggins Test, 457 • Complete Blood Count, 457 Chemistry Panel, 458 • Drug Testing Profile, 458	
Quarantine	458
Good Hygiene	459
Internal Parasites and Control	**459**
Effect of Internal Parasites on Performance	459
Types of Internal Parasites	461
Large Strongyles or Bloodworms, 461 • Small Strongyles, 461 • Ascarids, 462 • Stomach Worms, 462 • Pinworms, 463 • Intestinal Threadworms, 464 • Lungworms, 464 Tapeworms, 464	
Preventive Management for Parasite Control	464
Herd Management, 465 • Environmental Management, 465 • Deworming Products, 466 Recommended Deworming Schedules, 468 Administering Dewormers, 470	
The Meaning of Stress	**472**
Psychological Stress	472
Herd Instinct, 472 • Social Acclimation, 472 Isolation and Confinement, 473 • Stereotypic Behaviors, 474 • Relief from Boredom, 477 Changing the Environment, 477	
Transport Stress	**478**
Environmental Stress	478
Ambient Temperature, 478 • Air Quality, 479 Immune Function, 481 • Behavioral Adaptations, 482 • Muscular Fatigue, 483 • Particular Stress Features of a Traveling Horse, 483	
Protective Bandages	485

CHAPTER 16
The Eyes: A Horse's View of the World — 487

Mental Perception	**487**
Spooky Behavior	487
Anatomy and Function of the Equine Eye	**488**
Pupil	488
Corpora Nigra	488
Retina	489
Tapetum	489
Cornea and Lens	489
Third Eyelid	490
A Horse's Focus and Perception	**490**
Color Vision	492
How to Apply Vision Principles to Riding	492
Eye Injuries	**492**
Abnormal Ocular Discharge	492
Blockage of the Nasolacrimal Duct, 493	
Conjunctivitis	493
Eyelid Trauma	494
Corneal Ulcer or Laceration	494
Eye Irrigation, 496 • Types of Eye Medication, 496	
Managing a Painful Eye	496
Common Eye Diseases	**497**
Equine Recurrent Uveitis	497
Cataract	499
Eye Tumors	499
Anterior Segment Dysgenesis	500
Blindness	500

CHAPTER 17
The Neurologic System in Health and Disease — 501

Nervous System Function	**501**
Cranial Nerves	501
Balance and Proprioception	501
Strength and Posture	501
Testing for Neurologic Function	501
Infectious Neurologic Diseases	**504**
Viral Infection	504
West Nile Virus, 504 • Equine Encephalitis or Encephalomyelitis, 508 • Equine Herpesvirus, Neurologic Form, 508 • Rabies, 509	
Parasitic Migration	510
Equine Protozoal Myelitis, 510 • Parasite Damage, 513	
Bacterial Infection	513
Tetanus, 513	
Neurologic Irritation or Compression	**514**
Ear Inflammation	514
Otitis Media-Interna, 514	

Tick Paralysis	515
Headshaking	515
Horner's Syndrome	516
Cervical Vertebral Malformation aka Wobbler Syndrome	517
Equine Motor Neuron Disease	517
Shivers	518
Polyneuritis Equi	519
Narcolepsy	519
Syncope	520
Seizures	520
Neurologic Trauma	**520**
The Fallen Horse	520
Sweeney	524
Stringhalt	524
Nutrition-Related Neurologic Disease	**525**
Botulism	525
Moldy Corn Poisoning	527
Toxic Plants That Affect the Nervous System	527

CHAPTER 18

Reproductive Strategies and Health — 531

Promoting Genetic Improvement	**531**
Scientific Interference	531
Breeding Evaluation	532
The Stallion	**532**
Breeding Performance	532
Stallion Appraisal for a Mare Owner, 533 Booking to a Stallion, 534 • The Breeding Contract, 534 • Teasing Programs, 534	
General Physical Exam	535
Maintaining Stallion Health, 535 • Heritable Abnormalities, 535	
Reproductive Exam	535
The Testicles, 535 • The Penis, 536 • Venereal Disease, 536 • Semen Evaluation, 537 Siring Records, 538	
The Mare	**538**
Reproductive Cycle	538
Hormonal Manipulation, 539 • Artificial Lighting, 539 • Preventive Medicine, 540	
Estrous Behavior	540
Performance Aspects of Riding a Mare, 540 Hormonal Control of Estrous Behavior, 541 Mechanical Control of Estrous Behavior, 542 Acupuncture Control of Estrous Behavior, 542 Herbal Control of Estrous Behavior, 542 • Surgical Options to Eliminate Estrous Behavior, 542	
Abnormal Estrous Cycles	543
Performance Related, 543 • Anabolic Steroids, 543 Pain, 543	
Mare Pre-Breeding Exam	543
Preparing for Breeding, 543 • General Physical Exam, 543 • External Exam of a Mare's Reproductive System, 544 • Internal Exam of a Mare's Reproductive System, 546	
The Breeding Process	550
Natural Cover or Artificial Insemination, 550 Detecting Estrus, 550 • The Breeding, 551 Pregnancy Check, 552	
The Details of Artificial Insemination	553
The Expense of AI, 553 • Relative Value of AI, 553 • The Mare with a Foal by Her Side, 554 Breeding Several Mares at Once, 554 Frozen Semen, 554 • Embryo Transfer, 555	
Reproductive Diseases and Problems	**555**
Granulosa Cell Tumor	555
Mare Reproductive Loss Syndrome	555
Equine Viral Arteritis	555
Foaling and Complications	557
Fescue Toxicosis, 558 • Dystocia, 559 Retained Fetal Membranes, 560 • Passive Transfer and Antibody Protection, 561 • Umbilical Problems, 561 • Ruptured Bladder, 563 • Meconium Impaction, 563 • Dummy Foal, 563 • Neonatal Isoerythrolysis, 563 • Flexural Limb Deformity or Contracted Tendons, 564 • How Does a Sick Foal Present? 564	

APPENDIX A
Normal Physiological Parameters — 567

APPENDIX B
Common Drug and Supply Names, Uses, and Actions — 568

APPENDIX C
Common Toxic Plants — 571

APPENDIX D
Commonly Used Acupuncture Points in the Horse — 574

BIBLIOGRAPHY — 575

INDEX — 591

Note to the Reader

The scope of this book focuses particularly on the horse in exercise and work, no matter the athletic discipline, though specific riding pursuits are discussed when appropriate. Sound health management strategies are examined in depth and are applicable to any horse whether he stands idle in the field or is hard at work as a competitor. It is not possible to address every single situation that might occur in an athletic horse, but issues most commonly encountered are discussed. The breadth of topics arose out of my personal experiences over many decades as a horse owner and rider, from twenty years in the field as an equine veterinarian, and from questions commonly asked by horse-owning clients who have charged me with the responsibility of helping them do the best by their horses.

Ideas and suggestions herein are based on strategies that have proven successful in my hands or as described in the veterinary scientific literature, backed up by peer review. There may be various ways to achieve a similar end or instances where suggestions are not relevant within your own context. It is always advisable to confer with your veterinarian about health concerns of your own horse. In any situation, it is important to remember that each horse is an individual and every approach should be custom-tailored to suit each unique condition.

Within these pages, I have made reference to every horse as "he," but the reader should realize that this is meant to imply mares, as well. Similarly, a rider may be referred to as "he" when in fact, "he" may be a "she." This is not meant as a political incorrectness but rather to simplify the reading.

Instead of a glossary, I have briefly described a word or term the first time it is mentioned in the text—see the index for the page number. To read the main discussion of the disease or condition, refer to the page number indexed in *bold*.

I have included, in the appendix, information about the horse's normal physiological parameters; a compendium of common drugs along with their proprietary brand names, uses, and actions; a list of toxic plants and their effects; and a chart showing commonly used acupuncture points in the horse.

Nancy S. Loving, DVM

An Introduction

What used to be a necessity in travel over a century ago has formed the basis for our recreational pursuits. Time spent in the saddle assures us of the indomitable spirits of our horses. The human-horse bond intensifies with experiences of shared trust. When we partner ourselves with a horse, we assume a responsibility unique to any other form of competitive sports. Not only must we look after our own body and needs, but also we must attend to the basic requirements of our mount. It is the attention to the small details that allows a horse to give his utmost performance. To enable a horse to reach his athletic pinnacle requires a team effort by a rider/owner, a farrier, and a veterinarian. Every detail is addressed to improve a horse's quality of life, and to further soundness and health.

It is only after many years and many mistakes that seasoned riders come to grasp the subtleties that allow their horses to excel. With time and experience, a savvy rider is able to anticipate and respond to a horse's individual quirks, and to shape events to a favorable outcome. A horse speaks in a very fundamental language. Every nuance of excitement or discomfort or exhaustion is transmitted by a horse's body posture and attitude, if we look carefully. Knowledge gained from the study of exercise physiology has allowed insights into the tremendous physiologic capabilities and adaptations of an equine athlete. Natural talent plays a role in a horse's success, but without appropriate management, nutrition, training, and conditioning, a horse may not reach his potential. As more answers are unraveled, more questions arise. Whether one enjoys the wilderness as a competitive or recreational trail rider or develops skills in an arena setting, our common link is to help our horses complete their work with enthusiasm and safety.

As you delve deeply into this book, you will find discussions on each organ system within a horse's body and its influence on performance. Even when discussing each as a "stand-alone" system, its interaction to other organ systems should be obvious. But, at risk of only viewing the parts, we need also to make them a whole. The idea of viewing the body as a whole dates back to ancient times, most notably with the Oriental cultural view of medicine and of the cosmos: *The picture is a totality, and each detail takes on meaning only insofar as it participates in the whole* (Ted J. Kaptchuk, *The Web That Has No Weaver*, New York: McGraw-Hill, 2000). This concept aptly applies to developing a horse to be well prepared for any intended athletic pursuit.

A Horse's Body in Motion

To achieve a sense of the intricacies of interaction of all the body systems, let's imagine a working horse. Consider this animal to be robust and fit, in the peak of condition. He is cantering along; his ears pricked forward, his eyes scanning the surroundings for lurking dangers. As each limb reaches forward to cover the track, he is poetry in motion. His skin shines with damp sweat. With each contraction of his muscles, you feel his back lift beneath you, his body suspended briefly between strides. His balance and timing are perfect as he eagerly negotiates the course. You are poised quietly in the saddle, maintaining a steady, but gentle bit contact with his mouth, regulating his pace, guiding his direction. With a subtle glance you see each front hoof strumming the air beneath his nose, then settling back to earth. His breathing is rhythmic with each stride as he inhales the air that rushes past as the pair of you moves energetically along. This picture in your mind's eye seems entrancing, doesn't it? One could wax spiritual but the intention is to have you look carefully at the embodiment of what is occurring: a shared recruitment from all organ systems to propel this horse over the ground.

The Work of Movement

The muscles are doing the hard work of locomotion, fueled by food substrates (basic food components that are broken into energy molecules by metabolism) digested by the intestines and by oxygen consumed by the lungs. More than 60 percent of the energy generated by the metabolism of fuel sources in the muscles is "wasted" as heat. This heat must pass through a well-developed cardiovascular network of blood vessels and be pumped to capillaries in the skin. Sweat glands of the skin release this heat along with body water to cool the horse by evaporative cooling. With each beat of the heart, the blood vascular system in turn delivers oxygen (from the lungs) and nutrients to the muscles to sustain the effort of exercise. While the muscles of each limb are propelling the horse along the ground, these muscles are also dampening concussion and vibration within the tendons, ligaments, and joints. As long as muscles are not fatigued, then the soft tissue supporting structures can do their best job. Strong and active muscles relieve the load placed upon the supportive tissues so as to reduce the risk of injury to ligaments, tendons, and joints. In this fit horse, hooves and bone have been conditioned over seasons of training to withstand the impact stresses of the terrain as well as the weight of the horse descending on each of these systems.

Resting

You slow your horse as you near a resting place. Easing him to a stop, you evaluate his metabolic condition. His eyes are bright, and he surveys his surroundings with ears pricked and body erect. His heart rate drops quickly. His muscles feel pliable and he offers no resentment as they are gently kneaded with a hand. He gives no indication of pain as his back and girth areas are palpated by probing fingers. Mucous membranes are moist and pink, and capillary refill time is normal. Gut sounds are active in all quadrants and his appetite is greedy. He is eager to eat and drink, diving into green grass at his feet. Steam rises off his body in the brisk air as his circulatory system continues to move heat from the muscles to the skin. You help him continue to cool by sponging his neck and chest while he happily munches away. This is the picture of a contented, metabolically stable individual, one that is truly "fit to continue" in exercise.

The Composite Whole

In this scenario painted in your mind's eye, all the organ systems we will discuss are operating in full swing to produce a horse that is comfortable in his athletic endeavor. It is through diligent care and hard work that all the parts come together to produce a well-conditioned animal. Many techniques can be incorporated to derive the maximal performance from a horse for as long a time as possible.

Custom-Tailored Training

One key ingredient that is tantamount to success is to custom design an individually tailored program for each horse. To embrace only a template of general training principles without taking into account the peculiar idiosyncracies for an individual horse on a given day is to invite frustration and performance failure. Strategies that work for one person and horse may have no application to another situation. What has worked well in the past may need to be modified to suit a particular horse or a particular day. Success is in attention to the tiniest details.

Like people, horses have good days, bad days, sore days, and can't-do-anything days. Expectations need to adjust accordingly. A rider must be in tune enough with a horse and flexible enough to be able to make changes in both training and competition.

Talent

There is always an ingredient that is not directly under a rider's control: talent.

Talent is one feature that is indecipherable until a horse is put to the test. Raw talent comes in the form of an ambitious work ethic, physical strength, musculoskeletal soundness, effectiveness of gait, and metabolic efficiency. When these characteristics all work in harmony, a horse has the potential to excel as an elite athlete. Willingness and obedience to work as a team player with a rider are qualities that can be learned but are innate to a horse's disposition. A horse that stays calm in the face of adrenalin takes better care of himself. A horse's propensity to take care of himself on the road and during a competition can be taught, but in most cases, such a tendency toward survival is instinctive in an individual. A horse must eat and drink well en route to the venue and while on site. The physically exacting nature of athletic equine sports requires a horse to be in peak condition and to maintain himself in that state. The slightest energy deficit or component of dehydration is a liability in any competition.

A talented horse can carry a fair-to-moderately talented rider and achieve results in spite of a rider's mistakes. On the other hand, a talented horse enables a talented rider to excel, and to do so repeatedly. There are also instances of an excellent rider bringing an average horse to noteworthy achievements but the path to this end is a more difficult struggle.

How to find talent? The purchase price of a horse does not guarantee talent, and the pedigree of a horse does not guarantee talent. These factors are important in selecting a prospect, but just because a horse is expensive or of great breeding or the buyer is savvy about horse flesh does not mean the horse will have the heart or the stamina or skill to become an elite athlete. Luck, good horse sense, and diligent conditioning efforts will see a horse and rider team to great accomplishments.

Time Constraints

Success depends on dedication and commitment to the process of bringing a horse along. Developing fitness, for both horse and rider, takes time and care. Each competitor has a varied amount of time to devote to training and conditioning, depending on work and family commitments, weather considerations, and financial resources.

Management Strategies

Not all horse facilities are created equal. How a horse is stabled and managed has a lot to do with his mental happiness and physical health. Big turnout areas, preferably with pasture, and adequate social comingling amidst a herd are pleasures for any horse. Exercise and conditioning strategies become increasingly important for a horse confined to a small paddock as he does not receive the beneficial effects on legs and stamina that comes of wandering around the farm all day.

Diet and nutritional concerns have a lot to do with bloom and health of a horse. Horses involved in many athletic endeavors thrive on a high fiber, high fat diet. Excellent quality hay is important, however not all locales have access to good quality roughage and so must find substitutes in feed materials. This often becomes costly and quality may suffer. Ultimately, nutrition provides the staying power for an athletic horse to get the job done. No amount of conditioning will make up for deficiencies in feeding or general health care: vaccination and deworming strategies are critical to maintaining physical health of any horse. Preventing illness is a key concern for peak performance.

Farrier care is crucial to maintaining soundness. This element is not always within a horse owner's control. Scheduling of farrier visits to maintain hoof health is in the owner's hands, but much depends on who is available to shoe and how knowledgeable the farrier. Starting with a horse with excellent quality feet gives a competitor a keen advantage. (See chapter 3, *The Hoof*, p. 39.)

Terrain and Climatic Considerations

For riding disciplines that venture outside an arena environment, conditioning in varied terrain builds a versatile athlete. Living in an area that offers a diversity of terrain gives a rider multiple options, but this is not always possible. Some horses only have the option to train in deep sand whereas others are presented with exclusively mountainous terrain. Some horses never see anything other than flat ground that is useful for faster conditioning work or for equitation skills, whereas others exercise solely over difficult and rocky terrain that precludes training at speed or with precision. Each type of landscape lends its own peculiar strength to developing fitness. But, a horse trained on flat ground at fast speeds might not develop the stamina to encounter mountainous or rocky terrain without problems. A horse trained in mountainous and slower going has not developed the muscular and enzyme systems necessary to compete at faster speeds for prolonged periods. Tackling a rigorous course with too much relative speed imposes great risk to both the musculoskeletal structures and metabolic ability. It is important to condition a horse relative to the terrain where he will do his work.

Similarly, climatic factors should be considered. It is not so difficult for a horse already used to hot and humid weather to make a rapid adjustment to an arid climate. On the other hand, a horse acclimated to only a dry climate will have a difficult time dissipating heat in a hot and humid place unless properly acclimatized over at least three or four weeks.

Equipment

Saddling issues are pivotal in eliciting the greatest comfort for a horse while doing his work. An intelligent strategy is to have a saddle custom built for an individual horse's back;

this provides the best comfort for the horse and then the rider is both time and money ahead in moving forward in a training program. (See chapter 8, *The Horse's Back,* p. 203.) A well-fitting saddle enables a horse to work without having to guard himself from rubs and galls or pinching areas created by pressure points from poor saddle fit.

Horse and Rider Team

Skills of a rider dictate how efficiently a horse can move. A rider with soft hands mounted on a horse that does not brace against the rider or the bit has a distinct advantage. Cooperation between the two generates a more efficient gait with less muscular fatigue for both horse and rider. The rider should also have an adaptable and knowledgeable seat and have the ability to use hand, leg, and seat aids with precision. The horse should be trained to be responsive to these aids. A horse that is obedient will allow a rider to check his speed when necessary. A keen horse will increase his stride or speed when asked without pulling on the rider's arms to go too fast. The horse should be able to be rated in his pace so a rider can control progress rather than leaving this decision to the horse.

A rider should be tuned-in every step of the way, able to recognize subtle changes in a horse that might indicate fatigue or pain. Once a problem is recognized, it should be addressed immediately. Past experiences a horse may have encountered should be considered. If he has been allowed to work without constraint, this old habit is hard to modify. If he has suffered pain or abuse, or gotten sick doing his job, he is less likely to put forth a concerted effort. Researching a horse's history not only opens one's eyes to issues that need to be addressed but it also determines how well a horse and rider team may be able to work together. Knowing a horse's prior athletic history assists a rider in relieving a horse's anxiety and ensuring as calm and relaxed a ride as possible.

Sense of Humor and an Open Mind

Customizing a training strategy is only one part of any success story. The ability of a competitor to focus is essential to any task, but the ability to maintain a sense of humor is what provides joy in the outcome. Emotional angst brings anger and frustration when something goes awry. Remember that horses are sensitive to moods and body language. They react to subtle changes in our disposition. A tense rider may cause a horse to fret and worry. A horse that is not able to relax may not eat or drink well. A tense horse may display various signs of stress, leading to poor performance.

A talented rider maintains an open mind, open to possibilities and to continuous learning. As is often quoted: "The mind is like a parachute: it works best when it is open." Those who relate ideas and experiences to each other will find great pleasure in sharing similar passions. There is value in learning from each other so mistakes aren't oft repeated; this is to the benefit of horses.

Strategies to Optimize Performance

Strategies that enable a horse to perform to the best of his ability include:

- Preventive health management to ensure overall physical well-being. Good dental care, practical deworming strategies, regular immunizations, and excellent nutrition all enable a horse to maintain good body condition and an excellent immune system.

- Conditioning strategies that are applied with common sense over a period of years to develop a horse to peak form. Conditioning of the cardiovascular system and strength development of the muscles produce a metabolically efficient athlete. Joints, bones, hooves, tendons and ligaments are gradually and progressively trained over time to assume more load without overtaxing these structures.
- Not overtraining or excessively competing in a brief time span. Sufficient time is allowed between events to allow recovery and to enable a horse's body to develop and build on previous competitive or training experience. Sufficient time intervals between events prevent transport stress from taking a cumulative toll on a horse's system.
- Utilizing a well-designed trailer with adequate ventilation to ensure lung health and a comfortable traveling ambient temperature when hauling. Adequate numbers and length of rest stops along the road and prior to competition enable a horse to refuel with food and water to minimize dehydration effects.
- Use of tack designed specifically with a horse's comfort in mind, having a saddle custom built to fit a horse's back, if necessary. Sound dentistry practices and proper training techniques enable a horse to be ridden with a minimum of hardware in his mouth.
- Pursuit of professional riding instruction to better riding skills. A competent rider eases a horse's effort and minimizes fatigue of both horse and rider.
- Supportive care of the musculoskeletal system through use of appropriate joint therapies and with muscle maintenance of stretching and massage.
- Team efforts between rider, veterinarian, and farrier to provide the best foot care possible for a horse, using the newest technology and applications available.
- Recognition by a rider of subtle signs a horse offers in training and competition that alert to fatigue or pain. The horse is ridden at a pace appropriate to his level of conditioning and for the unique circumstances of each event.

All these strategies take time and patience to develop and to incorporate into a routine. The pursuit of riding becomes a lifestyle of its own. Those who place attention on these details will benefit from the sheer enjoyment of riding a horse with boundless energy and solid soundness, one that is up to the task at hand. Each organ system will develop to its peak and produce a vibrant horse of which you can be proud, a horse that will be your partner in your quest of dreams.

Conformation for Performance

As we strive for competitive excellence in a chosen equine sport, we are dependent on the talent of our equine partner. Talent derives from many factors, not the least of which is the conformational structure of the horse. Without the physical ability to perform in a particular discipline, no amount of mental desire or fitness can bring a horse to the leading edge. The ideal horse is an image to which we compare all others. There is no such thing as a perfect horse, but a horse with good conformation makes a durable athlete. Excellent conformation does not always guarantee excellence in performance; other talents such as temperament and trained abilities are necessary to create a superior competitor. Each horse has strengths and weaknesses in different areas, both physical and mental.

Ideal conformation is a debatable issue, but there is one thing all can agree on: it is difficult to find the ideal horse. It is said that the one horse that has come closest to meeting the imaginary embodiment of ideal has been *Secretariat*. His body-build and proportions meet all the specifications for excellence in performance in just about any riding discipline. A horse with excellent conformation is well suited to perform a variety of tasks, and is not just relegated to performing as one kind of sport horse. Our objective then, is to figure out what makes a versatile equine athlete. Many equine sports share some common threads: the horse needs to develop self-carriage and balance. He should be able to lighten his forehand and shift his center of gravity toward his rear haunches to distribute weight more equally between front and rear. This lends agility to his movement, while imparting the potential for power and bursts of speed. Depending on the particular sport, the haunches will assume varying amounts of the load. Along with strong haunches, many equine athletes require a strong back that well couples the fore and rear quarters. (For more discussion, see chapter 8, *The Horse's Back*, p. 203.) Athletic longevity relies particularly on correct limbs and strong hooves.

Anatomy and Function

A discussion of conformation is a study in anatomy and its relation to the function of each structure. Although various parts of a horse are isolated, scrutinized, and analyzed for their individual contributions to the abilities of that animal, each part influences the others as an interactive system. The interaction of muscles

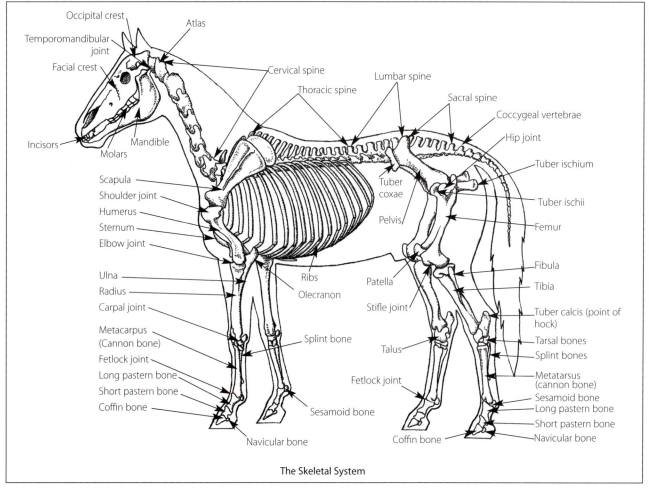

The Skeletal System

2.1 *The way the skeleton is put together, conformation, determines the strength and coordination of individual muscles.*

and tendons generates locomotion. Think of the musculotendinous units as levers and pulleys, moving different parts of the skeleton. The way the skeleton is put together, *conformation*, determines the strength and coordination of individual muscles. While different sports capitalize on strengthening some parts of a horse's body more than others, basic conformation principles apply in evaluating any equine athlete (figs. 2.1–2.4).

An Overview

To begin a conformation analysis, place the horse on a flat, level surface, and square him up. Stand back and survey the whole horse to gain an overall impression of his appearance and stance. Examine the horse's overall symmetry from front, back, and side.

His legs should be straight from chest to ground, with no signs of toeing-in or toeing-out, with no rotation of the cannon bone out from the knee. The knees should fit over the middle of the cannon bones, and all distal (lower) joints in the limbs should sit directly over the center of each bone. Limb crookedness creates a liability for an equine athlete; more stress will be felt on the sides of joints, bones, and hooves in a crooked leg. This can lead to degenerative arthritis, chronic ligament

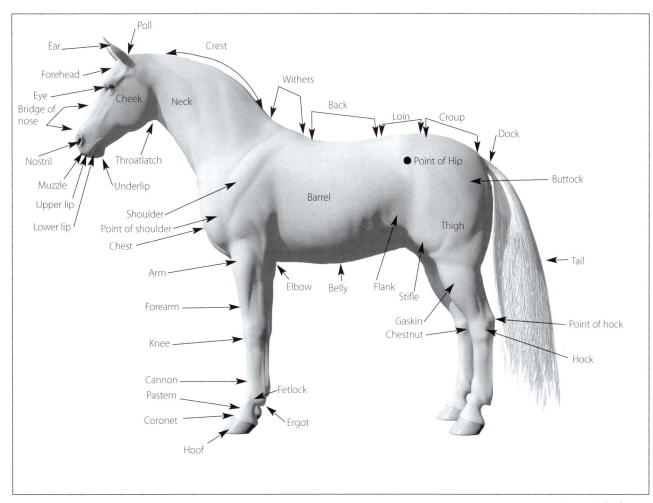

2.2 *Parts of the horse.*

injuries, or chronic foot pain. Also a crooked limb tends to paddle or wing in, contributing to muscular fatigue and the potential for interference injury of the opposite limb.

The same assessment should be applied when viewing a horse from the rear. The points of the hocks should point slightly outward but predominantly parallel each other. Each side of the buttocks should be symmetrical in height and proportion with good muscle development in the haunches.

From the side, the front legs should form a relatively straight column with the knees bent very slightly forward, while the rear legs should have some angulation between the stifle and the hock. The back portion of the rear legs should drop straight down with a plumb line running from the point of the buttock through the point of the hock, down the back of the cannon, and to the back of the heel bulbs.

An athletic horse generally has long forearms, short cannon bones, and a medium pastern. Bone is ample when there is at least 8 inches per 1000 pounds as measured at the circumference at the top of the cannon bone. Joints are large and strong in appearance to enable the pull of muscles and tendons across the joints. There should be no swelling over the joints that could denote inflammation within the joints.

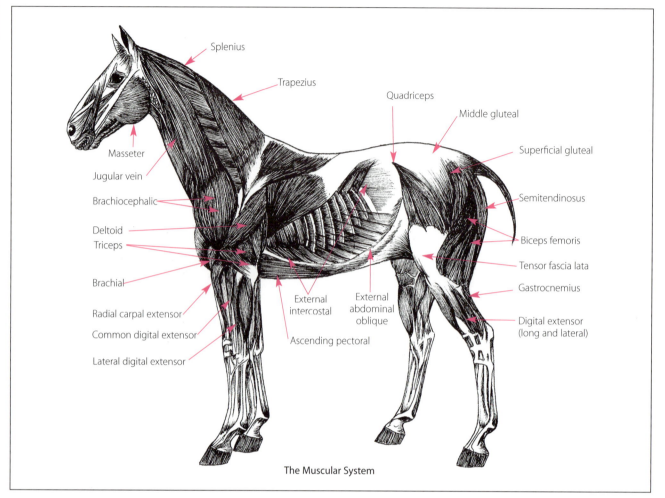

The Muscular System

2.3 *Each muscle and tendon unit works like a lever and pulley to move different parts of the skeleton from simple tasks such as eating and swatting flies to the grace and power of more complex athletic efforts of equine locomotion.*

Balance

Consider the balance of a horse as viewed from the side. Balance is determined by the location of a horse's center of mass. As a general rule, a horse with optimum balance is visually proportional into thirds:

- The front third encompassing the neck from the poll to the withers
- The middle third encompassing the back from the withers to the peak of the croup (at the lumbo-sacral joint)
- The rear third of the hindquarters encompassing the lumbo-sacral joint to the point of the buttocks

No horse can be divided into exact thirds, but a horse that comes close to these proportional guidelines will be well-balanced (fig. 2.5). The way to visualize the balance of a horse is by creating a "box": the height at the withers, the height at the hip, and the length of the body should be approximately the same. There are variations among breeds; for example, some Arabians have one less thoracic vertebra than other breeds. Thoroughbreds come closest to meeting the "box" guidelines.

Whichever method is used, imaginary dividing lines place the center of gravity of a well-balanced horse directly under a mounted rider with 60 to 65 percent of a horse's weight

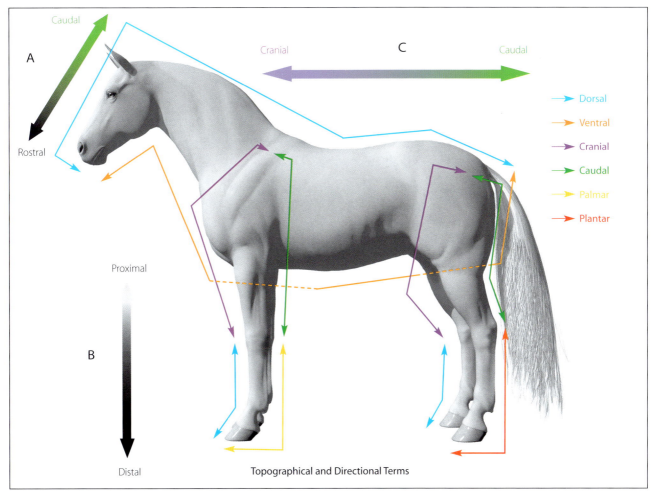

2.4 *Spatial terminology.*

falling on the forelegs. If a horse's head is too big or the neck is too long, it is difficult for the hindquarters to effectively counteract the extra weight up front. If the hindquarters are too small, there is no power to push the heavier front end. The haunches are the engine of locomotion that develops a horse's drive, impulsion, and thrust. It is the hind end conformation that enables a horse to rapidly accelerate, decelerate, turn, or jump. Any equine athlete needs well-developed musculature and proportion in this area for strength and speed. There may be differences in desirable back length, or shoulder length and angle depending on the sport a horse is asked to pursue.

Head

The head should be proportionate to the rest of the body, with ample length to provide room for strong teeth and the nasal passages. A head that is too large can create a heavy load on the front end, especially if attached to a relatively short neck.

Nostrils

The nostrils should be generous in size so a horse can breathe plenty of oxygen to fuel locomotion. A deeply dished face pinches the nostrils and nasal passages, and limits the performance of a speed or endurance horse.

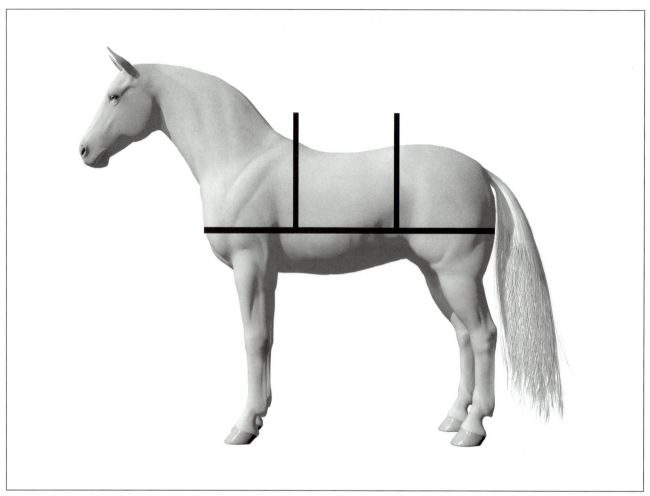

2.5 *No horse can be divided into exact thirds, but a horse that comes close to these proportional guidelines will be well-balanced.*

Jaws

A horse with narrow jaws may also have a narrow throatlatch, predisposing him to *laryngeal hemiplegia* or *roaring* (see p. 16 and p. 258). Sufficient space between the jaws allows for an active and open airway. The nasal passages are filled with a plexus of blood vessels that cool or warm incoming air to body temperature, preventing thermal shock to the respiratory system.

PARROT MOUTH

When the upper jaw extends past the lower jaw, the horse is referred to as having a *parrot mouth* (see photo 11.11 on p. 287). This trait is considered undesirable and is regarded as unsoundness. Because it is heritable, these horses are discouraged from becoming breeding animals. A horse with this condition gets along fine in acquiring feed and nutrition, but will require frequent and regular dental care.

Eyes

The eyes should be well placed for good vision. The ideal location is at the corners of the forehead. The eyes should have a soft expression, alert and interested.

Neck

Neck Function

The neck lowers a horse's head for grazing and drinking, and assists vision by swinging the head for accurate eye focus. A large range of motion of the neck enables a horse to shift and fine-tune his center of gravity to maintain balance of his massive body. As a biomechanical structure, a horse's neck is the ultimate in design. The triangular shape enhances its function as a cantilever beam to evenly distribute the weight of the head.

NECK AS A BALANCE

All equine athletes depend on using the neck to shift the center of gravity in the necessary direction to maintain balance and maneuverability. Consider the following examples:

- A roping horse as he slides to an abrupt stop, the neck raised as he sinks onto his haunches (photo 2.6).
- A dressage horse with an arched neck as he executes precision movements of pirouette or piaffe, which require collection and engagement of the hindquarters (photo 2.7).
- A trail horse with head and neck extended, maneuvering up a steep embankment (photo 2.8). As he descends a hillside, he raises the neck and head to lighten the front end, allowing the hindquarters to sink down for better stability on irregular footing.
- A racehorse at full gallop with neck and head extended to increase the length of stride and speed. This simple shift in the center of gravity enhances speed and also reduces fatigue.

NECK COUNTERBALANCE

Analysis of a horse's forward motion illustrates that the downward swing of the head and neck

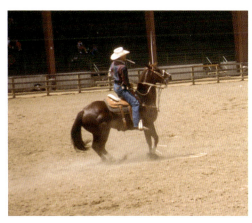

2.6 *A roping horse raises his neck to balance his mass as he sinks onto his haunches in a sliding stop.*

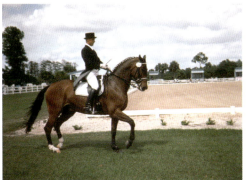

2.7 *An advanced dressage horse that has achieved this level of collection uses his arched neck to counterbalance his engaged and lowered hindquarters in movements such as pirouette and piaffe.*

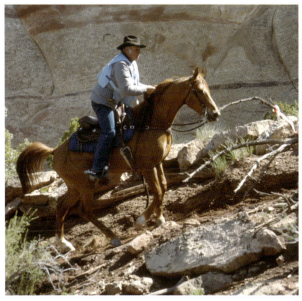

2.8 *A trail horse extends his head and neck to balance while maneuvering up a steep embankment. As he descends a hillside, he raises the neck and head to lighten the front end, allowing the hindquarters to sink down for better stability on irregular footing*

is accompanied by a forward pull of the back muscles. As the body moves forward, propelled from the hind legs to the forelegs, the hindquarters lift from the ground to advance to the next forward stride. As a horse steps under himself, the neck and head continue to work as a counterbalance. With the hind legs supporting the horse, the head and neck rise, followed by elevation of the forequarters and a forward swing of the forelegs to further advance the stride.

Bascule

A jumping horse must arch his neck into a *bascule,* which is an arc created by counterbalancing one end against the other, similar to a seesaw (photo 2.9). Bascule involves a series of steps: extending and lowering the head, arching the back, flexing the *lumbosacral joint* (L-S joint), and finally, engaging the hindquarters. In this way, a horse translates horizontal forward movement into vertical motion up and over a jump.

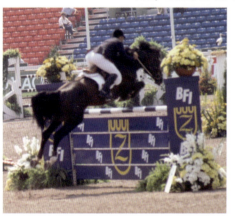

2.9 *A jumping horse must arch his neck into a bascule, which is an arc created by counterbalancing one end of the body against the other, similar to a seesaw.*

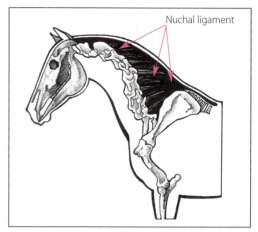

2.10 *The bony spine, buried deep with the muscles of the neck, provides a scaffold for ligament and muscular attachments. The fibroelastic nuchal ligament is an extensive fan-like structure forming the crest of the neck. This ligament passively supports the head and neck and assists extensor muscles of the head and neck.*

Neck Structure

The bony spine is buried within the muscular structure of the neck. It provides a scaffold for attachment of all other ligamentous and muscular parts (fig 2.10).

"YES" JOINT

The cervical spine is connected to the *occipitus,* or base of the skull, by the atlas vertebra, which is the first vertebra behind the skull. The joint formed at their connection, the *atlanto-occipital joint,* moves up and down like a hinge, earning it the name of the "yes" joint.

The head moves up and down without moving the rest of the neck or body, but the protrusions of the atlas vertebra restrict lateral, side to side movement of this joint. For riding purposes, the yes joint enables flexion at the poll to complete stretch through the topline that aids self-carriage to advance a horse to higher levels of performance.

"NO" JOINT

The *atlas* vertebra joins the *axis* (second) vertebra at the *atlanto-axial joint,* also called the "no" joint, because it rotates the head and neck side to side. The joint barely extends due to pressure against the atlas vertebra of another bony piece, the *dens.* The dens is the part of the axis vertebra that hooks under the atlas vertebra.

OTHER CERVICAL JOINTS

Other cervical joints are similar to each other in shape and range of motion. They are capable of flexion, extension, and lateral movement. Throughout a horse's life, the flexion and extension capabilities of these joints remain relatively constant. However, there is an age-related reduction in axial rotation in the middle section of the neck, leading to reduced suppleness in later years.

Neck Length and Shape

Every horse has seven cervical vertebrae, and it is the length of each of these that determines if a neck is long or short (fig. 2.11). A horse's neck can be compared to a gymnast's balancing pole as it moves to accommodate shifts in equilibrium of the body. There is more variety in the necks of horses than in other species due to changes in breed and conformational characteristics developed through centuries of controlled breeding. Ideally, a horse should have a medium-length neck that joins the chest just above the point of the shoulder and suits both his overall conformation and intended sport.

NECK MUSCLES AND STRIDE LENGTH

Neck muscles enable all body structures to synchronize to achieve balance. Interconnecting muscles between neck and shoulders swing a horse's forelegs through each stride. For the hindquarters to propel a horse forward, the shoulders and forelegs must swing freely. The length of a horse's stride is closely correlated to neck length; in extended gaits the forelegs can never reach past the point of the nose.

SHORT NECK

A short neck limits the range of flexibility of the head and neck, and is less able to adjust rapidly, which is necessary to fine-tune balance. A short neck is often thick and muscular, which not only reduces the neck's suppleness,

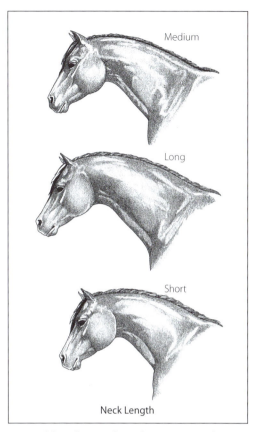

2.11 *Although every horse has seven vertebrae in the neck, the length of the neck is determined by the length of each vertebra. A short neck could slightly limit agility in some cases, while too long a neck creates added weight on the front end thereby increasing impact on the front legs.*

but also adds substantial weight. A thick throatlatch, often associated with a thick neck, limits airflow through the windpipe. It can also limit flexion of the head when a rider asks a horse to go "on the bit." A short neck limits the range of foreleg movement, with more wear-and-tear on the legs because more steps are required to move a distance across the ground. Short, choppy strides result in wasted energy for movement and cause limb fatigue.

LONG NECK

A horse performing at rapid speeds, such as a racehorse, event horse, or jumper, benefits from a moderately long and finely muscled neck. A neck that is too long is a disadvantage as it adds extra weight to the front end, shifting the center of gravity forward. This shift forces a horse to travel on the forehand, increasing stress on the forelegs.

Neck muscles contract and expand two-thirds of their natural length, and in so doing advance the shoulder and forelegs through a stride. Muscles in a neck that is too long may have greater difficulty developing strength and are prone to fatigue. The neck and head might droop, forcing the horse onto the forehand and reducing efficiency of movement. If a horse does not have the strength to support his own head and neck, he tends to pull on a rider's hands, depending on them for support.

As an example of the relationship of form to function, horses with very long, slender necks may be predisposed to *roaring* syndrome, or *laryngeal hemiplegia* (see p. 258). To breathe efficiently, the larynx at the top of the trachea must be able to fully open with inspiration. Nerve supply to muscles that open the *arytenoid cartilages* of the larynx comes from two branches (*recurrent laryngeal nerves*) derived off the *vagus nerve*. These branches are located on either side of the arytenoid cartilages. A longer neck is thought to increase tension on the vagus nerve, in most cases the left branch, leading to nerve damage and paralyzing the laryngeal muscle that opens the airway for breathing. The arytenoid cartilage controlled by this muscle then collapses into the airway on the left side. As air passes through the restricted opening it produces turbulence and creates a "roaring" sound. Exercise tolerance and stamina are compromised.

Neck Influence on Head Carriage

The shape of the neck and its connection to the head and withers determine normal head carriage in a horse (figs 2.12 A–E). Normal head carriage at a 45-degree angle to the ground optimizes a horse's field of vision while allowing the head and neck the mobility necessary to retain body balance. In this position, the larynx is open to promote efficient breathing. A rider has more control because the bit falls on the bars of the mouth rather than sliding into the cheeks as it would with the head held too high or too low.

Carrying the head at this natural angle enables the neck muscles connected to the shoulder to lift the shoulder so the forearm can swing freely, increasing limb advancement across the ground.

LOW-SET NECK

A low-set neck throws a horse onto the forehand by shifting the center of gravity forward and down, restricting shoulder movement and mobility as well as stride length. For a show hunter or Western pleasure horse, traveling "long and level" is ideal for competition, but this can compromise performance and coordination of a jumper, event horse, or dressage candidate.

Even in sports where a level neck is desirable, training a horse to carry his neck too low is dangerous to both horse and rider. The horse falls heavily on the forehand, increasing concussion to the forelegs. A low-set neck reduces the shoulder's freedom of movement, so the horse tends to shuffle and frequently stumbles.

The external shape of the neck depicts the internal configuration of the cervical spine. Over time, training methods build individual muscle groups, but the bony vertebral scaffold is unchangeable. The neck's actual *shape* has more influence on the way a horse travels than does its length.

HIGH-SET NECK

A horse may carry his neck and head held high due to a conformational tendency related to how high his neck comes out of his chest, or in response to training related to specific sport pursuits. A high neck carriage gives a fancy appearance important to many show ring endeavors, and to driving horses in harness. A horse engaged in higher levels of dressage will lift his neck and arch it to achieve collection from nose to tail.

In the extreme, high neck carriage could adversely affect a horse's gait efficiency and agility if the horse is not engaged in collection. If only his head and neck are held high, yet his back and hindquarters are disconnected from the front end, then the rider may experience a jarring ride, and be more challenged in controlling the horse. A high neck carriage may pose difficulty for a rider to see where he is going since the forward view may be obstructed by the horse's head.

EWE NECK

A horse with a *ewe neck* is predisposed to high head carriage, resulting in a hollow back and

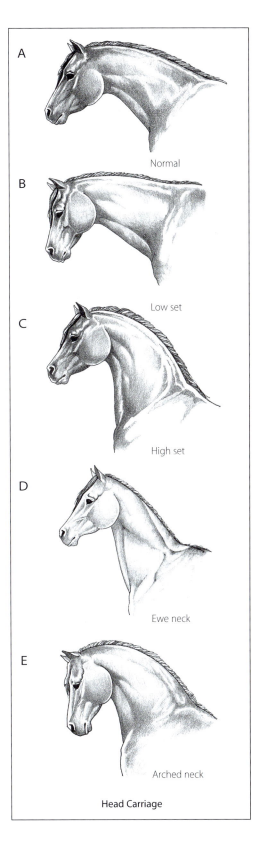

2.12 A–E *A horse with a normal head carriage has the best field of vision and mobility (A), while a head held too low puts the horse's movement more on the forehand with the propensity to stumble (B). If the head carriage is too high, it is difficult for a rider to control the horse or to engage the horse's hindquarters to perform collected movements (C). A horse with a ewe neck often carries his neck high and braces his back and body making it difficult to engage his hindquarters (D). A horse that carries his neck in an arched configuration more easily performs collected movements with freedom in the shoulders and forelegs (E).*

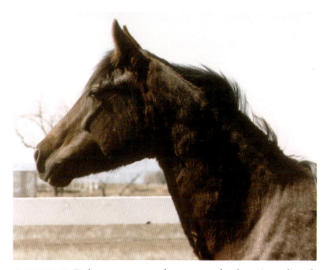 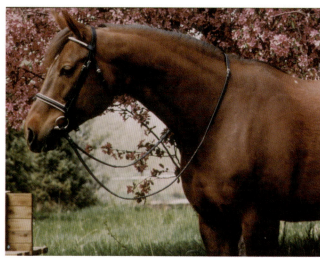

2.13 A & B *Before training and maturity, this horse's neck and topline is weak and undeveloped, giving her a ewe-necked appearance (A). After a few years of training, her neck musculature reveals that she is being ridden in a more collected frame, and that her basic conformation is of a normal curve to the cervical spine (B). Photos: Laurie Prindle.*

an inability to engage the hindquarters or move forward onto the bit. A horse with his head in the air is unable to move effectively because his front and rear ends are moving at odds with one another. Such a ride is uncomfortable for both horse and rider. With the head in a "stargazing" position, the bit does not properly contact the bars of the mouth. The situation is further aggravated as the horse throws his head higher to escape irritating bit pressure.

It is important to differentiate a conformational characteristic of a ewe neck from that of a neck that is undeveloped in musculature or one due to a rider incorrectly applying aids under saddle. The latter neck can be changed as muscles develop with maturity with strategic training techniques and correct riding (photos 2.13 A & B).

ARCHED NECK

If a neck is arched, the head is held in a vertical position that limits a horse's range of vision. The cervical vertebrae in the neck assume an "S" curve that functionally shortens neck length. These factors are important in advanced levels of dressage. A collected head carriage benefits performance of lateral, precision movements. Shortening the neck length moves the center of gravity toward the hind end. Shifting the center of gravity backward frees the head and neck to move up and down. Then, suppleness increases from side to side. The shoulders and forelegs also move with greater freedom.

Withers

Stretch through the Topline

For many equine athletic endeavors, the aim is to achieve longitudinal flexion (arching of the spine) through the entire back and topline. Stretched muscles are relaxed muscles. Consequently, they are less prone to fatigue and injury. Interactive use of muscle groups adds strength to a horse's movements. Stretch through the topline and neck starts at the withers. The withers are formed by the top portions of the 3rd through 8th thoracic vertebrae of the spine.

The Role of the Withers

The *scalenus muscles* of the neck connect to the first rib. As these muscles raise the base of the neck, an increase in the lever arm at the withers improves stretch through the topline. As the first rib is pulled forward, the rib cage expands and promotes respiratory capacity for speed and stamina.

The fibroelastic *nuchal ligament,* an extensive fan-like structure forming the crest of the neck, extends from the base of the skull and anchors onto the withers (see fig. 2.10). The nuchal ligament passively supports the head and neck to distribute the mechanical load, and assists extensor muscles of the head and neck. Additional neck muscles that raise the head and neck, or move them from side to side, anchor to the withers. Muscle groups that elevate the shoulder and extend the spine also anchor here.

A proper crest of the neck that carries well back over the withers enhances the fulcrum effect of the withers. As the withers rise when a horse stretches through his neck, the back and spine arch, engaging the hindquarters with hocks and stifles moving well beneath the body.

This specific arching movement is important not only to dressage horses, but to cutting, reining, jumping, and trail horses as well. Flexibility and suppleness are not only dependent upon conformational structure, but require conditioning.

HIGH WITHERS

The withers should sit about an inch higher than the horse's croup (fig. 2.14). Withers height permits a greater range of movement for

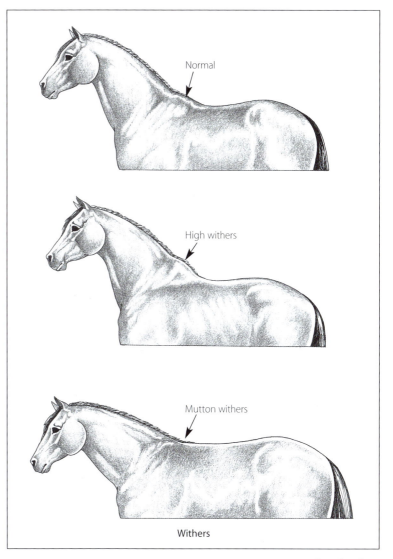

the neck and back muscles that attach to it. Like a seesaw, the higher the fulcrum point (withers), the more freedom both sides of the seesaw (neck and back) have to move up and down. A high, broad withers provides greater flexibility through the back and spine. As a horse lowers and extends the neck, the back rises. If the withers are too high, saddle fit may be a problem (see chapter 8, *The Horse's Back,* p. 203).

2.14 *Withers height permits a greater range of movement for the neck and back muscles that attach to it. Too high a withers creates a challenge for saddle fit, while a low, mutton withers allows the saddle to slide forward.*

LOW WITHERS

If the withers are too low, the saddle and rider slide forward, shifting the center of gravity forward and increasing impact on the forelegs. The saddle and weight of a rider may injure poorly muscled withers.

Chest

A good chest is deep and well-defined to allow for a large respiratory capacity and a well-developed heart. The depth of a horse's chest is more important than width. The ribs should have ample space between them and project backward to improve chest depth and allow for lung expansion during athletic pursuits.

Proper Width and Depth of Chest

A chest that is too wide, called *base-wide*, does not allow ample clearance for the elbows, and a horse is prone to girth gall. The greatest width of the barrel should lie behind the girth so shoulder movement is not restricted (fig. 2.15).

A narrow chest, called *base-narrow*, can result in limb interference like *plaiting* (placing one foot directly ahead of the opposite foot) or striking the inside of a leg with the opposite foot. A horse with base-narrow, toed-out conformation (the hooves are closer together than the shoulders) *wings* with his feet as he moves. If pigeon-toed, he would *paddle* instead. Limb interference results from winging, with potential injury to a splint bone. A base-narrow stance also creates pressure on the inside of the knee joints and inside splint bones, increasing the chance of developing *splints* (see p. 103).

Shoulder

Bones that are located higher in the leg have greater influence on the freedom of limb swing. It is actually the relationship of the shoulder blade (*scapula*) to the arm bone (*humerus*) that has the most influence on arm swing and stride length (fig. 2.16). Ideally, the angle between the scapula and humerus should be greater than 90 degrees, preferably nearing a more open angle of 105 degrees (fig. 2.17).

Stride Length

A horse's stride length depends on the conformational angles of his shoulder and foreleg. The longer a horse's stride, the faster he can cover ground, and the fewer steps a horse takes to get from point to point. The more steps a horse must take, the faster he may fatigue in addition to assuming more stress and strain on the limbs. The forelegs absorb up to 65 percent of the weight-bearing impact; shorter stride length increases the possibility of lameness.

SLOPING SHOULDER

A sloping shoulder anatomically moves the withers further back to relieve the shock of impact for a rider. A sloping shoulder distributes the attachment of muscles and ligaments over a greater area, thereby diffusing impact on a horse's musculoskeletal system. The slope of the shoulder is measured with a line running from the point of the shoulder to the top of the withers. The shoulder joint angle (that angle formed by the intersection of the scapula with the humerus) is optimal at 105 degrees. Looking at the actual inclination of the scapula itself, elite show jumpers tend to have a scapular inclination of 64 to 77 degrees, with most measuring 73 degrees. Although the scapula in these horses tends to sit more verti-

Conformation for Performance   21

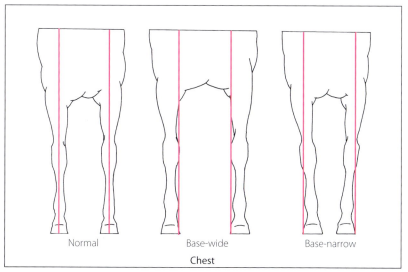

2.15 *A chest that is excessively wide (base-wide) restricts elbow clearance and may increase the chance of girth galls, while a narrow chest (base-narrow) may cause limb interference.*

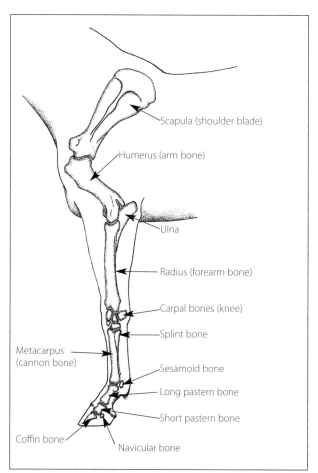

2.16 *A gently sloping shoulder with a long, vertical arm bone enables a horse to move smoothly. A horse with a more vertical shoulder is limited in his motion.*

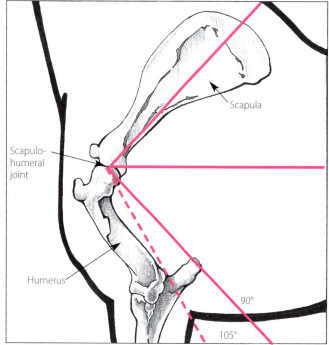

2.17 *Ideally, the angle between the scapula and humerus should be greater than 90 degrees, preferably nearing a more open angle of 105 degrees. The joint formed at the junction of the scapula and the humerus (upper arm bone) is called the scapulo-humeral joint. A relatively long humerus gives a more open joint to enhance a horse's agility and scope.*

2.18 *Viewed from the side, the foreleg should be a straight column from the elbow to the fetlock. A plumb line dropped from the middle of the shoulder blade and bisecting the fetlock should fall directly behind the heel. A horse's normal knee conformation is slightly sprung. If set too far back, it is a calf knee; if too buckled forward, it is a bucked knee. Tied-in behind the knee refers to a narrowness of the cannon bone and flexor structures just below the knee relative to a broader circumference of these same structures just above the fetlock.*

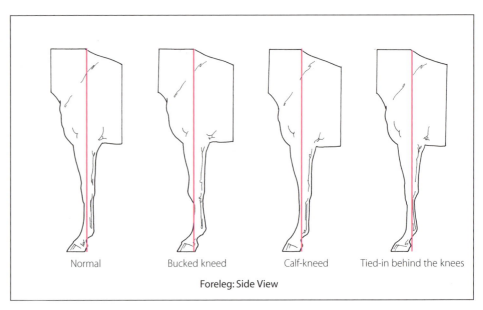

cally than expected, it is the open shoulder joint angle and the laid-back withers that improve athletic ability.

VERTICAL SHOULDER

An upright shoulder has a shoulder joint angle of less than 90 degrees and withers placed fairly far forward. This conformation predisposes to greater knee action. High-stepping knees create a rough, inelastic ride that transfers concussion to a rider while a horse covers less ground with each stride. The greater the number of steps a horse must take, the faster the onset of fatigue.

Forelimb Alignment

Viewed from the side, the foreleg should be a straight column from the elbow to the fetlock (fig. 2.18). Straightness of this column promotes equal-loading (axial compression) forces down a leg with weight bearing across the joints and bones. A plumb line dropped from the middle of the shoulder blade and bisecting the fetlock should fall directly behind the heel.

Any deviation from the straightness of the column predisposes to arthritis, known as *degenerative joint disease* (DJD). Abnormalities in bone growth plates lead to *angular limb deformities*, or ALD. *Valgus* refers to outward deviation; *varus* refers to inward deviation. These deformities predispose to DJD because of abnormal loading forces on the joint. Examples of ALD syndromes include: knock-kneed (*carpus valgus*), bowlegged (*carpus varus*), splayfooted (*fetlock valgus*), and pigeon-toed (*fetlock varus*) [fig. 2.19]. A pigeon-toed horse is at risk of developing *ringbone*, or DJD of the pastern or coffin joint.

Upper Arm

The *humerus* (upper arm) should be at least half as long as the scapula (see fig. 2.17, p. 21). If the point of the shoulder is high, the humerus is long and steep, creating a more open shoulder angle. A longer humerus enables a horse more freedom to move the elbow away from the body. Unrestricted elbow

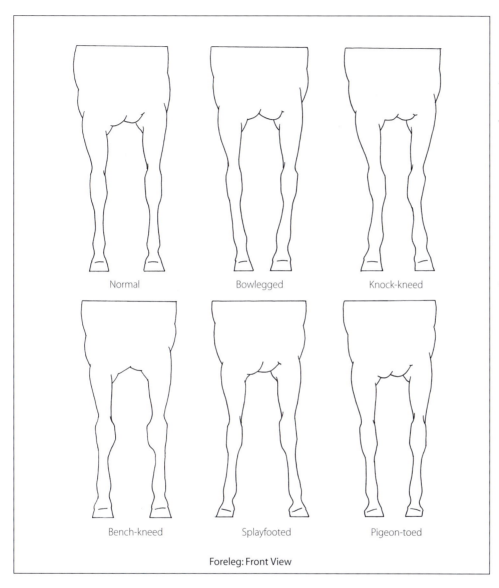

2.19 *Viewed from the front, each foreleg should form a straight column with the joints sitting in the middle of this column. Any deviation from this straightness is referred to as an angular limb deformity, which create various other knee conformations, like knock-kneed (carpus valgus) and bowlegged (carpus varus). A bench-knee is one in which the cannon bone sits offset to the outside of the cannon bone.*

movement improves athletic ability for speed and agility important to racing, jumping, or crouching as in cutting. If a horse can move the elbow without restriction, it is easier to execute lateral movements important to dressage, polo, and cutting.

A horse with a short humerus tends to have short, choppy strides, and does not easily perform speed or lateral work. If the humerus lies in a horizontal plane, the *scapulo-humeral* angle is more closed (see fig. 2.17, p. 21). The limbs cannot fold tightly, and a horse is less proficient at sports like cutting, barrel racing, jumping, or polo. The elbow should be located in front of the peak of the withers so the humerus does not tend to a horizontal alignment. A relatively horizontal humerus produces a *pigeon-breasted* horse that stands with the forelegs too far under the body. It is hard for a pigeon-breasted horse to be agile.

Forearm

Muscles in the forearm extend the limb forward and absorb the shock of impact. It is preferable to have strong, well-developed muscles. A long forearm increases the length of a horse's stride. A long forearm coupled with a short cannon bone and a medium length pastern provides structural stability in the limb, while achieving optimal leverage and strength of the *musculotendinous* attachments.

Knee

Normally a horse's knee *(carpus)* is slightly sprung and not entirely straight due to the normal curvature of the forearm bone *(radius)*. (See fig. 2.19, p. 23.) The front contours of the knees should be flat and shield-shaped, with well-defined corners. Injury to the carpal joints from conformational problems is most commonly related to high-speed activities like racing.

BUCKED KNEE
Excessive curvature of the radius leads to bucked knees or *over at the knee,* and potentially places strain on the flexor tendons. The tendon is caused to flex prematurely, assuming more strain with each stride. Such conformation places a horse at greater risk for developing tendon injury leading to a *bowed tendon*.

CALF KNEE
A knee that is set too far back is called a *calf knee,* or *back at the knee*. This is considered a major flaw that may lead to fractured knee bones in a racehorse, or degenerative joint disease in other athletes. An upright pastern and a long-toe low-heel (LTLH) foot (see chapter 3, *The Hoof,* p. 51) configuration create a functional calf knee, stressing the knee joints and flexor tendons, and delaying *breakover* of the foot.

OTHER KNEE DEVIATIONS
Knock-knee *(carpus valgus)* occurs when the knees deviate toward each other. Bowlegged *(carpus varus)* horses have knees that deviate away from each other. Both of these abnormalities predispose to DJD. The term b*ench-knee* refers to a knee that sits slightly offset to the cannon bone. This is a common conformational trait that in a mild form does not usually cause problems in low to moderate intensity athletics. (See "Offset Cannon Bone," below.)

Cannon Bone

For most equine athletics, with the exception of racing, the cannon bone should be short, particularly relative to the length of the forearm. The circumference all the way down the cannon bone should be the same width top to bottom. Bone is ample when there is at least 8 inches per 1000-pound horse as measured at the circumference at the top of the cannon bone, just below the knee (photo 2.20).

TIED–IN BEHIND THE KNEE
If the circumference measured at the top of the cannon bone is less than at the bottom of the cannon bone, this condition is referred to as being *tied-in behind the knees* (see fig. 2.18). The width of the flexor tendons and suspensory ligaments is smaller at the top of the cannon area, predisposing these structures to strain and injury.

OFFSET CANNON BONE
When the cannon bone is offset to the outside of the forelegs, a condition referred to as a *bench knee,* greater stress is placed on the inside of the knee joint (photo 2.21). This predisposes a horse to developing splints (see "Splints" in chapter 4, *Developing Strong Bones,* p. 103).

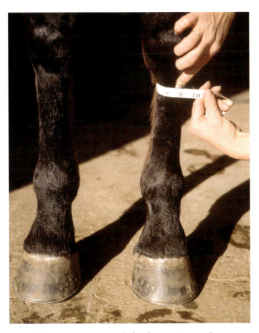

2.20 A measurement of the bone circumference at the top of the cannon bone, just below the knee, is considered ample when there is at least 8 inches per 1000-pound horse.

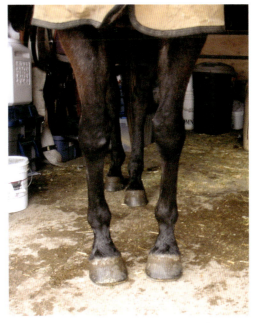

2.21 An offset cannon bone sits more to the side of the carpal joints. Such a bench-kneed conformation places more stress on one side of the joints than others, especially when coupled with an angular limb deformity like this horse's toed-in conformation.

Pastern

The angle of the pastern's slope to the ground is important to the stability of the joints in the lower legs and smoothness of stride. In general, the angles of the hoof, pastern, and shoulder to the ground should be the same and the pasterns should be of medium length (fig 2.22).

SHORT PASTERN

A short, upright pastern acts as a poor shock absorber. Not only does this configuration result in an uncomfortable ride, but also the horse receives added concussion to the rear third of each foot, predisposing to navicular disease. Short, upright pasterns also predispose to pastern joint arthritis (*ringbone*), especially in those equine athletes that engage in high impact sports like jumping, roping, cutting, reining, and polo.

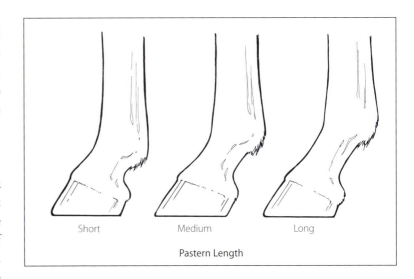

2.22 Evaluation of pastern length gives a rider an idea of what a horse's gait will feel like. A short pastern tends to create a shorter, choppier gait, while a long pastern gives more elasticity to the ride.

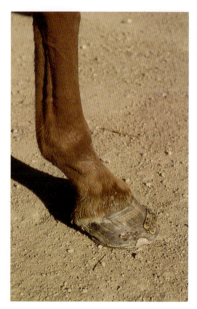
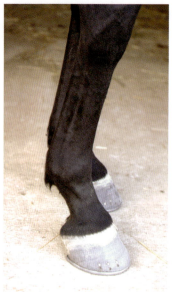

2.23 *This horse has a long and sloping pastern, which causes a greater range of movement through the fetlock. This gives a more elastic and comfortable ride.*

2.24 *In comparison to the previous photo of a long and sloping pastern, a long and upright pastern poses a greater risk for injury for horses engaging in high speed work because more stress is placed upon the flexor tendons and suspensory ligaments, as well as the fetlock joint.*

LONG PASTERN

A moderately long pastern with some slope to it enables a horse to have suspension (photo 2.23). A long pastern provides a comfortable ride; however, once it was thought that excessive fetlock drop associated with a long sloping pastern would predispose to tendon injury. Now, better understanding of biomechanics indicates that a long, upright pastern (photo 2.24) is more of a liability than a long, sloping pastern, particularly for horses that engage in speed activities.

A horse with a long, upright pastern often develops *windpuffs*, inflammation of the fetlock joint and flexor tendon sheath (see photos 5.6 and 5.7, p. 113). An upright pastern conformation also increases the risk for a bowed tendon, *sesamoiditis* (inflammation of the fetlock sesamoid bones), or *suspensory desmitis* (inflammation of the suspensory ligament). Refer to p. 186 for further discussion of these conditions.

Back

The way in which the muscles of the hindquarters connect to the back at the lumbosacral joint is called *coupling*. To achieve the greatest strength and flexibility, hindquarter muscles should be carried well forward into the back. The loin is unable to flex from side to side, therefore a *long* lumbar span creates a weak back. A *short* back (as defined by a short lumbar span) limits the range that a horse can move the legs and elbows vertically, which is referred to as *scope*. Scope is important in events such as racing, jumping, hunting, and cutting.

Back length also has to do with the relative size of the vertebrae: with the exception of some Arabian horses, which have one less vertebra in their spines, most horses have the same number of vertebrae, and it is the varied length of these that creates a relatively long or short back (fig. 2.25). A back that is too long may eventually develop a *sway back* as muscular attachments weaken with age and use. A sway-backed horse is often plagued with chronic back pain (see photo 8.12 on p. 212, and figs. 2.26 A–D). A long back also prevents a horse from executing lateral movements with ease, or achieving collection. Ribs and interlocking facets of lumbar vertebrae prevent a horse from rotating sideways in the area in front of the ninth thoracic vertebra. Maximum bending and rotation lie behind the area under the saddle and behind the rider's leg. (For more discussion, see chapter 8, *The Horse's Back*, p. 203.)

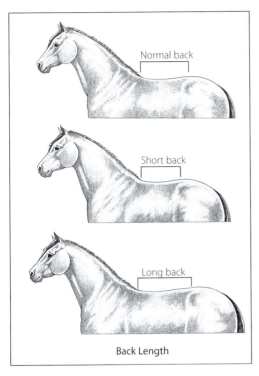

Back Length

2.25 *A horse with a short back may have limited scope, while too long a back can lead to back injury of muscles or spine, and a long-backed horse often has difficulty with collected or lateral movements.*

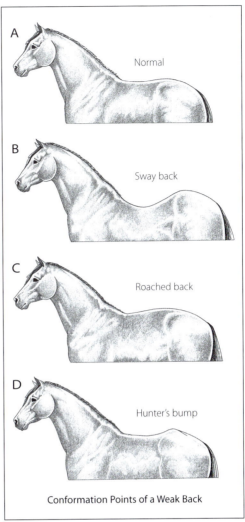

Conformation Points of a Weak Back

2.26 A—D *The strength of a horse's back is related to strength of the muscles and ligaments, and the conformation of the spine. Advancing age, poor conformation, athletic use, or trauma, may predispose a horse to back injury. Normal (A). A sway back is often a heritable, conformational defect of the spine but can also occur with weakening ligaments in an aging horse (B). A roached back is the result of enlargement of the vertebral processes of the lumbar region, due to conformation and/or injury (C). A hunter's bump on the croup is often a result of ligamentous strain, but can be a heritable conformational feature (D). Any of these conformational traits can limit performance by altering flexibility of the spine, and/or diminishing muscular development of the back, and/or by creating pain in the spine or back muscles and ligaments.*

Loins

Ideal loins are short and only encompass a hand span, or about 8 inches, between the last rib and the point of the hip (fig. 2.27). A horse that uses his loins well also has rounded hip (*gluteal*) muscles for upward thrust of the leg off the ground, and developed *quadriceps* muscles on the thigh that pull the hind leg forward. A long, weak loin reduces drive from the hindquarters, as evidenced by underdeveloped gluteals and quadriceps.

LOINS AND BODY CARRIAGE

As a horse carries his head and neck in the correct position for bit contact, he engages the hindquarters to relax and round the back. This allows efficient and fluid swing of the shoulders and forelimbs. Weight is distributed evenly fore and aft, and a horse in this frame is balanced and agile. A balanced frame permits shoulders to extend and flex to their full potential, not only lengthening the stride but also adding to suspension and smoothness of the stride.

Hindquarters

Many equine sports require quick turns, sudden stops, and perfect balance. A horse normally carries as much as 65 percent of his weight on the front end. Events like reining, roping, cutting, trail riding, polo, jumping, and dressage have at least one similar characteristic: these sports transfer a horse's center of gravity toward the rear end. Strong hindquarters improve the chance to perform well. The propulsive muscles of the body originate on the pelvis, so a strong hind end generates greater power and drive.

Effects of Exercise on Hindquarters

Just as calisthenic exercises for people strengthen attendant muscle groups, a horse in training improves muscle condition to retain balance through gait transitions and various movements. Collection of a horse begins in the hindquarters, specifically at the lumbosacral joint (L-S joint) at the top of the croup (see fig. 2.27 and photo 2.28), and is car-

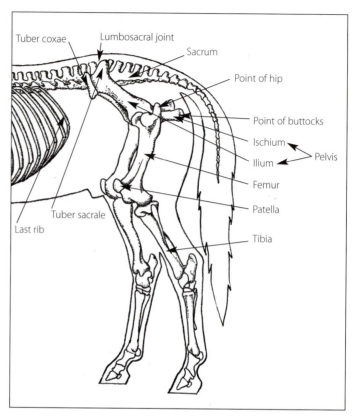

2.27 *Skeletal anatomy of the hindquarters.*

ried on through the back, withers, and neck, to the poll. If a horse's hindquarters are likened to an engine because they propel the horse into motion, then the L-S joint at the top of the croup is the transmission. The L-S joint pivots and rotates the hindquarters and pelvis forward beneath the body. The abdominal muscles help pull the pelvis forward to engage the hindquarters.

Angle of Croup and Pelvis

The slope of a horse's croup is determined by the slope of the pelvis bone from the point of the hip to the point of the buttocks (see photos 2.28 and 2.29). (The croup encompasses the lumbar and sacral vertebrae, but its slope is actually defined by the angle—slope—of the

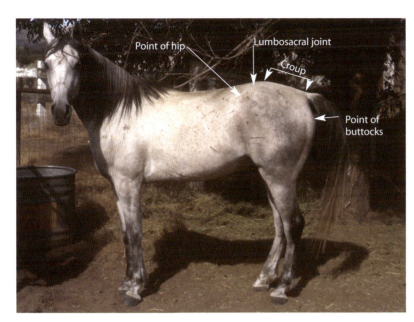

2.28 *The location of the lumbosacral (L-S) joint.*

pelvis.) Steeper slope and greater length of the pelvis enables more power in the hindquarters. A horse with a very steep pelvis generates a greater upward thrust, although his steps are small. This is an advantage to a working draft horse that uses power and push from the hindquarters to pull a load where speed across the ground is not as important as strength to move the load.

A pelvis and croup that incline toward the horizontal enhance *speed,* especially at the trot. A more horizontal pelvis allows the hip joint to lengthen when the hind leg is extended, allowing for greater forward push. This configuration gives a fluid, ground-covering stride as is seen with some Arabians with a flat, horizontal croup.

For the best biomechanical advantage for locomotion, the croup should incline about 25 degrees and be relatively long in proportion to the body (photo 2.29). Long muscles over the croup have a greater range of muscle contraction across the skeleton, improving speed. A short croup has shorter muscle contraction, resulting in less leverage and muscle power.

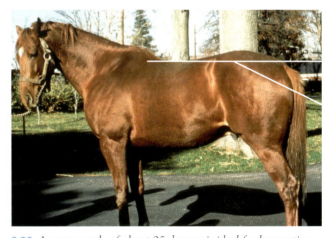

2.29 *A croup angle of about 25 degrees is ideal for locomotion.*

The hindquarters should have ample vertical depth as defined by a triangle formed by the point of the hip, the point of the buttock, and the stifle joint (photo 2.30). For an athletic horse, the best results are obtained with a long, relatively perpendicular thigh and a gaskin that is a bit shorter than the length of the thigh.

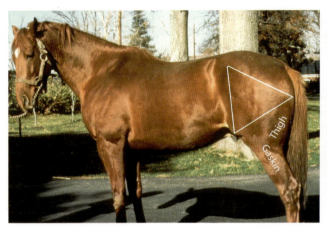

2.30 *The triangle formed by the point of the hip, point of the buttock, and stifle joint defines the vertical depth of the hindquarters, and the deeper, the better for performance. Also, it's best to have a horse with a long, perpendicular thigh and a gaskin slightly shorter than the thigh.*

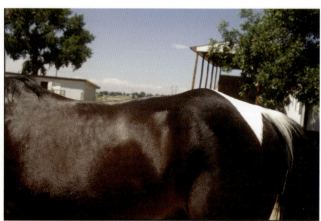

2.31 *A prominent hunter's bump is visible over the sacroiliac joint. This horse also has a roached back. Both of these conformational traits may limit athleticism.*

HUNTER'S BUMP

At the top of the croup lies the junction of the sacrum and the ilium. An enlargement may be visible in this location (see photo 8.5 on p. 208); this prominence may be a result of injury but is not necessarily related to ligamentous tearing or damage: it may simply be a heritable feature of larger than normal *tuber sacrale* of the pelvis (see fig. 2.26 and photo 2.31).

However, injury to the *sacroiliac ligaments* may occur when a horse is asked to negotiate a steep hill at a trot, or is repeatedly overfaced with a jumping obstacle beyond his ability or fitness, or when he slips while executing a sprint effort. Asymmetrical swelling in the location of the tuber sacrale should be examined for pain and injury. This enlargement may not be considered pathologic if there is no lameness, or soreness in the region of the bump (see chapter 8, *The Horse's Back*, p. 203).

ROACHED BACK

The coupling where the back and loins join the croup may appear to have an upward curvature in the spine. This conformational trait is referred to as a roached back (see fig. 2.26 C and photo 2.31). A roached back develops due to enlargement of the vertebral processes of the lumbar region, related to conformation and/or spinal injury. Since the vertebrae and spine of a roached back are somewhat diminished in range of motion, particularly if a result of injury, the loin muscles of a roached back may be less developed in substance and strength to preclude proper back lift and collection. Some horses are born with enlarged vertebral processes in this area of the back, and performance may only be limited relative to the degree of reduced flexibility in upward and downward movement and/or lateral bending. This has consequence to athletic pursuits that require agility and rapid changes in direction. Back pain may result, particularly in a short, roached back that develops *kissing spines* or vertebral impingement (see fig. 8.14, p. 213). A horse that holds his back rigid to protect against pain or discomfort presents a stiff or choppy ride, and has difficulty in achieving collection.

Limb Alignment

From the side, a plumb line dropped from the point of the buttocks to the point of the hock should fall along the back of the tendons to the fetlock.

Stifle

The stifle should sit at the same height as the elbow. The stifle is turned slightly out so a horse can move forward freely without physical interference from the flank. This preferred position of the stifle causes many horses to slightly toe out in the hind legs.

More than 80 percent of hind leg lameness develops in the hock or stifle joints; therefore, conformation of these structures is very important to continuing soundness in the performance horse. (For discussion on hock joints see below right, and see chapter 5, *Joints*, p. 119.) Any athletic pursuit (dressage, cutting, roping, reining) that moves the horse's weight toward the hindquarters amplifies the stress on these joints.

A relatively straight hind leg may be efficient at thrusting at the ground for push-off. This characteristic can be helpful for events such as jumping, Quarter Horse racing, or roping. However, if the limb is too straight, excess stress on both stifle and hock joints may lead to arthritis. These horses are also prone to *upward fixation of the patella* (a ligament of the stifle locks over the kneecap), and *thoroughpin* (windpuff of the Achilles tendon behind the hock).

In contrast, a long hind leg with some angulation of the gaskin helps a horse bring the hocks beneath the body, which is an important feature for dressage, cutting, and reining sports. A long thigh and short gaskin with good muscling are advantageous in any athletic endeavor except for the racehorse. For sprint horses, a long hip, gaskin, and thigh increase the muscle leverage for optimal stride length, power, and speed during a rapid and quick effort.

Stride length increases with a hind leg that is angled rather than being of straight conformation. However, a hind limb that is too angulated may create problems: a horse may be *camped-out* (the hind legs stick out behind) or *sickle-hocked* (the hind legs angle beneath the horse). (See text below and fig. 2.32.) Horses with these conformation problems are prone to:

- *Bog spavin*—excess joint fluid in the hock from inflammation (see photo 5.19 and text p. 120)
- *Bone spavin*—degenerative joint disease (DJD) of the hock (see photo 5.20 and text p. 120)
- *Curb*—strain of the plantar ligament on the back of the hock (see photo 7.8 and text p. 187)

If a rear limb is too long and angled, the croup may rise higher than the withers with each stride, resulting in a rough, uncomfortable ride.

Hocks

Between the tibia above and the cannon bone below, the hock forms a complicated mechanism of multiple joints. The hock joints alternately flex and swing and then extend the limb. This wide range of motion creates a mechanical advantage for support and push that produce drive and locomotion. The various positions accomplished by the hocks enable a horse to accelerate for forward propulsion, to turn sharply, to push off and launch into the air, and to brake for deceleration. Conformation of the hind limbs dictates the ability of a horse to rock back on his hocks

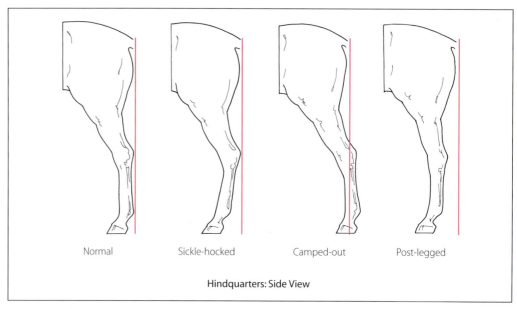

2.32 *From the side view, the rear legs should have some angulation between the stifle and the hock. A plumb line dropped straight down should go from the point of the buttock through the point of the hock, down the back of the cannon, and to the back of the heel bulbs. If the leg below the hock is in front of this plumb line the horse is considered to have sickle hocks, and behind is considered to be camped-out. A horse with limited angulation between the stifle and the hock through the gaskin is referred to as post-legged.*

to accelerate, suddenly change directions, to brake, or to suspend the body.

The hock of a horse is composed of multiple little bones and a series of several joints stacked one on the other: the *tibiotarsal* joint, the *proximal intertarsal* joint, the *distal intertarsal* joint, and the *tarsometatarsal* joint. The two lower joints (distal intertarsal and tarsometatarsal joints) are considered low-range motion joints that are arranged in a close-packed orientation to lend stability. As a horse accelerates, this close-stacked arrangement enables the force from the weight of the horse to maintain limb rigidity while the horse loads the limb. The hock and stifle joints act as shock-absorbing dampers along with the fetlock joints. The distal intertarsal joint is particularly affected by exercises that rely on hock flexion, as seen in dressage, cutting, reining, jumping, or draft-related pulling sports.

It is desirable to have open angles on the front face of the hind legs approximating 160 degrees. The hock joints should be well formed and large. Hocks that are *low set* (which results from a relatively short cannon bone) develop more power for pushing and quick turns. Sprint efforts benefit from this conformation.

Deviations from Normal

Any conformation that affects the angulation of the hocks as they attach to the gaskin will affect musculoskeletal efficiency. *Post-legged*, *sickle-hocked*, or *cow-hocked* conformation worsen loading pressures in the hock joints,

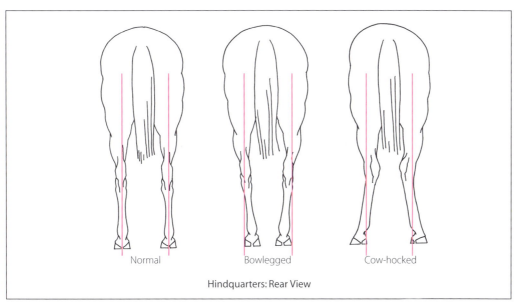

2.33 *From the rear view of a horse's hindquarters, the limbs should make a straight column with the hocks only very slightly rotated outward. When the hocks are rotated inward and the cannon bones outward, the condition is called cow-hocked. When the cannon bones rotate inward and the hocks rotate outward, it is called bowlegged.*

increasing the risk of developing degenerative joint disease (figs. 2.32 and 2.33).

POST-LEGGED

A horse with hind legs that are too straight (the angle is over 170 degrees) is post-legged (photo 2.34). This conformational flaw increases concussion and loading of the joints. The tendon sheaths have a tendency to develop windpuffs. A post-legged horse is predisposed to upward fixation of the patella, *thoroughpin* (see below), suspensory ligament injury, and bone spavin in the hocks or degenerative joint disease (DJD) in the stifles.

SICKLE HOCKS

Sickle hocks refer to hind limbs that tend to angle beneath the torso (photo 2.35). These are often associated with effusion of the hock joints and of *thoroughpin* of the Achilles

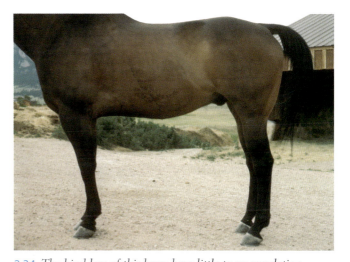

2.34 *The hind legs of this horse have little to no angulation between the stifle and hocks, giving the limb an appearance of a straight post, hence the term "post-legged" that describes this conformational trait. A post-legged horse is predisposed to upward fixation of the patella, thoroughpin, suspensory ligament injury, and bone spavin in the hocks or degenerative joint disease (DJD) in the stifles.*

The Lower Portion of the Rear Limb

Similar characteristics as described for the lower part of the forelegs apply to the hind legs to achieve mechanical efficiency. As in the foreleg, it is preferable to have short cannon bones in the hind leg to enable tendons to pull effectively on the point of the hocks to create drive. The fetlocks should be clean and tight, without bumps or nicks, and the pasterns should be strong, well-defined, and of medium length. Long, sloping pasterns of the rear limbs are undesirable as they are prone to suspensory ligament injury, and fetlock arthritis.

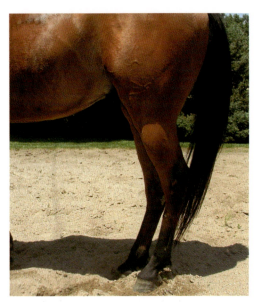

2.35 *Viewed from the side, this horse's hocks are angled slightly beneath his body when he is standing squarely at rest. This condition is known as sickle-hocked.*

tendon. Thoroughpin is a chronic inflammation or irritation to the tendon sheath around the deep flexor tendon where it attaches above the point of the hock. Continual compression or abnormal rotational forces on the joints elicit degenerative changes. Increased risk of *curb* (inflammation of the plantar ligament) is also a risk with sickle hocks.

COW HOCKS

A horse with true cow hocks (see fig. 2.33, p. 33) has limbs very different from the commonly seen toed-out conformation of Arabians and Trakehners. As visualized from behind, the fetlocks of a cow-hocked horse reach farther apart than do the point of the hocks. The hocks may sit fairly close together. In contrast, a *toed-out* horse has fetlocks placed directly beneath the hocks, yet the toes turn out from below the fetlocks. Cow-hock conformation places excessive strain on the insides of the hocks and stifles, predisposing to degenerative joint disease (DJD).

Conformation Related to Specific Athletic Pursuits

Breed, size, and disposition are important attributes that characterize the type of horse selected to perform an intended athletic pursuit. In addition, certain characteristics are desirable to meet the challenge of specific athletic endeavors such as jumping, dressage, eventing, cutting, or reining. Several features differentiate these various athletic disciplines.

The Western Performance Horse

Western performance sports like cutting and reining are high intensity sports. Not only that, but these horses generally start their training as 2 year olds to be competitive in their third and Futurity year; they must develop muscle power at an early age. These are sprinting athletics not too dissimilar to the muscular efforts experienced by human weight lifters. Western performance sports demand maximal or near maximal power in a very fast period of time, ranging from seconds to a minute or two.

Horses with a large degree of *fast twitch muscle fibers* excel in sprint activities (see chapter 6, *Muscle Endurance,* p. 143). Quarter Horses have nearly 90 percent fast twitch fibers in their rear-end muscles; Thoroughbreds and Appaloosas range between 80 to 90 percent; Standardbred horses possess a proportion of around 80 percent, while Arabians have less than 70 to 80 percent of their rear-end musculature devoted to fast twitch muscle fibers.

Besides having lots of "cow" sense, Western performance horses need to have extremely fast reaction times that are dependent upon central nervous system responses. This trait is heritable, but can be fine-tuned by practice and muscular conditioning. Most Western performance horses are small in stature, ranging from 14 to 15 hands high. Good size of bone is desirable as it implies strong joints and strong tendons. Unacceptable characteristics include any crookedness in the front limbs or a "downhill" frame in which the haunches sit higher than the withers.

The predilection for extreme maneuverability enables these horses to accelerate and decelerate rapidly with abrupt changes in direction. Just as a dressage horse needs the ability to collect his frame, a reining or cutting horse must be able to rapidly lighten his forehand and collect his frame while retaining flexibility and suppleness. An elite cutting horse moves the head and shoulders first to shift the center of gravity sideways. This allows limb thrust to be directed at an oblique angle to give the horse a fraction of a second advantage in acceleration. Faster time equates to a competitive edge. Studies have shown that a horse of "average" talent moves the lower portion of the front limbs before moving the head, neck, and shoulders. Talent to perform these sports with superior skill relies on heritable tendencies not entirely related to conformation.

The neck should be moderately short so as to limit weight over the forehand as the horse crouches for spins and turns. The withers should be relatively low so that sudden cat-like maneuvers do not cause the saddle to jam the spine or surrounding muscles. A moderately low withers allows the neck and shoulder muscles to blend nicely into the back and gives a broad surface area to distribute the movement stress beneath the saddle.

In addition to a need for agility, Western performance sports rely on abrupt stops, with reining horses making more dramatic sliding stops than cutting or roping horses. Nonetheless, all these horses spend a lot of time "sitting" and working off their haunches so they are particularly predisposed to rear end lameness and compensatory back soreness (see chapter 8, *The Horse's Back,* p. 203).

Cutting and reining horses should have "low" knees and hocks. This then provides them with short cannon bones, long forearms, long femurs, and moderately long gaskins. Elite competitors in these events have a measurable, optimal hock distance from the ground to the point of the hock of 22 to 23 inches. The optimal cannon bone length should be 9 inches. (Interestingly, these are the very dimensions of *Secretariat's* bone lengths despite the fact that he stood 16.2 hands.) All joints must be strong and large, and particularly the hocks. The hocks should be relatively straight without excessive angulation. Cow hocks are considered a liability because of the twisting forces exerted on the rear limbs during turns and slides. The hind feet should be set beneath the butt, but the horse should not be sickle-hocked. This rear-end configuration enables the cutting or reining horse to more easily "collect" the hind legs under his body, enabling him to make rapid maneuvers and to bolt forward or stop abruptly.

The loins should be short (that is, a short span between the last rib and the point of the hip) and broad, and the croup can withstand being moderately short. The stifle and gaskin muscles should be strong and well developed with pronounced muscular rounding, rather than appearing weak or "caved in." The fitter the horse, the bigger his chest and forearm muscles will be as these contract and pull the legs up and forward with each shift in direction.

The Jumping Horse

A jumping horse encompasses many shapes and sizes varying from the more sedately mannered show hunter to the speedy show jumper to the ambitious eventer. Additional jumping talents include the bold foxhunters, timber horses, and steeplechasers. One common characteristic applies to all these horses: the need for good, solid muscling of the hindquarters with the hindquarters comprising at least one-third of the overall body proportion. All jumping horses, possibly with the exception of a show hunter, need speed, agility, and strength to do their job. A jumping horse needs the ability to quickly collect for the agility to rapidly turn and bend, and accelerate and decelerate. The propulsive muscles of the haunches are used as brakes to decelerate forward momentum, so the horse must be able to bring his haunches well beneath him to slow down quickly.

Speed of acceleration and deceleration relies on how quickly a horse is able to put his feet down, not how quickly he picks his feet up. Since a horse's forward velocity cannot change in the air, the amount of time his feet spend on the ground influences his speed and change of direction. Each limb begins its deceleration before it hits the ground so by the time the hoof impacts terrain, it is going at a speed that is compatible with the ability of the limb to absorb the concussion and deceleration forces without blowing the limb apart.

The front end of a jumping horse works as both a support strut and a shock absorber so a jumping horse needs good musculature and big bone and tendons. The feet should be large and broad with a good cup (concave sole) rather than a flat sole (see chapter 3, *The Hoof*, p. 48). The frog and bars of the feet should be well developed. The pastern should be medium in length, and the cannon bones short with large tendons running behind the lower leg. Long cannons place extra stress on the knees and tendons, potentially leading to excess strain as the horse lands off a jump. Any limb crookedness amplifies concussive stresses on the joints and bones. Thus, pigeon-toed or toed-out conformation is frowned upon, and offset knees are a disadvantage.

The shoulder blade should be long and sloping and coupled to a long, sloping arm bone. The joining of these two bones should produce an angle of about 105 degrees, and certainly no less than 90 degrees. This enables a long, ground-covering stride while facilitating folding of the knees into a tightly tucked position (*scope*) that lends safety and beauty over jumps.

The loins should be short, strong, and broad as with the Western performance horse, to impart strength. However, a little longer back than what is seen in the Western performance horse makes it easier for a jumping horse to round his back over jumps and to develop thrust from his haunches. Too long a back is a detriment as it makes it difficult for a horse to activate his abdominal muscles to engage his hindquarters and compress and collect his frame. High and broad withers are desirable features to hold a saddle in position, and because the neck and back muscles join here. Like a seesaw, the higher the fulcrum, the greater the rise of the back and flexibility of the neck.

Remembering the previously discussed body proportions of one-third, one-third, one-third, too long a neck places too much weight on the forehand for a jumping horse, but some neck length is desirable for a horse to use his neck as a pendulum and balance over jumps, just as a tightrope walker uses a balance stick. The neck should carry back fully through the withers. In contrast, a preferred neck conformation for a show hunter is a lower neck carriage that is set more horizontal to the ground. This imparts the impression of a calm, relaxed horse. A jumper or eventer would have trouble negotiating sharp turns or the required speeds if the neck and head are set on low, and too much weight is transferred to the forehand.

The Dressage Horse

A dressage prospect and an event horse also rely on strong rear-end musculature. In these pursuits, the center of gravity is shifted equally between front and rear ends to achieve collection, smooth gait transitions, and more advanced levels of "gymnastics." The rear-end engine should be at least one-third of the overall proportion of the horse, but unlike a Western performance horse or exclusive jumping horse, there can be greater angulation to the hocks and stifles (see p. 31). This increases a horse's stride length, lending more brilliance to each movement while making gait transitions effortless. The hocks produce impulsion so these joints need to be large and strong, especially since nearly 90 percent of rear end problems in dressage horses occur in the hocks. The cannon bones should be short as with the other athletic disciplines so that tendons and muscles can pull more easily over the point of the hock to improve impulsion, drive, and suspension. Similarly, a long femur (thigh bone) and a shorter gaskin enable strength in locomotion from the hind end.

A dressage horse can afford to have a little more length in his back (not his loins) to simplify canter work and canter departs, but too long a back is a weak back, making it harder for the belly muscles to activate and develop in strength. A well-developed and fit dressage horse has a huge groin depth due to the extreme development of the abdominal ring of muscles along with a solid topline.

As with a jumping horse, a long, sloping shoulder coupled to a long, sloping arm bone improves the extension of the forelimbs and the brilliance and suspension of the length of stride. The ride is smooth and elastic, with minimal knee action, especially when a dressage horse possesses a long forearm, a short cannon, and medium pasterns.

Total correctness in the front limbs is not as great an issue for a dressage horse as for a jumping horse since much of a dressage horse's center of gravity is shifted toward the rear quarters, and dressage horses work in soft arena footing most of the time. Yet, in collected gaits, the front legs experience high forces and must increase in braking power. To counteract the downward movement of the body, the front legs try to push up while the body is sinking down. This results in suspension and an aerial element of each stride that is so desirable in collected gaits. As an example, in the collected canter, the front limbs push up like struts before the horse rolls forward over the front leg; the croup is lowered and the withers elevated, but both are about the same height in all phases of the canter. To achieve this end, the sling muscles of the shoulder must develop strength and tone to be able to counteract the weight of the horse's mass.

Strong feet are a must as any foot lameness results in an unevenness of gait that is highly penalized in dressage tests. In addition, if the front limbs are sore, stride length shortens, and the rear limbs have nowhere to go. The horse then demonstrates a short, choppy stride that veers away from the elastic, fluid stride so desirable to an elite dressage competitor.

In Summary

It is no surprise that many of the desirable features described for each discipline cross the boundaries of the type of sport, whether it be an English or Western event. A well conformed horse knows no limitations and can take up the challenge of a multitude of equine sports as varied as driving, or endurance, or jumping. If you've ever watched a demonstration of a dressage horse and a reining horse executing similar moves at the same time in an arena, you will be stunned by the similarities of these seemingly dissimilar disciplines. The horses may be ridden with different tack and the riders wear different clothing, but the physical movements are comparable, and both resemble a combination of gymnastics and ballet.

In critique of a current or potential riding prospect, follow the basic principles for conformation, basing your selection more on breed, size, disposition, and inbred talent for your intended equine athletic discipline.

The Hoof 3

There is probably no truer adage, "No hoof, no horse." Without this solid foundation, a horse cannot perform to potential no matter how well trained, how fit, or how athletic he may be. A horse's hoof is a marvel in design. Although seemingly a covering of "dead" tissue, the tissues just beneath the hoof wall are quite alive, constantly remodeling to accommodate changing stimuli.

Nourishment of a horse's hooves comes from within, dependent on good genetics, a good quality diet, and adequate exercise. The type of exercise a horse performs and the terrain over which he is ridden stimulate surface changes of the outer hoof. Movement across the ground toughens the soles and cleanses debris from the bottom of the feet. Excellent shoeing techniques are important to maintaining healthy and sound feet.

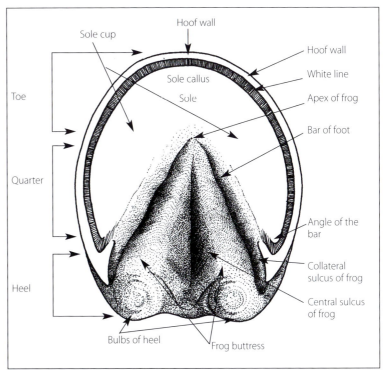

3.1 *Parts of the hoof.*

Hoof Structure and Growth

As an equivalent body part to a human, a horse's hoof corresponds to the last digit of our middle finger. It has evolved to support the full load of a horse as he propels himself across broken ground, over jumps, and as he spins and turns (figs 3.1 and 3.2).

The Hoof Wall

HOOF GROWTH

The hoof wall, composed of *keratin*, is a modified extension of the skin. Much in the same way fingernails grow out from the cuticles, a horse's hoof continuously grows down from the *coronary corium* of the coronary band (fig. 3.3). A young horse grows hoof faster than a mature horse: a foal may grow ½ inch of hoof per month, while a mature horse grows hoof at the rate of about ⅜ inch per month. An adult horse completely grows out the toes within a year and the heels within 4 to 5 months. Hoof grows at different rates throughout the year, depending on season and climate. It grows fastest during periods of warm temperatures and moisture, corresponding with springtime and lengthening daylight hours.

Succeeding *basal cells* arising from the coronary corium push older cells downward to achieve growth. Collections of cells (*keratinocytes*) are organized into *tubules* that reach continuously from the coronary band to the ground (fig. 3.4). *Horn tissue* forms perpendicular to these tubules to produce an intertubular composite that provides strength and stiffness against impact forces that are transmitted up the hoof wall. The tubules reinforce this horny material, but it is the intertubular horn that provides toughness to the hoof wall, not the tubules. With continuing maturity of the cellular components into *corneocytes*, intercellular cement fills around each cell to

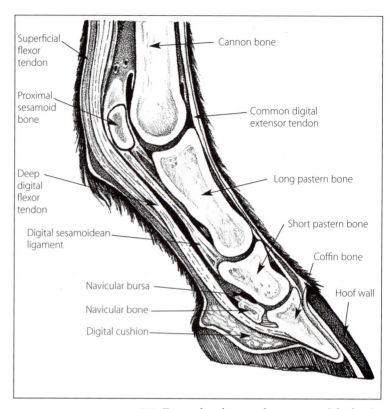

3.2 *External and internal structures of the hoof.*

anneal one to another. Mature corneocytes join together as *hoof wall* to support the weight of the horse while creating an impregnable barrier to external elements. The horny part of the hoof is tissue that has keratinized to form the hard hoof shell and *insensitive laminae*. The hoof capsule, then, can be viewed as a "laminated composite," with differing zones along the hoof imparting various qualities of stiffness and elasticity. Energy is absorbed through the interfaces between zones of the hoof.

Healthy hoof horn is resilient, expanding at the heels by as much as ¼ inch with each step. As the heels of the foot spread, blood and oxygen are pumped throughout the hoof. At the same time, impact energy is absorbed by the inner components of the foot, such as the *horn tubules*, the *frog*, the *digital cushion*, the

The Hoof

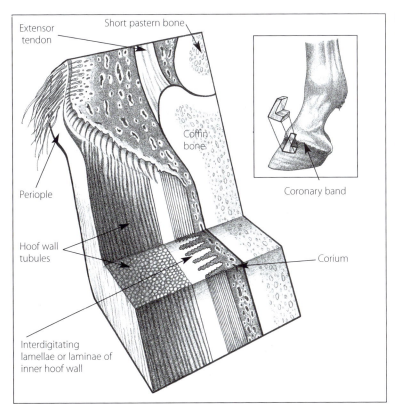

3.3 *The vast surface area provided by interwoven leaves of lamellae (or laminae) stabilizes the attachment of the coffin bone inside the hoof capsule. The epidermal lamellae lining the hoof wall interdigitate with an expansive network of connective tissue, nerves, and blood vessels, called the corium or "quick." These lamellae also interdigitate with the lamellae of the hoof wall to improve stability.*

3.4 *The lamellae (or laminae) of the hoof wall are folded and interwoven to form a large surface area of connective tissue interlaced with blood vessels that arise from the corium. The primary lamellae are layered in parallel rows on the inner surface of the hoof wall, while the secondary lamellae project off the primary lamellae to increase the surface area, all lamellae serving to suspend the coffin bone within the hoof capsule by connection through the basement membrane (not visible here). The corium of the hoof, known as the "quick," is filled with blood vessels, and is responsible for nourishment of the inner hoof structures and it connects the basement membrane to the coffin bone. The tissue elasticity of the laminae along with the interwoven blood supply from the corium serve to absorb energy within the foot. The hoof tubules additionally dissipate energy concussion and the intertubular material that connects them further imparts strength to counteract the impact generated by each hoof strike.*

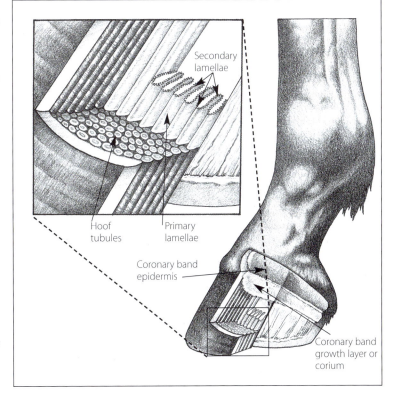

sensitive laminae, and the *lateral* (or *ungual*) *cartilages* to reduce concussion to the coffin bone and joint (fig. 3.5). By the time ground impact forces rise to the level of the fetlock, more than 90 percent of impact energy has been dissipated through the internal layers of the hoof wall.

THE CORIUM

The inner surface of the hoof wall folds into extensive leaves, called *lamellae,* or *laminae.* The vast surface area provided by interwoven leaves of lamellae stabilizes the attachment of the coffin bone inside the hoof capsule. The *epidermal lamellae* lining the hoof wall interdigitate with an expansive network of connective tissue, nerves, and blood vessels, called the *corium* or "quick." Not only does this layer provide nutrition to the hoof, but it also interlocks with lamellae of the hoof wall (see fig. 3.3).

A tough, connective portion of the corium forms a *basement membrane,* the junction between the connective tissue of the surface of the coffin bone with the hoof lamellae. The basement membrane suspends the coffin bone within the hoof capsule. At contact points between the basal cells of the lamellae and the basement membrane are "spot-welds" called *hemidesmosomes. Anchoring filaments* bridge the hemidesmosome attachments to the basement membrane to further improve coffin bone stability. (*Laminitis,* as described on p. 74 in detail, is caused by failure of the basement membrane and its anchoring points.) Coronary corium attaches the coronary band to the top of the coffin bone to intricately connect these structures, another feature that is important in pathology of laminitis.

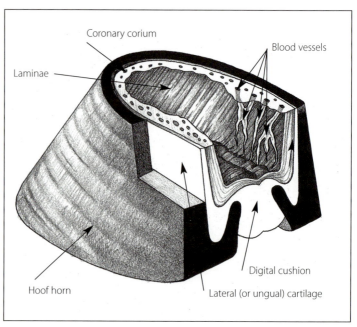

3.5 *The lateral (or ungual) cartilages in a "good" hoof are well-developed and thick, each base extending toward the midline and blending with the digital cushion, as seen in this diagram.*

REMODELING OF THE HOOF IN GROWTH AND IN RESPONSE TO STRESS AND INJURY

The hoof is a continually growing tissue. In order for new cells to migrate and proliferate downward, some attachments to the basement membrane must be loosened to allow controlled growth of the hoof wall. Part of the normal process of hoof growth relies on enzymatic activity of *matrix metalloproteinases,* or MMPs. As a normal consequence of hoof growth and replacement, or when there is minor injury to the hoof wall, this process occurs with careful, localized cellular organization. The basement membrane forms a template over which new cells migrate to reconstruct fresh lamellae. In summary, MMP activity on a daily basis facilitates:

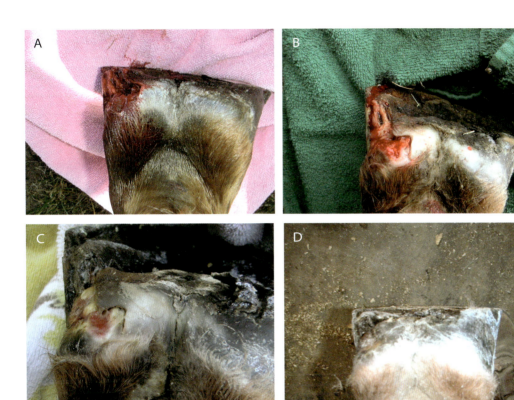

3.6 A–E This horse tore a large piece of hoof away after getting it caught in a pasture hazard (A). At 6 days, the hoof is showing signs of repair (B). At 13 days, new hoof wall has filled in some of the defect (C). At 30 days, the hoof repair is stable and non-painful (D). At 68 days, there is little sign of the previous hoof injury (E).

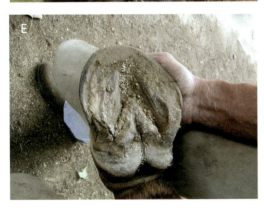

- Hoof growth
- Maintenance of lamellar orientation as the hoof grows down
- Repair of local areas of injury (photos 3.6 A–E)

MMP activity is orchestrated by opposing activity of *MMP inhibitors* that keep this process in check to retain structural stability of the foot. Cellular detachment from the basement membrane only occurs in small portions at a time so the coffin bone remains safely suspended within the hoof capsule. (This process can be likened to the pulling apart of a portion of Velcro with the rest of the Velcro holding everything together while a small, separated piece of Velcro is "repaired.")

3.7 *The white line is visible from the bottom as a rim of white around the perimeter of the hoof. In this picture, you can see a small deviation at the left-hand side near the toe where an abscess had caused a defect in the white line.*

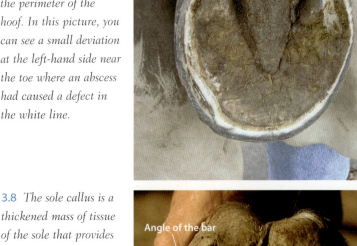

3.8 *The sole callus is a thickened mass of tissue of the sole that provides weight-bearing support to the normal foot. Farriers tend to remove this layer of sole, with the result that the sole is thinned and the horse more susceptible to deep bruising. You can also see the bars that provide stability and strength to the hoof. The bars are formed as the white line curls in toward the frog.*

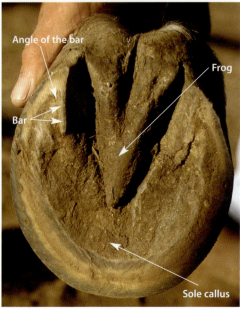

ample hoof density and strength. A white line that has points of separation, has a tendency to flake apart, and/or is very thin usually indicates some underlying structural weakness in the laminae (see "Laminitis," p. 74).

The Sole

SOLE CALLUS

In an unshod hoof, just behind the white line is a tough layer of sole tissue called the *sole callus* (photo 3.8). This dense sole "pad" contributes to protection and support of the coffin bone. It is important for a farrier to leave the sole callus intact by trimming the hoof wall to the same height as the sole callus. The sole callus is one of the weight-bearing structures of the hoof.

The Bars

The *bars* are the area on the bottom of the foot where the white line curls in at the heels toward the frog (see photo 3.8). On a good, solid foot, the bars are well developed and lay at an oblique angle to the white line. The bars of a contracted foot lie in an upright or vertical position. Healthy bars should not be pared away by a farrier as they are also weight-bearing structures of the foot.

The White Line

The *white line* forms at the junction between the tubular horn of the sole and the soft horn (*epidermal lamellae*) of the hoof wall (see fig. 3.1). The white line demarcates the meeting of the *sensitive* and *insensitive laminae* within the hoof. Thickness of the *white line* is visible in an unshod foot (photo 3.7). Typically, it has a uniform thickness along its curvature of 3½ mm. Normal thickness of the white line indicates

The Frog

The frog should be firm and resilient, similar to the feel of a rubber eraser. The frog should be well developed and in contact with the ground surface. The *frog buttress* is the callused portion of the rear of the frog, and it functions to distribute limb load. A poorly conformed foot has a receding frog with little ground contact; most of the load support occurs on the perimeter of the hoof wall rather than allowing the frog and sole callus at the toe to contribute to weight bearing.

The *central sulcus* (crevice) should be shallow. There should be no offensive odor to the bottom of the foot, especially from the frog and the *sulci* (crevices) beside it. The frog should be centered in the bottom of each foot (see photo 3.8). A frog that sits off to one side may be accompanied with flares in the hoof face related to an imbalanced hoof strike: such asymmetrical features imply that one side of the hoof repeatedly receives more impact than another (photo 3.9).

Interactive Structures of the Foot

COFFIN BONE SUPPORT

In an unshod hoof, support of the coffin bone comes from the weight-bearing load assumed by the hoof wall, the buttresses and apex of the frog, the sole callus at the toe, the bars and heels, and by dirt compacted into the frog *sulci* (see fig. 3.1).

NAVICULAR STRUCTURES

Seated beneath and behind the coffin bone is the *navicular bone* (see fig. 3.2 and photo 3.10). This bone and its associated flexor tendon create a functional increase in the surface area of the coffin joint, reducing the impact of landing. The *deep digital flexor tendon* runs behind the navicular bone and attaches to the back of the coffin bone. The position of the navicular bone places the deep digital flexor tendon away from the center of the coffin joint, creating a larger range of motion of that joint.

CONCUSSION ABSORPTION

Internal structures of the foot absorb downward compressive forces by the body and gravity. Ideally, the load should be distributed equally across all weight-bearing parts of the

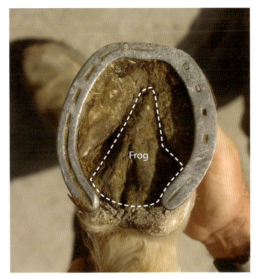

3.9 *The frog should sit in the center of the sole as seen in photo 3.8. In this picture, the frog is deviated to one side, indicating uneven loading of the hoof from one side to the other, also noticeable as worn nail heads and shoe on the right side of the photo.*

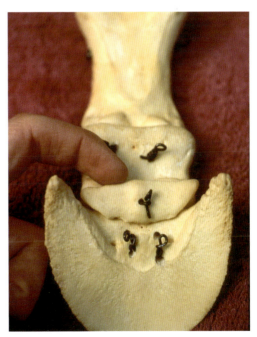

3.10 *Looking at the bones from the bottom of a skeleton, the finger is pointing to the shuttle-shaped navicular bone that lies above and behind the coffin bone.*

hoof to minimize twisting forces on the legs and to prevent bruising within the hoof structures. Optimal biomechanical function of the foot is determined by the:

- Balance of the foot
- Conformation
- Horseshoes
- Contour of the terrain
- Impact surface of the ground

Foot Health, Genetics, and Performance

Exercise and ground-contact stimulation of the frog, bars, and solar (pertaining to the sole) surface are critical ingredients in developing a "good" foot. The objective is to increase the surface area contact, particularly in the rear portion of each hoof. Interaction of the hoof with its environment elicits adaptive responses to develop hoof quality. Each region of the hoof responds differently depending on its peculiar interaction with the ground.

The ultimate factor dictating response of a foot to environmental influences is the genetic predisposition of a horse. An anatomical structure will only be as good as its genetic potential. Exercise and balanced nutrition maintain foot health and restore diseased feet to normal. Conformational shape, size, and hoof wall thickness are controlled by genetics, whereas improper shoeing, lack of stable hygiene, and environmental dehydration may adversely alter genetic propensities.

LATERAL OR UNGUAL CARTILAGES

Internal components of horse hooves are similar until age 4 to 5 years, regardless of breed, unless there has been injury or disease. After that time, environmental stimulation may develop strong structures within the hoof, creating a template for sound feet. Weak and diseased feet may develop from lack of exercise and inadequate hoof stimulation. Dissection of "good" feet compared to "bad" feet points out certain features. A good foot has the following characteristics (see fig. 3.5):

- *Lateral cartilages,* also called *ungual cartilages,* are well developed and relatively thick.
- The base of the lateral cartilage extends toward the midline, blending into the *digital cushion.*
- The digital cushion forms bundles of *fibrocartilage*, which unite with the lateral cartilages to provide ample rear foot support and dissipation of impact energy.
- A stout (chondroungular) ligament is present that connects the lateral cartilages with the deep digital flexor tendon at the level of the navicular bone.
- An abundance of vascular channels and microvessels (the blood vessels in fig. 3.5) courses within the lateral cartilages and digital cushion.

"Poor" hooves are not as well developed in any of these structural areas. Thin cartilages lack many important elements: limited numbers of microvessels, less developed base, sparse array of fibrocartilage in the digital cushion, and a thin ligament connection of cartilage to tendon. These deficits result in greater energy transfer to bones and ligaments of the hoof, leading to lameness issues.

Sidebone

Sidebone, or ossification of the lateral cartilage, has been implicated as a cause of lameness (photo 3.11). However, there is no correlation between sidebone and lameness. Some horses have a heritable tendency to develop sidebone, while in others this may develop due to excess hoof concussion over

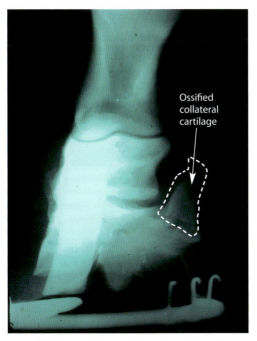

3.11 *Sidebone refers to a lateral cartilage that has cartilage replaced with more mineral. This shows up best on an X-ray view, although it can be felt as a very firm, unmovable structure when pushed with a finger on the side of the lower pastern just above the coronet band.*

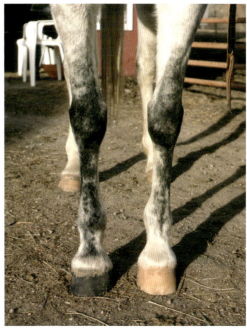

3.12 *This horse has one black hoof and one white hoof, yet based on biochemical studies, both feet should have the same strength and durability despite the difference in coloration.*

time. It is a phenomenon commonly seen in draft horses and is also noted in Warmblood breeds. On a rare occasion, an ossified lateral cartilage may fracture; in that situation, a horse may be lame.

Hoof Characteristics

Hoof Wall Integrity
Studies have repeatedly demonstrated that there are no differences in the relative elasticity, tensile strength, percent moisture, or mineral composition due to color or pigmentation of the hoof wall. Hoof wall characteristics are markedly influenced by seasonal variations as well as nutritional and management strategies, with seasonal variations having the predominant impact on hoof wall structure.

Hoof Color
It has been claimed that hoof color (white versus black) affects the strength and durability of a hoof (photo 3.12). Many believe that white feet are softer, more crumbly, and more predisposed to bruising and injury than black feet. However, a scientific study (Landeau, 1983) on the mechanical properties of equine hooves found *no* difference in the stress and strain behavior or ultimate strength properties between black and white hooves.

Hoof Size

Toe length is best evaluated with a horse standing with all four limbs square on a firm surface. A measure of toe length is taken from the middle of the coronary band to the tip of each toe. Compare front feet to each other, and back feet to themselves. Are the feet similar in size?

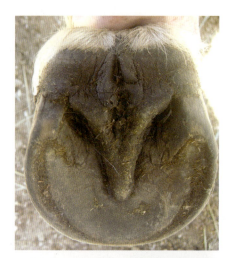

3.13 *A foot with concavity to the sole is considered to have a good "cup." This raises the sole off the ground, which limits trauma to the bottom of the foot.*

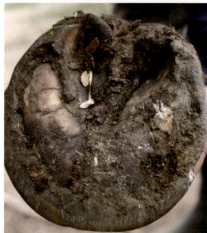

3.14 *This hoof has a flat sole without any concavity. A flat-soled horse bears more weight on the sole so is more prone to bruising and trauma of the inner structures of the hoof.*

Hoof width is measured across the widest part of the bottom of the hoof. The concavity of the bottom of the sole is referred to as the *cup*. A normal hoof has a moderate cup to the bottom of the foot (photo 3.13). A flat sole, with no cup, may be continually traumatized by contact with the ground during limb loading (photo 3.14). A farrier should only remove loose, exfoliating material in order to preserve depth of the soles. Flat feet, with little sole depth are prone to bruising, and to developing collapsed heels and dropped soles. A foot that is too small for a horse's overall mass lacks shock absorptive ability; then, excess concussion is absorbed in the feet and up the limbs.

Feet with *contracted heels* (narrow heels) and *straight walls* have little flexibility under loading (photos 3.15 A & B). The presence of a foot with contracted heels suggests that a horse doesn't bear as much weight on that limb as the other. A horse with persistent discomfort or chronic lameness protects the leg by not loading it or the hoof as much as normal. A contracted heel is a symptom of relative disuse of a limb, and in itself is not a disease.

Not all horses have pairs of feet that are exact mates in size and shape, and this may be normal for some individuals (photo 3.16). Yet, any difference in size should be viewed with suspicion as a sign of disease and/or pain. Slight deviations are expected, but large differences should be addressed by veterinary evaluation (see "Understanding Diagnostic Tests," p. 88).

Hoof Angle

Hoof angle describes the geometric relationship of the hoof to the ground. Hoof angle is measured by the angle formed at the junction of the dorsal (front) hoof wall and the ground surface of the foot. When examining a horse's feet, create a mental picture of what hoof angles are normal for that individual. Studies (Gene Ovnicek) on wild horses found that the hoof angles of the front feet range between 50 to 65 degrees, with most horses' front hooves measuring 54 to 58 degrees. Other sport medicine physiologists have found that most horses prefer a front hoof angle of around 54 degrees, with a range of 48 to 55 degrees. General rules are only guidelines; each horse's con-

The Hoof

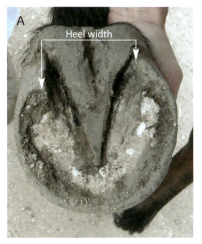 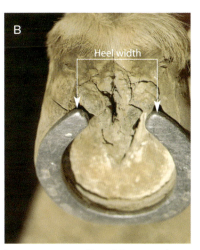 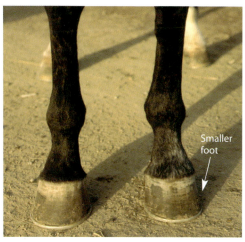

3.15 A & B *Although the sides of the heels are uneven in "length" in (A), this hoof shows an overall correct "width" of heels—within a normal range—as contrasted with the hoof, that has contracted heels (B). This is a sign of an underlying problem, and not a disease in itself. When a horse favors a limb due to discomfort or pain, the heels tend to narrow and contract.*

3.16 *In this photo, you can see that the horse's left front hoof is smaller than his right front, reflecting that he is not putting his full weight on the left one when he is moving, probably due to some degree of pain.*

formation is unique and must be addressed accordingly. Ideally, the feet should be trimmed so that the slope of the front of each hoof wall is parallel to the slope of the pastern of that limb, this alignment being a normal and desirable *hoof-pastern axis* (see further discussion, p. 50).

BREAKOVER AND HOOF STRIKE

Breakover is important to a discussion on hoof dynamics (photo 3.17). Breakover relates to the phase of the stride that occurs between the time the heel lifts off the ground to the time the toe lifts off the ground. The heel rotates around the fulcrum of the toe, and the degree of tension necessary to achieve this action is dependent upon the pull of the deep digital flexor tendon (see fig. 3.2). Ligamentous structures of the navicular bone are also stretched during the breakover phase of each stride. Any foot configuration that makes it difficult to lift the heel also increases tension on the flexor tendon and navicular structures.

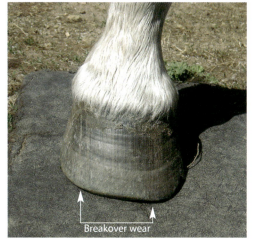

3.17 *As a horse moves forward across the ground, his heel will rotate over the toe, and the point at which the hoof wears at the toe is called the breakover point of the hoof. The wear pattern seen in this photo, with the breakover to the outside of the toe, is typical of most horses with normal foot flight.*

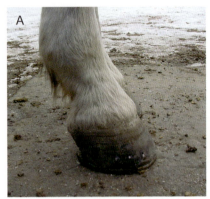 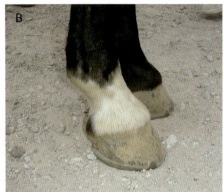 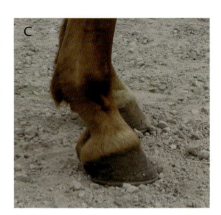

3.18 A–C *Alignment of the hoof-pastern axis is achieved when the slope of the front of the hoof wall is parallel to the slope of the pastern, as seen in these photos.*

The angle of a hoof affects the position of the hoof when it lands, but has no effect on stride length or the flight path of the foot. The position of the coffin bone within the hoof capsule dictates how a horse's hoof will strike the ground. Some specific features related to hoof angle have strong implications for foot health:

- The lower the angle (acute angle), the more likely the hoof will strike toe first, which is undesirable.
- The lower the angle, the more tension will be placed on the deep digital flexor tendon and the greater the compression felt by the navicular structures.
- The lower the angle, the greater the circulatory congestion leading to reduced blood flow to the heels and higher pressures in the marrow of the navicular bone.
- Lower hoof angles increase weight bearing on the heels, leading to an increased incidence of *caudal* (rear of the foot) heel pain and poor performance. The more load the heels assume, the slower will be their growth. (See "Long-Toe Low-Heel Syndrome," p. 51.)

Breakover can be improved by "backing up the toe" (rasping or squaring it back) with trimming and applying a shoe that is set slightly back from the toe, or a shoe with a rolled or "rockered" toe. On surfaces that permit the toe to dig into the ground, breakover is facilitated.

BROKEN-BACK HOOF-PASTERN AXIS

Examine the slope of the hoof and its relationship to the axis (a straight line passing through the pastern relative to the hoof) of the pastern. To properly evaluate the hoof-pastern alignment, place a horse on a flat, level surface and square him up as best as possible. Then stand to the side and analyze the alignment of the pastern relative to each hoof. Ideally, the slope of the front of the hoof wall should be parallel to the slope of the pastern (photos 3.18 A–C). This is a critical objective for a farrier to achieve with trimming. If this axis is *"broken-back,"* the pastern angle appears steeper (or more upright) than the hoof face (photo 3.19). A low hoof angle creates a *broken-back hoof-pastern axis*. This amplifies stress on the rearmost structures of the feet, including the navicular apparatus, as well as resulting in a toe-first landing. Repetitive overload of the heel structures of the foot is detrimental to any athletic horse.

The Hoof

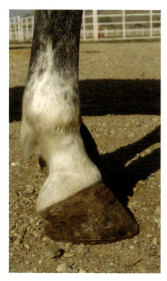
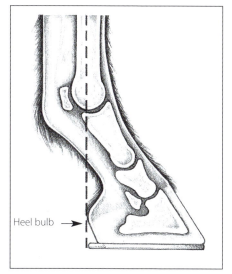
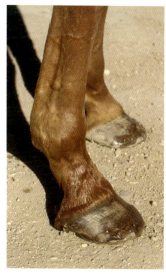

3.19 *When the slope of the pastern is steeper than the slope of the front of the hoof wall, this is referred to as a broken-back hoof-pastern axis, as seen in this picture.*

3.20 *Viewed from the side, the heel bulbs should fall directly beneath an imaginary line drawn through the center of the cannon bone.*

3.21 *Both a long toe and a low heel create an acute angle of the hoof relative to the pastern.*

LONG-TOE LOW-HEEL SYNDROME

Viewing the horse from the side, the heel bulbs should fall directly beneath an imaginary line drawn through the center of the cannon bone (fig. 3.20). The heel should have a slope similar to the front face of the hoof wall. A horse is considered to have an underrun heel if the heel bulbs fall in front of the ideal line bisecting the cannon bone, and/or if the slope of the heels is more acute than the front hoof face.

A horse with a broken-back hoof-pastern axis typically has underrun (low) heels and long toes. Both a *long toe and low heel* (LTLH) cause the hoof to assume a low (more acute) angle relative to the pastern (photo 3.21). This amplifies the steepness of the pastern and concentrates significantly greater stress on the navicular structures and the coffin joint while also stretching the deep digital flexor tendon. The hoof tubules are compressed with a LTLH con-

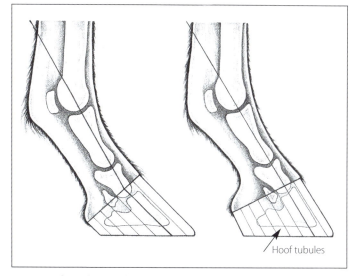

3.22 *On the right, a well-trimmed foot shows proper alignment of the hoof tubules (represented by the angled lines drawn on the hoof surface). On the left, a foot with a long toe and low heel. Note the hoof tubules extended in a more horizontal direction and at a more sloping angle.*

figuration, and over time, much like collapsed springs on a car, they lose their shock-absorption ability (fig. 3.22 and see photo 3.44, p. 63). A long toe makes it more difficult for a horse to

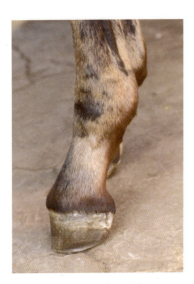

3.23 *A club-footed horse has a hoof angle that is steeper than the pastern. In this case, the hoof-pastern axis is broken forward.*

break over the foot with each stride, thereby increasing the muscular effort of each limb lift. More strain is applied to the tendons and ligaments in a foot with LTLH configuration. A delay in breakover also increases the tendency for a horse to *forge* (striking of a front foot with a hind.)

The bottom of the surface of the coffin bone normally assumes a 5 to 10 degree angle relative to the ground surface. And normally, the heel contacts the ground before the toe as an attempt to have the coffin bone directed toward the ground in a flat position. This allows the heel to sink into the ground for increased traction and push-off. A long-toe and low-heel configuration lowers (relative to normal) the heel of the coffin bone inside the hoof capsule. As a result of forming an acute angle (less than 90 degrees) between the ground surface of the coffin bone and the ground surface of the terrain, a long toe strikes the ground first so the coffin bone surface can be directed in the preferred manner: flat. Toe-first contact makes it more likely that a horse may trip and stumble, while also increasing concussion on the foot.

LTLH creates other problems during loading of the limb: ground contact of the hoof is moved forward beneath the coffin bone rather than remaining beneath the highly supportive lateral cartilages. Normally, the hydraulic effect of microvessels of the lateral cartilages and digital cushion serves to dissipate energy impact felt through the hoof. With the lateral cartilages distanced from the loading point by a LTLH hoof configuration, energy dissipation is diminished, resulting in a greater amount of hoof and limb concussion.

CLUB FOOT

A horse with long, steep heels and a "coon-footed" appearance to the hoof has a *broken-forward hoof-pastern axis*, and is often termed *club-footed* (photo 3.23). Usually, this problem is evident because one foot is shaped differently than the other. The hoof angle of a club foot is generally greater than 61 degrees. A high hoof angle elicits heel-first landing. A club foot may have a dished appearance to its hoof face due to shearing stresses within the sensitive laminae created by the steep hoof angle. A young horse that develops *flexural contracture* develops a club-footed appearance. If not corrected early in life by special shoeing or with surgery, the foot will remain this way for the rest of the horse's life. (See "Flexural Contracture," p. 198, in chapter 7, *Strong Tendons and Ligaments*, and "Flexural Limb Deformity or Contracted Tendons," p. 564, in chapter 18, *Reproductive Strategies and Health*.)

Not all club-footed horses are lame, or will become lame. However, the coffin bone inside the hoof capsule rarely sits in a "normal" position in a club-footed horse. A high heel and short toe, as seen with a club-footed horse, increases the angle of the surface of the coffin bone related to the ground, and such a horse will strike the ground with an exaggerated heel-first contact. This makes the coffin bone, navicular apparatus, and structures of the sole more susceptible to bruising and strain. Clinical significance of a club foot can be evaluated with X-ray films (*radiographs*) to measure the alignment of the coffin bone within the hoof wall (capsule).

Problems often develop if overzealous attempts are made to trim a club foot to "look" normal. Caution should be applied to lower the heels only as much as necessary to relieve tension on the deep digital flexor tendon when the opposite limb is held off the ground. When adjusting the heel angle, the objective is for tension on the deep digital flexor tendon to be less than that of the superficial flexor tendon and suspensory ligaments.

Hoof Balance

It is important for a horse to land equally on both sides of each hoof. A farrier attempts to achieve this through *geometric balance* by trimming the bottom of the hoof so that it is perpendicular to the long axis of the limb. However, it is the horse in motion that determines hoof landing, or *dynamic balance*. This is dependent on conformation and a horse's unique quirks of limb movement. The objective is to achieve symmetrical landing of the bottom of each foot with every step. Without the use of a treadmill to evaluate dynamic balance, it is difficult to achieve perfect side to side (*mediolateral*) hoof balance at all times (photos 3.24 A & B).

Not all hooves are created equal, but if left to do their own thing, most horses' barefoot hooves will wear to a natural shape compatible with a horse's structural conformation and movement. However, an equine athlete often needs the protection of shoes to withstand the rigors of exercise. Shoeing and trimming errors are frequently implicated as the foremost causes of lameness. Problems both within the foot and higher in the limb often start at the ground level, with the hoof. Hoof imbalance puts a horse at risk for developing lameness. Imbalances of a horse's feet may derive from heritable conformational tendencies to toe-in (*varus*) or toe-out (*valgus*). (See chapter 2, *Conformation for Performance*, p. 22.) Similar imbalances may be created artificially by poor trimming and shoeing techniques.

A healthy hoof is not just about quality of the hoof horn, resiliency of the frog, or lack of odor or debris in the frog clefts. A healthy hoof depends on good trimming and shoeing techniques, appropriate dietary management, and exercise compatible with a horse's level of fitness.

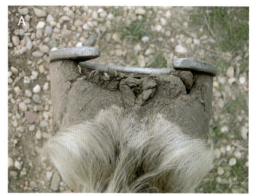

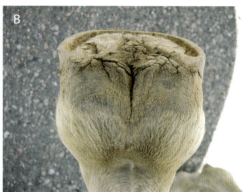

3.24 A & B *The left side of photo (A) has a longer heel than the right side, leading to a severe side-to-side imbalance. The longer side of the hoof will strike the ground first, causing the hoof to then roll over to the shorter heel. This creates torque and vibration in the joints and soft tissue structures, potentially leading to lameness. The hoof will record these imbalances by developing sheared heels, hoof flares, and an asymmetric coronary band. The hoof in (B) appears level from side-to-side when viewing the bottom of the foot sighting down the heels. Compare this medial-lateral hoof balance to the unbalanced hoof in (A).*

The Hoof as a Visual Record of Stress

The clip-clop sound of each foot striking the ground has a musical cadence of regularity. A steady rhythm gives a sense of well-being as each hoofbeat chimes aloud that a horse is sound. But, when that cadence becomes irregular in its timing, something might be wrong. In general, over 90 percent of lameness in the front legs of a horse results from a problem in one or both feet. Lameness is detectable by watching a horse in motion, by listening to his footfalls, and by visually appraising hoof structure. Examination of the appearance of the hoof reveals how concussive forces are directed across the foot to identify specific problems. Although some changes are internally subtle, over time they will produce a visual record on the face of the hoof. By recognizing structural changes that are recorded in a horse's hoof walls, measures can be taken to prevent development of a debilitating problem.

Abnormal Hoof Contours

A normal hoof wall is smooth with no signs of imperfections. Fine, longitudinal lines running from the coronary band to the ground show the position of horn tubules as they grow down from the coronary corium. If the growth rate increases or slows in different areas of the foot, a change is visible. If toe and heel of the hoof wall grow at different rates, the hoof wall assumes a wavy contour (photos 3.25 A & B). Rings develop in the hoof wall as the growth plates diverge between heels and toe. Just as growth rings of a tree chronicle seasonal and climatic variation in the development of a tree, so does the hoof reflect internal and external stresses on its face.

Ripples, ridges, or *dishing* (concavity) in the face of the hoof wall may reflect underlying ill health of the hoof tissues and laminae. Irregular contours are not always significant, but do warrant further investigation. Ripples may be visible in the hoof wall as a consequence of previous laminitis. Or, these ridges could result from seasonal variations in hoof growth, dietary changes, or a previous fever that temporarily altered hoof growth. Anything that interferes with blood flow in the foot directly affects the rate of hoof wall growth.

Asymmetric ridges in the hoof wall also reflect localized impact stress created by hoof imbalances. Hoof horn grows more quickly in areas of a foot that receive increased impact; this leads to a rippling effect in the horn. The side of a hoof that impacts the ground more quickly develops a steeper wall, while the other side of the hoof often develops a flare (see figs. 3.26 A & B and "Hoof Wall Flares," p. 56).

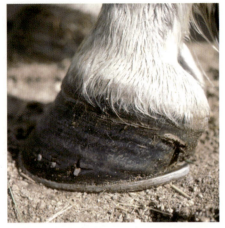
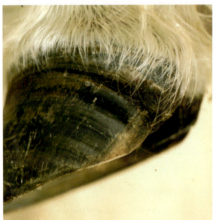

3.25 A & B *Differing growth rates of the toe and heel create waves or ripples in the face of the hoof wall. Variations in growth rate occur due to an inflammatory event like laminitis, or due to fever, changes in diet, and seasonal effects.*

Dishing in the front face of the hoof wall may develop due to shearing forces created in the hooves by too long a toe (photo 3.27). Long toes increase leverage within the foot, with resultant shearing of the laminae. A dish in the hoof wall is commonly related to subclinical (disease present but as yet undetected) or chronic laminitis. Any inflammatory event within the hooves may elicit laminitis; this will be recorded on the horse's hoof wall as the feet grow out. Excess concussion trauma to the feet and ensuing inflammation are credited with the development of horizontal hoof cracks along the front of the horn (photo 3.28). Any irregularities in hoof contour warrant radiographic (X-ray) examination to determine if there are underlying problems with the coffin bone (see "Laminitis," this chapter, p. 74).

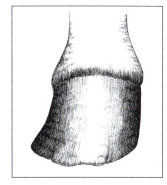 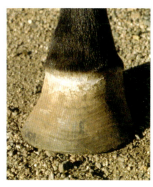

3.26 A & B *Hoof flares develop when one side of the hoof impacts the ground before the other. The side with the greatest impact steepens, while the other side develops a flare. In this drawing and photo, the left side is flared, while the right side, which receives the more concentrated impact, is steeper.*

IMBALANCED TRIMMING AND SHOEING
If a foot is unbalanced side to side or the shoes fitted too tightly, stress lines appear on the hooves as irregularities or ridges at the points of abnormal shoe pressure. A flare develops on the side with the least loading while the side of the hoof that receives more impact will grow a steeper wall (see photos 3.24 A and 3.26 A & B).

CHANGE IN DIET
Not all hoof wall rings indicate disease in the foot. A change in diet or quality of nutrition also alters the growth and chemistry of keratin, and may create ridges in the hoof wall. As the hoof grows, an abnormal ring moves toward the ground, followed by healthy and smooth hoof wall.

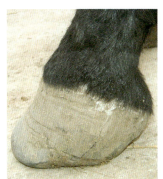

3.27 *A dish to the front contour of the hoof often indicates some bout of inflammation within the hoof, or shearing forces created by too long a toe from improper trimming.*

SEASONAL EFFECTS
Seasonal variations produce a similar effect on hoof growth, when the warmth and moisture of lengthening spring days stimulate a growth surge. Growth spurts appear as several ridged rings across the hoof wall.

FEVER
A fever may also stimulate a transient growth spurt in the feet, and rings may be evident weeks later. Elevated body temperature increases heart rate so circulation is increased to the feet.

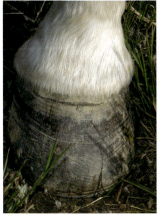

3.28 *A previous bout of concussion trauma to the foot will result in horizontal hoof cracks like these, which will move downward as new horn grows from the coronary band.*

INFLAMMATION

Any inflammation of the foot or coronary band creates rings in the hoof wall. Increased circulation through the coronary corium causes a rapid growth of the wall, possibly leading to divergent growth planes at the toe and heel.

Hoof Wall Flares

The hoof wall as a malleable tissue continually remodels in response to impact and weight-bearing stresses, and so assumes a shape directly reflective of those stresses. As said earlier, a steeper appearance develops on the side of the hoof wall that receives more concentrated impact with increased circulation. Growth rate of the hoof on that side speeds up relative to the other side. The portion of the hoof that receives less stress develops a *flare* (see photo 3.26 B). The foot breaks over the side with the steeper slope: a flare is perpetuated as the weight-bearing load remains concentrated on the side of the hoof with the steeper wall. Configuration changes in the hoof wall can be traced back to deviations in hoof balance, either due to trimming or to conformation. Shoeing imbalances may be rectified in time, but conformation is there to stay.

Studies note that 80 percent of adult feet have a steeper medial wall with a slight flare on the lateral side, indicating that, in most cases, breakover is not dead center. Only 5 percent of horse hooves were found to possess a round shape with no asymmetry.

Coronary Band Response to Uneven Stresses

In a normal foot, the coronary band forms a relatively straight line across the front of the hoof in a plane parallel to the ground and perpendicular to the long axis of the leg. It slopes away slightly toward the quarters of the heels, equally on both sides. Alignment changes of the coronary band reflect alterations in the circulatory tissue nourishing the foot or uneven stresses on the foot. If impact is repeatedly felt on one side of a foot more than the other, the coronary band will be "driven" upward directly above the impact area. The coronary band realigns itself with an asymmetrical slope (photo 3.29). Such a configuration may signal imbalance of the feet related to incorrect hoof trimming or due to uneven loading created by poor conformation.

Sheared Heels

By studying each foot and its changes over several months, the effects of trimming and shoeing may be appreciated. As one side of the foot persistently hits the ground harder than the other, eventually the heel bulb on that side is "driven" upward relative to the other. This phenomenon is known as *sheared heels* (photo 3.30). If allowed to persist, the heels become unstable, in some cases enough so that they may be displaced with hand pressure. Such heel instability results in pain and lameness. Similar asymmetric loading forces experienced

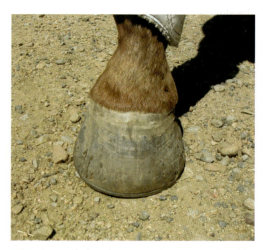

3.29 *An angled and asymmetric coronary band is indicative of uneven hoof strike due to hoof imbalances.*

by the foot are felt throughout the limb. The side of the foot (and limb) that receives added concussion may develop *quarter cracks* (see below), sidebone (see p. 46), or navicular disease (see p. 85).

Hoof Cracks

In a healthy hoof, crack propagation is prevented from reaching sensitive tissues interior to the hoof wall because of high water content within the inner layers of the hoof wall. Also, crack propagation tends to move vertically from the ground surface of the hoof upward along the tubular plane, which is weaker than the horizontal plane of intertubular horn. Location dictates how a crack is named: *toe crack* (photo 3.31), *quarter crack* (photo 3.32), or *heel crack* (photo 3.33). An injury or defect in the coronary band often results in a permanent crack in the hoof wall created by interruption of horn tubule growth from the coronary corium.

Cracks in the hoof horn reflect the presence of an unbalanced foot. Improper trimming and excessively dry or thin walls contribute to hoof cracking upon impact. A hoof with LTLH foot configuration is prone to dehydration and the development of multiple, superficial cracks known as *sand cracks* (photo 3.34). A more serious and deeper hoof crack may start at the bearing surface and work toward the coronary band. There may be pain if sensitive tissue moves with weight bearing. Hoof cracks also provide an avenue for infection to invade inner structures of the foot. Daily inspection identifies cracks before they become a simmering problem.

SELENIUM TOXICITY
Selenium toxicity stimulates the development of horizontal hoof cracks, in one or more hooves (photo 3.35). Chronic consumption of selenium-rich plants is referred to as *alkali disease*. In excess, selenium alters the normal chemical

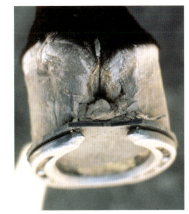

3.30 *Sheared heels result when one side of the foot impacts the ground harder than the other such that the hard-striking heel is driven upward relative to the other heel. This is visible in this photo as the left side of this hoof is considerably higher than the right side. Deep clefts develop in the frog, and pain and lameness ensue.*

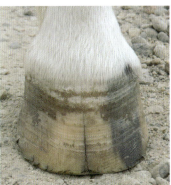

3.31 *Central toe crack.*

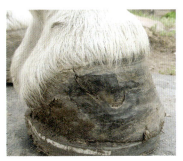

3.32 *Quarter crack.*

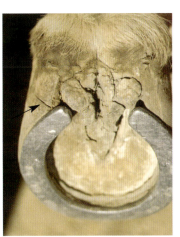

3.33 *This heel crack (on the left side of the photo) developed from point loading by a shoe that is fit too small for the foot both in length and width.*

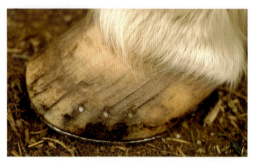

3.34 *Dry, brittle hoof horn is likely to develop fissures in the face of the hoof wall, called sand cracks. These are usually superficial, but can extend deeper into sensitive tissue.*

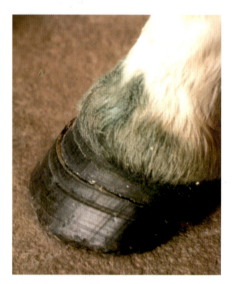

3.35 *Horizontal hoof cracks resulting from selenium toxicity may lead to sloughing of the hoof capsule away from the coffin bone, a painful and potentially fatal condition.*

bonding of the keratin that forms the hoof. Because selenium is substituted for sulfur in the amino acids of body proteins, keratinized structures (hair and hoof) are most affected. Hair loss and thinning of the mane and tail may occur before lameness develops. Any horse suspected of selenium toxicity should receive veterinary evaluation and dietary modifications. Should a horse continue to ingest a diet excessively high in selenium, the poisoning may progress to the point of complete separation of the hoof wall from the foot. Such a predicament is excruciating for the horse and is life threatening. Certain geographic areas have selenium-rich soils while other areas are deficient in selenium. It is important to know the selenium constituents of local pasture and of hay fed, and best to consult with your veterinarian before adding supplements to the diet. (See "Selenium," p. 162, and "Selenium Toxicity," p. 374).

Shoes and Pads

Shoeing: Injury versus Protection

DYNAMIC FORCES IN AN UNSHOD HOOF

In an unshod foot, the heel impacts the ground slightly before the toe, expanding the heel outward. As a limb bears weight, the short pastern bone compresses against the digital cushion. The digital cushion then pushes against the lateral cartilages, and downward against the frog that absorbs only a small degree of impact shock. Compression of the digital cushion dissipates energy as heat, transferring it to a profuse network of blood vessels in the digital cushion. The bloodstream removes the heat energy up the leg, away from the foot.

As the toe hits, an upward compressive force is relayed through the horn tubules that comprise the hoof wall and through the microvessels of the lateral cartilages. These cells absorb energy by their spiral, spring-like configuration. The vascular network and laminae "glue" the coffin bone to the hoof wall to further resist downward forces of limb loading

ALTERATIONS CAUSED BY SHOEING

A horseshoe has an intrinsic value to support a hoof from ground contact and to minimize bruising and contusion. A shoe may be protective on one hand, while injurious to a foot, on the other. Shoes change the dynamics of the foot and musculoskeletal structures in many ways:

- Shoes add weight to the limbs, which hastens fatigue.
- Weight of a shoe forces the flexor muscles of the elbow to work harder to raise and protract the limb, adding to fatigue.

- A shoe increases flexion of the knee and fetlock, resulting in a higher hoof flight arc, with more concussion incurred in the foot and joints.
- Horseshoe nails weaken the hoof wall.
- The protective *periople* (hoof coating) is often removed with a farrier's rasp, modifying moisture retention properties of the hoof (see also p. 66).
- A shoe affects normal flexibility of the hoof wall and its spread at the ground surface.

Heel expansion is possible because the hoof wall is thinner at the heels and quarters than at the toe. The heels can expand and rebound with weight bearing. According to biomechanical stress studies, the extent of heel expansion is unaffected by a shoe. However, a shod foot expands faster than a barefoot hoof, which modifies the shock absorption ability of the foot, especially the horn tubules. A shoe causes the hoof to absorb concussion rather than dissipate impact through the limb. Heel bruising, sole bruising, coffin bone inflammation (pedal osteitis), and laminitis may develop. It is imperative to fit and size a shoe to accommodate the foot. Long-term, improper balancing of a foot or improper fitting of a shoe leads to foot pain, sprains, tendon injury, or degenerative joint disease.

SHOEING FOR PROTECTION

Within 3 to 6 weeks following the pulling of horseshoes, an unshod hoof widens, the frog becomes more prominent, and depth to the sole and sole concavity (cupping) increase; all of these features improve ground contact of the hoof. Although these are highly desirable features, unshod horses often cannot withstand the athletic exertions asked of them. The hoof wall wears to the point that a horse assumes excessive loading on the sole, while stones and rutted ground may bruise the feet. Shoes chosen for hoof protection should be as light as possible, yet should achieve the objectives of protection, traction, and foot support. As few nails as possible should be placed in each hoof to hold a shoe; nails should only be placed forward of the widest part of the foot.

Boot Alternatives to Shoes

Current technology has provided a rider with many choices of hoof gear. Rubber boots have been designed with the performance athlete in mind. These boots (Old Mac Boots® or Easy Boots®, for example) fit over the entire hoof, and in some cases may be applied over shoes to provide added protection (photos 3.36 and 3.37 A & B). These plastic or rubber boots withstand rocky terrain and miles of abuse, including successful use on 100-mile endurance horse competitors. Each boot should fit the

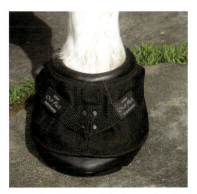

3.36 *An Old Mac Boot® is made of rubber and Cordura, designed for durability and good traction. Its integrated design includes a component that wraps around the pastern to keep the boot from twisting or falling off. It is a popular alternative to using horseshoes.*

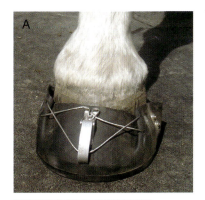

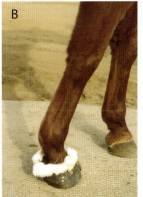

3.37 A & B *An Easy Boot® is a useful protective boot to use on a barefoot or shod horse (A). Cotton keeps gravel and debris from falling into the boot (B).*

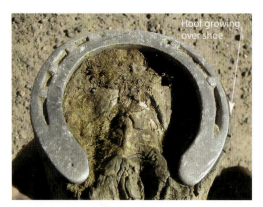

3.38 *This shoe was fit too small for the hoof, and the hoof is growing down over the side of the shoe (visible on the right side of the photo).*

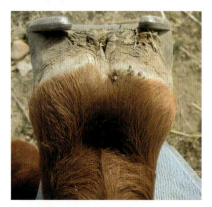

3.39 *The branches of the shoe on this foot are pinched inward. This places pressure on the heels, which are contracted. This can lead to corns or heel lameness.*

foot well and not contact or abrade soft skin tissue such as the coronary band or the heel bulbs. Caution should be taken if using rubber or plastic boots for jumping or galloping sports, as they could be slippery on grass or wet ground.

IMPORTANCE OF PROPER SHOEING

Besides attention to detail to achieve proper hoof angle being paramount, specifics related to shoe size and application also influence hoof dynamics. A hoof wall loses flexibility if:

- A shoe is too small for the foot (photo 3.38).
- The branches (the long sides) of the shoe pinch inwards (photo 3.39).
- The branches do not extend far enough back under the heel to provide weight-bearing support (photo 3.40).

A hoof fit with too small a shoe often develops stress rings at the heels and quarters, or hoof cracks form at the point of compressive loading (photos 3.41 A & B). Stress rings and cracks are evidence of improper shoeing techniques, or poor conformation, or both, resulting in unequal load distribution across the foot.

An appropriately sized shoe applied wide enough at the heels encourages heel expansion (photos 3.42 A & B). A shoe may also be *slippered* (beveled) to encourage the heels to expand with impact. Nails should only be placed in front of the widest bend in the quarter of the hoof to limit restriction of heel expansion.

SOUND SHOEING PRINCIPLES

Customized hoof care needs to be individualized to each horse. This includes balancing each hoof side to side, i.e. medial to lateral, so the horse lands as flat as possible on all aspects of the hoof (photo 3.43 and see also p. 53). Landing on one side of the hoof wall, even infinitesimally sooner than the other side, elicits abnormal stresses. The foot will feel asymmetrical impact concussion along with excess tension in supporting tendons and ligaments, while the uneven loading creates damaging shearing forces in the foot. As mentioned previously, it is essential to eliminate long toes, underrun heels, and a broken-back hoof axis. The toes should be *backed up* (shortened) and/or rolled to facilitate breakover. (Backing up the toe is accomplished by using a rasp on the front of the toe to square it back.) Low or collapsed heels should be supported temporarily with a wedge if necessary to elevate the heels to promote more normal growth of the hoof tubules (photo 3.44 and see photo 3.48, p. 65). Most importantly, the hoof and pastern axis angles should parallel the alignment of each other (see photos 3.18 A–C, p. 50). This is not new

The Hoof   61

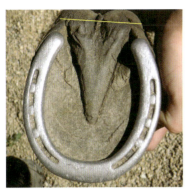

3.40 This horse's foot has been shod with too small a shoe, thereby creating a condition known as "short shod." Also, the heels of the shoe branches are pinched in so much that hoof wall has grown over the edges of the shoe. The yellow, horizontal line at the top of the photo marks the rearmost end of the buttress of the frog, which is where the branches of the shoe should extend to give adequate support to the heels.

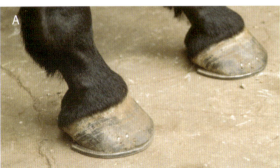
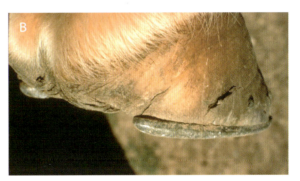

3.41 A & B When the branches of the shoe do not extend far enough back under the heel to provide weight-bearing support, it is referred to as "short shod" (A). In this photo you can see that the ends of the shoe do not reach as far as the heel bulbs. Looking at the foot from the bottom, the branches should extend to the widest part of the frog in order to provide the best support for the rear of the foot (see photos 3.42 A & B). The short-shod hoof in (B) has the branches ending way too short, resulting in point loading at the heel with crack formation just under the tip of the shoe. This causes pain and lameness.

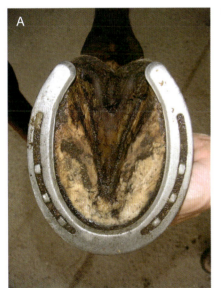
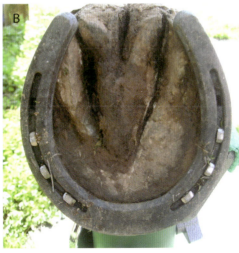

3.42 A & B The concept of shoeing to the widest part of the frog means that the branches of the shoe extend to the buttress of the frog. This provides ample support to the rear of the foot, prevents point-loading pressure on the hoof wall that might form cracks in a short-shod foot, and promotes correct alignment of the growth of the hoof tubules. A well-shod hoof with an aluminum shoe (A) and a steel shoe (B).

wave thinking; such basic principles of farrier care were documented in the 1800s in horse manuals as techniques useful in keeping horses sound.

"CORRECT" SHOEING OR CORRECTIVE SHOEING?

As equally important as aligning the hoof-pastern axis, balance of the foot from side to side, and fore and aft corrects many shoeing problems and lameness issues. The goal is to encourage equal distribution of weight across all weight-bearing surfaces of the foot, and to provide ample support to all structures of the foot to accommodate loading with each footfall. With compressive forces evenly loaded across the foot, no single side of a joint or a ligament receives excess strain.

Once a horse has matured in skeletal growth, "corrective shoeing" for poor limb conformation can only attempt to balance and level each foot as best as possible. Filing one side of a foot shorter than the other worsens an already less-than-perfect situation, adding torque (twisting) and strain across the joints. The objective is to allow each hoof to land as flat as possible, without it twisting side to side on hoof strike.

TRACTION DEVICES

It seems logical to apply some sort of traction device to the bottom of a horseshoe when conditions are slippery or icy. Such devices include hard-surfacing materials such as borium caulks or metal studs that are applied to the heels and/or toe of the shoe (photo 3.45). The objective in using these is for the shoe to grab the ground if a horse's foot starts to slip. There is an inherent problem in using traction devices: surfaces a horse runs over are not always slippery in entirety. If a horse's hoof grabs on a surface with ample traction, there is the likelihood of lower limb injury as the

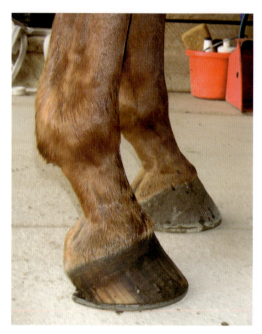

3.43 *This horse has been shod with ample heel support, with the branches of the shoe extending to the widest part of the frog. If you dropped a plumb line through the middle of the cannon bone with the horse standing square, the plumb line would drop directly down the back of the heel bulbs, and the end of the branches of the shoe would touch that line. This is desirable when attempting to provide good heel support with a shoe. The hoof-pastern alignment seen here is reasonable, although the toe could be "backed up" just a bit more.*

horse's body continues while the limb sticks in place, even briefly. (For more discussion, see pp. 97, 184, and 211.)

To minimize the risk of injury if borium is used, it should not be applied as large projections sticking off the bottom of the shoe, but rather should be spread as a thin layer of sequential spots at the heels and/or melted evenly along the toe area. Studs can be used as an alternative traction device. These can be

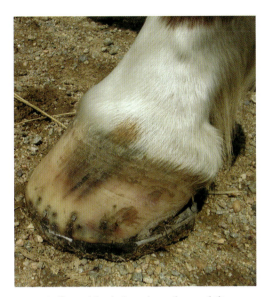

3.44 Collapsed heels lose their elastic ability to flex and expand to dissipate impact concussion due to hoof tubules growing in a more horizontal direction rather than more vertically. The foot seen here is typical of a horse with collapsed and under-run heels. Bruising is visible on the hoof wall as a pink discoloration, indicating inflammation in the hoof.

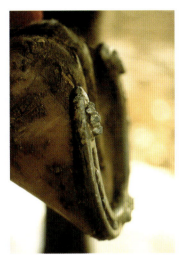

3.45 Caulks or toe grabs are devices used to increase traction on slippery surfaces. However, a horse could incur limb injury due to excessive traction as the caulked shoe sticks on non-slippery ground.

driven into drilled holes in a shoe as a permanent feature, or they can be added or removed as screw caulks as surface conditions dictate. Studs come in various sizes to provide a choice of traction ability relative to the size of the horse and the slipperiness of the surface. Another traction alternative is the use of *ice nails*, which are horseshoe nails coated with a thin layer of borium. *Frost nails*, with their wedge-shaped nail heads, were the original traction devices. Traction nails are useful until the nail head wears down and loses contact with the ground.

A practical compromise to using heel caulks or toe grabs relies on the application of *rim* shoes that have a groove in the center of the shoe, making them less slippery than *keg* shoes. To further increase traction, the large crease of a *fullered* or *full-swedge* shoe extends all the way around the shoe, improving its grab. Polo horses and barrel horses need to turn suddenly and rapidly, and so are often fitted in these types of shoes for added traction.

IMPORTANCE OF DAILY CARE

Successful shoeing practices depend on foot care and hygiene by the farrier and by the daily caretaker. Daily cleaning of the soles and frogs removes collected wads of manure and pebbles that might bruise the foot. Cleaning the hooves thwarts overgrowth of bacteria, preventing *thrush* and *canker* (see p. 73). Removal of snowballs in cold, winter climates limits bruising of the sole from snow and ice that pack in the bottom of a horseshoe. During periods of excessive wetness, check that horseshoes are firmly affixed. The sucking action of mud can loosen the nail clinches or cause twisting of a shoe, resulting in *abscesses* (see p. 70) or *corns* (see p. 71). A lost shoe leaves the sole unprotected and at risk of bruising.

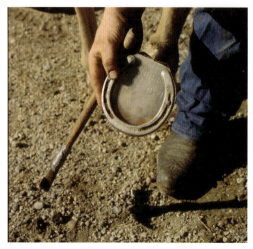

3.46 *A full pad placed between the hoof and the shoe may provide some protection against bruising in a tender-footed horse.*

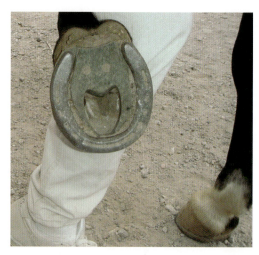

3.47 *A heel pad is an option to give some added protection to the rear of the hoof without covering the entire sole.*

Padding the Foot

A dilemma often exists: to pad or not to pad. A pad is usually placed beneath a shoe to serve as a protective barrier between the ground and the sole (photos 3.46 and 3.47). Packing material applied beneath the pad prevents dirt and pebbles from collecting between the pad and the sole. A pad limits normal expansibility of the foot by adding rigidity to an already rigid shoe. On the other hand, some horses have naturally tender or flat feet, and therefore need sole protection. Overzealous use of hoof nipper, knife, or rasp may remove too much foot, leaving behind a very thin sole that is then in need of padding.

In some cases, it is necessary to do more than just apply a standard shoe to cover the bearing surface of the hoof wall. A horse with laminitis (see p. 74), navicular disease (see p. 85), chronic heel pain, or a horse that is prone to bruising due to genetically flat feet, may need to wear pads continually. In these cases the benefits may outweigh any detriments. Pads may also serve as therapy and protection for short-term problems, such as:

- Sole abscess
- Nail puncture
- Bruise
- Corn
- Laminitis

EFFECTS OF LONG-TERM PADDING

Weakened Foot

A full pad minimizes focal bruising of the subsolar corium (sensitive tissue beneath the sole). Some pad materials provide a limited amount of concussion reduction. However, there is a trade-off: padded feet become pad-dependent. The sole of a padded foot softens and lacks support from the ground surface, promoting sole flattening and weakness. Even a foot that starts out properly cupped and concave may flatten with time under a pad. When pads are later removed, soles are susceptible to trauma. Or, when a shoe is lost, the previously padded sole is soft, making it vulnerable to injury and bruising. Nails tend to loosen easily through a pad, so shoes are lost more easily.

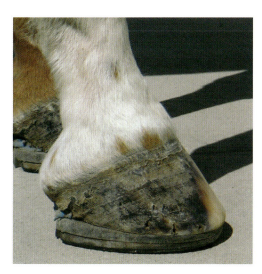

3.48 *A wedge pad lifts the heel on a low-heeled horse, however such a wedge may increase pressure on the heels and lead to worsened collapse of the heels and lameness.*

Wedge Pads

Wedged pads are applied to lift the heels of a horse that has low heels (photo 3.48). However, over time, this strategy may be counterproductive: wedge pads increase pressure and wear on the hoof wall at the heels, leading to worsened collapse of the heels.

Thrush, Bruising, or Abscess

Moisture beneath a pad promotes bacterial growth, potentially resulting in thrush (see p. 73). An inadequate seal of the packing material (commonly used are polyurethane, silicone, oakum/pine tar, or foam) allows dirt or debris to seep in under the pad. Local pressure points of dirt or pebbles create bruises or abscesses, accompanied by lameness.

ALTERNATIVES TO FULL PADS

Consider alternatives before padding a horse's feet. Inactive or stall-confined horses develop weak feet that are easily bruised. Over time, turnout and regular exercise strengthen and toughen such feet. Just as bones in the body strengthen with appropriate stress, the hoof responds to external stimuli. Not only does a foot conform to internal stress, but the hoof also builds stronger horn to accommodate hard ground surfaces. Although not applicable to all, horses turned onto rocky pastures may develop tough feet with stronger soles and hoof walls that are resistant to bruising. Sometimes it is practical to leave a horse barefoot and then apply rubber boots only when he is ridden (see p. 59).

Application of tincture of iodine (7 percent solution) or similar sole products to the bottom of the sole helps toughen the foot. Use a squeeze bottle to carefully apply strong iodine solutions to the sole and frog without contacting skin where it may be irritating.

Wide-Web Shoes

Wide-web shoes increase protection to the bottom of the foot without the ill effects of a pad (photo 3.49). However, the wide web of the shoe should not contact the sole; shoe support should rest only on the weight-bearing hoof wall. If any part of the shoe rests on the sole instead of the hoof wall, misapplied stress can bruise the foot.

Rim Pads

A pad placed between the hoof wall and a shoe is called a *rim pad*. Some feel that rim pads minimize concussion transmitted by a metal shoe up the legs; however, such a pad does not provide the same energy dissipation offered by an unshod foot. A rim pad can serve as a lightweight "spacer" that raises the sole farther from the traumatic ground surface. Rim pads do not exert negative effects on the sole as would a full pad, but nails may tend to loosen, and a shoe is more easily lost—as with any pad.

3.49 *A wide-web shoe may provide extra protection to the foot, but care must be taken to prevent contact of the sole with the shoe.*

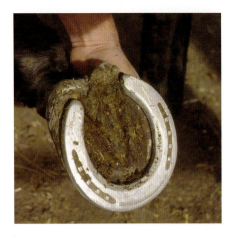

The Use of Hoof Dressings and Supplements

Horse owners are proactive people, hoping to "do" things to improve a horse's athletic ability. One such management strategy promotes the use of dietary supplements or hoof dressings to improve the growth or quality of hoof horn. Many commercial products are available, and many horse owners are convinced they get results. By examining physiologic properties of hoof growth and quality, a personal decision can be made as to whether such supplements have value.

Reasons for Moisture Loss in the Hoof

The hoof wall is actually an extension of the outermost layer of the skin, the *epidermis*. The function of the hoof wall is to protect the internal structures of the hoof from drying and from environmental insults. Because the hoof capsule is impermeable to water-soluble substances, it forms such a protective barrier. A very dry hoof is defined as having moisture content of 19 percent, while an extremely dry hoof is defined by moisture content of 30 percent. The percent of moisture in the hoof wall is not necessarily associated with *hoof strength*, i.e. the ability of the hoof to deform under a load without incurring chips, cracks, or bruising. A study of permeability features of the hoof has illuminated some interesting results: normal hoof horn that was immersed in water for two weeks did not change its permeability barrier whereas immersed brittle hoof horn did. In another test, when baked in an oven at 140° F (60° C) for two weeks, neither normal nor brittle hoof horn showed any alterations in permeability. Another trial used acetone to disrupt the lipid layer of the horn to create hoof horn of poor quality. Following acetone treatment, the permeability barrier was breached with immediate loss of moisture. The conclusion: the permeability barrier in horn of poor quality is compromised while normal hoof horn can withstand extremes of heat and wet.

GROUND ABRASION AND MOISTURE

Harsh environmental effects of heat and moisture do not alter normal hoof horn. Moisture of the hoof comes from within; once it is wicked away, there is little one can do to put it back in from the outside. Abrasive ground wears away the protective hoof coating, called the *periople*. Wet pastures or paddocks adversely affect feet with poor quality hoof horn. The combination of poor hoof quality and moisture softens the hoof horn, and then subsequent drying of the ground causes the hooves to dry out excessively.

LONG-TOE LOW-HEEL CONFIGURATION

Correct trimming technique is *the* single most important feature to maintaining natural moisture within the hoof. As discussed earlier, feet that are allowed to grow a long toe or develop a run-under heel (LTLH) tend to have compressed horn tubules. As the heels compress and the toe runs out, the horn tubules run in a horizontal direction rather than retaining the more optimal vertical orientation as in a normal hoof (see p. 51 for earlier discussion and fig. 3.22). The more horizontal the horn tubules grow, the more they lose their shock-absorption capabilities. The tubules also lose their moisture-retention properties. The hoof horn becomes weak and dry, and cracks result.

SAND CRACKS AND THIN WALLS

It is not unusual for a horse to be afflicted with dry, brittle horn of the hoof wall, or to see a hoof that is littered with sand cracks (see photo 3.34, p. 58). The surface features of poor hoof quality extend into layers of the hoof capsule due to hoof dehydration. It is difficult to affix a shoe to shelly, thin walls; horses with thin walls are predisposed to lameness.

Hoof Dressings

Hoof dressings come in the form of an oil or grease base, often with the addition of rosin (pine tar) or lanolin. Although hoof dressings are thought to minimize moisture loss from the hoof by serving as a "temporary" periople to reduce evaporation of internal moisture, there is little benefit gained from their application. Even with frequent application, the dressing wears away as did the original periople. Hoof moisture comes from internal sources with only a very small amount gradually assimilated by osmosis from the environment. Some hoof dressings are astringent and dehydrate the foot. Examples of harsh dressings include those containing turpentine, bleach, formalin, or phenol. Such compounds applied occasionally to a moist frog or sole will control bacteria that thrive in wet conditions, but persistently repeated applications may be overly drying and cause the sole to flake.

MASSAGE OF CORONARY BAND

While hoof dressings do not necessarily impart moisture into the hoof, massage of the coronary bands stimulates hoof growth. This stimulation is accomplished by applying sheepskin coverings saturated with lanolin over the coronary bands, or by daily massage with vegetable or mineral oil.

Feed Supplements for Hoof Nutrition

ORGANIC NUTRIENTS

Minerals are involved in activation of enzymes that are needed for forming keratin in hooves. In horses, no association has been linked between zinc supplementation and tensile strength or relative elasticity of the hoof wall. Some minerals, such as sulphur, copper, and calcium, may play an important role in hoof quality yet further studies are necessary to elucidate the significance of micro and macro minerals to equine hoof wall integrity.

Biotin

Biotin is a water-soluble B vitamin important to glucose and fat metabolism. It also has an essential effect on growth and maintenance of epidermal tissues such as skin and hoof wall. Original studies on the effect of biotin on hoof growth were performed on pigs subjected to long courses of antibiotics that killed off normal intestinal flora and thereby eliminated the body's natural ability to produce biotin. The results were extrapolated to horses with recommendations to feed 30 mg/day of biotin to enhance hoof growth. Subsequent studies have found that biotin has some effect on improving hoof horn quality, specifically by increasing hardness of the quarters and toe. Hoof growth rate is affected by biotin, albeit minimally, with the most reported change being 15 percent increase in hoof growth. This amounts to an extra growth of 4.6 mm of hoof in biotin supplemented horses over a 5-month period. (Supplemented horses achieved a hoof growth rate of 0.19 mm per day as compared to 0.16 mm per day for horses not receiving additional biotin.) To appreciate noticeable effects from biotin supplementation it is necessary to supplement for at least 5 to 8 months, and may require "super" supplementation of 60 milligrams (mg) per day for a 1200-pound horse.

A normal horse commonly produces biotin in his intestines at a high enough content that supplementation is not deemed necessary. Most foodstuffs, especially corn, provide ample biotin in a horse's diet. Biotin products may be helpful to a horse with reduced intestinal function, such as an older, debilitated horse, a horse with an intestinal illness, or one that has been on long-term antibiotic medications. Dehydration and decreased intestinal motility are certain features of prolonged exercise. The assault of rigorous and extended exercise on the equine intestinal tract may impair synthesis of some essential components such as biotin. If the hindgut of a horse is kept healthy, there should not be a requirement for biotin supplementation but supplementation will not cause harm. Because biotin is water-soluble, the kidneys excrete any excess fed.

D-L Methionine

D-L methionine is a precursor to the sulfur molecules that contribute to growth of the hoof tubules. Similar to biotin, this product may be helpful to a horse experiencing or recovering from an intestinal illness. In any event, neither product is harmful as a daily supplement, and in unique cases may yield results. Follow package recommendations or consult a veterinarian.

ISOXSUPRINE HYDROCHLORIDE

Isoxsuprine hydrochloride is a medication used to treat navicular syndrome and laminitis in an attempt to improve circulation within the foot. A convenient, albeit anecdotal, side effect that has been noticed in horses on this medication is that hoof horn grows out faster and with improved condition. It is noteworthy that horses on this medication usually start out with a malady within the hoof, and as a consequence hoof circulation is impaired. Isoxsuprine may not stimulate as pronounced an effect in a normally healthy hoof. Because this is considered a medication rather than a feed supplement, isoxsuprine is banned from use in a horse during competition and must be withdrawn at least four days prior to an event.

Maintaining Healthy Hooves

EXERCISE

The importance of exercise to a horse's feet cannot be overemphasized. Exercise stimulates the expansibility of the hoof, increasing the surface area and reducing concussion during a performance effort. It increases blood circulation to the feet, promoting health and elasticity of the hoof wall, and stimulates new growth of all foot structures. The sole toughens with repeated use, making it less vulnerable to bacteria and bruises. The scrubbing action of soil clods as they are flung from moving feet contributes to foot hygiene by removing dead pieces of sole and frog. Exercise encourages the circulation of tissue nutrients throughout the limbs, and reduces stagnation often seen as "stocked-up" legs. Exercise also strengthens ligaments and tendons that support the joints and act as shock absorbers to cushion the load on the joints and feet.

"FEED FOR A BETTER HORSE"

Abnormal concussion forces on a horse's foot make for irregular and asymmetrical hoof horn. Uneven loading creates the possibility of crushed heels, underrun heels, long toes, a broken-back hoof-pastern axis, fissure cracks, thinning of the white line, thrush, corns, sheared heels, laminitis, navicular syndrome, and the list goes on. The genetic template with which a horse begins defines the extent of issues that may develop over time. Constant concussion can cause even a genetically superior horse to go lame. Excellent farrier care cannot be overemphasized as a powerful contributor to athletic longevity of an athletic horse. Feed supplements and hoof dressings are only one small part of the overall equation to maintaining a horse's foundation. A piece of advice worth following: "It is better to feed for a better horse than to focus on feeding supplements for a better hoof."

The Many Faces of Hoof Lameness

Any noticeable lameness or stiffness should receive veterinary attention as soon as possible. Due to the complexity and interaction of many internal structures of the foot, inflammation or trauma of one area may create a problem in neighboring tissues. Pain in the feet, along with mechanical damage, adversely affects future performance capabilities.

Identifying a Beginning Problem

Early identification of subtle problems or gait inconsistencies is instrumental in maintaining athletic longevity. Put the horse on the longe line periodically to check his gaits. Longing on asphalt or concrete surfaces emphasizes gait abnormalities related to the foot or joints. A hard surface allows one to hear inconsistencies in the way a lame foot strikes the ground. Videotape of a horse's movement on serial occasions allows comparison of one day to another. Slow motion videography enables evaluation of how each foot lands, and measurement of the length of stride of each limb. It is worthwhile to schedule veterinary examinations at intervals to monitor a horse throughout a season. Subtle behavioral changes also hint at problems. Refusal or dislike of work in a horse that normally likes to work may indicate pain or discomfort. Attitude problems associated with pain include:

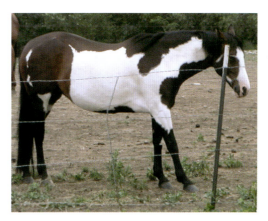

3.50 *A horse that regularly stands with a leg extended in front of him is often afflicted with throbbing foot pain.*

- Tail wringing
- Head tossing
- Bucking
- Refusal to pick up a lead
- Grumpy behavior when being saddled

Watch a horse at rest in the paddock. Does he stand with legs camped out in front as if he's trying to lighten the load on his front feet? Does he point one foot more than another (photo 3.50)? Does he shift his weight from foot to foot trying to get comfortable? And, under saddle, how does he behave? Does he insist on walking on the soft grass or dirt rather than the gravel road? Does he shorten his steps as he descends a hill? Does his stride shorten?

All these behaviors and expressions are a horse's way of communicating that his feet hurt. Possible reasons behind foot pain are many and varied, but should not be ignored. Learn to feel the digital pulses behind the fetlocks to determine the presence of a bounding pulse that might indicate inflammation within a foot.

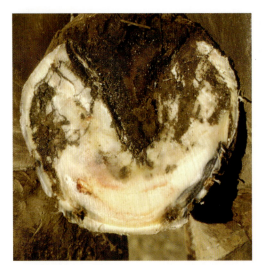

3.51 *Pink or red discoloration to the sole or hoof indicates bruising with bleeding into the tissues. This discoloration will remain until the injured hoof grows out.*

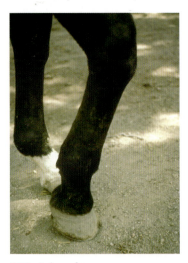

3.52 *A foot abscess may cause a horse to appear fracture lame and unwilling to step on the limb at all. In this picture, the horse is painful in the rear of the foot and so tips the heel off the ground to relieve pressure over the abscess. When he is asked to walk, he barely touches his toe to the ground, and mostly hops on the other front limb.*

Sole Bruises, Abscesses, and Corns

SOLE BRUISE

Any localized concentration of abnormal impact on the hoof puts a horse at risk of going unsound. Injury to underlying tissues of the sole may take the form of a deep bruise (photo 3.51). Not all sole bruising results in lameness, although performance may suffer. Bruising occurs from:

- Thin soles
- Overly worn hoof
- Shoe contact on the sole
- Too small or too tight a shoe
- Unbalanced hoof and unlevel hoof impact
- Rocky terrain or point loading from a stone or pebble

Persistent point loading and associated deep bruising may form blood or serum pockets beneath the sole. A *subsolar abscess* (see below) or *corn* may develop; a fluid pocket or necrotic area in the sensitive tissues can cause lameness. *Laminitis* is also a potential consequence of deep solar bruising (see "Laminitis," p. 74).

Treating Sole Bruising

Management of a sole bruise requires patience. Most horses respond within a couple of weeks to hoof protection, anti-inflammatory drugs, and rest. Others require 3 to 6 months to recover. Crushing of the subsolar corium leaks red blood cells that stain the horn. As the hoof grows out, this stain may be visible as a pinkish area on the underside of the foot, or along the side of the hoof wall. Not all sole bruises are visible, especially in a dark hoof.

HOOF ABSCESS OR GRAVEL

Potentially, bruised hoof tissue may develop a *subsolar abscess,* which is a pocket of serum or infection that forms beneath the sole. Abscesses may develop from bruising and trauma to the sole, from a nail puncture, infection of the white line, or a misplaced ("hot") horseshoe nail seated too close to sensitive lamina (see "Hot Nail," p. 72). An abscess that migrates up the white line is referred to as *gravel.*

A horse with a foot abscess is profoundly lame, at times reluctant to step onto the foot at all (photo 3.52). Foot pain usually elicits a peculiar stance, with the horse "pointing" the limb (see photo 3.50, p. 69). In some cases of hoof abscess, the lower limb will swell, giving a mistaken impression of a pastern or cannon injury. There may be a notice-

The Hoof

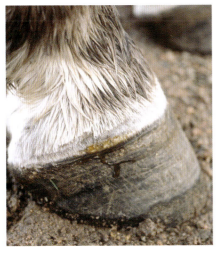

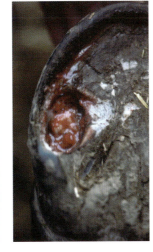

3.54 *This foot abscess developed due to a nail puncture. Infection in this foot undermined the overlying sole; all necrotic tissue and pus debris needed to be dug out of the injured area to allow healing to proceed. Pink, healthy granulation tissue is visible in the depths of the hole.*

3.53 *Not all abscesses are created by a puncture to the solar surface. An infection in the white line, or a deep internal bruise may form an abscess that breaks open at the heel bulb or along the coronary band, as seen here.*

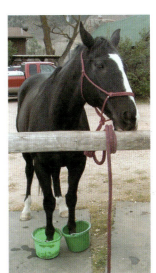

3.55 *A hoof abscess often responds well to foot soaks in Epsom salt baths.*

able increase to digital pulses of the affected limb, related to inflammation within the hoof. Hoof tester examination is helpful to identify the specific location of an abscess. It is sometimes possible to identify a smoldering abscess by pushing on one of the heel bulbs or along the coronary band, and eliciting a pain response from the horse. An abscess tract follows the path of least resistance, often popping out at the heel bulb or along the coronary band (photo 3.53). Once the pressure is relieved, lameness immediately subsides. Identification of the exact location of a subsolar abscess allows a veterinarian to pare it out from the bottom of the sole before the infection migrates through soft tissues of the foot (photo 3.54). Foot soaks twice a day in warm Epsom salts help draw an abscess to the surface (photo 3.55), or a poultice bandage may be applied to the hoof (photo 3.56).

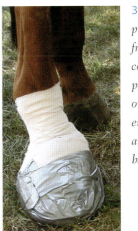

3.56 *A foot bandage protects an abscess from dirt and fecal contamination. A poultice pack applied over the abscess also encourages drainage and medicates while bandaged.*

CORNS

Another manifestation of deep tissue bruising within the foot is the formation of a *corn*. A corn is an area of pressure *necrosis* (tissue death) that develops at the *angle of the bars* formed where the walls of the heel

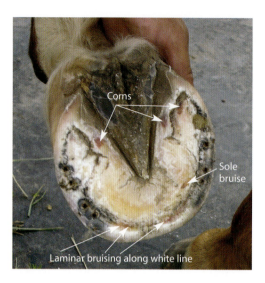

3.57 *The circular red spots on this horse's heels are known as corns. These are areas of bleeding related to pressure points created by a poorly fitting shoe coupled with repetitive impact incurred during athletic demands. Although a corn usually develops at the angle of the bar, this horse has developed multiple pressure points that have formed corns around the bars. A corn is not always visible until it moves toward the bottom of the sole with hoof growth. As the corn grows out, a horse's lameness will resolve provided the problematic shoeing issues are addressed. This foot also shows other signs of concussion with a visible sole bruise, and bruising of the laminae reflected as a pink discoloration along the white line.*

meet the bars (photo 3.57). A corn may be created by abnormal pressure from the heel of a poorly fit or too small shoe. A shoe that pinches too tightly at the angles or the heels, or a loose or twisted shoe that persistently presses on a spot with each step can also create a corn. Bruised tissue dies back, forming a *dry abscess*. Corns are painful because they create a pressure point beneath the sole. Often, they take weeks to months to resolve and grow out.

Treating Corns

Generous fit of width and length of a shoe at the heels eliminates pressure at the angle of the bars. Shoeing appointments should be scheduled at 6 to 8 week intervals. (Some horses in hard work may need to be reshod every 4 to 6 weeks.) Employ a competent farrier who will fit the foot with a properly sized and applied shoe. Sole bruises or corns can put a horse out of action for a time, and then it may be advantageous to pad to provide mechanical protection to the bottom of the foot.

HOT NAIL

A "hot" nail refers to any nail that has irritated the sensitive lamina within the hoof sufficiently to create an inflammatory response. A nail does not necessarily have to be driven into the sensitive laminae of the white line to cause a problem. Sometimes a portion of a nail is seated against the sensitive part of the white line; over a few days, constant pressure of the nail at this location elicits an inflammatory process or infection. If a nail is inadvertently driven directly into the sensitive tissues, the horse shows immediate discomfort. Sometimes the response is no more than a "knee-jerk" reaction of flinching or pulling the leg away. Sometimes the horse will put the foot down and point the hoof in front of his body, or he may pick the leg up and down persistently, due to discomfort.

Nails that are driven high up the face of the hoof wall are more likely to create a hot nail condition as the white line thins out higher up the hoof face. Thin-walled horses are more prone to developing a hot nail due to the thin white line with which a farrier has to work. Horses that fidget and move while being shod also increase the risk of a nail missing its target. And, a hot nail can develop if a shoe twists on the foot allowing the nail to wiggle within the white line. The shoe may still remain on the foot, but in a twisted condition; or, the shoe may tear loose, with the damage already done before the horse throws off the shoe.

Thrush, White Line Disease, and Canker

THRUSH

Thrush (pododermatitis) results from moist and unhygienic conditions. Accumulation of manure, rotten straw, or mud on the bottoms of the feet encourages growth of anaerobic bacteria within the crevices (*sulci*) of the frog. Often, a thrush infection travels deep into the sensitive layers of the frog, causing considerable pain and lameness, adversely affecting the horse's performance. A foul odor is associated with thrush, and the frog becomes dark and discolored by discharge. Normally, the frog should be firm, but pliable like a rubber eraser; a thrush-affected frog feels spongy as it degenerates.

Treatment of Thrush

Thrush is preventable with good hygiene: picking out the feet daily and housing in a clean environment. If a horse lives in a damp environment, medicate the bottom of each foot a couple times a week with tincture of iodine or copper sulfate products. If pads are worn, regularly squirt these solutions beneath the pads as antiseptics. If a problem remains chronic, then it'll be necessary to remove the pads to allow air contact and drying of the bottom of the feet. The abrasive action of the ground also peels away shedding tissue that harbors bacteria. Frequent trimming every 6 to 8 weeks removes dead tissue that traps debris. Athletic horses may need trimming and shoeing every 5 to 6 weeks to maintain foot hygiene.

WHITE LINE DISEASE

A hoof with a problem that weakens the white line is at risk for developing *white line disease*. Separation of the white line allows invasion of bacteria or yeasts to create a smelly, painful infection within the sensitive laminae. Abnormal foot conformation, such as a long toe with underrun heels, or a club foot, makes a foot more susceptible to white line separation. Attention to hoof integrity and good hygienic practices minimize hoof degradation. High urea concentrations from urine weaken keratin proteins of the hoof wall. Fecal moisture further degrades intercellular cementing substance between horn cells. Such alterations in horn quality allow invasion by bacteria or fungi. Horses stabled in muddy, wet conditions are most susceptible. Hot shoeing has also been implicated in development of white line disease. Burning the shoe into the hoof may occlude a weak spot, trapping infectious organisms within the white line. Pads may have a similar adverse effect.

CANKER

Another inflammatory condition of the hoof is known as *canker*. Canker develops in unusually moist and warm climates. A horse with canker develops a foul smelling, moist infection of the frog and sole. Frog tissues proliferate quite dissimilar to frog degeneration seen with thrush. Affected foot structures turn white with a cottage-cheese consistency, in contrast to the black, decaying appearance of thrush. Canker invades deeper into the horny tissues than does thrush, with thrush confined primarily to the frog. Successful treatment of canker depends upon aggressive surgical removal of all affected tissue along with application of appropriate topical medications.

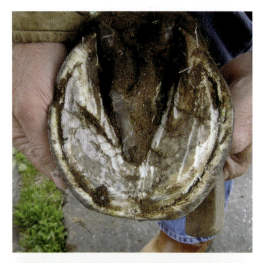

3.58 *Laminitis (inflammation of the sensitive laminae within the hoof) has many causes, among them obesity, rich nutrition, grain overload, concussion, and hormonal problems. Weakness in the sensitive laminae of the hoof from inflammation often leads to separation of the white line, as seen here in this hoof.*

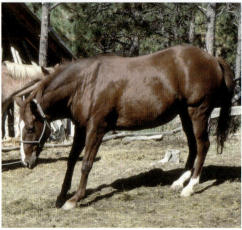

3.59 *This is the typical stance of a laminitic horse, weight shifted toward the hindquarters, front feet extended out in front. When the horse is asked to move, he shifts his weight further to the hind end to pivot around the painful and throbbing front feet.*

Laminitis

Laminitis is an all-encompassing term that denotes inflammation of the *lamellae* (sensitive laminae) within the hoof, no matter the cause. For horses, it is a crippling disease, and is potentially life threatening. Typically, laminitis develops as a result of metabolic disturbances related to a rich diet, obesity, or hormonal imbalances. Laminitis can also develop as a consequence of dehydration, electrolyte imbalances, colic, systemic infection, or exhaustion syndrome. And, laminitis may occur as a mechanical complication of excess foot concussion or trauma, particularly on a thin-soled horse.

The hoof wall records an inflammatory event by forming ripples, ridges, or dishing on the front face (see photos 3.25 A & B, p. 54). Another telltale sign of inflammation in the hoof laminae is often seen as separation of the white line (photo 3.58). Radiographic examination of the internal coffin bone yields information as to the consequences of this disease to a horse's athletic future.

CHARACTERISTICS OF LAMINITIS

An affected horse appears "stiff" in the front end, or shifts his weight from foot to foot. The horse is often reluctant to move, and places both hind legs far beneath his body to shift weight from the painful front feet to the rear (photo 3.59). This weight shift is amplified as the horse is asked to turn. A laminitic horse appears to be "walking on eggs." A perceptive owner may appreciate warmth in the feet, or hoof temperature can be measured. Bounding pulses may be felt in the digital arteries located just behind the fetlock. Rapping on the front face of the hoof wall often causes an affected horse to flinch and pick up his painful foot. Some horses react to hoof pain by sweating, acting anxious or colicky; others spend a lot of time lying down.

In most cases, laminitis usually only occurs in the front limbs. Laminitis is a true emergency condition; immediate damage must be attended promptly and an underlying problem corrected (see p. 81).

Grading of Severity of Laminitis

The degree to which a horse exhibits pain correlates well with the extent of microscopic lamellar damage. Pain response is graded on an Obel scale.

- Obel Grade 1: A horse will move freely but shifts weight from one foot to the other.
- Obel Grade 2: Lameness is more obvious, particularly when asked to turn. The gait is stilted and mincing. The horse is able to stand on each affected foot when the other leg is lifted.
- Obel Grade 3: The horse is reluctant to move and refuses lifting of the opposite limb because of pain felt when standing on the affected foot.
- Obel Grade 4: The horse refuses to move or lies recumbent.

WHAT IS LAMINITIS?

The process of laminitis might be considered an element of a natural physiologic process gone awry. Laminitis occurs when there is failure of the lamellar attachments. When enzyme activity of metalloproteinases (MMPs—see p. 42) proceeds unchecked without normal inhibition of its effects, devastating destruction occurs: affected lamellar tissue loses contact with the basement membrane, resulting in tissue separation and laminar "disorganization" with potentially irreversible damage. Think of what happens when a knit sweater starts to unravel: one strand begins to pull apart, and all attaching knitted fibers pull loose. The laminae of a laminitic hoof disintegrate into incongruous parts much in the same way that an unraveled sweater shreds into a disarray of fibers that no longer connect to one another (figs. 3.60 A & B).

Before clinical signs are appreciated, a *developmental phase* lasting about 40 hours occurs, with progressive separation of the lamellae. It is at this point, before a horse becomes appreciably painful, that aggressive treatment measures may avert a crisis before it becomes irreversible. In many cases, an owner is unaware of the occurrence of this developmental phase. However, in instances of known carbohydrate overload from rich pasture or feed, or when a horse has accidentally gotten into the grain bin, strategies can be implemented to arrest the developmental phase (see "Therapy for Laminitis," p. 82).

METABOLIC CAUSES OF LAMINITIS

Circulatory Compromise

Previous thinking about the inciting cause of laminitis has focused on explanations about circulatory compromise in the hoof. Internal parts of a horse's foot receive oxygen through a branching network of blood vessels. The main vessels run down the leg toward the foot. At the coronary band they branch into smaller divisions heading deep into the hoof. The *dorsal laminar arteries* feed the front of the foot through branches of the *circumflex artery* that runs around the bottom of the coffin bone (fig 3.61). A latticework of tissue and blood vessels (lamellae or laminae) supports the coffin bone within the hoof wall. For blood to reach the sensitive laminae in the front of the foot, it must flow against gravity, with blood moving upward from the circumflex artery at the bottom of the foot. Development of laminitis has been suggested to be a consequence of reduced blood flow (vasoconstriction) due to shunting and compression of circulation elicited by chemical mediators of inflammation. These vascular events do occur, but recent information redefines the progression of events to suggest that by the time vasoconstriction occurs in the hoof, laminitis is well under way. It is possible that circulatory compromise is a consequence of laminitis, rather than the sole cause (see fig. 3.60 B).

3.60 A & B *Laminitis Disintegration:* The upper two images show the orientation of the laminae in a normal hoof, as compared to the crushing of the laminae in a laminitic hoof with coffin bone rotation (A). The bottom two images illustrate the normal circulation of the circumflex artery and dorsal laminar arteries in the hoof, as compared to circulatory occlusion with coffin bone rotation in laminitis (B).

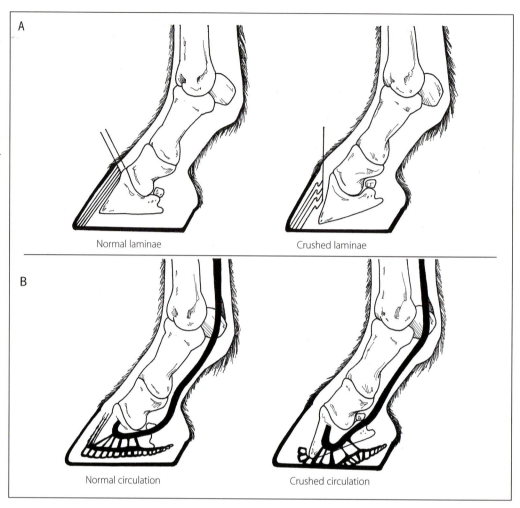

3.61 The blood supply to the hoof runs down the leg with multiple branches along the way. For blood to reach the sensitive laminae in the front of the foot, it must flow against gravity, with blood moving upward from the circumflex artery at the bottom of the foot.

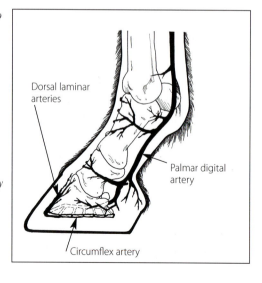

Rich Pasture Consumption or Grain Overload

Research (Dr. Chris Pollitt) has identified a plausible explanation of what occurs in the hoof tissues when a horse is afflicted with laminitis. Carbohydrate overload illustrates the role of dietary starch in stimulating a laminitic attack: this research model mimics what happens to a horse that consumes too much rich pasture grass, a source of a complex sugar known as *fructan*, also called *oligofructose*. Fructan is present in abundant concentration in grass stems in spring and fall when ground temperatures are low. In certain conditions dependent on sunlight, temperature, moisture availability, and species of grass, a horse

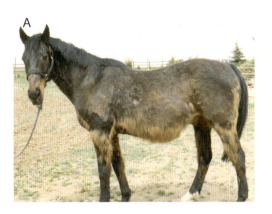 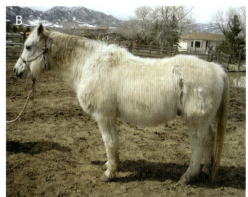

3.62 A & B *A horse with Cushing's disease grows a long and wooly hair coat that sheds out erratically in spring (A). The horse in (B) has the hair coat and body shape that is highly typical of this disease.*

grazing on fructan-rich pastures is able to consume twice the amount of starch that is known to induce laminitis.

Classic grain overload situations exist: horses are adept at breaking into areas where they don't belong, like the feed shed, and there they overeat. Sometimes it is difficult to tell exactly how much grain a horse has eaten. If treated aggressively within the first 8 to 12 hours, most cases of grain overload do not develop into a problem. If several horses have access to the grain, all should be treated even if one is seemingly less dominant in food acquisition.

The danger in high fructan or carbohydrate ingestion is based on the simple fact that a horse (and other mammals) does not possess digestive enzymes to metabolize fructan; it passes into the cecum of the large intestine in a relatively undigested form. In the cecum, rapid fermentation of fructan by bacterial microbes promotes proliferation of Gram-positive organisms (*Streptococcus bovis*, *Streptococcus equinus*, and *Lactobacillus* spp.), along with pH changes to acidify the cecal contents. Massive overgrowth of these bacteria in the cecum releases factors that trigger laminitis. At the same time, damage to the lining of the hindgut promotes uptake of bacteria along with laminitis trigger factors into the systemic circulation; there they elicit activation of specific enzymes, notably *matrix metalloproteinases*, or MMPs, which cause separation of the *basement membrane* of the laminae. In the developmental phase of laminitis, clinical signs of fever, elevated heart rate and respiratory rate, and diarrhea may appear in response.

Pituitary Disorder

A common disease of an older horse is called *Equine Cushing's Disease* (ECD), also known as *pituitary pars intermedia dysfunction*, or PPID. Abnormal function of the pituitary gland (that resides in the brain) results in hormonal imbalance, leading to altered glucose and cortisol metabolism. It is documented that 70 percent of horses over the age of 20 show some obvious or subclinical signs of dysfunction of the pituitary gland, and signs may appear as early as 15 years of age. Clinical signs of ECD include any of the following:

- Long, shaggy fur coat that doesn't fully shed out in the spring (photos 3.62 A & B)
- A pot-bellied appearance that results from a loss of muscle mass and tone
- Fat deposited around the orbits of the eyes make them seem puffy and protrusive (photo 3.63)

3.63 *One hallmark sign of Cushing's disease is the puffiness of the eye orbit in a middle-aged or older horse. Fat deposited around the orbits of the eyes makes them seem puffy and protrusive, whereas a normal, older horse is sunken in over the eyes.*

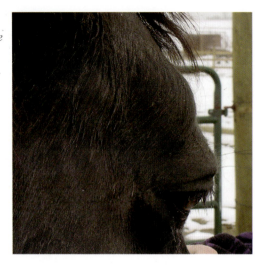

- Low energy
- Increased appetite with no apparent weight gain
- Tendency to drink as much as 3 or 4 times more than usual and excess urination accompanies excess thirst
- Vision problems related to associated pressure on the optic nerve in cases where the pituitary gland enlarges
- Personality changes
- Poor immune response
- Laminitis

Because of high circulating levels of *corticosteroids* created by abnormal feedback from a diseased pituitary gland, these horses often have poorly functioning immune systems. (Corticosteroids are potent anti-inflammatory hormones that suppress inflammation, pain, heat, swelling, and the immune system.) Despite regular deworming schedules at frequent intervals, an ECD horse may appear unthrifty due to persistent gastrointestinal parasitism. Some ECD horses are slow to heal wounds. Frequent viral and/or bacterial infections occur, with one common development being a chronic sinus infection that responds poorly to antibiotics. Oral ulcerations and gum disease are also frequent findings in horses affected with ECD.

One of the biggest problems seen with ECD is the eventual development of chronic laminitis as a result of the influence of persistent high levels of corticosteroids, and also related to changes in carbohydrate and fat metabolism. Glucocorticoids have multiple adverse effects when found in excess in the circulation. One adverse effect is interference with oxygen delivery to the tissues due to inappropriate reactivity of blood vessels. Another effect is atrophy and weakening of skin tissues; hoof and skin are different parts of the same organ. Laminitis is an indirect consequence of overabundant glucocorticoid production.

Management of ECD

Medications such as *cyproheptidine* or *pergolide* are available to control the effects of ECD in affected horses; these medications have their best effect before laminitis develops so it is of benefit to recognize the early warning signs of this problem.

Once laminitis has occurred in a Cushing's horse, the prognosis is poor for continued quality of life since it is difficult to resolve the problems in the feet while the metabolic derangements persist. Feeding a high fat and high fiber diet improves glucose and insulin metabolism in ECD horses. Avoid feeding these horses grain or molasses that upset an already altered carbohydrate metabolism.

Equine Metabolic Syndrome (Peripheral Cushingoid Syndrome)

Although diagnosis of a horse with recurrent laminitis may be suspicious for Cushing's disease, instead of being a primary problem within the pituitary gland as is seen with Cushing's, high levels of circulating corticosteroids may originate from enzyme activity in local intestinal sources. These sources include liver or the fat cells within the abdomen, including the *omentum* that covers the bowel. Fat cells are responsive to endocrine signals; the more fat cells present as occurs with obesity, the greater the risk of hormonal irregularities.

This malady is recognized as *equine metabolic syndrome,* also referred to as *peripheral cushingoid syndrome*. The age of horses affected by metabolic syndrome generally ranges between 8 to 18 years, but geriatric horses are also at risk. Such a horse is overweight in body condition, with a body condition score of 7 to 9 on a scale of 1 to 9. (See chapter 12, *The Digestive System: Nutritional Management,* p. 346.) An owner finds it difficult to slim down such an "easy keeper" (photo 3.64).

Any breed may be affected but breeds most prone are those body types that readily lay down visible fat pads. (Examples include Morgan horses, Peruvian Pasos, Paso Finos, Spanish Mustangs, as well as pony breeds.) Fat deposits are distributed in the crest of the neck, in the rump areas, and within the *prepuce* (sheath) of male horses. Affected horses are often difficult to breed due to infertility issues. Many fat horses are erroneously diagnosed as being hypothyroid. Although there may be some degree of diminished thyroid hormone levels, the problem is not within the thyroid gland itself but rather is related to irregular hormonal feedback as a result of high circulating levels of corticosteroids.

An overweight horse is predisposed to laminitis. "Obesity-associated laminitis" may develop slowly and without overt symptoms of pain that would be noticed by an owner. The hoof wall may demonstrate characteristic signs of laminitis such as diverging growth lines and ridging in the face of the hoof wall (see photos 3.25 A & B, p. 54).

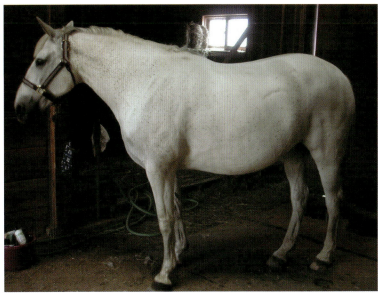

3.64 A horse with equine metabolic syndrome is an easy keeper, with a body condition score of 7 to 9, and he is difficult to trim down despite dietary modifications and exercise. Fat deposits develop in the crest of the neck, the rump, and in the prepuce of male horses.

Insulin Resistance

In any age or breed of horse, overconsumption of fructan or of daily amounts of carbohydrate-rich supplements (grains or legume hays) may lead to *insulin resistance.* Insulin resistance is the reduced ability of insulin to promote uptake of glucose by peripheral tissues, otherwise known as *glucose intolerance*. Insulin resistance is known to occur as a consequence of obesity, equine metabolic syndrome, gastrointestinal disease, uterine infection, or systemic disease. Persistently elevated concentrations of insulin in the circulation lead to muscle wasting, and potentially may lead to laminitis. Pain from laminitis is a stressor in itself, acting as a trigger for insulin resistance, making it difficult to resolve metabolic problems that are self-perpetuating.

Normally, the pancreas secretes insulin as a response to glucose derived from food ingestion. Insulin enhances uptake of glucose by skeletal muscle, fat cells, and the liver. Factors that create interference with the normal action of insulin cause blood glucose levels to increase (*hyperglycemia*); insulin continues to increase in response. Yet, in spite of excess glucose in the circulation, there is insufficient glucose delivery to target cells dependent upon glucose, as for example, structures in the hoof. This results in damage to the linking attachment points (*hemidesmosomes*) that adhere the lamellae to the basement membrane (see p. 42); this disruption leads to clinical laminitis. At the same time, other tissues that do not depend upon glucose for metabolism, such as red blood cells, are presented with toxic levels of glucose, so red blood cells succumb and die. This results in *oxidative stress* in the circulation of many tissues, including the hoof.

Management of Equine Metabolic Syndrome

Despite dietary restriction, it is difficult to reduce the weight on horses afflicted with equine metabolic syndrome. At the current time, there is no approved medical treatment of this condition other than strict dietary management and reduction of caloric intake. Dietary strategy relies on feeding only grass hay (7 to 10 percent protein) at amounts 1½ to 2 percent of body weight. (Hay analysis can evaluate carbohydrate content.) It is suggested that soaking hay may reduce the level of soluble carbohydrates.

It is important to eliminate *all* grain products as well as molasses, other high carbohydrate feed, or high fat feeds, as these exacerbate insulin resistance. Green pasture should also be eliminated as a feed source, as green grass often contains high levels of *fructan*, which can trigger physiologic events leading laminitis (see p. 76). Fast growing, short grasses contain the highest concentrations of fructan sugars so a pasture need not be full and lush to pose a risk of developing laminitis.

Chromium supplementation has been used to address insulin resistance, although there is no agreement as to its effectiveness as a treatment. *Chromium tripicolinate* can be fed safely at a dose of 3 to 5 mg/day. Antioxidants such as vitamin E (up to 10,000 IU per day) may have a role in treatment of red blood cell dysfunction related to insulin resistance.

MECHANICAL CAUSES OF LAMINITIS

Plant-Related Toxicity

Black walnut (*Juglans nigra*) shavings exert life-threatening effects on horses stalled in bedding composed of at least 20 percent of this material or from ingestion of the bark or nuts of live trees. Within 10 to 24 hours of exposure, the legs swell and laminitis develops. Respiratory problems also develop from this tree when pollen sheds in the spring.

Ingestion of *hoary alyssum* (*Berteroa incana*) hay is known for its effect of limb swelling and laminitis, as well as onset of fever and diarrhea. In both cases, removal of the offending plant product allows for recovery (see *Appendix C*, p. 571).

Road Founder

Laminitis is also caused by mechanical concussion. *Road founder* develops from trauma and bruising of the laminae from vigorous exercise on hard, concussive surfaces (photo 3.65). Feet that are excessively trimmed or worn are easily traumatized. Stone bruises or nail punctures that result in infection or foot abscesses can also cause laminitis.

Support Founder

Support founder results from a leg injury, like a fracture, that renders a horse inactive for months at a time. Blood flow stagnates in the opposite, uninjured limb with excessive weight bearing, setting up conditions for laminitis to occur in the "good" foot. A period of only 2 to 3 days of full weight on a limb is sufficient to create lamellar damage (photo 3.66).

Prevention relies upon application of an effective support shoe, and provision of ample

The Hoof   81

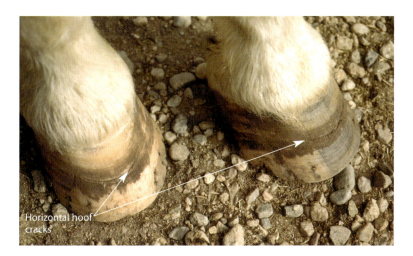

3.65 Horizontal crack lines as seen here indicate a period of acute inflammation of concussion laminitis. These cracks indicate that the time of insult occurred a few months prior to this photo, and they are being pushed down the hoof as new, healthy horn grows out. In this case, the horse had experienced a fast, long distance ride and immediately became foot sore and lame. Once the initial crisis resolved, he was allowed to heal by having his shoes pulled and turning him out to pasture.

bedding to encourage a horse to lie down to relieve excess load from the foot to restore hoof circulation.

CONSEQUENCES OF LAMINITIS

An inflammatory crisis develops within the hooves due to any systemic disease that elicits overgrowth of intestinal bacteria or affects blood flow to the feet. Following the developmental onset phase of laminitis described above, the acute phase is accompanied by pain and lameness. Reduced blood and oxygen supplies in the tissues are accompanied by vascular hypertension, which is felt with finger pressure as a pounding arterial pulse in the lower limb. Decreasing oxygen circulation in the foot worsens laminar swelling. As laminar tissues swell, pain is similar to what one might feel when a blood blister develops beneath a thumbnail. For the horse having to walk on such injured feet, the pain is excruciating.

Enzymatic activity of MMPs proceeds unchecked to worsen structural loss of the basement membrane. As the basement membrane separates from the lamellae, there is nothing to counteract the weight of the horse and the pull of the deep digital flexor tendon that attaches to the back of the coffin bone.

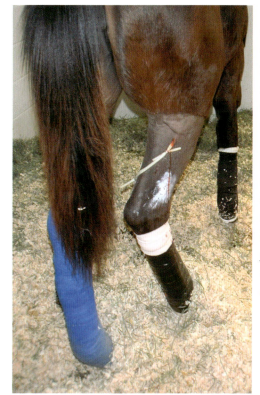

3.66 A serious Strep infection in the muscles of the right rear limb forced this mare to support her full weight on the left rear for an extended period of time. In spite of aggressive surgical and medical procedures and preventative hoof support, she developed supporting-limb laminitis (support founder) in the left rear and had to be euthanized.

The toe creates a lever effect, further amplifying pull from the tendon. The coffin bone may detach from the hoof wall, in part or in whole. Without its supportive laminar attachments, the coffin bone can rotate or sink to the bottom of the sole. It is possible to see rotation as soon as 3 hours after the laminae begin to swell (figs. 3.67 A–C). In a very severe case, the bone may perforate the bottom of the foot. Immediate action must be taken to halt the progression of damage.

PREVENTION OF LAMINITIS USING CRYOTHERAPY

Dr. Pollitt's research elaborates suggestions about first aid measures that may be taken in a horse with a known carbohydrate or fructan overload. He advocates the use of cryotherapy before clinical signs become obvious: immersion of a horse's front limbs to the level of the knees into an ice water slurry (36 to 41° F or 2 to 5° C) for 48 hours to elicit vasoconstriction of hoof circulation. (As said earlier, enzymatic separation of the basement membrane from the lamellae occurs 36 to 48 hours prior to the appearance of clinical signs, during the *developmental phase*.) Unlike humans, horses do not appear to have receptors to cold in their hooves so are not bothered by the application of cold for a prolonged period. This strategy is beneficial for several reasons:

- Tissue metabolism within the hoof is reduced.
- Reduced circulation minimizes delivery of laminitis trigger factors that would otherwise activate MMP enzymes.
- Enzymatic activity of MMPs is reduced by 50 percent for every 17° F (or 10° C) decrease in temperature.

Every few hours a horse's hooves normally vacillate between periods of vasoconstriction (decreased blood flow) and vasodilation (increased blood flow). In the study, all horses that were left untreated to experience vasodilation cycles of the hooves did develop laminitis. The feet of horses receiving cryotherapy only suffered minor cellular changes. Based on historic theories that poor blood circulation and reduced oxygen delivery to the hoof tissues were the causes of laminitis, we then would expect vasoconstriction with ice therapy to cause more harm than good: this was not the case. Favorable results achieved with cryotherapy validate the proposed theory that matrix metalloproteinases and laminitis trigger factors elicit profound damage at the cellular level.

THERAPY FOR LAMINITIS

There is no single recipe for therapy for laminitis; each case must be tailored to the severity of the crisis and the unique metabolic problem of the horse. Upon recognition of a crisis:

- If known carbohydrate or fructan overload exists, foot-soaks in ice water prior to the onset of clinical signs have shown favorable effects in reducing laminar damage by reducing delivery of matrix metalloproteinase enzymes or laminitis trigger factors to the hooves.
- Call a veterinarian to attend the cause, e.g., grain overload, retained placenta, intestinal disease, or concussive trauma.
- Eliminate rich feed (grain, alfalfa, pasture) from the diet.
- Implement dietary strategies for an overweight horse to reduce metabolic upset, and to reduce weight on compromised feet.
- Use of nonsteroidal anti-inflammatory (NSAIDs) drugs (*ketoprofen, flunixin meglumine, phenylbutazone*) counteracts pain and inflammation, and flunixin meglumine is beneficial against the effect of endotoxin.
- *DMSO (dimethyl sulfoxide)* given systemically (intravenous or oral route) has antioxidant effects on tissue, and may have value in an acute case of laminitis (see p. 127).
- Stomach tubing with mineral oil is useful to treat cases of grain overload to prevent grain fermentation and subsequent overgrowth of intestinal bacteria, and to limit

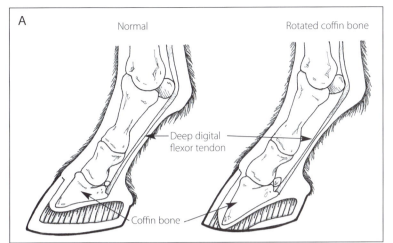

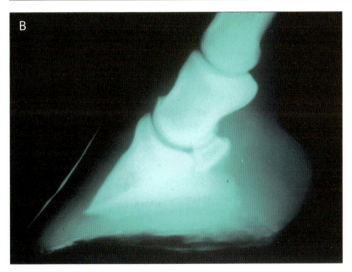
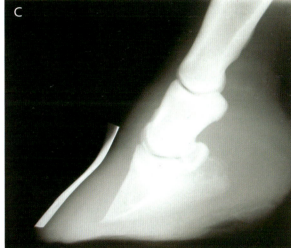

3.67 A–C Appearance of a normal vs rotated coffin bone (A). The radiographs show the coffin bone in parallel alignment with the front of the hoof wall as in a normal hoof (B), and a good example of a coffin bone rotation within the hoof capsule caused by laminitis (C).

the absorption of toxins from the bowel.
- Application of frog support, like blue Styrofoam, to the bottom of the foot provides support to the coffin bone (photo 3.68). Or, sand bedding provides a supportive cushion beneath the sole.
- Confine the horse so movement does not continue to damage the laminae through the pull of the deep flexor tendon. Exercise *must* be restricted.

Other controversial therapies address improvement of circulatory blood flow within the hooves, using vasodilators like *nitroglycerine*, and *pentoxyfylline* or *isoxsuprine hydrochloride*. *Acepromazine* has proven to be of value. In addition to being a potent vasodilator, acepromazine also increases insulin secretion and makes glucose available to hoof tissues.

Once a horse is stabilized in an acute crisis, serial radiographic (X-ray) evaluations enable therapeutic trimming and shoeing to provide coffin bone support. In addition to elimination of pain and discomfort, a few other elements associated with desirable healing progress include productive sole growth and recovery of the concave cup to the sole.

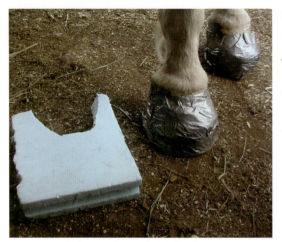

3.68 *One of the best means of providing coffin bone support is to apply blue Styrofoam to the bottom of the foot. The hoof outline is traced on the foam with a Sharpie pen, and the foam is cut to fit the outline. Duct tape is used to affix the Styrofoam to the foot; care should be taken to avoid application of tape to the coronary band or above, otherwise this compresses hoof circulation, compounding the problem. The foam moulds over a few hours into a form fit of the bottom of the foot, and provides a cushion to the sole, while also placing upward pressure on the frog to stabilize the coffin bone in the hoof capsule.*

RECOGNIZING CHRONIC LAMINITIS

Acute laminitis means a horse experiences a new or sudden occurrence. *Chronic laminitis* refers to internal changes within the hoof that have occurred in prior and/or multiple acute attacks that create an ongoing condition. A horse with chronic laminitis may seem pain free for a while after a bout of the disease, only to relapse later into an acute crisis of pain and lameness. A horse with chronic laminitis has damage within the hoof, and these changes are usually recognizable externally.

The presence of a dished contour to the hoof wall, or the presence of "laminitic rings" indicates that a horse has experienced prior inflammatory incidents. Horn tubules of the foot normally grow in a straight, nearly vertical line from the coronary band. When the coffin bone is compressed downward or rotates within the hoof wall during a laminitic crisis, the horn-generating coronary corium is compressed and trapped between the hoof wall and the extensor process (see fig. 3.60 A, p. 76). (The extensor process is a bony protrusion at the top of the coffin bone to which the extensor tendon attaches.)

Horn tubules at the top of the hoof wall bend at steep angles, further crushing the sensitive coronary tissue and reducing the blood supply (see fig. 3.60 B, p. 76). Once the coronary corium is compressed and its blood supply is limited, oxygen deprivation of the tissues alters growth of the hoof wall in the front third of the foot. Horn tubules then grow out deformed. Toe growth slows considerably due to misalignment of the horn tubules from the coronary corium. The result is divergent growth planes in the hoof wall, seen as rings or ridges in the hoof wall (photos 3.69 A–D). Extensive collateral circulation in the heels allows them to grow at a normal rate. Altered blood flow and accompanying hoof dehydration, along with reduced weight bearing from pain inevitably lead to contraction of the entire foot, as well as a deformed appearance of the wall. The front of the hoof wall develops a dished shape, also reflecting an internal deformity in the coffin bone (see photo 3.27, p. 55) If affected hooves are allowed to grow unmanaged, the horn will curl up at the toes in the appearance of Arabic slippers.

The sole often drops and bulges in chronic laminitis cases or with those affected with downward displacement of the coffin bone; the sole loses its concave form. Removal of a thin layer of the sole reveals red, bruised tissue beneath, reflective of internal trauma related to pressure of the coffin bone against the solar corium (photo 3.70). Sterile hoof abscesses may develop at the toe due to damage to the solar tissue.

The Hoof

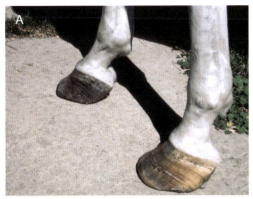 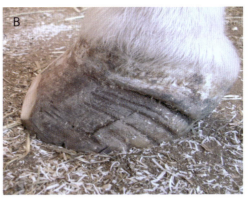
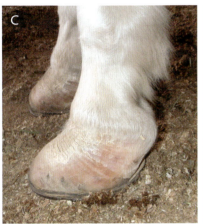 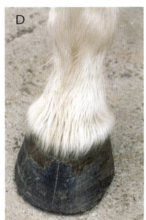

3.69 A–D An incident of laminitis causes the horn tubules to grow out at irregular rates, leading to deformity of the hoof wall with dishing of the front face of the hoof wall, and rings of irregular hoof growth (A). This hoof demonstrates typical hoof wall deformation and rings associated with chronic laminitis (B). The dishing, ridging and long heels of the horse's hooves in (C) are typical of a severe case of laminitis of many years duration. Although his laminitis is reasonably under control, he has repeated bouts of inflammation within the hoof, which perpetuate growth of abnormal hoof wall. Divergent growth planes of the hoof wall may also lead to shearing of the internal laminae, resulting in a central vertical toe crack (D).

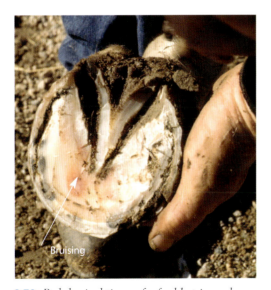

3.70 Red, bruised tissue of a freshly trimmed sole reflects internal trauma related to pressure of the coffin bone against the solar corium in a horse with laminitis. Staining of the tissue from bleeding causes a pink or red discoloration.

Navicular Syndrome

WHAT IS NAVICULAR SYNDROME?

Navicular syndrome refers to a degenerative condition within the navicular apparatus that includes multiple structures: the *navicular bone* (also known as the *distal sesamoid bone*), the *navicular bursa*, the deep digital flexor tendon as it courses beneath the navicular bone, and the supporting ligaments of the navicular bone.

In most cases of navicular disease, the condition affects both front feet with lameness. The typical stride of a "navicular horse" is short and choppy to reduce the impact upon sore heels. The horse stumbles frequently. Some horses try to land toe first, instead of landing with the normal placement of heel

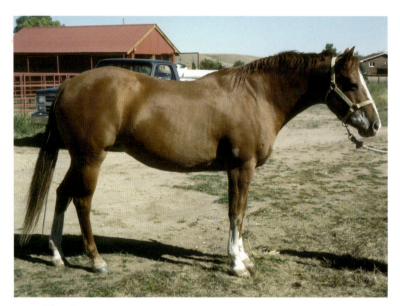

3.71 *This Quarter Horse with his fine bones, steep shoulder, upright pasterns, and small feet is typical of a horse with the potential to develop navicular disease.*

first. These individuals are prone to bruised toes, with the potential for development of recurrent sole abscesses.

As the disease progresses, one or both forefeet may appear noticeably smaller, with the heels contracted. The frog loses its robust appearance and appears shrunken. It is sometimes hard to tell if a foot is contracted if both forefeet are affected. A contracted heel (see p. 48) represents underlying pain in the foot that forces a horse to reduce the normal weight-bearing load on that foot.

Horses most at risk are those that have certain heritable conformation features such as upright pasterns and small foot size relative to body mass (photo 3.71). Horses that are subjected to sports with front-end impact such as cutting, reining, roping, or jumping are also at greater risk for developing navicular disease. Horses that are frequently worked on hard-packed surfaces have increased risk. Certain breed types tend to develop this syndrome more than other breeds. While Arabian horses rarely develop navicular disease, Quarter Horses, Appaloosas, Paint horses, Thoroughbreds, and Warmblood breeds are most often afflicted. This syndrome typically shows up in horses aged 7 to 14 years, but early athletic stress can bring this on in younger horses as well.

STRUCTURE OF THE NAVICULAR APPARATUS

The navicular bone is a shuttle-shaped bone wedged between the coffin bone and the deep digital flexor tendon in the foot. The flexor tendon passes behind the navicular bone, attaching to the back of the coffin bone. Between the navicular bone and the tendon is a bursa that provides a smooth gliding surface for the tendon (figs. 3.72 A–C). The bottom (also called *flexor*) surface of the navicular bone is also smooth, and enhances the gliding effect. The top (*articular*) surface of the navicular bone increases the surface area of the coffin joint and thereby decreases the concussive load on it as the limb impacts the ground. Ligaments that anchor to the wings of the navicular bone support the top of the coffin bone. These ligamentous supports, along with the deep digital flexor tendon below, maintain the position of the navicular bone within the foot.

ETIOLOGY

Historically, there have been multiple explanations for how this syndrome develops:

- *Bursitis* as a result of inflammation from concussion and pressure between the flexor tendons and the navicular bone
- *Thrombosis/Ischemia* due to local trauma and inflammatory mediators creating circulatory disturbance to the navicular bone with resulting pain (a vascular theory that has been discounted due to no supporting evidence of its occurrence)
- *Bone remodeling* caused by abnormal pressures from the deep digital flexor tendon as it is pressed against the bone subsequent to increased loading in the heels

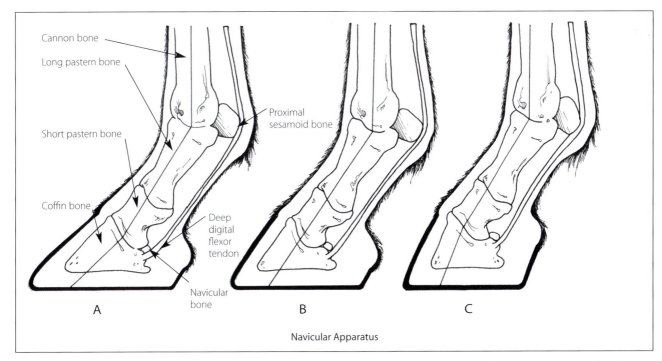

3.72 A–C *A hoof with a long toe, low heel configuration amplifies tension and strain on the navicular structures, even when the horse is at rest* (A); *a hoof with a good hoof-pastern axis alignment showing minimal tension on the navicular structures is shown in* (B); *and* (C) *is a club foot or high-heeled hoof that has the least tension on the navicular structures.*

As of this writing, a more complex theory based on recent anatomical discovery has provided plausible explanations for many of these consequences. It has been concluded (Dr. Robert M. Bowker) that navicular syndrome is a problem within the entire foot, involving more structures in the foot than just the navicular bone. It is noted that clinically healthy feet have a more substantially developed *collateral cartilage* complex within the hoof. It is thought that an increased vascular system associated with thicker collateral cartilages may improve dissipation of stress forces within the foot. Sensory nerve endings associated closely with blood vessels are known to course through the collateral cartilages. The sensory nerve supply to the navicular bone courses through the supporting ligaments. Locomotion and movement of the coffin joint forces the navicular bone to assume some of the weight-bearing load; stress is transferred from the pastern bone to the *suspensory ligaments* of the navicular bone. (The weight-bearing load on the navicular bone is at its maximum during breakover when the solar surface is perpendicular to the ground surface, just before the toe leaves the ground.) Pull on the deep digital flexor tendon creates shearing forces between the deep digital flexor tendon and the *distal suspensory impar ligament* of the navicular bone. Repeated and abnormal tensions ultimately lead to inflammation.

Adaptive responses within the navicular structures and ligaments are related to stress during the stance and impact phases of locomotion and not solely to age of the horse. In horses afflicted with navicular disease, significant changes have been identified in the distal suspensory impar ligament and in its attachment to the coffin bone where it intersects the attachment of the deep digital flexor tendon. It is at this "bottleneck" that sensory nerves and blood vessels course on their way to other areas of the foot. Sensory nerves in this area serve to maintain blood flow within the soft tissues of the foot when it encounters loading during locomotion. Increased circulation stimulated by the sensory nerve signals serves as a hydraulic cushion to guard against impact concussion.

No matter the theory, it is recognized that an upright pastern exacerbates concussion within the heel region. Additionally, Bowker's theory lends an explanation as to why underrun heels and long-toed feet are afflicted with heel and foot pain due to reduced concussion dissipation (see fig. 3.22 and "Long-Toe Low-Heel Foot Configuration," p. 51). The digital cushions of healthy feet may dissipate concussion better than feet with weak and collapsed heels (see photo 3.44). About 70 percent of horses diagnosed with navicular disease have a long-toe and low-heel (LTLH) foot configuration. Almost 60 percent of navicular horses have an unlevelness of the hoof from side to side, referred to as *medial to lateral hoof imbalance*. If trimmed and shod incorrectly, even horses with excellent feet can develop this syndrome. Prevention is essential: every attempt should be made to avoid a LTLH foot configuration, a broken-back hoof axis, or foot imbalances.

UNDERSTANDING DIAGNOSTIC TESTS FOR HEEL PAIN

The gait that comes to be associated with a footsore horse is quite typical of many problems ranging from heel soreness to laminitis. In general, a footsore horse moves with a short, choppy gait; is reluctant to negotiate downhill inclines; or walk or trot on hard or uneven terrain. On uneven or inclined surfaces, a moderately lame horse appears to be tentative, mincing along with each step. A heel-sore horse, as one would be with navicular syndrome, tends to land toe first in an effort to relieve loading of the heels. Ironically, this rapid unloading of the heels in response to heel pain increases the force exerted on the navicular bone by the DDFT. Each time a horse quickly unloads his heels, disease progression is exacerbated by extra compressive stress on the navicular structures.

Before a horse is labeled as having navicular syndrome, it must be identified if heel pain is generalized through the hoof, or if it is associated specifically with navicular disease. No single diagnostic test gives the exact answers. It is important to combine a thorough clinical exam with the findings of multiple tests as described below, and then to corroborate all the information with the clinical picture of the horse. In this way, an accurate diagnosis can be made.

Hoof Tester Exam

In addition to gait analysis, other tools used to identify the source of pain include the use of a *hoof tester* exam of the bottom of each foot. These plier-like devices are squeezed over the frog in an attempt to elicit a reaction from pressure on painful navicular structures inside (photo 3.73). However, this test has been found to be the "least sensitive manipulative test for navicular pain." A horse truly suffering from navicular syndrome is only positively responsive 48 percent of the time to a hoof tester exam. Response is dependent on the structural location of the degenerative disease, as well as the difference in how the limb is loaded by the horse's weight as compared to squeezing of the bottom of the foot with the limb suspended in the air.

Flexion Tests

Another commonly used test for localizing navicular pain relies on flexion tests of the lower limb. This test yields accuracy of only 53 percent and has trouble differentiating between exclusively navicular pain versus other syndromes that create generalized heel pain. A *frog wedge test* places a wedge beneath the frog with the horse's full weight standing on the wedge for a minute, and then he is trotted off. This gives a positive response only 53 percent of the time. Similarly, in a *hoof extension test*, a wedge is placed beneath the toe in an effort to increase strain on the rearward structures of the foot and after holding the other limb in the air for a minute, the horse is then trotted off; this is only 49 percent accurate. (For more on flexion testing, see p. 115 text and photos.)

Diagnostic Nerve Blocks

Diagnostic nerve blocks are invaluable in localizing pain to a specific area (photos 3.74 and 3.75). A common nerve block used to anesthetize the heel region of the foot is the *palmar digital nerve* (PDN) block. Nerves that innervate the back third of the foot are anesthetized with a small amount of local anesthetic infused over these nerve branches low down in the pastern. However, there are problems with this block in its specificity:

- A PDN block may numb the sole, yielding a false positive result if the horse goes sound because of lameness associated with a bruised sole or a problem associated with pain from structures local to the solar region.
- On occasion, accessory branches of this nerve course across the front of the pastern and so are not anesthetized by local anesthetic injected over nerves in the back of the pastern, hence giving a false negative result if the horse does not go sound.
- Fibrous adhesions may create mechanical restriction to limb movement; although pain is numbed, the horse still appears lame.

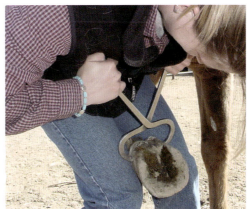

3.73 *A hoof tester is a pliers-like device that exerts pressure across areas of the foot so the examiner can attempt to elicit pain to localize the source of a musculoskeletal problem*

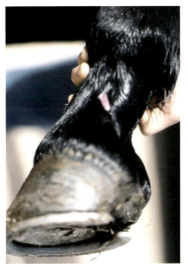

3.74 *A diagnostic nerve block is a useful tool to identify the location of pain. In this photo, a needle is placed along the palmar digital nerve (PDN), which provides the nerve supply to the rear third of the hoof and the sole. A small bleb of anesthetic is deposited over both this nerve and the nerve on the other side of that limb in the same location. If the horse's lameness improves after a few minutes, the diagnosis suggests a problem in the rear third of the foot, and/or in the sole of the foot, all areas which are numbed by the regional anesthesia.*

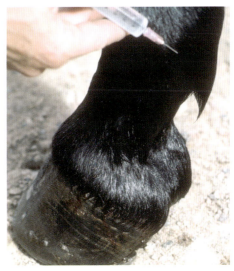

3.75 *Another diagnostic nerve block further up the limb is used when previous lower blocks fail to improve lameness. In this photo, anesthetic is being placed in one of the abaxial nerves behind the fetlock. Once both sides of this area are numbed out, any improvement in lameness confirms that one problem lies in a region of the pastern or below.*

- There may be another concurrent lameness issue such as coffin joint arthritis or a problem elsewhere, again yielding a false negative response to the nerve block.

A valuable diagnostic procedure to isolate navicular pain from other causes of heel pain is that of anesthesia injected directly into the coffin joint. This diagnostic nerve block would not necessarily be the first to try since there is value in gaining information without invading a joint when possible. This procedure is about 90 percent accurate for navicular disease although instances of sole pain can be blocked out with anesthesia into the coffin joint. Coffin joint arthritis often develops as a sequel to navicular disease; in fact, over half of horses with navicular disease also have pain associated with the coffin joint. However also keep in mind that there are cases of coffin joint arthritis that occur due to a joint-specific injury unrelated to the navicular structures. Ultrasound of the navicular structures and coffin joint is also useful to identify structural changes.

Nuclear Scintigraphy

Another test that has been used to localize pain to the navicular region is that of *nuclear scintigraphy*. Nuclear medicine is a form of imaging that relies on injection of radioisotopes into the bloodstream, and then a specialized computer camera scans the horse's bones or soft tissues to identify locations where there is uptake of the radioisotopes in areas with increased circulation, such as is seen with injury or pathology. However, this has a predictive value of only 67 percent because not all reasons for navicular pain are associated with uptake of the radionucleotide in that region.

Radiographic Evaluation of Navicular Structures

Although it is tempting to read a lot into navicular X-ray films, a radiographic exam is not always conclusive. Much discussion amongst veterinary practitioners hinges on the significance of increased number, size, shape, and location of *synovial invaginations* in the bone, or the presence of *cysts* (demineralization) or *sclerosis* (increased mineralization) within the navicular bone, or flattening or erosion of the central ridge of the bone, or the presence of *enthesiophytes* (bone spurs) on the edges of the navicular bone (photos 3.76 and 3.77). All these are telltale signs of bone remodeling (see p. 96) and changes in the navicular bone. These may or may not be related to a clinical problem. In one study, only 34 percent of horses with navicular disease evidenced radiographic lesions of three of the "changes" mentioned above. In addition, many painful issues that stem from disease of the navicular apparatus have to do with soft tissue inflammation of the bursa, tendon, or supporting ligaments. Such soft tissue injuries will not show up on a radiographic examination.

It is generally accepted by the veterinary community that radiographs of the navicular bone correlate less than 40 percent of the time with clinical disease. In other words, horses with navicular "changes" on X-ray exam do not always have clinical disease, while many horses with severe clinical disease will not show radiographic "changes" within the navicular bone because the bulk of the problem lies in the soft tissues. Caution should be taken in overinterpretation of navicular radiographic findings in a lame horse or in a horse being examined for prepurchase.

Magnetic Resonance Imaging

The advent of sophisticated technology has improved diagnostic skills, particularly of foot problems. Magnetic resonance imaging (MRI) units are currently available in many equine referral hospitals. The MRI is very sensitive to enable detection of bone changes, providing

The Hoof

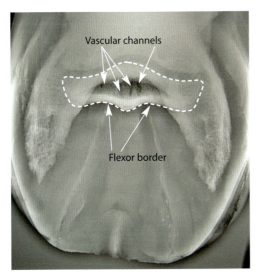

3.76 A special view of the navicular bone, taken by holding the machine behind the hoof, and aiming the X-ray beam forward and down while the horse's foot stands on the X-ray plate. This enables visualization of the shuttle-shaped navicular bone and any cysts, fractures, spurs, or abnormal mineralization of the bone.

3.77 This X-ray view is taken by holding the machine in front of the horse and then aiming the beam downward at a 60-degree angle while his foot stands on the X-ray plate. The flexor border of the navicular bone is evident here, showing irregularities and erosions of the bone along what should be a regular and smooth border.

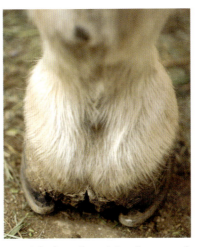

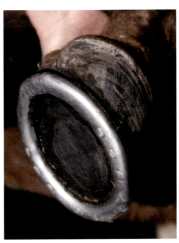

3.78 The branches of this shoe extend just beneath the heel bulbs, and the horse is shod to the widest part of the frog to provide ample caudal heel support.

3.79 An egg bar shoe provides caudal heel support, which is helpful to a horse with heel pain or navicular disease. The advantages must be compared to the disadvantage of its heftier weight.

images at high resolution. Anatomical detail is well visualized and instrumental in defining obscure foot lameness and in corroborating findings from other diagnostic techniques.

PALLIATIVE TREATMENT FOR NAVICULAR SYNDROME

Farrier Care

The most important element of returning a foot-sore horse to comfort is to trim and shoe him correctly to relieve the abnormal stresses within the foot. In addition to application of basic shoeing principles, it is important to provide a heel-sore horse with support to the rear structures of the foot (photo 3.78 and see photo 3.43, p. 62). The use of egg bar shoes is not only a legitimate treatment option to increase the rear support of the foot and to reduce loading on the heels, but these shoes may be useful as a preventive measure, in some cases (photo 3.79). Past studies have indicated that 57 percent of heel-pain horses respond favorably to application of egg bar shoes.

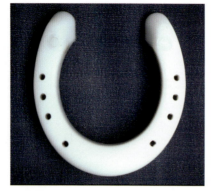

3.80 *This Mustad Nail-Shu is an example of an aluminum shoe that is embedded in synthetic plastic materials. Plastic materials like polyurethane, which is commonly used in synthetic shoes, are good at absorbing the shock of impact concussion.*

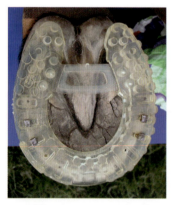

3.81 *There are many synthetic, flexible shoes similar to this Equi-Flex shoe. This one incorporates a small bar (across the frog) that can be lengthened or shortened slightly to vary the width at the heels, while providing stability to the*

Synthetic horseshoes play an important role in both treatment and prevention of footsore and joint-sore horses. Anti-concussion properties of polyurethane impregnated aluminum shoes have been well recognized in sport horses for years. The varieties and brands are plentiful; experiment and find which style of synthetic shoe works best for each horse (photos 3.80 and 3.81). The ideal strategy is one of prevention, and these shoes may be a great adjunct in a preventive strategy.

Medical Therapy

Oral Isoxsuprine or Pentoxyfylline

Over the years, oral supplementation with *isoxsuprine hydrochloride* has been a mainstay in treating navicular horses. Another product that works similarly for the same purpose is *pentoxyfylline*. Currently, these products are held in debate as to how effective either is for this application. In theory, circulation should increase in the foot with either of these medications; if the theory of thrombosis/ischemia is partially to blame for pain associated with navicular syndrome, then such medication may play an important role. A study (1996) on 6 horses given isoxsuprine or pentoxifylline demonstrated that neither medication elicited an increase in blood flow to the feet of healthy horses. It was also mentioned in that study that it is possible that these medications may be beneficial in diseased feet while having no effect on healthy feet. In addition, the study only administered the medication for 10 days, yet it has been recognized that at least 3 to 4 weeks of treatment has been necessary to notice clinical improvement. It is the author's experience that many horses with navicular syndrome have benefited from treatment with isoxsuprine. Attempts to discontinue this medication in horses that have responded favorably have resulted in lameness relapses. If a horse is placed on isoxsuprine therapy for 6 weeks with no signs of improvement, then this medication probably has no role in treatment of that individual. If a horse is medicated with isoxsuprine, check with medication control at horse shows for withdrawal time of this drug prior to competition.

Tiludronate

Clinical studies using *tiludronate* (1 mg per kg) have demonstrated clinical improvement and reduction of lameness of navicular horses. Based on the pharmacology of this medication, which inhibits bone resorption, there is evidence that bone remodeling is part of the navicular disease complex.

Polysulfated Glycosaminoglycans or Hyaluronic Acid

Other systemic medications that have been used to manage navicular pain include *polysulfated glycosaminoglycans* given intramuscularly or *hyaluronic acid* (see chapter 5, *Joints*, p. 125) given intravenously. Polysulfated glycosaminoglycans have been found to be most useful in navicular lameness that has been present for less than a year. It is thought that systemic medication may work by inhibiting enzymes involved in the breakdown of the cartilage matrix.

Intra-Articular Anti-Inflammatory Medication

Direct treatment of the navicular region entails injecting anti-inflammatory medications such as *corticosteroids* and hyaluronic acid directly into the coffin joints. Such intra-articular injections have provided excellent success in managing the chronic lameness of navicular disease. Generally, these horses require intra-articular injections once or twice a year to maintain athletic comfort.

Nonsteroidal Anti-Inflammatory Medication

In cases that do not respond well to the above-described treatments, it may be necessary to keep horses comfortable by using a low dose of nonsteroidal anti-inflammatory (NSAIDs) medications such as phenylbutazone, flunixin meglumine, or ketoprofen.

Surgical Options

Palmar digital neurectomy is a salvage option when medical and mechanical strategies fail to eliminate pain and lameness. A neurectomy involves cutting of the palmar digital nerves that feed the navicular region. A neurectomy eliminates sensation of pain from the back third of the foot. It should be understood that this is strictly a palliative treatment intended to keep a horse as comfortable as possible for as long as possible. Favorable results from this surgery may extend for as little as a few months to as long as many years. Adverse consequences can occur such as development of a painful *neuroma* or rupture of the deep digital flexor tendon, but in most cases failure of this surgery to relieve pain is due to either incomplete removal of all the nerve branches at the time of surgery or due to regeneration of the severed nerves. In one report, 74 percent of horses undergoing a neurectomy remained sound for one year, while 63 percent remained sound for two years.

Desmotomy of the navicular suspensory ligaments is another surgical option that has received mixed reviews. In some reports, 50 percent of horses having this surgery experienced symptomatic improvement.

In all cases of medical and/or surgical intervention for navicular syndrome, appropriate shoeing techniques are still critical to success.

Additional Management of a Heel-Sore Horse

Many sore-footed horses have spent a bit of time moving with a guarded gait. Muscles in the neck and shoulders are often tight and restricted since the horse attempts to land more softly on sore feet, and so holds his body relatively rigid in front. Over time, *myofascial* tissues of the upper body tighten, causing muscles to contract and shorten. Even though shoeing management and foot therapy relieve the immediate foot pain, these horses may continue to move with a short, choppy stride despite alleviation of the original source of the problem. Concurrent with treating the feet, it is helpful to gather an excellent support team of skilled people to address the soft tissue restriction within your horse's shoulders and back. Find a capable acupuncturist who can improve circulation and energy flow through these tissues, and have massage or myofascial release techniques applied as necessary to further free up your horse's movement.

Exercise and turnout are important to maintain lubrication and nutrition of cartilage within the joints and navicular structures. Blood flow is improved within the hooves. Regular movement minimizes formation of adhesions between the navicular bone and flexor tendon.

Developing Strong Bones 4

Like the composition of a story, or like the size and shape of the canvas of a painting, the shape of a horse's skeletal frame determines his beauty, and more importantly his function. The alignment of bones within this frame tells the story of an individual's conformation (photo 4.1). And, it is conformation that dictates the mechanics and efficiency of locomotion.

But at a more microscopic level, the strength of the bones that comprise the skeletal structure is an important feature to athletic longevity in a performance horse. Bone is an organ, in the same way that the heart or liver or skin is an organ. It may seem that bone is a hard structure with no visible appearance of change, but bone tissue does continually adapt and change in response to stimuli related to movement and training.

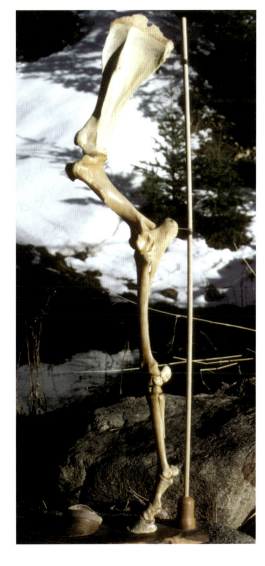

4.1 *The skeleton of the front limb of a horse (from the scapula down) demonstrates how although the muscles flesh out the bones, structural conformation takes on the shape and size of the underlying skeleton.*

Bone as a System

On the surface, bone feels hard and unforgiving in its content, but it is a tissue that is well supplied with blood vessels. Besides being the structural scaffold for attachment of muscles and tendons, bone serves an important metabolic function. Mineral within bone is able to be retrieved in time of need, as for example calcium or phosphate are mobilized according to hormonal response to the fluctuating metabolic status of a horse. Bone is important as a calcium reservoir to replenish losses in sweat, particularly in equine disciplines that require extended efforts, such as endurance sport activities. Calcium is lost in large quantities in sweat at a time when it is most needed for efficient muscle contraction, not only of skeletal muscle, but also of cardiac muscle and smooth muscle of the intestines.

As dynamic, everchanging support tissues, the cellular constituents of bone continually respond to loading stresses in a process known as *remodeling*. It is this feature of bone, that is the ability of cells to remove bone and then replace it with new bone tissue, that render it able to grow, and capable of repair.

The Remodeling Process

Looking through the eye of a microscope, we can see that bone cells called *osteoblasts* secrete molecules that organize into collagen fibers arranged in a very specific pattern; this material is called *osteoid*. As the skeleton matures, mineral is deposited within the osteoid to form the substance we recognize as bone. In response to external stress, either loading of the skeletal column or injury created by twisting or overloading forces, bone is removed or added along its surfaces in this remodeling process.

Persistent turnover and repair of bone tissue within its depths and along its edges is an active response in the growing skeleton and also occurs due to training. *Osteocytes* respond to mechanical loading by increasing their metabolic activity. Cells continually modify bone architecture to accommodate external stimuli. Bone can only model and remodel within its genetically predetermined architecture that is specific to each bone in the body. Training may develop a horse's athletic potential, but will not enable an individual to surpass his inborn capacity.

An example commonly cited to describe bone's remodeling response to stress is that of the arm bone (humerus) of a professional tennis player: The bone of the playing arm is more developed and thicker than the bone of the nonplaying arm. In contrast, a bone that is immobilized in a cast loses mineral density over time due to being "protected" from an adequate loading stimulus. Once a cast is removed, bone regains its density and its strength with slow reintroduction of exercise.

FORCES THAT STRESS BONE

Bone has the capability of deforming under a mild to moderate load without breaking. The elastic rebound of a load applied within its physiologic limits allows bone to return to its original shape and configuration. One can't visibly see "deformation" of bone, but it is measurable and defined. In physical terms, *strain* is considered to be a measurement of the amount of deformation that occurs in bone (fig 4.2). Bone is continuously exposed to different strains:

- *Tensile strain* results in elongation of bone: much like the rebar within concrete, the collagenous fibers of bone impart tensile strength; this is important as the levers and pulleys of musculotendinous and ligamentous structures "pull" on bone to move it to create locomotion.
- *Compressive strain* (created by loading of a limb with a horse's weight) results in shortening of bone: *hydroxyapatitie crystals* (or mineral), analogous to concrete, impart compressive strength.
- *Flexural strain* creates bending forces leading to compression along the concave surface, and tension along the convex

surface; bone remodels accordingly, referred to in physics as *Wolff's Law*, by increasing its mass in areas of compression, and resorbing mineral and hence bone from areas under tension.
- *Shearing strains* (tissue is displaced in a plane parallel to itself) are mostly abnormal and have the potential to create injury.
- *Torque or rotational strains* are similarly damaging to bone if too forceful.

Compression and Tension

Collagen, the connective tissue of bone, accounts for tensile (stretch) strength while the mineral content determines compressive strength and stiffness. Bone mineral content provides maximal strength to a bone since it is most adept at resisting compressive forces. Excessive and repeated concussion to a limb results in progressive loss of stiffness and decrease in strength, inviting bone fatigue, lameness, and failure.

Torsion (Twisting)

An equine limb can withstand large amounts of compressive force, but the torsional strength is only one-third as strong as the compressive strength. Torsion or twisting on the bony column puts a horse more at risk of injury. Torsion results from:

- Abnormal conformation
- Angular limb deformities
- Irregular ground contours
- Inconsistent composition of the ground surface
- Lack of uniformity in the moisture content and cushioning features of the ground
- Caulks or toe-grabs on horseshoes (see photo 3.45, p. 63)

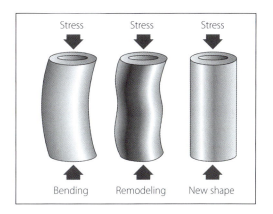

4.2 *Internal remodeling proceeds without changing the observable shape of the bone or skeleton. Bone remodels according to the direction and intensity of the stress created by limb loading and impact with locomotion.*

Propulsive Forces

At a walk, most limb strain occurs in the *swing phase* when the foot is off the ground. The predominant force on the limb is tension created by tendon pull. At a gallop, reaction forces from the ground contribute to bone strain. These strains occur as the limb is loaded when the foot hits the ground.

Multiple Forces

A bone is not uniform in cross-sectional area. Its shape varies along the shaft, and *cortical* (outer) walls vary in thickness. Because of these variations, different forces are applied simultaneously within a single bone. Stresses and strains on bone result from multiple forces at one time:

- Pull of tendons, ligaments, and muscles
- Effect of weight-bearing and support of body mass
- Forces created from impact with the ground

BONE STRENGTH

Governed by the principles of Wolff's Law, in the most simplistic terms bone deforms beneath a load, and remodels to accommodate that load. As an example of the geometric properties that impart strength to bone, let's look at the shape of the cannon bone since it has been studied extensively. Shape of the bones of the lower limbs tends to be eccentric rather than shaped like a true cylinder (photo 4.3). This concentrates bone mass on the front surface (*dorsal cortex*) so that it has increased stiffness in one plane. As a result, bending forces are less likely to cause the bone to deform during loading under conditions of normal gaits. This eccentric "design" develops with age; the most dramatic changes in cannon bone circumference occur during the first and second years of growth, and continue in the modeling process until a horse is about 4 years of age. After that age, geometric properties of the cannon bone tend not to change much at all. Bone density may change until about age seven, but by age four, the geometric configuration matures to provide the best design to withstand normal loading forces on the limb.

Abnormal loading forces include fast speeds, like a gallop at 16.6 meters per second (m/sec) or 37 mph. A fast trot (5.5 m/sec or 12 mph) lies within a safety range of loading, but repetitive strain at any speed may create cumulative damage. Because low speed training does not elicit appropriate remodeling changes to sustain high speeds, it then becomes important to integrate interval training with bursts of speed to encourage the remodeling process to improve bone density.

Importance of Bone to Performance

Bone Size

Most elite-caliber equine athletes have a large circumference of the cannon bone. Circumference of the cannon bone is measured just below the knee. Ideally its circumference should be at least 8 inches in a 1000-pound

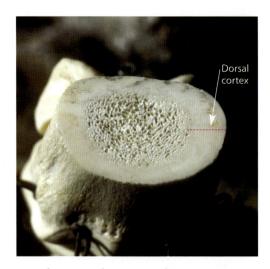

4.3 *The cannon bone as seen here in cross-section demonstrates the eccentric shape of the bones of the lower limb. Note the thicker bone of the dorsal cortex (on the front of the leg). This increased thickness adds stiffness to the bone, and the bone is less likely to deform with loading of the limb with weight bearing.*

horse. For horses of various sizes, use the following formula:

Ideal circumference = 0.008 x body weight (in pounds) of horse

This size is genetically predetermined, and its importance lies in the sturdiness of the bone when loaded, as well as the efficient pull of large attaching ligaments and tendons with muscular contraction.

In aerobic, low-to-moderate intensity sports, like distance riding, dressage, or eventing, big bones are favored, whereas in anaerobic, high speed sports like horse racing, thinner bone size has a slight advantage due to less weight. About 50 percent of the power used by a horse galloping at 15 m/sec (33 mph) is used to accelerate and decelerate the bones of the lower limb. A reduction in bone mass of 10 percent may reduce a horse's mechanical work effort by 5 percent. Hence, thinner bone is lighter and requires less muscular work to propel the horse across the ground at speed. Speed horses are bred for finer frames for this reason when fractions of seconds determine winning or losing. In contrast, in sports where stamina and endurance are key to success, durability of bone and support tissues are key to performance longevity.

Nutritional manipulation or exercise regimens cannot hasten growth and maturation. Genetics and breed determine skeletal maturity, and these factors are dictated by time. Yet, conditioning programs can improve ultimate bone strength and build a durable athlete.

Bone Density

Unlike changes seen in developing musculature, adaptive responses in bone are not visible to the naked eye. Training will not visibly increase the size of bone, but it does improve the ability of bone to withstand loading forces by increasing its mineral density over time. Much like concrete in a rebar and concrete construction, the mineral components impart compressive strength to bone so it is more capable of sustaining the pounding of concussion and the bending forces created by angular rotation of limb movement. As bone matures, minerals (calcium and phosphorus) are deposited into the bone at the expense of *cellular fluid* to occupy up to 65 percent of the space. By the time a horse is fully mature, minerals make up 95 percent of the bone. The amount of these minerals in a bone determines its *bone mineral content*). Internal remodeling proceeds without changing the observable shape of the skeleton. However, these invisible changes in the bones greatly affect intrinsic strength and skeletal maturity of a horse (see photo 4.3).

Bone in different parts of the limb has different properties. As an example, cannon bone is stiffer than that of the long pastern bone, but subsequently it is not as able to absorb as much concussion energy. This works well in that the cannon bone, being further distant from the point of ground impact undergoes more bending forces, while the long pastern bone needs to be able to absorb impact loading. Being closer to the ground, the pastern bones more directly feel the energy of concussion.

Interaction of Bone with Tendons, Ligaments, and Muscle

Of all the structural tissues in the body, bone takes the longest to develop to maximum strength. Integrated movement of muscles, tendons, and ligaments dictates how bones receive loading stress. At different gaits, muscles and tendons oppose bending forces on bone to improve the centering of weight-bearing forces through the long axis of bones. Tendons store elastic energy when stretched and this makes it easier for muscles to move the long bones (bones of the limbs) to propel a horse across the ground. This type of energy storage occurs with each limb loading cycle. In the stance phase when the limb supports the horse's full weight, the fetlock hyper-extends; this stretches the flexor tendons and suspensory ligaments. Once the limb moves past midstance, stored elastic energy within the tendons and ligaments is responsible for raising the fetlock and flexing the joints of the lower leg to assist each limb in lift off. This improves gait efficiency and minimizes bending, compressive, and tensile strains on bones and joints.

Muscular activity is also critical to integrity of the blood supply within bone. As muscles contract, venous channels are temporarily occluded and the vascular pressure within the bone marrow increases to achieve a kind of pumping action to improve circulation. The configuration and strength of interactive and ever-developing muscular and skeletal systems directly determine stride efficiency and time to fatigue. These systems require years to develop to peak.

Conditioning Bone to Reach Peak Strength

Many elements comprise a strategy to develop bone to its peak strength. Careful attention to nutritional balances of minerals (calcium and phosphorus), energy, and protein is important to ensure proper development of the growing skeleton. In addition, the weight of a rider should be proportional to the size of a horse. A general rule dictates that the weight of the rider and tack should not exceed 20 percent of the horse's body weight. Training skills should be introduced at a time appropriate to skeletal maturity. For example, the bones and joints of a two-year-old are inadequately prepared for strenuous athletic efforts, such as jumping or distance riding.

The objective in any training program is to increase the strength of the skeleton while minimizing the risk of injury. The road to peak strength is built upon a *long slow distance* (LSD) program that provides a solid structural foundation of all the systems (see p. 226). LSD conditioning takes at least one or two seasons to reach peak cardiovascular and muscular ability. Once this base is built, *interval training* improves bone density, up to a point (see p. 227). Adaptations achieved by exercise will be different for each horse depending on his age as well as the duration and intensity of his training program. The cannon bone of two-to-three-year-olds takes on a more oval shape in response to aging and training. A mature horse's cannon bone flattens and the rear surface becomes concave, resembling a leaf spring in a truck and similarly more able to withstand normal bending forces.

High-Speed Training

An incremental training strategy that includes short gallops of 200 to 400 meters (⅒ to ¼ of a mile) distance can elicit a controlled bone remodeling response. Research originally done (Lanyon and Rubin) on bones of turkey wings demonstrated that only a small number of rapid cycles are necessary to stimulate and maintain remodeling responses. In the horse, a loading stress repeated about 30 or 40 times is sufficient stimulus to elicit a training response, however nothing more is gained with an increased number of loading cycles. Once a horse has been legged up with LSD conditioning, a bone-training program starts with slow gallop speeds, incrementally increasing speed over 4 to 6 weeks. Steady increases in the increment of applied stress gives bone sufficient time to adapt, minimizing the risk of injury during the training period. Once prepared, bone strength develops best with the application of short sprints as opposed to extended work at long, slow gallops.

Research done on young racetrack Thoroughbreds detected that to elicit an adaptive response in bone, speed should exceed 12 m/sec (26.8 mph) even for brief periods of just a few minutes applied at intervals. For conditioning of non-racing horses, this type of speed work should be reserved for a horse's second or third year of training, and in some cases may never be attained if the performance goal does not depend on speed. The objective with interval work is to gallop for either 2 minutes or over a distance of about a mile, targeting a heart rate of 180 to 200 bpm (beats per minute). Most horses in non-racing pursuits will not reach a speed of 27 mph, but short, fast speed bursts do generate response by bone. Following interval work, a horse is recovered at a slow trot or walk to bring the heart rate down to 90 to 100 bpm.

High-speed training elicits a small increase in bone density by encouraging more mineral deposition within bone. In a mathematical model, strength of bone is directly proportional to the cube of its density. Bending forces around the dorsal (front) cortex of the cannon bone during galloping stimulate enlargement in the cross-sectional area by building more bone along the dorsal cortex. This phenomenon is true to some extent even in adult horses. A greater cross-sectional area of bone effectively decreases stress to the bone in that area.

In young horses, although high-speed exercise encourages deposition of bone to increase the cross-sectional area, this bone is initially low in mineral density since mineralization is a slow process. Without being fully mineralized, bone is liable to deform under loading with the potential for shearing forces to occur between newer, less mineralized bone and older, more densely mineralized bone. Then, microfractures and inflammation occur from fatigue at these junctions. In racehorses, this phenomenon results in *bucked shins* (see p. 103).

In youngsters, only very short periods of high-speed exercise are necessary to stimulate both an increase in bone mass and density as long as the strategy is intelligently applied over time. At the same time, any form of exercise (fast or slow) improves alignment of collagen components to contribute to building compressive strength within long bones.

The importance of achieving a specific strain rate cannot be overstated. Months or even years of *submaximal* exercise (aerobic exercise at walk, trot, slow canter—see p. 220) does not modify either the mass or density of cortical bone of the cannon bone once a horse has reached full maturity (by 7 years of age). Even a fast, extended trot does not sufficiently generate adequate bending forces to elicit an adaptive response; only with galloping speeds will bone achieve that end. Simply put, bone tissue must recognize this stimulus to make its adaptive response. Bone training is a process of "informing" bone cell populations to increase strength by adjusting bone mass to accommodate the stresses.

Skeletal Strength

The best way to achieve maximum skeletal strength is to expose the tissue to a variety of stresses. If only one kind of stimulus is recognized by bone, it only achieves strength in response to that and will less safely accommodate added stress. As an example, a horse trained only to walk and trot is not adjusted to the high-speed demands of a gallop. Not only does the skeletal tissue need to "see" this type of speed work in order to minimize the risk of injury, but so do other supportive structures (like ligaments and tendons). Muscle endurance particularly benefits from repetitive exercise demands over time. If the objective is to only ride at slow, steady speeds, then training only needs to target that level of low intensity. Yet, maximal bone strength is achieved by interspersing short, fast workouts amidst a diversity of gaits and speeds over varied terrain.

In the high-speed track world, fatigue of bone is continually considered, but in distance sports, a horse's long bones rarely meet these kinds of stresses and strains. So the primary concern in sports involving moderate or prolonged aerobic exercise is in generating an environment that encourages adaptation and strength to give a competitive horse a solid foundation to withstand years of rigorous exercise. Only after three years of conditioning do bones achieve maximal density related to the remodeling process in response to moderate, submaximal exercise. A strategy to develop a durable equine athlete should consider the necessary dedication of time to develop strength of all parts of a horse's body relative to the intended sport.

EVALUATING THE STATUS OF BONE STRENGTH

Realistically, there are no practical means to evaluate a horse's bone strength or density. High tech tools are available to evaluate bone mineral content. One such method is *photon absorptiometry* to measure transmission ultrasound velocities of bone. Gamma nuclear *scintigraphy* is useful to appreciate the presence of fatigue fractures or microfractures within long bones. *Infrared thermography* may have a more applicable role in determining if there is excessive circulation denoting inflammation, or impaired circulation within a localized area. However, thermography is not specific for bone, but also includes evaluation of all the surrounding soft tissue structures. Radiographic evaluation is useful to detect problems within the joints, but does not inform of very subtle problems within the long bones or damage to joint cartilage.

Skeletal Maturity

Different breeds mature at different rates. One long bone, the distal radius (lower part of the forearm) located at the top of the knee, has previously served as a monitor for the entire body. Most growth plates of the limbs are "closed" by age 2 to 3 years, which means that longitudinal growth of the leg bones ceases, and now metabolic energy is targeted toward depositing mineral within the skeletal system, and remodeling to conform to biomechanical stress. Closure of the growth plates of the long bones is not the only criterion used to determine the age at which a horse can begin competitive athletics.

As examples of the importance of structural strength in athletic pursuits, some sport-horse organizations recognize the need for skeletal maturity before engaging in demanding competition. The American Endurance Ride Conference (AERC) and various Competitive Trail organizations require that a horse be a minimum of 5 years of age before competing in distance events of 50 miles (80 km) or more. The Fédération Equestre Internationale (FEI) requires horses to be 8 years or older before undertaking 100 mile (160 km) endurance events. Years are required to develop all the organ systems to peak strength to ensure athletic longevity, with bone taking the longest.

Specific activities should be avoided or carefully controlled to protect young horses from significantly increased biomechanical stress on bones and joints:

- Weight-bearing stress of carrying a rider at too young an age
- Longeing, even in large circles, exerts twisting forces on bones and particularly on immature bone and joints
- Jumping a young horse overloads the limbs
- High speed exercise is detrimental to a growing skeleton

Musculoskeletal Stress from Exercise

Effects of Overtraining

To achieve optimal strength of bone, stimulation must come from loading it at specific strain rates. High speeds increase the risk of injury from concussion, but some concussion is necessary to strengthen bone. However, once a repeated loading strategy is "recognized" by bone, additional and subsequent repetitions won't affect the magnitude of the adaptive response. Bone architecture does not modify further once bone has adapted to a certain load. Beyond a threshold, excess deformation creates irreversible damage. This may occur during a single exercise period. Or, it may occur subsequent to repeated loading and deformation over time that elicits cumulative damage such as seen with too many miles or days of training. Ultimate failure occurs in the form of a bone fracture. However, in horses engaged in low to moderate exercise intensity, "failure" is commonly recognized as bone changes within the joints. With excess training, bone undergoes an internal remodeling process that involves replacement of damaged areas with new, but weaker bone. This "new" bone has less mineral density and therefore is less stiff and less resistant to compressive loading.

Overtraining of young horses may result in disastrous consequences. The growth plates feel the effects of too much speed and concussion. Growth plates are responsible for elongation of the long bones, a necessary part of growing. The *periosteum* (the nutrient fibrous covering of bone) is responsible for the thickening of bone to widen the circumference. Normal range of loading on growth plates increases compression to accelerate the growth of the plate on that side, yet loads in the abnormal range retard the growth of the plate. *Angular limb deformities* may result with alterations to the conformation of the individual (see chapter 5, *Joints*, p. 134). A crooked leg further amplifies rotational strain on the bones of the limb (see chapter 2, *Conformation for Performance*, p. 22).

BONE FATIGUE

When bone begins to lose elasticity after being deformed by loading and unloading cycles, it has reached its fatigue state. An illustration of how differently applied loads on a limb affect its strength can be appreciated in the following example: if a Thoroughbred runs at top speed on a straight line, assuming all else is normal, it can run for 19 miles before fatigue failure of the cannon bone. Yet, running through a turn dramatically increases the load per unit area. Instead of 19 miles, bones subjected to uneven loading in the turn can travel only ¼ mile before fatigue develops. There is a level of exercise that brings bones past a fatigue state, into an overload range, with subsequent disaster.

BUCKED SHINS

Excessive and repetitive stresses to young limbs cause failure, particularly with high-speed work. Of three-year-old racing Thoroughbreds, 70 percent suffer from *bucked shins*—microfractures in the cannon bone along the front and inside surfaces (photo 4.4). In humans, a similar phenomenon called *shin splints* occurs along the lower tibia. Initially, microscopic fractures appear in the bone *cortex* (outermost portion of the bone), but with an eventual overload, a saucer fracture or a total stress fracture may result, with catastrophic breakdown. In milder cases that recover, once the bones adapt to stress, bucked shins do not seem to recur. High speed applied in small doses may improve bone adaptation with less risk of bucked shins. Galloping speeds increase the risk.

Initial signs include pain, heat, and tenderness along the front of the cannon bones. Visible swelling may or may not be present in this location. An affected horse is usually lame, or moves with a short-strided gait.

SPLINTS

Nestled on either side of the cannon bone of each leg, two slender bones are "splinted" to the cannon bone by a fragile ligament. At first glance, the pencil-thick splint bones may not

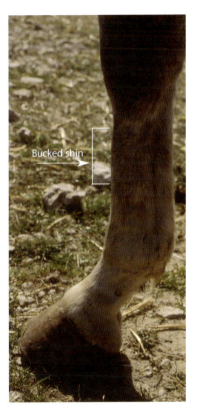

4.4 *Bucked shins develop from microfractures along the front of the cannon bone, and the active inflammatory process is visible until the injury repairs and the bone remodels.*

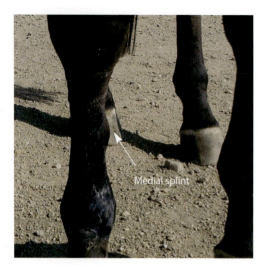

4.5 *A splint commonly develops along the medial side of cannon bone due to conformational imperfections or due to trauma from being hit by the opposite limb. This may remodel to some degree with time, but the horse will always have a cosmetic blemish of a lump in this location.*

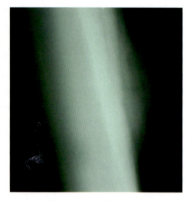

4.6 *Radiograph of the irregular appearance of an acute splint with active bone reaction.*

seem more than vestiges of digits that the dawn horse, *Eohippus*, once used for running. But, just as "reinforcement bars" strengthen concrete, "splint" bones add structural strength to the central cannon bone. The splint bone on the inside of each front leg is particularly susceptible to mechanical injury. Not only does it assist in supporting the load through the carpal (knee) joints, but also it can be struck by interference from the other leg. Certain conformation characteristics predispose a horse to splints. As viewed from head-on, an ideal set of front legs emerges straight out of the center of the carpal (knee) joints in perfect alignment. Viewed from the rear, similar symmetry should be appreciated for the rear limbs as they emerge from the center of the hocks. Obvious defects, like bench-knees (cannon bone set to the outside of the knee joint), calf-knees (knee joints set back too far), or knock-knees place added load on the inside of the limb, with the inside splint bone forced to assume too much stress (see chapter 2, *Conformation for Performance*, p. 24).

Although referred to as a "popped" splint, the tiny splint bone does not actually pop away from the cannon bone. The firm bump visible on the horse's leg is a reflection of underlying inflammation within the periosteum overlying the bone. Inflammation may occur within the *interosseous ligament* that normally stabilizes the splint bone against the cannon bone, or in associated bone. As a horse ages, the interosseous ligament is eventually replaced with bone to fuse the splint bone to the cannon bone. Beginning at about age 3, this process continues to completion by 10 years old. A younger horse is at greater risk of tearing the still-present ligament along the inside splint. Any age horse can suffer a traumatic impact injury to the splint bone. The initial injury is sometimes referred to as a "hot" or "green" splint. It is accompanied by tenderness, swelling, and often lameness (photos 4.5 and photo 4.6).

In most cases, not only is there soft tissue inflammation at the trauma site along the interosseous ligament, but the bone or periosteum of the bone also becomes inflamed. This is especially true for those splints resulting from external trauma from a kick or interference injury. Splint fractures generally heal well if given sufficient time, 6 to 12 weeks (photo 4.7). Once new bone growth forms along a splint, little can be done to permanently reduce newly deposited calcium. Attempts at surgical removal (with a bone chisel) only incite the bone to repeat the calcification process with unsatisfactory reduction of the cosmetic blemish.

Prevention involves the use of protective "splint" boots to prevent accidental interference trauma (photo 4.8). Frequent hoof care with balanced trimming encourages level hoof landing to minimize interference. Limit longeing in tight circles to a minimum as this places additional load on the inside of the legs. Train a horse to be efficient and strong when spinning, turning, or executing sudden stops. Try to train on surfaces that are not excessively hard. Build a horse slowly in fitness before asking for speed work. One of the most common causes of splints is overexertion past a certain level of fitness. Be careful not to overfeed a horse as extra weight additionally overloads the limbs with exercise.

Inactivity and Layup

No additional benefits are gained by repetitively pounding a horse's legs into the ground at speed. It only requires a few loading cycles each day to improve or maintain skeletal strength. Horses in confinement are at increased risk of losing mineral density in their bones if not regularly given the opportunity to exercise. In all cases it is important to properly warm a horse up well and to cool him down. This maximizes efficiency of muscles, tendons, and ligaments, and reduces the risk of injury to those structures.

DISUSE

Demineralization occurs when the skeleton is subjected to weightlessness or reduced gravitational loading. The extreme case occurs in the human example of space flight and to a lesser degree with bed rest. These specific phenomena are of no concern in caring for the equine athlete. However, application of a cast or disuse of an injured limb for an extended period similarly decreases bone strength. Bone mineral content diminishes as cells dissolve existing bone while bone-forming cells remain quiescent. With this caution in mind, rehabilitation of an injured horse must proceed slowly.

MENTAL STRESS AND CORTICOSTEROIDS

A loss of bone, or lack of development, can also result from administering excessive amounts of corticosteroids. Similar problems result when a body produces excess corticosteroids due to persistent stress and anxiety. Mental stress (see p. 472) develops from:

- Chronic pain
- Overtraining
- Anxiety
- Travel
- Competition
- Overcrowding

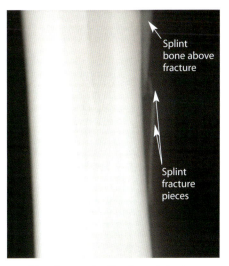

4.7 *This fractured splint bone is broken into three small pieces. Months of rest allowed these to fuse and resolve completely.*

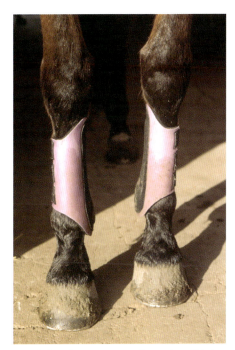

4.8 *Splint boots protect a horse from hitting himself with an opposite limb, and protect against trauma from external hazards.*

Extracorporeal Shock Wave Therapy

A noninvasive technique for treating chronic lameness problems relies on pressure waves generated by the discharge of a high voltage current; these waves are "focused" on a particular location within the tissues. Originally, this therapy was developed to break up kidney and urinary tract stones in humans with great success. The theory behind *extracorporeal shock wave therapy* (ESWT) as applied to lameness is that pressure waves have their main effects where there is bone and soft tissue interface; it is here that impedance changes for the pulsing waves. At these changing interfaces, the shock waves develop gas bubbles that create "jet streams" or waves to impact hard tissues in the body, like bone or where ligament meets bone. The machine pulses 2000 waves to the tissues in a span of 5 to 10 minutes. Any shock wave machine is called "extracorporeal" because it is applied "outside the body" as a noninvasive procedure.

Different Machine Types
There are different types of shock wave machines, one type being a radial form of energy impulse in which the shock waves concentrically ripple into the tissues, much like the ripples created by a stone thrown into water. A more focused form of shock wave machines (Wolf, Storz, or Equitron) delivers waves to a specific area, and the waves emitted are more powerful than those from the radial machines (Swiss Dolorcast) that rely on mechanical concussion rather than actual shock waves.

Although the focused machines are larger and more expensive than the radial devices, both types emit pressure-gradient waves that impact the tissues. The waves emitted by a radial shock have no focusing system so the waves lose energy as the distance from the source increases. With the loss of wave energy further from the probe source, more of the energy is delivered to the skin instead of into deeper tissues. It is thought that since there is relatively little tissue overlying bone in equine limbs and that because most orthopedic injuries are located fairly superficially, the radial shock wave machines are able to emit sufficient energy to create a therapeutic effect. To date, there are no direct comparisons between results achieved with focused vs. radial machines. More machines are constantly entering the market, confusing the picture even further. The type of shock wave device used is important in achieving results. It would be a good idea to discuss the value of different shock wave machines with your veterinarian, and the relevant application to your horse's orthopedic problem.

What Does ESWT Do?
It is suggested that ESWT has a stimulatory effect on bone metabolism and because of this property, this treatment has been applied to orthopedic problems in the human field such as heel spurs, tennis elbow, and non-union fractures. Shock waves elicit cellular production of nitric oxide that can increase bone remodeling. The degree of response is dose-dependent.

Studies have been undertaken to evaluate the effect on bone and associated soft tissue structures in the horse. It has been determined that blood vessels within the bone remain intact during shock wave treatment, and in some cases these vessels actually dilate to deliver more oxygen and nutrients. Although there are no soft tissue changes created by the therapy, there is some hemorrhage along the periosteum of the bone. Scott McClure, DVM, applied focused ESWT on equine cannon bones and concluded that treated bone does not undergo any structural changes, nor do any microfractures occur. Instead, cortical (outermost layer) bone thickens and subchondral (beneath the cartilage) bone strengthens with ESWT (see chapter 5, *Joints*, p. 130); these changes are proportional to the energy level of the treatment. There is a transient and mild swelling and sensitivity at the treatment site that abates within a couple of days. Shock wave treatment should not be used in areas afflicted with infection or cancer, around growth plates of a young horse, over large nerves or blood vessels, or in areas where there is an air/tissue interface, such as wounds or around the lungs.

Shock wave treatment elicits some analgesic effects that transiently reduce pain for about 48 hours. Caution must be taken in using a horse for an intense athletic endeavor immediately following treatment. Transient reduction in pain may have no direct correlation to tissue healing. The injury remains but perceived relief from pain could give false impressions that the horse is better when in fact he is not. The horse may not hurt as much as before treatment and so no longer protects an injured limb. For a racehorse or a jumping horse, this could result in catastrophic breakdown injury.

Nutritional Disease of Bone

Nutritional Secondary Hyperparathyroidism

Also referred to as *Big Head Disease*, this syndrome is caused by a diet that is too high in phosphorus or too low in calcium. Feeding excess amounts of bran (rice or wheat) or grain provides an overload of phosphorus in the diet. With a relative deficiency of dietary calcium, *parathyroid hormone* stimulates mobilization of calcium from the bones as well as increasing re-absorption of calcium from the kidneys and excreting excess phosphorus from the kidneys. The overall result is skeletal depletion of calcium.

Signs of this problem include shifting leg lameness, a stilted gait, distortion of the facial bones, broadening of the face across the bridge of the nose, and loosening teeth. Supplementation with legume hays along with removal of grain and bran products from the diet can resolve this disease if caught early before permanent skeletal damage occurs.

Joints: Health, Problems, and Therapies 5

The equine industry has witnessed a revolution in ways to manage lameness in athletic horses. Of the many problems that plague an athletic horse, joint injuries are among the top offenders. Joint injury takes many forms, ranging from a mild and transient inflammatory insult to more serious and career-threatening *degenerative joint disease* (DJD), otherwise known as *traumatic arthritis* (see p. 116). Many joint problems stem from trauma incurred over time and miles of exercise. One goal is to enable a horse to withstand years of athletic wear and tear. Even in the face of degenerative joint disease, a joint may continue to function sufficiently so a horse can continue his athletic career. Yet, it is the nagging pain associated with the degenerative process that hinders performance or causes a horse to be too lame to ride. One of the greatest challenges faced is that of finding ways to fend off the ravages of arthritis and to maintain our equine partner in as pain-free a state as possible.

Parts of a Joint

A *synovial* joint is a complicated organ structure and a marvel in design. Although at a brief glance it would appear a joint does nothing more than bridge a span between two bones, it is actually comprised of many different parts (fig. 5.1). Each joint is stabilized by a series of ligaments and a fibrous *joint capsule* to maintain its movement in an expected plane. Some joints have a large range of motion and are able to move away from, or across the body (such as

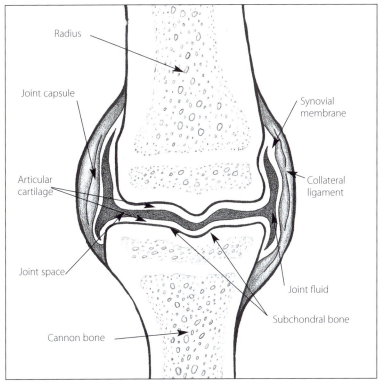

5.1 *Parts of a joint.*

the hip or shoulder), whereas most joints only bend or flex and have limited or no rotation side to side. The joint capsule is well supplied with nerves and blood vessels. Within each joint, the *synovial membrane* produces a viscous hydraulic layer called *synovial fluid* that is rich in *hyaluronate* (also called *hyaluronic acid*.) The *articular cartilage* is the glistening surface at the end of bones that allows bones to glide across each other for efficient movement. (*Articular* refers to "joint.") Cartilage is bathed in synovial fluid. *Subchondral bone* is the tissue at the end of the bone; it blends into the articular cartilage that covers it. This bone is rich in blood vessels and nerves but does nothing to supply nutrients to the joint itself.

Properties of Articular Cartilage

Articular cartilage imparts special characteristics to a joint:

- A network of collagen makes up a large part of the cartilage matrix and provides resistance to tension forces within the joint.
- Proteoglycan components of cartilage impart stiffness to the cartilage to withstand compression and shearing forces between two joint surfaces; proteoglycans are made up of proteins with side chains referred to as *GAGs* or *glysoaminoglycan* molecules, each GAG chain having an electrical charge that repels each other but does attract water.
- Water content of articular cartilage is 70 to 80 percent.
- Nutrients for the cartilage are derived from synovial fluid and the "water" exchange within the cartilage matrix.

Areas of cartilage that receive the most stress have the highest content of proteoglycans and are stiffer than surrounding areas. Compressive loading of a joint squeezes the proteoglycans and exudes water from the articular cartilage. As a joint is loaded with each stride, the cartilage elastically deforms in relation to the distribution of collagen fibers. The cartilage also "creeps," meaning compressed cartilage expresses water and forces it to the surrounding uncompressed cartilage. This process of creeping is dependent on the proteoglycan content of the cartilage. As the limb lifts up and loading is relieved, the pressure is removed; the cartilage rehydrates and expands due to contribution from the synovial fluid. As the limb is unloaded, proteoglycans in previously compressed areas of cartilage once again imbibe "water." Such a constant exchange of synovial fluid into and out of the cartilage is important for maintaining healthy metabolism and nutrition of the joint cartilage.

Based on these physiological principles, it is easy to understand why it is important for a horse to move around to establish and maintain normal joint function and health. Cartilage metabolism and integrity are dependent upon repeated loading of the joints that comes with walking, short sprints, and field play. Stalled and confined horses are more at risk of developing degenerative joint disease (DJD) than horses turned out to pasture.

Joint Function

Joints serve multiple functions:

- Minimize frictional forces between bones and thereby impart range of motion to each limb and the spine
- Stabilize the skeletal structures during the loading phase as the horse fully bears weight on each limb

As a limb swings during locomotion, each joint acts as a "hinge" to allow rotational forces to move a horse forward, sideways, or backward, or in some cases, up and down. Each joint is regulated in the extent of its movement by the pulley levers created by muscles, tendons, and ligaments. Articular cartilage does not act as a shock absorber for the joint. Rather, it is the bone and soft tissue support structures around the joint that absorb impact concussion and diffuse the load on the cartilage.

CONFORMATIONAL EFFECTS ON JOINTS

Efficiency of biomechanical movement depends on a horse's conformation, his skeletal structure, and the configuration and balance of each foot. Joints that are busy in their movement (paddling or winging) such as seen in a crooked-legged horse will experience more wear and tear than joints that move through a small arc to push off and then set the limb on the ground. To prevent ligament strain, joint capsular sprain, or injury within a joint, hooves should be shod to encourage sliding of each foot and to prevent abnormal torque and twisting of the limbs.

EFFECTS OF EXERCISE ON JOINTS

Bone is known for its incredible ability to adapt and remodel to accommodate progressive loading achieved with the conditioning process. Joint surfaces respond to a far lesser degree. The most important time for physiologic adaptation of cartilage in response to exercise appears to be during the first 5 months of life. A young foal that has been withheld from exercise may experience delayed adaptation of cartilage. Provision of regular periods of submaximal loading (aerobic exercise) is an important element to cartilage development in a young horse. On the other hand, short bouts of heavy exercise following stall confinement exert negative effects on the ability of cartilage to resist injury.

Moderate exercise (trot and canter), in both a young and older horse, elicits a phenomenon known as *enhanced cyclic loading*. This loading increases the proteoglycan content of cartilage to increase stiffness of cartilage so it is more capable of withstanding the stress of moderate exercise. Greater limb loading brings more surface area of the articular cartilage into play to diffuse stress across the joint. Excessively strenuous exercise injures cartilage. Smooth, gliding joint surfaces degenerate when irritated by overload. Loading of a joint increases:

- When a horse has to carry more weight (his own and/or a rider's)
- When worked at greater speeds or over greater distances
- As a result of changes in the irregularity or firmness of the ground surface

It has been difficult for scientists to measure and analyze joints in motion, but certain elements are known. Any exercise beyond a moderate level sets up conditions for cartilage irritation and trauma of the soft tissues associated with a joint, as for example *synovitis* or *capsulitis*. As will be discussed, it is the inflammatory process within the synovial membrane or joint capsule that creates an environment conducive to cartilage degeneration. Repeated concussion trauma may create microfractures within subchondral bone. Eventually, this bone stiffens and looses some shock-absorbing ability. Then, the articular cartilage incurs more trauma as loading increases with each step.

An athletic horse potentially suffers from "wear and tear disease" that exacts its toll on the joints, even in the most perfectly conformed horse. Dressage horses, reining horses, cutting horses, roping horses, and Standardbred racers are examples of athletes with amplified punishment on the hocks. Horses with high impact work on the front end (jumpers, reiners, cutters, ropers) also experience a high incidence of DJD

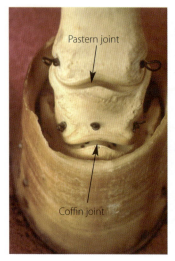
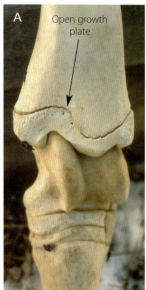
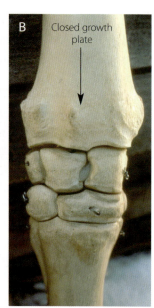

5.3 A & B *This bone of the tibia shows an open growth plate just above the hock (A), while this bone of the radius shows a closed growth plate just above the carpus, or knee (B).*

5.2 *The coffin and pastern joints of the lower limb contribute to a high proportion of musculoskeletal problems from injury and athletic use.*

in the pastern and coffin joints (photo 5.2), also known as *ringbone* (see p. 121). For a distance horse, the bulk of joint problems develop in the fetlocks, with the pastern and coffin joints following behind in frequency.

EFFECTS OF AGE ON JOINTS

Age and skeletal maturity are important to develop a horse's ability to withstand compressive loading associated with consistent exercise demands. Growth plates in the limb joints are closed by 2 years of age, but impact on joints should be applied carefully until a horse has reached full maturity at age 6 to 7 years (photos 5.3 A & B). Light riding is appropriate for ages 3 to 5 to develop the cardiovascular and muscular systems, but persistent riding over longer distances or arduous demands should be reserved for horses over the age of 6 to 7 years. By then, joint cartilage will have developed sufficient compressive stiffness and subchondral bone will have reached maximum strength to better withstand accumulated miles and speed over distances, effort, and time. It is not just joint trauma acquired during a competition that takes its toll; it is the training and conditioning efforts leading to an event that stress the overall system, and particularly the joints and hooves. Appropriate development of these structures may take several years to acquire peak strength.

Signs and Symptoms of Joint Injury

Lameness and Pain

Not all joint injuries show obvious signs of heat or swelling. In most instances, the horse with a joint problem will be lame, or at the very least show some change in stride length and/or willingness to perform. These indications may be so subtle as to be barely detectable; poor performance may be attributed to a horse having an "off" day.

Often, an affected joint has a reduced range of motion and/or the horse displays pain when the joint is manipulated with the limb off the ground.

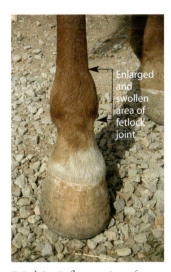 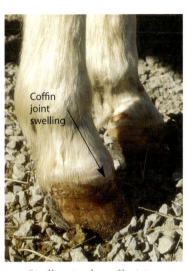 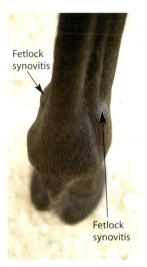 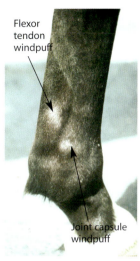

5.4 *Joint inflammation often causes a joint to appear enlarged, particularly as seen on the inside of this fetlock.*

5.5 *Swelling in the coffin joint related to osteoarthritis causes a protrusive appearance on the front of this pastern just at the hoof line.*

5.6 *The windpuffs seen here are related to excess fluid in the fetlock joint (synovitis) that causes the joint capsule to puff out.*

5.7 *The windpuffs seen here are located in two places: the fetlock joint (synovitis) and the flexor tendon sheath (tendinitis).*

Heat and Swelling

Occasionally, skin warmth is felt overlying an inflamed joint. But, this is an unreliable and subjective interpretation depending on who is examining the tissues. An *infrared thermography* unit may be useful to detect true temperature gradients.

Other cases of injury may be more obvious as a joint distends with excess synovial fluid that is produced in response to inflammation (photos 5.4, 5.5, 5.6, and 5.7). The resulting puffy appearance is clinically referred to as *joint effusion,* also known as windpuffs. A joint exhibits this response particularly when there is damage to the synovial lining (*synovitis*) or of the joint capsule (*capsulitis*). Joint pain is associated with inflammation to these structures and/or because of distention (stretching) caused by excess production of synovial fluid. Since synovitis and capsulitis often precede DJD, aggressive treatment is necessary to prevent further joint deterioration (photo 5.8).

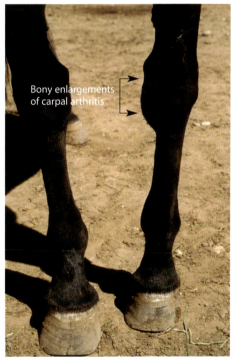

5.8 *The carpi (knees) of this horse are affected by advanced degenerative arthritis, visible as knobby bone spurs and enlargements.*

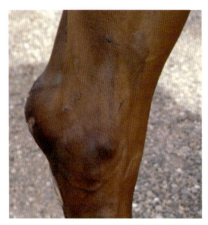

5.9 *Injury to the point of the hock may result in a swelling known as a capped hock. Unless this becomes infected, it is usually only of cosmetic significance.*

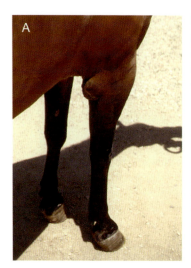
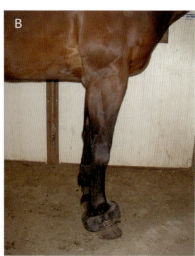

5.10 A & B *Repeated trauma to the elbow may lead to a capped elbow (A). This often occurs when a horse lies down and the foot and/or shoe persistently hits the elbow. Shoe boil rings can protect the elbow from this trauma (B).*

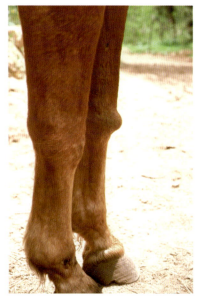

5.11 *Swelling of the bursa of the extensor tendon over the carpus (knee) is called a hygroma, which tends to be only of cosmetic significance.*

Soft Tissue Injury Over Joints

Injury to the *bursa* (a soft tissue sac formed in areas of friction, such as a prominence where a tendon passes over a bone) may result in swelling, with or without a potential infection. Typically, such a swelling (*capped hock, capped elbow,* and *hygroma*) is non-painful, and is of concern primarily as a cosmetic blemish.

CAPPED HOCK

Trauma to the point of the hock may result in irritation to the Achilles flexor tendon running behind the hock. This may only form a cosmetic swelling, known as a *capped hock* (photo 5.9).

CAPPED ELBOW

Trauma to the point of the elbow may occur when a horse lies down and bumps the elbow with the hoof or shoe. This results in a swelling, and potentially an infection, known as a *capped elbow* or *shoe boil*. Shoe boil rings, shaped like donuts, can be placed on the pasterns to provide a spacer to eliminate further elbow trauma (photos 5.10 A & B).

HYGROMA

On the front of the knee is an extensor tendon bursa that may become traumatized from a kick injury or a fall. Swelling here results in another cosmetic blemish known as a *hygroma* (photo 5.11).

Joints: Health, Problems, and Therapies

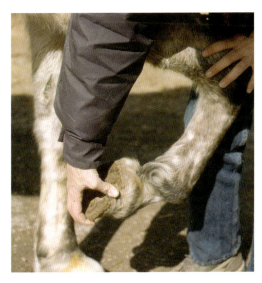

5.12 *A flexion test of the lower structures of the limb yields information about pain and lameness. One or more joints are flexed for 1 to 2 minutes, and the horse is asked to trot off in a straight line. Degree and duration of lameness achieved with flexion are evaluated. A normal horse trots off sound, whereas a horse with a problem may take several to many lame steps.*

Flexion Tests

To further the hunt for joint pain, a helpful diagnostic tool includes the use of *flexion tests*. A horse's joint is held in a tightly flexed position for 1 to 2 minutes and then the horse is asked to trot off (photo 5.12). A "positive" flexion test is associated with a noticeable lameness for at least several strides. Lame steps following the flexion are graded according to intensity and duration of lameness, which will vary depending on the nature of an injury. To bring this to a personal context, imagine how it would feel were you to squat on your heels with your bad knee scrunched tightly for a couple minutes, and then take off in a jog. You might feel pain for the first several steps, feeling compelled to limp until the joint "loosened" up as you ran. This is comparable to the response seen with a positive flexion test in a horse. Radiographic evaluation of an affected joint may shed light on the cause of an injury if bone is involved and particularly in cases of long-standing arthritis.

Injurious Effects of Inflammation

Avoiding joint trauma is a management goal, but unlikely to be successful with an equine athlete. Training and competition take their toll, but fortunately there are strategies that can improve athletic longevity. Ensuring sufficient warm-up time, stretching a horse at the start of a ride, cooling down at the end, and avoiding maneuvers that are beyond a horse's level of fitness and training are many ways to minimize a horse's chances of injury. However, once initial trauma has occurred, the key to limiting damage to joint cartilage is to arrest an inflammatory process (photo 5.13). Harm to cartilage is created by active inflammation that

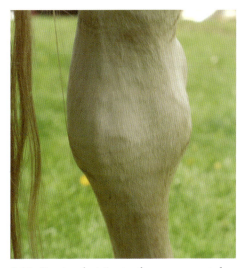

5.13 *Sprain of a joint is often accompanied by diffuse swelling as seen in the hock in this photo. The inflammation that occurs within a joint elicits enzymatic damage that is injurious to joint cartilage.*

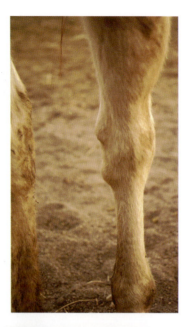

5.14 *Degenerative arthritis of the hock joints is a common problem for sport horses. Signs include poor performance, reduced hock flexion, and toe dragging. There may be an observable enlargement on the inside of the hock as seen here.*

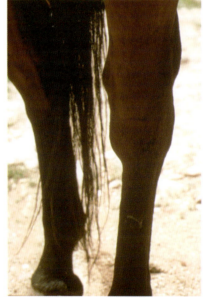

5.15 *This horse's hocks are afflicted by advanced degenerative arthritis. The formation of extensive bone spurs makes the condition visible, although in many cases of hock DJD, a more overt problem is best identified with a good physical exam and radiographs.*

releases inflammatory enzymes from the synovial membrane, along with prostaglandins and free radicals that degrade cartilage. Many of these destructive components are also released from white blood cells that are summoned to the area to clean up an injury as a body's natural response to inflammation.

Chronic inflammation or irritation within a joint may cause a permanent loss of articular cartilage. This creates pain as cartilage is frayed away and bone rubs on bone. Cartilage is *not* replaceable; once it is lost from a joint, options for treatment are limited. The end result is *osteoarthritis*, also known as DJD (photos 5.14 and 5.15), which is best identified with radiographic exam (photos 5.16 A & B). In this crippling process, a chronic, painful condition develops due to ongoing degeneration of the joint cartilage, the underlying subchondral bone, the joint capsule, supportive ligaments of a joint, and/or the synovial membrane lining the joint. It is irreversible, but for low-range motion joints such as the pastern or lower hock joints, there is one final option to manage pain: surgical or chemical fusion to freeze all motion and eradicate pain affected with cartilage loss. High-range motion joints, which include all the other joints of the legs, require a different therapeutic approach to minimizing pain.

Long-Term Expectations for Osteoarthritis

There is no complete cure for arthritis. Once a degenerative process has begun, it continues whether or not a horse is ridden. A common question often asked is "Will I hurt my arthritic horse by continuing to ride him?" Light work can be beneficial by maintaining tone of supporting muscles and ligaments. In some cases, it is necessary to use anti-inflammatory medications to minimize pain. Diligent attention should be paid to trimming, and shoeing when appropriate.

An arthritic horse communicates how much work he is able to do comfortably. Listen to his behavioral cues, and watch his body posture. If he seems grumpy, or has a stance protective of a sore leg, forego an anticipated ride. If he doesn't warm out of his soreness, stop riding before he is hurt more. Because an arthritic horse is in a state of chronic discomfort, consider a change in his athletic career to

Joints: Health, Problems, and Therapies

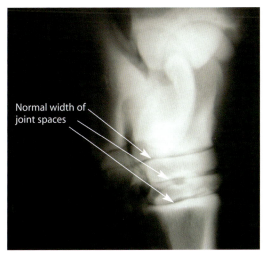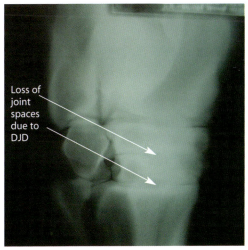

5.16 A & B *Normal hock joints with wide joint spaces (A). Radiographic views of a hock may reveal evidence of degenerative joint disease as in (B). The two lower joint spaces are almost entirely obliterated due to erosion of cartilage. The result of this degree of degeneration is loss of the joint space; loss of this cushion leads to apposition of bone on bone, which is accompanied by significant lameness (see also photos 5.22 A & B, p. 121).*

a pursuit that is less physically demanding. Consider purchasing a younger, more nimble horse to ride in precision sports that require sharp turns and quick stops. An arthritis-afflicted horse can often be turned into a reasonable trail horse, or used in light schooling sessions for a novice rider. For more intense activities, expectations for performance should be lowered. Work demand on the horse also needs to be lessened in frequency and time under saddle. Workout periods may need to be limited to 30 to 40 minutes, 2 or 3 times a week, if that. It is important for an arthritic horse to be brought to a level of fitness and maintained there with a minimum of rigorous exercise. Extended periods of rest make it harder to bring him back to his previous level of condition.

It is possible for a well-trained horse to continue to compete with a minimum work program. Since he already knows the skills, he'll need only an occasional tune-up to sharpen his mind. Prepare to pull from a competition at a moment's notice if a horse is having a bad day due to arthritis.

Gait Considerations of Specific Areas with Joint Pain

SIGNS OF STIFLE PAIN

Some horses with stifle pain will stand knuckled over on the fetlock, allowing the stifle to hang in a relaxed position. This relaxes many of soft tissue structures of the stifle. Most horses with stifle pain stand without the knuckling, but the limb may be held slightly to the side.

In movement, a horse with stifle discomfort is reluctant to flex the stifles. On the forward excursion of the hind limb, the stride is shortened, and the flight of the hoof is low to the ground. Many horses with hind limb pain will wear away the front of their toe as they drag the limb to protect it from pain. This is visible

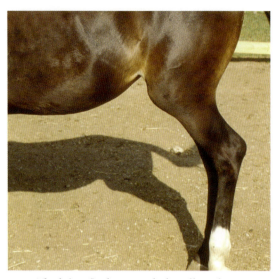

5.17 *The left stifle shows marked swelling that is created by excess fluid distention in the joints. Pain causes this horse to hold the limb in a flexed position. Many horses with stifle pain will hold the limb slightly rotated and away from the body as well.*

as a "dubbed off" (worn) toe, and should be a reason to look deeper for a subtle problem. A horse with stifle pain often rotates the limb outward away from the body when in motion.

Some horses with stifle pain prefer to canter rather than trot, and they may demonstrate a "bunny-hopping" gait with both rear limbs striking the ground together. This takes the stress off one or both painful stifles. Often, a stifle-sore horse has difficulty in taking canter leads because the action required to pick up a lead necessitates bringing a rear limb across the midline so it can assume his body weight as he makes the gait switch. On turns, a stifle-sore horse tends to get rough in his stride. On inclines, gait abnormalities become more striking.

Standing behind a horse trotted out in a straight line, it may be apparent that there is a hip hike on the side with the affected limb. This is due to a rapid excursion of the leg and a horse's desire to unload the limb as quickly

as possible. So, the hip on the affected side remains higher than the limb on the unaffected or less affected side. A chronic condition of rear limb lameness may cause the hip and quadriceps muscles to appear atrophied or less developed than the "normal" side. In an effort to protect a painful leg, the horse quickly unloads it when possible. Atrophy is a result of reduced muscle tension and lessened use relative to the normal limb.

An upper-limb flexion test held for 1 to 2 minutes may elicit an increase in lameness when a horse is asked to trot off. This would be considered a positive flexion test. It is difficult to discern with this test whether a horse hurts in the hock joints, stifle joints, hip joint, or proximal suspensory ligament because anatomy dictates that all these structures are flexed simultaneously.

Typically, a diseased stifle has *effusion* (filling) of the joint capsule with extra fluid (photo 5.17). Such distention is visibly apparent, or it may be felt by placing a hand over the joint. There may be thickening within the supportive ligaments of the joint.

Delayed Patellar Release or Upward Fixation of the Patella

The kneecap (*patella*) can become locked in place by the *medial patellar ligament* that runs across it in a slightly oblique direction. *Delayed patellar release*, also referred to as *upward fixation of the patella*, occurs just as the rear leg begins to flex. In a mild case, what is seen is an intermittently "sticky" limb motion; in a severe case, the ligament locks over the tibia and the upper limb is stuck in an extended position, the horse unable to move (fig. 5.18). Repeated sticking of the ligament over the patella makes some horses sore and lame as a result.

Deep footing or fatigue may precipitate delayed patellar release. A very hard ground surface also poses a risk since the toe cannot cut into unforgiving ground for push-off, and so the stifle must flex more. Downward transitions are noted for rapid flexion of the stifle, and so pose an opportunity for locking. A conformational trait of a straight stifle predisposes to this syndrome, particularly when coupled with a low heel. Young horses may grow out of the problem as the long bones eventually catch up to their genetic potential.

An adult horse that develops upward fixation may require physical therapy and planned exercises to strengthen the quadriceps muscles in the haunches to minimize locking of the stifle. It is also important to ease hoof breakover by squaring the toe and setting the shoe back. Some veterinarians advocate the use of *intramuscular estrogen therapy* to elicit ligament relaxation. Such treatment may help some cases of delayed patellar release. Historically, surgeons would cut the medial patellar ligament to relieve the problem; however, some horses develop fragmentation or osteoarthritis of the patella subsequent to the surgery. If 3 to 5 months of rest follows this surgery, adverse effects are lessened. Another procedure that has been useful is medial patellar ligament splitting. This technique irritates the ligament so that it thickens and then is less likely to catch over the bone.

There are instances of upward fixation of the patella that are related to a neurologic problem and associated weakness of the quadriceps muscles. A thorough neurologic exam should be done on horses with a locking patella to rule out neurologic disease.

SIGNS OF HOCK PAIN

Horses with hock pain do not always demonstrate an obvious lameness. Sometimes, a horse simply performs poorly: he refuses to jump, runs out, stops slowly, refuses to pick up his leads, bucks, or refuses to engage in collection. Some hock-sore horses wring their tails

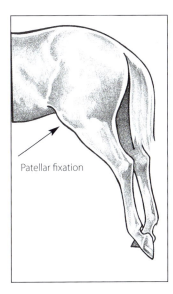

5.18 *Upward fixation of the patella locks the stifle in an extended position. This is caused by a ligament "catching" over the top of the kneecap.*

and act cranky. In motion, there may be a noticeable lack of pelvic swing as the horse holds his torso rigid to avoid pain. Performance issues are often gradual in onset, becoming more obvious as discomfort increases.

Features of Hock Soreness

A horse with a mild degree of hock discomfort will appear to have reduced flexion as he loads the limb. In addition, the forward swing of the leg is diminished. Problems become most noticeable in activities where the limb is heavily or suddenly loaded, such as in collected gaits of dressage, or in reining, cutting, and roping activities. Weight bearing is reduced on both the lame rear limb and on the diagonal front limb, as well. However, contrary to what might be expected, there is no increase in weight bearing on the compensating diagonal legs. Instead, a horse with sore hocks moves with less bounce in his stride and a flatter gait in an attempt to decrease concussion on the limbs. The compensating limbs assume no additional load. What a rider might notice prior to recognition of an overt lameness is deterioration of the quality of the gait.

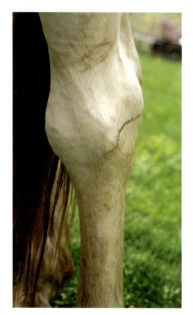

5.19 *Bog spavin refers to fluid distention of the hock joint. Often it is only of cosmetic significance however, a "boggy" hock may also be associated with osteochondrosis, necessitating surgery (see p. 133).*

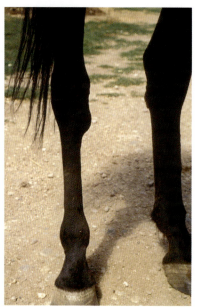

5.20 *Bone spavin refers to bony enlargement of the hock joint(s) related to osteoarthritis, also called degenerative arthritis. Cartilage erosion or thinning of the joint space renders the joint less stable than normal; the body's reponse to stabilize the area is to lay down new bone. Bone spavin is not always externally visible as what is seen in the advanced case in this photo and often requires radiographic evaluation to give an accurate diagnosis.*

Effects of Advanced Hock Soreness on Gait

A horse afflicted with degenerative arthritis of the hocks is less inclined to normal flexion of the hind legs, especially in the swing phase of the stride. The horse does not appear to fully lift the limb from the ground. The gait appears stiff and stilted. The hooves are not lifted as high as normal, leading to an obvious wearing away (dubbing) of the front aspect of the toes of the hoof. Some horses with hock pain shorten the forward phase of the stride. Others move with a noticeable "stabbing" appearance to the gait. Because the horse tends to land more on the toe first, eventually he wears back the front of the toe, polishing it to a smooth and shiny glow. There is often increased wear on the outside aspect of the hoof wall. Another tip-off that there may be hock pain is a recurrence of chronic back pain. Horses with hock or stifle pain assume an abnormal load in their backs due to efforts to protect themselves by moving oddly. The tension is carried through into the back.

A horse that is uncomfortable in his hind end often demonstrates a noticeable hip "hike" on a straight-line trot. The gluteal muscles on the non-painful side appear relatively higher in the trot. The painful limb is unloaded quickly to avoid pain. Viewed from the side at the trot, the horse may appear to drop his head during the *stance phase* of the lame rear limb. A horse's gait is described relative to location of a limb at a given point:

- The *stance phase* occurs when the hoof is in contact with the ground.
- The *swing phase* occurs when the limb is in flight, beginning at toe-lift until the next hoof-strike.

Many horses with degenerative hock arthritis may start out sticky in their gait, and then warm up slowly and appear normal. One means to determine if there is pain in the upper portion of the rear limbs is to perform flexion tests (see p. 115). A horse with osteochondrosis (see p. 133) of the tibial-tarsal joint usually has distention of that joint, referred to as *bog spavin* (photo 5.19). Swelling of the joint may be present long before clinical signs of lameness appear. In more advanced cases of hock DJD (bone spavin), there may be visible signs over the joint and/or obvious changes on radiographs (photos 5.20, 5.21 A & B, and 5.22 A & B).

Joints: Health, Problems, and Therapies

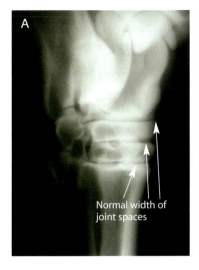
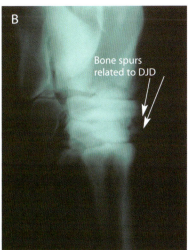

5.21 A & B *A normal hock joint (A). There are clearly demarked joint spaces and no signs of bone spurs or deposits. An arthritic hock joint showing evidence of advanced disease (B). Bone spurs and extensive bone deposition are telltale signs of osteoarthritis, called bone spavin in the hock.*

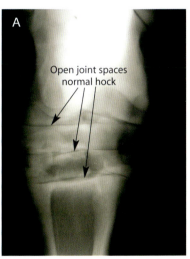
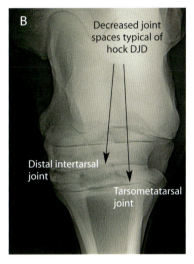

5.22 A & B *An X-ray of a normal hock taken with the beam perpendicular to the limb, i.e. the X-ray machine faces the front of the hock and points at an X-ray plate positioned along the back of the hock (A). An X-ray of a hock with degenerative arthritis taken from the same radiographic view (B). (For a different view, see photos 5.16 A & B, p. 117.)*

RINGBONE

The lowest two joints in a horse's limb (the coffin joint and the pastern joint) are at risk of developing arthritis because they take an intense amount of punishment during athletic use. The term "*ringbone*" aptly describes the buildup of bone around one of these two joints due to DJD, or to trauma around the joint. Development of a "ring of bone" around the pastern joint is referred to as *high ringbone*: it is sometimes visible as a firm swelling about one inch above the coronary band (photo 5.23 A & B). Involvement of the coffin joint is called *low ringbone*. This is

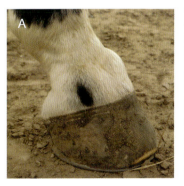
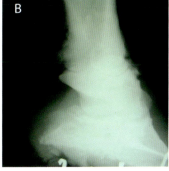

5.23 A & B *An obvious sign of high ringbone is the enlargement around the pastern joint (A). Radiographic evidence of osteoarthritis of the pastern joint (high ringbone) is apparent on this X-ray film (B). The horse in (A) may have radiographic changes comparable to this.*

rarely seen with visual inspection because the overlying top portion of the hoof hides bone changes. Radiographic exam is diagnostic for advanced stages of ringbone.

These two joints in the horse are only capable of forward and backward movement, just as the lower joints of your fingers cannot move sideways or in a circular fashion. Bracing ligaments on the sides and back of each joint prevent side to side or rotational motion. Normal bone protuberances and ridges also prevent rotation of these joints. The pastern joint is particularly limited in its range of motion; even in its normal movements, it hardly flexes or extends as compared to other joints in the body.

If ligaments that stabilize the coffin or pastern joint are strained or torn, a horse's body responds with damage control by building new bone around the injury. When bone proliferates in an area that does not impinge on a joint, it is referred to as *non-articular ringbone*. This usually occurs at areas of ligament attachment on the bone. Abnormal bone that forms directly around the joint space is known as *articular ringbone*; it signifies a more serious arthritic condition, involving degenerative changes in the joint.

Warning Signs of Ringbone

One way to be attuned to the beginning of a problem is by paying close attention to a horse's way of going. Ringbone is a difficult problem to identify without a full veterinary exam, but be on the alert for symptoms, and call your vet if you notice one or more of the following:

- Initially, a horse shows a subtle lameness that has no obvious source
- A horse's stride may shorten as he guards against the pain in his leg
- He may be reluctant to perform difficult movements, like sharp turns, quick stops, or rollbacks
- Lameness may be intermittent, appearing one day and not another, and may occur only with specific exercises, or may be particularly noticeable on turns
- Rest improves both the horse's soundness and disposition, but the odd steps and bad attitude resurface once he is put back to work
- A horse with *high ringbone* tends to slap his heel down first, similar to the peculiar gait movement seen with mild laminitis
- Heat, swelling, or sensitivity to finger pressure may be present around the pastern or coronary band, but these signs are not always present

Prevention and Management of Osteoarthritis

Controlling Inflammation

The first approach to managing a joint injury and preventing a downward inflammatory spiral involves controlling further mechanical trauma to the joint. A horse won't take care of himself, put his leg up, or rest in bed, so exercise has to be restricted to confinement in a stall or small paddock. Rest, in its fullest sense, is the operative strategy. This means the horse should have no exercise of any kind (free or forced) for at least 2 to 3 weeks while a joint rests and then begins to "heal." (Cartilage cannot heal back to normal, but inflammatory effects should subside to give relief.) Concurrent with rest, strategies are integrated to control pain and inflammation with the use of medications and cold therapy as damage control.

An ideal treatment strategy involves removing the degradative enzymes from an injured joint. This is not always practical and is usually reserved for very serious cases by flushing the joint with sterile solutions also containing anti-inflammatory medications. Such a technique is employed when a wound has penetrated into a joint or tendon sheath, or if a joint tap reveals watery or bloody looking synovial fluid.

For traumatic injury caused by persistent concussion impact or twisting motions (*strain* or *sprain*) on a joint, medications are used that inhibit the production, release, and function of degradative enzymes within the joint. (These medications will be elaborated in detail further in this discussion.)

In a chronic condition of a painful joint, many therapeutic strategies can only treat the symptoms but not serve as a cure. At best, the objective is to limit the progression of joint deterioration such that a horse maintains a useful athletic career yet remains relatively pain-free. In cases where chips or *osteochondrosis* fragments persist in a joint, *arthroscopic surgery* should be pursued to remove the pieces when possible (photos 5.24 and 5.25). If fragments are not removed, ongoing inflammation renders most medical treatment temporary at best, and the joint will continue to degenerate despite best-intentioned efforts. Arthroscopic surgery is also indicated to remove excessive synovial membrane that develops in response to chronic inflammation, particularly in a fetlock joint where it is known as *villonodular synovitis* (photo 5.26).

Shoeing Strategies to Minimize Joint Pain

Proper shoeing strategies are very important not only in preventing joint injury (see chapter 3, *The Hoof,* p. 62), but during rehabilitation of a horse coming off an injury. Feet should be trimmed level and balanced to limit abnormal twisting forces on the joints. Toes should be squared back to ease breakover, while a rocker or rolled-toe shoe also helps the horse lift and break over each limb. Shoes should be fitted full so the rear branches extend beneath the heel bulbs to give adequate support to the rear of the foot. All efforts should be made to balance the foot so that with each step, both sides of each foot land simultaneously. It is useful to videotape a horse's forward movement and play it back in slow motion. This gives the horse owner, the vet, and the farrier visual information helpful to balance each foot while it is in motion.

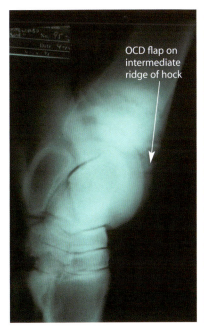

5.24 *A common location for an osteochondrosis lesion in the hock is on the distal intermediate ridge. Here you see a flap of loose cartilage that was successfully removed with arthroscopic surgery.*

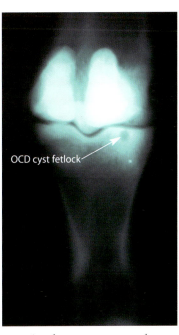

5.25 *Another common osteochondrosis lesion is a cyst as seen here on the long pastern bone in the fetlock.*

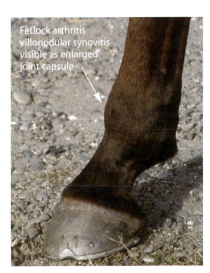

5.26 *A horse with villonodular synovitis has inflammation in the synovial lining of the fetlock, often visible as fetlock distention on the front face of the joint, as seen here.*

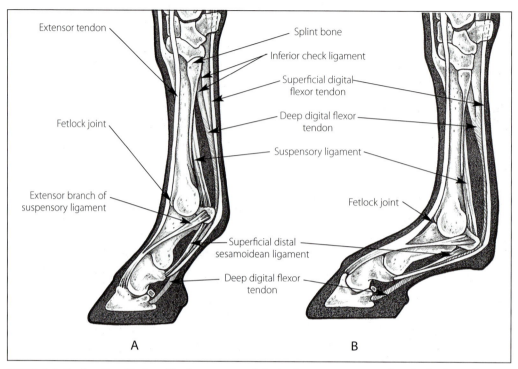

5.27 A & B *Tendon Dorsiflexion: The lower joints of the limb support a tremendous load when a horse moves at speed or lands on a single limb. In this figure, you can see the extreme range of motion through the fetlock joint as it is drops in dorsiflexion. Tissue damage can occur when the fetlock cycles through this extreme range. The parts marked on (B) are under particular stress.*

- One important feature of maximizing soundness is to schedule a regular and correct shoeing program, arranging to have a farrier come at about 6 week intervals so a horse's toes do not grow overly long.
- Prevent a long-toe, low-heel foot configuration that creates an upright and/or broken-back pastern conformation (see p. 50): the toe should be shortened with trimming and rasping.
- An egg-bar shoe, or a shoe with extended branches may be affixed to the foot to increase the length of support for the back of the foot, and to prevent excessive dorsiflexion (fetlock drop leading to stress on other portions of the joints) of the lower joints with weight-bearing (figs. 5.27 A & B and see photo 3.79, p. 91).
- The foot should be encouraged to break over at the point that promotes a straight flight of the foot through the air to prevent excessive winging or paddling of the foot that over-rotates the lower limb.

Medical Treatment of Degenerative Joint Disease

Confer with a veterinarian to work out the best program or combination of therapies for a horse, and an affordable financial strategy. Any of the treatment regimens discussed on the following pages (either singly or in combination) is far less expensive than replacing a beloved horse, provided the strategy gives a horse some relief. The objective in managing any chronic lameness problem is to enable a horse to continue his riding career as comfortably as possible and for as long as possible.

HYALURONIC ACID

Hyaluronic acid, also known as *sodium hyaluronate* or *hyaluronan* and nicknamed HA, is a normal component of joint fluid. The compressive stiffness of cartilage is dependent on the integrity of the proteoglycan components of the cartilage, of which HA is a main ingredient. These aggregated proteoglycans (*glycosaminoglycans*) give cartilage resiliency and tensile strength to withstand loading of the joints. Just as importantly, HA serves as a lubricant of the synovial membrane, allowing a joint to flex, extend, and rotate (when appropriate) with ease.

When a joint suffers an injury, inflammation and disease processes deplete the normal supply of HA within the joint. Glycosaminoglycan (GAG) components of the cartilage also decrease in degenerative joint processes, creating decreased cartilage elasticity; damage continues, as the cartilage is less resistant to exercise stresses.

HA injected into a joint is referred to as "acid." It associates itself with the synovial membrane to exert continued beneficial effects that persist even after HA has cleared from the joint, generally within 96 hours. In a joint that is inflamed, clearance of HA may be more rapid than that, yet favorable effects continue. By injecting HA directly into a joint, normal production of hyaluronic acid is stimulated from the cells of the synovial membrane that line the joint. In addition, HA exerts anti-inflammatory properties such as:

- Inhibiting the movement of white blood cells to the area where they would subsequently release degradative enzymes
- Scavenging of free radicals to minimize their deleterious effects
- Inhibiting the release of prostaglandins that exacerbate the inflammatory process

An approved form of hyaluronic acid is available as an intravenous injection (see *Appendix B,* p. 568). Although its mechanism of action is uncertain, when given intravenously hyaluronic acid seems to localize within the synovial membrane lining joints. There it continues to exert anti-inflammatory effects for as long as 50 days following a series of 3 injections at weekly intervals. Because this membrane is well supplied with blood vessels, HA reaches the joint through the blood circulation, making this an effective means of treatment of acute synovitis or capsulitis.

INJECTABLE POLYSULFATED GLYCOSAMINOGLYCANS

Polysulfated glycosaminoglycans are referred to as PSGAGs or GAGs. An approved product is currently available in both an *intra-articular* (into the joint) form and an intramuscular (IM) form (see *Appendix B*, p. 568).

One of the claims about this product that makes it so useful for managing joint injuries is that it has *chondroprotective* properties, meaning that it protects cartilage against further damage. This is especially indicated when cartilage has already suffered damage in a chronic condition, or as a preventive strategy when cartilage damage is anticipated with an upcoming competition. Prophylactic (preventive) use of this drug in its intramuscular form may help prevent day-to-day loss of cartilage components during persistent trauma incurred with training. Using a PSGAG in its IM form makes it a convenient means of managing multiple joint problems.

Ideally, chondroprotective drugs are used to prevent, retard, or reverse cartilage destruction.

As a chondroprotective agent, a PSGAG inhibits the release and production of destructive enzymes within the joint, as well as inhibiting the release and production of prostaglandins and other inflammatory substances. And, it also stimulates the production of naturally occurring hyaluronic acid within the joints. Whether an injectable PSGAG is administered directly into the joint or given by intramuscular route, it diffuses into the articular cartilage within hours, reaching its peak therapeutic concentration in the joints within 2 hours, remaining there for up to 96 hours. An increase in HA concentration elicited by PSGAGs within the synovial fluid occurs within 24 hours, and this effect is also sustained for 72 to 96 hours. Joint pain is decreased by this medication, and range of motion of an affected joint is improved.

The protocol for the IM form of PSGAGs as a treatment for pre-existing joint injury is to give a vial (500 mg) every 4 days for 7 injections. By the third or fourth injection, some favorable results should be evident, whereupon it is worthwhile to pursue the entire series of 7. Then as continued treatment, a horse should receive 1 injection every 4 to 6 weeks to suppress the inflammatory cycle within a joint (or joints) that may ultimately lead to irreversible DJD. As prophylactic use in an uninjured horse to limit wear and tear disease, it is wise to give an injection monthly, especially prior to a competition. At competitions and events with strict, drug-free regulations, this injection should be given no less than 96 hours prior to an event.

ORAL GLYCOSAMINOGLYCANS

Popular as a feed supplement, oral glycosaminoglycans are sold with claims of preventing and minimizing joint damage and pain. The theory behind administering oral GAGs to a horse to manage joint health is based on studies performed on man and laboratory animals such as rats. To date, studies continue to scrutinize evidence of effectiveness of oral forms of GAGs. Information is still being examined as to how well these products are absorbed from the gastrointestinal tract of the horse or if they are able to localize within equine joints to exert chondroprotective effects. (The reader should take caution when reading efficacy studies to bear in mind that a nutraceutical company might be funding the research on a particular product. Favorable findings are consistently reported when the companies manufacturing an oral joint supplement product are the ones sponsoring a study.)

Glucosamine

Some oral GAG products contain *glucosamine* that is a precursor component of GAGs. As a small molecule, glucosamine appears to be capable of absorption from the small intestine. In rats, dogs, and man, this substance is found to be 87 percent absorbed; absorption from equine intestines is thought to be as high as 60 percent. The latest evidence indicates that the glucosamine-3-sulphate form has beneficial effects on joints whereas the n-acetyl-glucosamine form does not.

Glucosamine is important for synthesis of glycosaminoglycans. It has properties that inhibit the production of degradative enzymes and oxidative damage of cartilage. It also seems to exert some anti-inflammatory effects for preservation of cartilage. As a supplement, glucosamine must be fed for at least 2 to 3 weeks before realizing clinical improvement. At least 10 grams per day for a 1000-pound horse is required to achieve positive effects.

There is some concern that glucosamine supplementation for osteoarthritis may contribute to insulin resistance. This may be worthy of consideration when managing horses afflicted with equine metabolic syndrome.

(For more discussion, see "Laminitis" on p. 74 in chapter 3, *The Hoof*.)

Chondroitin Sulfate

Other oral GAG products contain *chondroitin sulfate*, which is the predominant GAG component of articular cartilage. In man, this substance is absorbed 70 percent by the oral route, whereas only 14 percent is absorbed in horses. There is no evidence of any active beneficial effect of this product for use in joint therapy.

CORTICOSTEROIDS

An effective strategy to curb inflammation within a joint is to directly inject the joint with a *corticosteroid*, or a combination of corticosteroid/hyaluronic acid (known as "*white acid*"). Steroid medications exert powerful anti-inflammatory effects, with rapid onset of between 12 to 24 hours. Steroids suppress pain within a joint, but their use should not be misconstrued as a cure. In the best case, an intra-articular injection of a corticosteroid or "white acid" may give a horse relief for months and even years by breaking the inflammatory cycle. The main action of steroids is to inhibit the movement of inflammatory cells into the site of injury, and in so doing, this limits the amount of ongoing cartilage destruction.

NONSTEROIDAL ANTI-INFLAMMATORY DRUGS

These medications, commonly known as NSAIDs, are the old standbys used to manage musculoskeletal injuries for decades. Examples include phenylbutazone, flunixin meglumine, and ketoprofen. These drugs give relief from inflammation and pain within a short 4 hours by inhibiting *prostaglandins*, which are an active part of the inflammatory cycle (see p. 442). However, because NSAIDs mask pain in an injured joint without providing any other therapeutic effects, a horse may "ignore" the problem and cause himself further damage. There is also evidence that NSAIDs may contribute to cartilage destruction by interfering with normal metabolism of the cells that regulate cartilage maintenance and nutrition. NSAIDs also reduce concentrations of PG E2, which is known to sensitize nerve endings to mechanical stimuli and to chemical activation of pain receptors. By reducing pain "sensation" in an injured area with NSAID administration, a horse is likely to do himself harm by not protecting the damaged part.

The strategy when using NSAIDs should be to use the least amount possible so as to prevent adverse gastrointestinal effects, such as stomach or intestinal ulcers, or kidney damage. It may only require 1 to 2 grams per day of phenylbutazone to have an effect on inhibiting prostaglandin synthesis within the joint so there would be no reason to use more than this dose. In some cases, every-other-day treatment with a low dose may effectively manage a painful arthritic condition.

NSAIDs can be dangerous when given to a dehydrated competitor. Only administer these drugs once a horse has had ample time to restore fluid losses after a ride or competition, otherwise kidney damage or intestinal ulcers may develop. In addition, NSAIDs should not be administered to a young horse less than 8 to 9 months of age unless treating concurrently with anti-ulcer medications; foals are highly prone to developing gastric ulcers. Also, be cautious in treating older or debilitated horses since liver and kidney function may be compromised in these animals, potentially leading to NSAID toxicity. (For detailed discussion, refer to this topic in chapter 14, *Equine First Aid, Medication, and Restraint*, p. 445.)

DMSO

Dimethyl sulfoxide (DMSO) is a potent anti-inflammatory medication (see p. 195) that scavenges

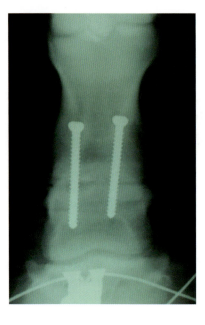

5.28 *A surgical process, called an arthrodesis, fuses an arthritic joint by drilling away remaining cartilage and then affixing the bones together with screws. Surgical fusion of this pastern joint renders it immoveable, but with no movement, there is no pain.*

free radicals and suppresses prostaglandin synthesis, both of which are features of the inflammatory cascade within a joint. Rubbing a light layer of DMSO over a joint and placing a support wrap over the area may help a horse's acute joint injury feel better. In more serious injuries, a veterinarian may elect to give liquid DMSO by stomach tube or through intravenous fluids to gain a systemic anti-inflammatory effect. Or, in a penetrating wound to a joint, DMSO would be added to the flush solutions to limit damage done to the cartilage by degradative enzymes. Whenever working with DMSO, remember that it penetrates skin, human as well as horse, so wear protective gloves.

Surgical Options for Joints

LASER-FACILITATED JOINT FUSION

For those horses that do not respond to medical treatment strategies, it is feasible to surgically fuse (*arthrodese*) the distal hock joints, the two lowest rows of the hock joints. Historically, this procedure has relied on a highly invasive process that drills away the cartilage and then screws the joints together. An alternative procedure uses a laser to destroy the cartilage and fuse the joints. The horse is put into daily work 2 weeks following laser surgery; a successful outcome is dependent upon continual exercise during the rehabilitation period. This technique is still in investigative stages but shows great promise as being a solution to chronic hock pain of the distal joints.

SURGICAL FUSION FOR RINGBONE

In the ideal situation, it is desirable for a case of articular ringbone of the pastern joint to advance on its own to complete fusion (*ankylosis*) of the joint without any intervention. The horse's pain is eliminated as the joint is immobilized by an encasement of new bone growth. This process can occur unnoticed, or it may progress in fits and starts with periods of extreme discomfort for the horse. Ankylosis of a joint can take many years, and it is not a reliable process: it may never completely develop to a pain-free level.

In addition to management strategies and medical therapeutic options as discussed above, some forms of ringbone are amenable to surgery. Besides removal of impinging bone spurs of *non-articular ringbone*, there is another surgical procedure for a horse diagnosed with *high articular ringbone*, a procedure to hasten fusion of the pastern joint. Surgical fusion of a joint is called an *arthrodesis* (photo 5.28). The horse is placed under general anesthesia and the cartilage surfaces of the joint are removed as much as possible with a drill, and then the joint is screwed together. Ample new bone forms to completely immobilize the pastern joint.

A rehabilitation period with return to full use is expected to take up to an entire year. Seventy percent of horses undergoing this surgery successfully return to athletic function. Because the pastern joint is a low motion joint to begin with, its fusion does not interfere with a horse's movement abilities.

Involvement of the coffin joint casts a poor prognosis: a continued athletic life is rarely possible. This joint has a far greater range of motion than the pastern joint, and never successfully fuses on its own, nor can be surgically fused with any expectation of athletic ability. Coffin joint arthritis is persistently painful; the horse would do better to be permanently retired or turned out to pasture as a breeding animal provided the problem is not conformationally heritable.

Alternative Therapeutic Options for Joints

Besides the conventional treatments discussed above, there are more possibilities available to manage painful joints than only relying upon pharmaceutical management. Following is a brief list of alternative therapies that may be instituted as pain-controlling measures.

THERMAL THERAPY

Ice therapy is an adjunctive treatment for minimizing inflammation following an exercise bout. (For more detail, see "Thermal Treatment" in chapter 7, *Strong Tendons and Ligaments*, p. 192.) Joints cool slowly and may remain "cooled" for up to two hours. If a joint can be safely moved, intermittent flexion during cold therapy hastens the cooling process. In deeper structures such as muscles and joints, cold deters swelling, but *edema* (swelling of cells with fluid) may develop beneath the skin (*subcutaneous*) at temperatures less than 59° F (15° C). However, a light pressure bandage can control this mild swelling and the benefit derived from cold therapy far outweighs mild, superficial edema.

ACUPUNCTURE

For millennia, *acupuncture* treatment has been used to break the pain cycle in humans and animals, as well as improve circulation within meridian channels that are involved with the painful limb. Acupuncture is effective in accomplishing these ends especially if a horse is managed initially with several acupuncture treatments spaced 4 to 7 days apart.

MASSAGE AND STRETCHING

Massage is another useful vehicle to relieve cramping and constriction created by sore muscles that have tightened in response to protecting a painful limb. Likewise, stretching exercises further release tension in taut muscles, also improving flexibility and suppleness of the horse (see chapter 6, *Muscle Endurance*, p. 153).

THERAPEUTIC ULTRASOUND

Therapeutic ultrasound is effective in managing soft tissue injuries (see p. 197); since soft tissue components (joint capsule, synovial membrane, and supportive ligaments of a joint) are often injured concurrent with cartilage trauma, this can be an adjunctive means of promoting healing. Pulsing of sound waves into an injured area stimulates cellular responses. These include improvement of circulation to the area and delivery of oxygen and nutrients to the area of injury, while also whisking away metabolic waste products produced subsequent to inflammation.

SOFT LASER

Similar in theory to the reported benefits gained from therapeutic ultrasound, soft laser therapy is often incorporated into treatment of soft tissue injury. It is thought that the laser light stimulates acupuncture points to improve circulation and promote healing. Currently, there is no scientific documentation that laser light will do as claimed, but anecdotal reports attest that favorable results are appreciated with laser treatment.

MAGNETS

Reportedly, magnets exert favorable effects on tissue by eliciting improved circulation within the area to which magnets are applied. A wealth of information has been written on the beneficial effects of magnets, but not all magnets are created equal. Prior to purchase of these expensive devices, request documentation from a manufacturer in support of therapeutic claims.

IONTOPHORESIS

Iontophoresis, often used in human physical therapy, has made its way into the veterinary field as a means of "driving" small molecules of pharmaceutical compounds into an injured area, using an electric current applied for 10 to 20 minutes. Medication molecules pass through pores, sweat glands, and hair follicles to enter deeper tissues. As a bonus, skin retains some of the drug, acting as a reservoir to allow extended release of a treatment. Examples of medications used with iontophoresis include NSAIDs and steroids, each of which diminishes the inflammatory cycle.

EXTRACORPOREAL SHOCK WAVE THERAPY

ESWT has been applied to refractory (do not yield to treatment) cases of *bone spavin* (degenerative arthritis of the lower hock joints—see p. 000) that neither respond to direct injection of the affected joint(s) with anti-inflammatory medications, nor are relieved with other surgical procedures. In one study of joints (139 horses) treated with ESWT, 80 percent improved *at least* one lameness grade while 18 percent improved to sound. No horse's lameness worsened with the treatment, although 20 percent did not improve at all with a single treatment. With a second treatment, a quarter of them improved slightly.

The best results were found treating the tarsometatarsal joint, the lowest joint row in the hock (see photo 5.22 B, p. 121). The treatment did not encourage fusion of the afflicted joints, although pain was certainly diminished. It is possible that remodeling of subchondral bone and its strengthening help to "maintain joint shape and contribute to shock absorption to spare the cartilage from damage." Clinical results are the best means of identifying if a treatment is working because no changes are visible on radiographic (X-ray) exam.

Shock wave therapy is being tried on other areas of musculoskeletal problems, such as for navicular disease, foot pain, splints, back pain, bucked shins, and various tendon and ligament injuries. Improvement in lameness for these other syndromes is not nearly as consistent as the results found in hock or proximal suspensory treatment (see chapter 7, *Strong Tendons and Ligaments*, p. 187). Navicular syndrome is a plaguing lameness entity that results from pathology developing in a variety of soft tissue and bony structures within the heel (see chapter 3, *The Hoof,* p. 85). ESWT will have variable results dependent on which of the many anatomical structures are affected by the degenerative disease.

Although there remains some debate in exactly how the shock waves achieve results, no side effects have developed with application of ESWT. Its pain-reducing properties make it an attractive alternative and adjunctive treatment for notoriously chronic and debilitating lameness conditions. (For a more comprehensive description of ESWT, see chapter 4, *Developing Strong Bones,* p. 106.)

Management Strategies for Joint Problems

In addition to the medical and surgical strategies discussed, management of a horse in his environment and his work are important to joint health. Recommendations include:

- Do not confine a horse to a stall, but rather allow self-exercise in a large paddock or pasture; the slow movement of wandering and walking helps lubricate joints, and reduces pain and stiffness that develop with stall confinement.
- Pay careful attention to an ample warm-up and cool-down period of 10 to 15 minutes to improve a horse's athletic longevity: a warm-up increases circulation to the musculoskeletal structures to improve flexibility and joint lubrication, and it also prevents ligaments and tendons from overstretching prematurely.
- Following a workout, ice an injured area of a limb for 20 to 30 minutes to retard inflammation that threatens to flare in a sore leg: immerse the lower leg in a bucket of ice water, or direct a stream of cold water with a hose over the area of concern, or use ice boots, wetting the fur and skin before application.

Ongoing Research into Joint Therapy

GENE THERAPY FOR TRAUMATIC ARTHRITIS

A strategy that holds great promise for future application is that of preventing osteoarthritis rather than simply managing inflammation after the fact. This strategy involves injecting a *gene transfer vector* directly into a joint at the time of joint trauma.

The scientific study model used to evaluate effectiveness of this therapy was based on creation of an osteochondral fragment in the carpus (knee) with arthroscopic surgery. (This same bone-fragment model is the one often used to test many types of intra-articular therapies.) In the study protocol, a newly injured joint was "treated" by administering the gene transfer vector directly into the joint. A total of 16 "control" horses (these received no treatment at all) and treated horses were exercised on a treadmill at trot and gallop to simulate athletic race training. After humane destruction, the joint cartilage of each horse was evaluated. This study concluded that IL-1Ra (gene transfer vector) has a protective effect on osteochondral fragment-induced proteoglycan loss. The researchers also found that the therapeutic expression of IL-1Ra significantly decreased signs of joint pain as measured by degree of lameness. The amount of *synovial effusion* (joint filling with excess joint fluid) associated with an osteochrondral fragment was also significantly decreased in joints that received the gene transfer vector.

Extrapolation and experience have shown that joint response to therapy is similar for synovitis, capsulitis, and/or osteoarthritis as it is with the osteochondral fragment model. Gene therapy holds promise not only for preventing arthritis in an injured joint in a horse, but also as a means to discover additional anti-arthritic gene sequences for use in managing equine joint disease.

Joint Diseases

Developmental Orthopedic Disease

It is relevant to an equine athlete that during the developmental stages of his life, his bones and joints should mature without problems. Some developmental orthopedic problems may not appear until a horse is in steady work as a three-to-six-year-old. *Developmental Orthopedic Disease* (DOD) results from a variety of multi-factorial issues but nutritional imbalances are known to predispose a young, growing horse to this malady. Many of the developmental problems seen involve the bones of the joints. DOD is linked to an imbalance of calcium and phos-

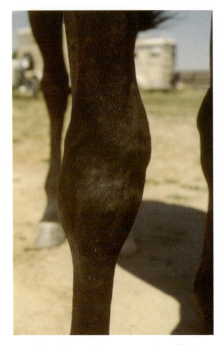

5.29 *Epiphysitis (more correctly called physeal dysplasia) is an abnormality in the development of the growth plate that often creates lameness, and can result in permanent damage to the joint if not corrected early on. Epiphysitis of the carpus makes the knees look knobby and enlarged.*

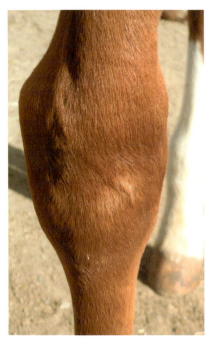

5.30 *Another example of a knobby and enlarged knee afflicted with epiphysitis.*

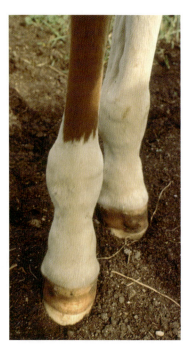

5.31 *Epiphysitis of the fetlock gives the joint a telltale hourglass shape.*

phorus, and/or a deficiency in microminerals such as copper, zinc, and manganese. *Epiphysitis* is one manifestation of DOD; other problems that develop due to nutritional inconsistencies during growth include *osteochondrosis* (OCD—see p. 133), *Wobbler syndrome* (see p. 517), and *flexural contractures* (see pp. 198 and 564). In many cases, DOD remains undetected until a horse is introduced into steady work. The complex of DOD has significant consequences to future performance.

EPIPHYSITIS

Epiphysitis is a term that describes defects in the ossification of the growth plate (*physis*) at the ends of long bones. The syndrome should be more correctly called *physeal dysplasia* since it is the growth plate and metaphysis that are affected. (The growth plate is responsible for growth in length of the long bones). A young horse of 4 to 6 months of age typically exhibits problems in the fetlocks, while a yearling up to 2 years of age is susceptible to epiphysitis around the carpal joints (knees). Affected carpal joints or fetlocks exhibit an hourglass-shaped, firm swelling just above the joints: the joints appear "knobby" and enlarged (photos 5.29, 5.30, and 5.31). Only one limb may be affected, but usually there will be signs of change in similar joints on two or more limbs. A horse with epiphysitis may be lame, but not always.

Dietary imbalances of copper, zinc, calcium, and/or phosphorus are linked to epiphysitis. Overfeeding is just as likely a cause as imbalanced nutrition in stimulating this disease. Rapid growth due to excess energy intake is implicated in causing epiphysitis. Epiphysitis also may occur from "crushing" of the physeal plate by trauma due to excessive loading of the limb as a result of too much exercise, or if a growing horse is carrying too much flesh on his frame for young bones to support. Abnormal conformation may overload one side of a growth plate to create this condition, while trauma from a kick or fall can also cause damage. Although seemingly innocuous, epiphysitis is often the tip of the iceberg in the complex of DOD.

OSTEOCHONDROSIS

Another component of the syndrome of DOD is called *osteochrondrosis* or OCD. A defect in *endochondral ossification* at the joint surface causes displacement of an area of abnormal cartilage as a fragment or as a flap, or as a cyst that remains just beneath the surface of the joint (see photos 5.24 and 5.25, p. 123). Eventually, OCD in any of these forms can lead to lameness and arthritis. More than 60 percent of horses diagnosed with OCD show symptoms prior to their first year birthday. Such symptoms include varying degrees of lameness, distention of the affected joint, or reluctance to flex the limb, particularly when OCD develops in the hocks and/or stifles. Some horses may have difficulty getting up or down. In over half the cases, OCD is present in bilateral joints although obvious symptoms may only show up in one. Delay in noting the presence of a problem is dependent on the age at which a horse is introduced to regular exercise.

Rapid Growth

OCD is considered a multi-factorial problem although diet is highly implicated. Excess energy intake (120 percent of National Research Council nutrient requirements) has been correlated to OCD as has a high protein diet. Too rich a nutritional supply enables a growing horse to become fat with subsequent overload of developing joints. Hormonal changes associated with a rich diet also may affect joint metabolism.

Adverse effects of an imbalanced diet are amplified by other high risk factors. The potential for rapid musculoskeletal development is dependent on genetics as well as on nutrition. Rapid growth adds stress to the growing bones of the skeletal system and joints when they can least withstand the added body mass. OCD as a developmental problem occurs by virtue of joints being more susceptible to damage during specific times in their development. The stifles and hocks are most at risk from between 6 to 8 months of age. Risk increases if the youngster overly stresses the limbs with exercise, causing damage to bone and to the blood supply within the joints. Conformation has a role to play in OCD development. Crooked limbs and less than perfect conformational traits contribute by overloading susceptible joint surfaces; this potentially leads to cartilage damage.

Role of Exercise

One controversial, yet significant, stressor to joint development is that of confinement. Youngsters that are limited in their daily exercise may not have sufficient development of the subchondral bone to support their body weight. Then, when the horse is turned out, he may overload the joint cartilage abruptly.

Microminerals

Mineral imbalances have deleterious effects on joint cartilage development. It is known that high phosphorus (and relatively low calcium) levels may cause cartilage defects. A diet that is low in copper may also increase the prevalence of OCD. Copper is essential for synthesis and maintenance of elastic connective tissue, and for copper-related enzyme systems responsible for "digesting" cartilage before its conversion to bone. High zinc levels may suppress copper absorption and result in a diet that is relatively deficient in copper. Microminerals in the feed should be analyzed to determine if the diet is properly balanced for both pregnant mares and growing foals.

Treatment for OCD

For OCD lesions, the treatment of choice is arthroscopic surgery to remove a defective piece of cartilage or cyst. This is followed by 3 months of rest. The overall success for return to athletic function is about 65 percent. The chance of surgical success is dependent on the size of the lesion in a joint, with smaller cartilage defects leading to better results. Subsequent injections of anti-inflammatory medications into the joint may be necessary to achieve the best possible outcome.

WOBBLER SYNDROME

Cervical vertebral malformation (CVM) is another manifestation of DOD. This occurs when the joint surfaces of the spinal vertebrae develop OCD lesions. Instability in affected cervical vertebrae and narrowing of the spinal canal may lead to compression of the spinal cord to elicit subsequent neurologic disease, known as *Wobbler syndrome*. Cervical radiographs may be a useful diagnostic predictor of animals affected with developmental orthopedic disease. (For more discussion on Wobbler syndrome, refer to *The Neurologic System in Health and Disease*, p. 517.)

ANGULAR LIMB DEFORMITIES

An *angular limb deformity* (ALD) in a foal may create a crooked-legged horse. A commonly seen problem is knock-kneed conformation, a condition known as *carpus valgus* (photo 5.32). In this case, the carpal joints (knees) touch or are too close together and one or both of the lower front limbs are splayed out. This type of outward deviation of the legs can also occur in the hocks, there known as *tarsus valgus*. In either case, the problem may have begun as a collapse of the carpal or tarsal bones in a very young foal due to being incompletely formed at birth. The best means of evaluating condition of these bones in the joints is by radiographic examination. Another type of ALD is that of *fetlock varus* which results in a toed-in conformation. An additional form of ALD results in *windswept* rear legs that are both abnormally angled, but in the same direction (photo 5.33).

Congenital Factors for ALD

Many factors elicit a *congenital angular limb deformity*, or one that

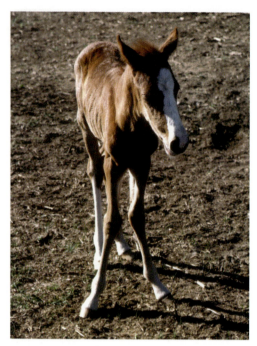

5.32 *An angular limb deformity (ALD) such as carpus valgus (knock-knee) as seen here can render a horse incapable of performing high level athletic demands.*

develops *in utero*. These malformations are often associated with external factors:

- Overfeeding of a mare in the last half of gestation
- Ingestion of locoweed by a pregnant mare
- Intrauterine malposition of the foal
- Ligament laxity at birth with resulting soft tissue injury (photo 5.34)
- Incorrect development of a foal's growth plates due to bone infection, or inflammation of the growth plates
- Incomplete ossification of the tarsal or carpal bones

Some of these situations can be controlled through attention to management details: feed a balanced ration to a pregnant mare, and eliminate access to toxic plants, weeds, or medications that are known to cause birth defects. The other factors in this list are often out of one's control, and can only be managed rather than prevented.

Acquired Factors for ALD

There are innumerable situations that lead to *acquired limb deformities* in the horse:

- Incorrect conformation placing abnormal stress on the growth plates
- Overfeeding of rich supplements and feeds, and/or imbalanced nutrition during periods of growth
- Excessive exercise leading to musculoskeletal fatigue and soft tissue injury
- Lameness that causes more of the weight-bearing load to be assumed by the opposite limb
- Growth plate trauma due to an injury or infection

In these cases, human intervention has a role in preventing a few of these scenarios: select only proven athletic stock for breeding, concentrating on horses with minimal conformational flaws. Eliminate the overfeeding equation by paying close attention to providing a balanced ration. Similarly, foals can be restricted from overzealous exercise. Limb injury or infection can only be addressed once these have occurred.

Treatment Options for Angular Limb Deformities

Initially it is helpful to try some therapeutic measures for correction of an ALD before considering surgical intervention. Exercise must be restricted to minimize stress on the incorrectly aligned joints. A cooperative effort by a veterinarian and farrier may improve some of these

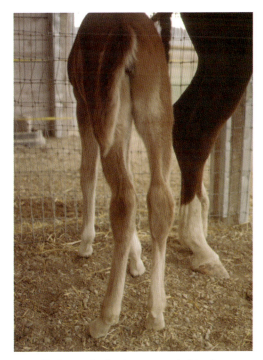

5.33 *Both rear limbs that are angled in the same direction are referred to as "windswept." This is another form of angular limb deformity that can last into adult years to preclude high levels of performance.*

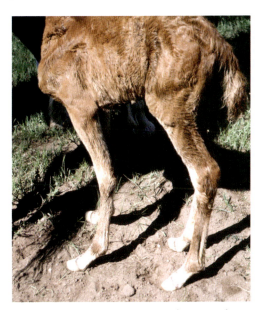

5.34 *Ligament laxity at birth, such as carpal hypoflexion seen here, can create lasting soft tissue injury to the joints.*

cases easily. Corrective trimming and shoeing of the young foal is a prime strategy. A glue-on extension is applied beneath the medial aspect of the hoof for a foal that has a valgus deformity. Some foals also need the benefit of splints or tube casts to "straighten" the limb.

Surgery initially relies on a procedure known as *hemicircumferential periosteal transection with periosteal stripping*. An inverted T-shaped incision is made into the periosteum (sheath covering the bone) on the concave side of the leg. This technique relies on increased growth at the physis due to mechanical release of tension forces created by the periosteum. As this incision in the periosteum heals, the other side of the limb catches up in its growth; then both sides continue to grow at the same rate, with a straightened limb as the result. If satisfactory results do not appear within 4 to 6 weeks following this surgery, a more aggressive surgical procedure is recommended. For initially severe deformities or cases that don't respond to conservative management, screws and wires (*transphyseal bridging*) may be placed on the convex side of the limb to retard its rate of growth. These metallic implants need to be removed when the leg straightens to a more correct alignment.

The important issue with any surgical intervention is its timing. An ALD associated with fetlock growth plates must be corrected within 2 months of age; these growth plates are closed by 4 months old so surgery must be performed while there is still growth to achieve correction of the crooked limb. The knee and hocks should receive surgical intervention no later than 4 to 6 months of age to achieve results.

Lyme Disease

Lyme disease is caused by a spirochete called *Borrelia burgdorferi*. This organism is transmitted by *Ixodes* ticks commonly found on deer and some rodents. Most of the time, transmission of the disease requires the tick to be attached to the host for at least 24 hours. (For further discussion on ticks and their removal, see chapter 13, *The Skin as an Organ,* p. 387, and on tick-caused paralysis, see "Neurologic Irritation or Compression," p. 515.)

CLINICAL SIGNS

Signs of infection are variable in the horse, but joint pain is one of the most prevalent signs. Lameness or stiffness occurs in more than one limb, with the dominant lameness often shifting between different legs. Behavioral changes are another common sign of Lyme disease. Other clinical signs include joint swelling, a low-grade fever, muscle pain or tenderness, increased sensitivity in the skin, skin lesions, lethargy, decreased appetite, and in a rare case, inflammation within the eye. These are fairly non-specific clinical problems that can be attributable to various systemic diseases.

LABORATORY TESTING

Blood tests are necessary to confirm the presence of the spirochete, testing for antibodies specific to *Borrelia* infection. A lab test may not show positive results until 3 to 10 weeks following infection.

TREATMENT OF LYME DISEASE

The antibiotics of choice are intravenous tetracycline or oral doxycycline. It is often necessary to maintain treatment for at least a month.

Muscle Endurance   6

Depending on one's point of view, each person has a particular prejudice about which body structures are considered the most critical to the making of a superior equine athlete. Arguments abound that the heart is the most important organ in the body, while another exclaims that the hooves are the most important system to performance. Yet in the encompassing view of the concept of "organ," without efficient working muscles an athletic horse cannot perform at an optimum level for very long.

Each chapter of this book isolates each body system to investigate its parts in detail, to describe impacts on performance, and how to condition that system to reach its peak. However, each system is intricately linked to each other system of the body so that all parts work in harmony: a strong muscular system cannot be developed without concurrent development of the cardiovascular system; without muscles, tendons do not strengthen nor is efficient locomotion achieved; without strong joints, muscles cannot exert maximal force to move the bones.

Muscle mass of a horse comprises about 45 percent of the horse's body weight, so it is a ponderous organ in its own right. Whereas some organ systems are genetically predetermined in their strength and development, muscle is a highly malleable tissue, capable of responding to training. With fitness and conditioning, muscle architecture and metabolism adapt to applied stresses to improve the efficiency of locomotion and muscular work.

The "Nuts and Bolts" of Muscle Tissue

Levers and Pulleys

Let's review how muscles do their work of moving a horse's body across the ground. Each muscle is attached to bone by some fibrous component, either tendon or *fascia* (a fibrous sheet of tissue beneath the skin that envelops muscle—see fig. 2.3 on p. 10 and fig. 6.1 on p. 145. As a muscle contracts, it applies tension to the spots of tendinous attachment where it inserts on bone. This in turn, creates locomotion. The fulcrum for the muscles (and tendons) to pull against is often located at or near a joint. Like a series of levers, long muscles contract over a long distance, while shorter muscles have a large cross-sectional area to provide maximum contraction strength over a short distance, "Short" muscles maintain postural positions such as positioning of the head, while "long" muscles move the long bones to initiate and maintain locomotion. The geometric design and position of the long muscles enables them to move the bones with minimal shortening of the muscle fibers.

Muscles of the limbs join their respective tendons and insert at an angle to the direction of the force. This creates an optimal mechanical advantage by maximizing the cross-sectional area of the muscles to improve both power and efficiency of contraction. Similarly, a rock climber is held on belay on a safety rope that is positioned more or less at right angles to the position of the climber. Following the principle applied to the mechanics of a block and tackle, the right angle created by the belay rope enables a person to hold a fallen climber through a huge force but with minimal muscular effort or strain. In a similar way, the geometric configuration of lengthy thigh muscles brings their tendinous attachments at right angles as the Achilles tendon runs over and inserts behind the point of the hock.

Muscle Contraction

An equine muscle is composed of thousands of individual fibers. Organized contraction of stimulated muscle fibers creates movement of a muscle. A tendon connects a muscle to a bone. Movement of a muscle moves the complementary bone and joint. Large muscle groups working together propel a horse into motion or slow him down. Muscle control and coordination improve with practice and training to produce greater precision, power, and speed.

Muscles are composed of spindle-shaped skeletal muscle cells that overlap and connect in an orderly arrangement of fibers, with most muscle fibers being about 5 to 10 cm in length. Motor neurons (a nerve or bundle of nerves through which impulses travel to excite activity) are abundant throughout muscle tissue. Nerve fiber branches invaginate (fold-in) into each muscle fiber at a "terminal" referred to as a motor endplate. Here, electrical and chemically induced nerve impulses are propagated across the cell membrane to elicit a muscle contraction.

Muscles possess unique properties that ensure their ability to sustain work:

- Within each muscle cell is a registered alignment of contractile proteins called myofibrils extending through the entire length of the muscle cell.
- The cell membrane propagates an electrical potential (called an action potential) to stimulate contraction and/or relaxation of a muscle.
- Calcium concentrations and ATP (adenosine triphosphate energy molecules—see "Muscles Produce Energy", p. 140) within muscle are regulated through energy-generating biochemical reactions to elicit a process of excitation-contraction coupling, which stimulates muscular movement.

In resting muscle, calcium concentrations are at a low level. Muscle cells contain relatively high concentrations of potassium and low concentrations of sodium and chloride. An increase in free intracellular calcium is a trigger for muscle contraction. As a nerve signal passes across the cell membrane, calcium is released from its storage within the *sarcoplasmic reticulum* to then pool within the muscle cells. The change in electrical charge within and surrounding the muscle cell sets off an action potential and a contraction. Like a ratchet, the muscle fiber filaments slide over each other to shorten the tissue, and form a contraction that moves the skeleton. The muscle relaxes again when the calcium ions are actively "pumped" (using ATP energy) back into their storage areas.

Not all muscle fibers are recruited at one time within a given muscle, as rarely does a muscle need to generate maximum tension. The pattern and quantity of fibers that are selectively recruited depend on a horse's gait, his speed, and the duration of the performance effort. Muscular tension is increased by recruitment of additional muscle cells. This occurs by increased intensity of electrical stimulation that exceeds the threshold for contraction and that approaches the maximal stimulus necessary for greater speed or power.

CONCENTRIC CONTRACTION

Concentric contractions shorten the muscles. Let's compare a muscle contraction with a ladder. In this analogy, a fully elongated extension ladder represents a relaxed muscle fiber. A muscle contraction shortens the ladder as the rungs slide over one another. As parts of the ladder overlap, it thickens as it shortens; so does a muscle fiber in concentric contraction. Pulling apart the extension pieces once again lengthens (or relaxes) the ladder (or muscle fiber). Pulling a ladder apart or pushing it together requires work, as does moving a muscle to flex a joint.

ECCENTRIC CONTRACTION

Another common type of muscle contraction is an *eccentric* contraction that lengthens the muscle. It is used to overcome the pull of gravity as a limb supports a horse's full weight. Extensor muscles protect joints from overflexion and damage. A horse that travels down a steep hill uses eccentric muscle efforts to slow the descent.

ISOMETRIC CONTRACTION

Some muscle fibers do not change length with contraction. If the length remains the same because of an opposing pull from another muscle, this is called an *isometric* contraction. Isometric contractions occur in a horse that is on the verge of moving. For example, a roping or event horse that is tensely poised in the start box, or a racehorse ready at the gate, is using isometric contraction. A cutting horse, when hunkered down anticipating movement of a calf, is also using a form of isometric contraction.

Food for Muscle Energy

A horse involved in a rigorous conditioning and training program must be fueled with high-energy food. Food becomes fuel for everyday living and normal biological functions, as well as for hard-working muscle. The main types of fuel derived from food are carbohydrates, fats, and proteins. Protein is a metabolically expensive food source to generate energy. It costs more energy to metabolize than other food fuels, while at the same time creating little energy for working muscles as compared to carbohydrates and fats. Its use as a muscle fuel therefore has limited application to an adequately fed performance athlete. The most important fuels for working muscles are derived from carbohydrates and fats.

Muscle Fuels

GLUCOSE AND GLYCOGEN

Glucose is obtained from digestion of carbohydrate sources such as grain, hay, and forage. Glucose enters the circulation and is either used immediately by muscle tissue to produce energy, or is stored as *glycogen* in skeletal muscle and in the liver. Glycogen is a connected chain of glucose sugar molecules. To be used by muscle cells, stored glycogen must be broken back down into sugar molecules.

FATTY ACIDS

Fiber from hay and other sources of roughage is digested in the large intestine to form *volatile fatty acids,* or VFAs (see p. 292). Because VFAs provide less than 10 percent of the energy requirement of resting muscle, working muscle needs a more rapidly available source of fuel for performance. Energy is obtained from glucose and fatty acids that are absorbed into the bloodstream following digestion of food from the intestinal tract. Blood glucose is readily available for working muscle to use; however, there is a limited supply because insulin drives glucose into the liver and muscle cells following a meal.

Fat from dietary sources (such as vegetable oil or rice bran) is digested, and formed into *triglycerides*. VFAs that are not needed immediately to fuel muscles are stored in fat reserves *(adipose tissue)* as triglycerides. (A triglyceride is composed of 1 molecule of glycerol joined to 3 molecules of fatty acid.) When a horse needs more fuel, triglycerides are released from the adipose tissue into the bloodstream, and then they are called *free fatty acids*. Exercise improves the ability of muscle to use stored fat reserves. (For more discussion of feeding fat, see chapter 12, *The Digestive System: Nutritional Management,* p. 330.)

Energy Production

MUSCLES PRODUCE ENERGY

For a muscle to provide locomotion, it must contract, which requires energy. And, it must relax, which requires even more energy. Muscles cannot store enough energy for more than a few seconds of forceful contractions. Using glucose and fatty acids, muscle cells produce and consume millions of energy molecules called ATP *(adenosine triphosphate)*. An ATP energy molecule consists of an amino acid attached to 3 phosphate molecules. To create energy, muscle enzymes break apart the bond between two of these phosphate molecules. This action creates energy for muscle contraction. What remains is ADP *(adenosine diphosphate,* an amino acid attached to 2 phosphate molecules) plus the unattached, free phosphate molecule.

To produce more ATP energy molecules, the above process is reversed. Muscle cells use glycogen and fatty acids as fuels to reattach a free phosphate molecule onto an ADP, creating ATP. These processes occur within the muscle cells thousands of times every microsecond. Without fuel, phosphate molecules cannot be reattached. ATP would not be formed, so there would be no phosphate bond to break, and no energy for muscle contraction.

METABOLISM

As muscle fibers contract and relax, they consume large amounts of energy. The processes of energy production and consumption are called metabolism. How the muscles produce and consume energy distinguishes certain muscle fiber types from each other. There are two basic types of muscle metabolism: *aerobic* metabolism uses oxygen to produce energy, while *anaerobic* metabolism proceeds in the absence of oxygen.

Aerobic Metabolism

Aerobic metabolism means the muscle cells burn fuels using oxygen and enzymes to produce energy. Both fuels, glycogen and fatty acids, can be used in aerobic metabolism. This form of metabolism is the most efficient way of producing energy because fuel substrates (basic food components that are broken into energy molecules by metabolism) are "burned" completely and without generation of toxic by-products. Muscle cells that function in the presence of oxygen produce energy in specialized cellular "factories" called *mitochondria*. Mitochondria break down energy sources of fatty acids and glycogen to form energy along with by-products of carbon dioxide and water. These by-products are harmless to the tissues and are easily transported from muscle by the circulatory system.

The complexity of the aerobic metabolic process only permits slow production of energy. With more rigorous exertional demand on the muscles, energy must be generated more quickly, using anaerobic metabolism.

Anaerobic Metabolism

In the absence of oxygen, energy is created rapidly through an anaerobic pathway. Anaerobic metabolism produces energy faster but less efficiently than aerobic metabolism. While 36 molecules of ATP are created by aerobic metabolism for every molecule of fuel substrate consumed, only 2 molecules of ATP are produced by anaerobic metabolism. In addition, anaerobic metabolism produces by-products of heat and lactic acid.

Fatty acids cannot be "burned" anaerobically, but glycogen can be used through either the aerobic or anaerobic pathways. There are two types of anaerobic metabolism, each using a different fuel: *phosphocreatine* or glycogen.

Sudden, High Intensity Work

The first type of anaerobic metabolism occurs as a horse accelerates with a burst of speed as from a starting gate or roping box. During an initial energy burst at the start of an exertion, muscles are fueled by *phosphocreatine*. High-energy phosphocreatine supports high intensity work required of sprint acceleration or jumping efforts. Breaking apart the bonds of each phosphocreatine molecule provides energy; this process does not require oxygen. It also does not produce toxic by-products. But it can only support efforts lasting a few seconds.

Although great thrust and rapid speed are possible when muscles are fueled by phosphocreatine, its supply is extremely limited. After several seconds, muscle supply of phosphocreatine is depleted; the muscles then depend on aerobic metabolism or the second type of anaerobic metabolism for continued sprint performance. Phosphocreatine is replenished in about 3 minutes, but by then the sprint activity (such as Quarter Horse racing, calf roping, or barrel racing) is finished. Neither conditioning nor dietary strategies can increase phosphocreatine stores in the muscles.

Lack of Oxygen During Strenuous Work

A second form of anaerobic metabolism occurs when a horse cannot breathe in enough oxygen to support strenuous work. Muscle enzymes break down glycogen into energy in the absence of oxygen. The toxic by-product of this type of anaerobic metabolism is lactic acid, which if produced in excessive amounts will depress enzyme systems and limit the amount of ATP that is produced (see p. 147). With a limited energy supply available for contraction, muscles rapidly fatigue and performance suffers.

CONSERVING GLYCOGEN

Fatty Acids versus Glycogen

Fatty acids, both VFAs and free fatty acids, are more efficient at generating ATP energy molecules than glycogen, which is why fatty acids are the preferred fuel for muscle contraction. A fat-supplemented diet improves the efficiency of energy production within muscles during exercise.

Using Fatty Acids as Fuel

Energy stored in a horse's fat depots is 30 times greater than all the glycogen reserves found in the skeletal muscles and liver. The primary benefit of aerobic conditioning is that it promotes the use of fatty acids as an energy source. Fatty acids are released into the bloodstream from adipose tissue storage, and carried to the muscles for fuel. The metabolism of fatty acids conserves glycogen stores and delays muscle fatigue so a horse can perform for a longer time without accumulating *lactic acid*. An aerobically trained horse can better convert fatty acids into energy instead of using glycogen as fuel.

However, fatty acids cannot provide an exclusive energy source because their rate of uptake by muscle tissue is limited. In situations where exercise demand intensifies or oxygen supplies decrease, then the muscles must rely on glycogen as a fuel source. Depletion of glycogen reserves leads to exhaustion. This lack is what ultimately limits an endurance athlete's performance.

Increasing the fat stores in the horse by allowing it to gain weight does not improve a body's ability to use fatty acids for energy production. Only aerobic conditioning can accomplish this goal. In fact, extra body weight is detrimental because a horse uses more energy to carry the extra weight around, and a layer of stored fat prevents heat dissipation from working muscles. Both of these factors lead to fatigue.

Increased Glycogen Storage

Not only do a horse's muscles learn through conditioning to more efficiently metabolize fatty acids as an energy source, but conditioning also creates more glycogen stores in the muscles. Glycogen reserves may increase as much as 33 percent over a 10-week conditioning period.

USE OF ENERGY

Working muscle does not exclusively use a single energy form; however, the longer the muscles can use fatty acids to fuel exercise, the more glycogen is spared for later use, and the longer fatigue is delayed. Depending on blood circulation and oxygen supply in the muscles at any given moment, fats or carbohydrates (fatty acids, glucose, and glycogen) will be used as needed. Oxygen supply depends on the horse's level of fitness and the type of activity. Some sports are primarily aerobic, others are primarily anaerobic, and some depend on interplay between the two types of metabolism.

Endurance Type Activities: Aerobic Metabolism

Endurance type sports consist of prolonged activity at steady, moderate paces of walk, trot, and slow canter averaging 8 to 12 mph. Horses involved in these activities primarily use aerobic metabolism, relying on fatty acids and glycogen as energy sources. They include:

- Dressage
- Pleasure and competitive trail riding events
- Endurance riding
- Combined driving
- Roads and tracks phase of eventing
- Hunter classes
- Show pleasure and performance classes
- Show equitation

Sprint Type Activities: Anaerobic Metabolism

Sprint type activities demand intense efforts of short duration (up to 1 minute) at or near maximum speed. A horse depends heavily on anaerobic metabolism during a short sprint. The muscles are fueled from sources that do not require oxygen for metabolism, such as glycogen and phosphocreatine. Examples of sprint activities include:

- Calf roping
- Barrel racing
- Quarter Horse racing

Combination Activities

Many activities involve both aerobic and anaerobic metabolism. A combination of endurance and sprint activities include:

- Reining
- Cross-country phase of eventing
- Show jumping
- Cutting
- Flat racing
- Harness racing
- Steeplechasing
- Polo

In combination activities, portions of each effort depend on anaerobic metabolism using the phosphocreatine method of immediate energy production. As the activity progresses, a horse relies on aerobic metabolism of fatty acids and glycogen. When aerobic metabolism is no longer sufficient for energy needs or bursts of speed or effort, anaerobic metabolism again comes into play, using glycogen for fuel. These processes happen simultaneously in the muscles but at any one point in an event a horse may depend more on one form of muscle metabolism than another.

Muscle Fiber Types

Three types of muscle fibers are found in skeletal muscle:

- Slow twitch high oxidative, or ST, or Type I
- Fast twitch high oxidative, or FTH, or Type II A
- Fast twitch low oxidative, or FT, or Type II B

Slow Twitch High Oxidative Muscle Fibers

Postural needs and low intensity exercise rely on recruitment of Type I muscle fibers which are also known as *slow twitch high oxidative* (ST) muscle fibers. This muscle fiber type is a more slowly contracting and more slowly relaxing muscle tissue than the *fast twitch* fibers. ST muscle fibers have a greater resistance to fatigue, but are dependent on an abundant oxygen supply. ST muscle cells contain large numbers of *mitochondria,* the energy-producing factories within the cells that require oxygen to convert fuels to energy for sustained contractions. Also, lipids are stored within Type I fibers, contributing to the efficiency of using fat as an energy source for aerobic work.

The diameter of the ST muscle cells is smaller than other muscle types, enabling more blood and oxygen to reach these cells. Due to a greater number of capillaries within ST fibers, this type of muscle tissue appears red. A protein called *myoglobin* that readily binds oxygen for use by the mitochondria imparts this color. Arabians have a large preponderance of slow twitch muscle tissue compared to other breeds like Thoroughbreds, Standardbreds, Quarter Horses, or Warmbloods. This is one reason why Arabian horses are well suited to the demands of long distance work. Such highly oxygenated muscle tissue is capable of prolonged and sustained contraction, using fats and glycogen as energy to fuel locomotion in the presence of oxygen in the tissues. These slow contracting fibers are most often found deep within the muscle belly.

Fast Twitch High Oxidative Muscle Fibers

Most skeletal muscle is composed of all types of muscle fibers to enable a coordinated and gradated contraction as work demands increase. With the need for faster speed, more tension is necessary to supply adequate power to each muscular contraction, so a different muscle fiber type, Type II A, is then recruited. These are also referred to as *fast twitch high oxidative* (FTH) fibers. Such muscle tissue type is located more superficially within a muscle group. As an intermediate form, these muscle fibers contract more quickly than ST fibers, but not as quickly as Type II B or *fast twitch low oxidative* (FT) fibers.

Fast Twitch Low Oxidative Muscle Fibers

During periods of effort involving rapid acceleration, jumping, or maximal speeds such as experienced in racing, steeplechase, or sprinting activities, Type II B fibers will be recruited. These are glycolytic fibers that depend strictly upon anaerobic metabolism. Initially, Type II A high oxidative fibers will fire, then the Type II B glycolytic fibers will come into play. Type II B fibers shorten ten times more quickly than ST fibers. There is a price to pay for improved mechanical power that imparts short bursts of speed: at maximal output, muscle looses its metabolic and locomotor efficiency, and it fatigues rapidly.

Measuring Fiber Types with a Muscle Biopsy

Attempts have been made to measure a horse's athletic potential by evaluating a muscle biopsy. A core sample of tissue taken from the middle gluteal muscle of the hip should give a representative sampling of the types of muscle fibers present in an individual. Proponents of this tool feel that muscle biopsy profiles may select horses with a high proportion of Type I and Type II A fibers. However, elite talent in a horse is determined by a multitude of factors (see p. 3), so reliance on a muscle biopsy profile is misleading as to a horse's true performance abilities. Also, with training, muscles can be conditioned for optimum performance for specific athletic disciplines to allow even the least genetically gifted animals to develop a competitive edge.

Response of Skeletal Muscle to Exercise

General Training Responses

IMPROVING NEUROMUSCULAR REFLEXES

Conditioning improves neuromuscular reflexes, which in turn improves muscle coordination and efficiency of motion. Muscles work together to prevent strain on a muscle, or damage to a joint. To prevent excessive exertion and damage in early stages of conditioning, *agonist* muscles have opposing *antagonist* muscles to counteract them. For example, as an agonist flexor muscle flexes a joint, an antagonist extensor muscle opposes it. This system protects muscle movement to remain within a safe range (fig. 6.1).

A young, awkward horse does not always possess fine-tuned coordination of the agonists working in concert with the antagonist muscles. If too much demand in the form of speed or distance is placed on an undeveloped musculoskeletal system, an unfit horse becomes muscle sore and is at risk of ligament or tendon damage as the muscle groups work contrary to one another. Repetitive exercises coordinate movement and improve neural signals to the muscles over time.

NUMBERS OF MUSCLE FIBERS

A horse's muscles may appear bulkier as he develops condition. This is created by a training-induced *hyperplasia* of the muscle, meaning the numbers of muscle fibers increase, rather than an increase in the size of individual fibers. A larger cross-sectional area of the fiber is an advantage for a galloping horse as it imparts greater maximal force output to give speed, acceleration, and increased stride length. Bulkier muscle that is achieved by an increase in cross-sectional area of the muscle fibers limits oxygen delivery to muscle cells, and so would be a disadvantage to a distance horse.

Muscles adapt to the type of stress applied to them. A horse that exclusively performs aerobic exercises does not build power or bulk in muscle. An example of the effect of aerobic exercise is the flat muscling typical of Arabian endurance horses. Aerobic exercises are low resistance but highly repetitive, like trotting along a level trail at the same rhythm and speed for miles. This exercise improves stamina, neuromuscular precision, and economy of movement. Range of movement and muscle elasticity also improve. Slow twitch fibers benefit from aerobic conditioning by improving their use of oxygen.

Aerobic Skeletal Muscle Adaptations

SIZE OF MUSCLE FIBERS

One of the most widely adaptable tissues in the body is skeletal muscle. It is capable of responding to training over time. The most noticeable changes over time are appreciated in muscles of horses that start in an untrained state rather than those already seasoned.

For a young horse, over 80 percent of his growth occurs in the first 18 to 24 months, with 70 percent of muscle-fiber size achieved by the time the horse is a long yearling (about 18 months old). A mature horse achieves minimal increase in muscle-fiber area with aerobic training. Aerobic training stimulates the higher oxidative muscle-fiber types such as ST and FTH, which have smaller cross-sectional areas. This characteristic provides an advantage to a distance horse since the smaller the cross-sectional area of each muscle fiber, the easier it is for blood and oxygen to reach the fibers and for metabolic waste products to be removed through the circulation.

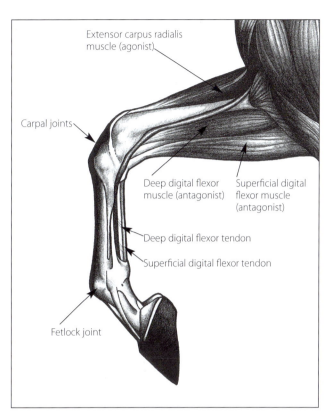

6.1 *Each muscle is attached to bone by some fibrous component, either tendon or fascia. As a muscle contracts, the skeleton moves due to muscular tension applied to the tendon or fascial attachment point where it inserts on bone. As an agonist flexor muscle flexes a joint, an antagonist extensor muscle opposes it to prevent overflexion. Similarly, as an agonist extensor muscle extends a joint, an antagonist flexor muscle prevents hyperextension.*

FIBER TYPE CONVERSION

During aerobic training, the proportion of Type II A (fast twitch high oxidative) muscle fibers may increase although there is a limited transformation (up to 7 percent) of Type II B (fast twitch low oxidative) to Type II A. Some studies speculate that the proportion of Type I (ST or slow twitch high oxidative) fibers changes dramatically either from transformation of Type II A to Type I fibers or because there is a loss of Type II fibers with age.

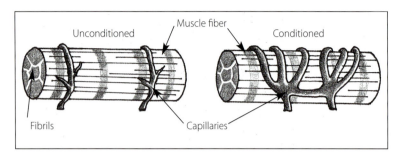

6.2 *With conditioning, capillaries enlarge in size and number within the muscle beds to bring more oxygen to the tissues.*

METABOLIC CAPACITY FOR AEROBIC EXERCISE

Training accomplishes its best effect by stimulating an increase in the oxidative capacity within muscle. Well-conditioned muscle increases its aerobic enzyme activity over twofold from where it started in an untrained condition. Mitochondria increase in volume density. More capillaries develop within the muscle beds to bring more oxygen to the tissues (fig. 6.2). Although the proportion of muscle-fiber types is a genetic feature, it can be modified slightly with training. The proportion of Type II A relative to Type II B fibers may increase, giving a greater proportion of FTH fibers with greater resistance to fatigue.

Oxidative changes occur quickly during the first few months of training with most metabolic changes peaking during the first 1 to 2 years of training. With improved aerobic capacity of the muscles, more efficient production of ATP energy molecules is forthcoming to sustain aerobic work. Also, a horse's muscles improve in their capacity to use free fatty acids during submaximal (aerobic) endurance exercise, thus having a glycogen-sparing effect. This is once again attributed to the enhanced production and activity of metabolic enzymes appropriate to aerobic exercise.

While all these changes develop on a microscopic level, the muscles improve in their ability to store glycogen for energy. This becomes critical for the demands of long distance performance, and is especially important at longer durations of distance competitions where the longer that glycogen stores can be retained, the greater will be a horse's resistance to fatigue.

Sustained Aerobic Exercise

With sustained submaximal activity, exercising muscle relies on free fatty acids derived from intestinal breakdown of fiber as well as glycogen stores in liver and muscle to fuel locomotion. As aerobic efforts persist in endurance-type events, liver stores of glycogen become depleted, unable to support ATP turnover that is needed to utilize lipid stores or to oxidize free fatty acids. Plenty of fat may still be available as an energy substrate, but the muscles may not be able to make use of it with the depletion of glycogen.

As glycogen stores diminish, more muscle fiber types are necessarily recruited. Initially Type I and Type II A fibers maintain low intensity work; then progressively all fiber types are recruited as others fatigue. Muscle glycogen supplies are used up and then the horse is only capable of very low intensity exercise fueled by free fatty acids within oxidative fibers. In such an instance, a horse demonstrates serious performance deterioration, leading to exhaustion.

IMPROVING HEAT DISSIPATION

Biochemical reactions that burn fuels for energy also produce heat as a by-product. Conditioning improves a horse's sweating mechanisms to efficiently dissipate heat from the working muscles. Reducing heat buildup further delays the onset of fatigue. (For more discussion, refer to "Skin's Role in Thermoregulation" in chapter 13, *The Skin as an Organ*, p. 355.)

Anaerobic Skeletal Muscle Adaptations

Anaerobic exercises are high resistance efforts with fewer repetitions, lasting up to 30 seconds. Short, brisk gallops or rapid, hill climbs are examples of anaerobic drills. During each intense exercise, muscles are quickly depleted of stored energy, and then rested between bouts. Such exercises increase the bulk and substance of fast twitch muscle fibers.

At almost all intensities of exercise, a horse eventually dips into anaerobic metabolism using Type II A and Type II B fibers, with the production of lactate (or lactic acid) as a by-product. Higher speeds or protracted exertions generate more of this material. Usually at low intensity aerobic exercise, there is little rise in blood lactate since its removal remains comparable to its rate of production. Under normal situations, the circulation removes lactic acid to the liver where it is converted to glucose. Glucose is then delivered by the bloodstream to working muscles; there it is used as an energy source. When the rate of production of lactic acid exceeds its rate of removal, blood lactate levels rise to levels exceeding 4 mmol (millimoles) per liter in the bloodstream. This is referred to as the *anaerobic threshold* or the limit of a horse's *aerobic capacity*. The point at which this occurs depends on the fitness of the horse, the terrain over which he is working, the duration of the effort, and the climatic conditions. In sports of prolonged exercise duration, heat and humidity greatly increase the risk of dehydration, electrolyte depletion, excess tissue temperature, and energy depletion.

INCREASED MUSCLE MASS

Anaerobic conditioning builds muscle mass because the cross-sectional areas of the fast twitch muscle fibers increase to improve muscle strength and power. Increased cross-sectional area of muscle fibers creates strength for the fast, explosive acceleration so vital to a successful sprint horse. An increase in the area of each individual fiber increases muscle mass as a whole. Most affected are the hip and thigh muscles, the chest, and the forearm muscles. For example, compare the heavy muscling of a Quarter Horse to the lean, flat muscling of an Arabian. The large hindquarter muscles of a Quarter Horse athlete develop from anaerobic muscle conditioning in addition to genetics.

LACTIC ACID TOLERANCE

During intense bursts of exercise, anaerobic metabolism of muscle glycogen is the main source of energy. Because energy demands increase 200-fold during these intensive exertions, the high rate of energy production provided by anaerobic metabolism is essential to a sprinting horse. During most anaerobic metabolism, glycogen is broken down into energy and lactic acid. At first, this toxic by-product is carried away from the muscle by the bloodstream. With increased energy demands, more lactic acid is produced than the circulation can remove. Lactic acid accumulation in the muscles slows energy production and weakens the contractions of muscle fibers. Accumulating lactic acid causes fatigue and muscle soreness so it is important to train the muscles to develop lactic acid tolerance.

Anaerobic training teaches a horse's muscles to tolerate the anaerobic state. Muscles learn to store more glycogen, increase in mass, develop enzyme systems to neutralize lactic acid, and produce energy from lactic acid to a small degree. Muscle tissue normally contains protein buffers that neutralize lactic acid. Sprint conditioning stimulates the production of these proteins, which increases the buffering capacity of muscle cells, and therefore delays fatigue.

Anaerobic Threshold

The *anaerobic threshold* is the point at which

lactic acid begins to accumulate in the muscles and bloodstream with blood lactate levels exceeding 4 mmol per liter. Sprint conditioning can raise the anaerobic threshold by making anaerobic energy production more efficient. It also trains specific enzyme systems to buffer, or neutralize lactic acid. Raising the anaerobic threshold delays the onset of fatigue. With a higher anaerobic threshold, a horse can travel at faster speeds or an endurance athlete can travel longer distances before excessive lactic acid accumulates in the muscles.

Using Lactic Acid as Fuel

The stamina of the sprint horse also depends on the availability of glycogen supplies. If glycogen is depleted, the muscles run out of fuel, and muscle contractions weaken. A sprint horse works so quickly and for such a brief duration that lactic acid cannot be immediately flushed from the muscles. Some of this lactic acid can be metabolized by FT Type II A muscle fibers that use oxygen to produce energy. Any lactic acid that can be converted to energy by FT Type II A fibers improves a sprint horse's stamina.

Muscle Conditioning

LONG SLOW DISTANCE TRAINING

The basis of developing the best muscular and cardiovascular endurance is dependent upon *long slow distance* (LSD) training (see p. 226). As a horse's cardiovascular system develops conditioning, the muscles respond similarly to exercise stress (see chapter 9, *Cardiovascular Conditioning and Health,* p. 225). Because muscle responds quickly to conditioning, reaching its peak within six months of strategic training, there is often a premature conclusion that a horse has reached top strength. Yet bone, tendons, ligaments, and joints take years to develop to peak (see p. 224 and fig. 9.3, p. 225). To develop the kind of strength it takes for a horse's muscles to perform over arduous jump courses, or over 50 and 100 miles of trail, or at higher levels of dressage training relies on more than aerobic conditioning techniques of long, slow distance work. Both strength-training and interval-training techniques should be applied to develop muscle.

STRENGTH TRAINING

Strength training for horses is similar to what human body builders do when lifting weights or jogging stairs. It has been demonstrated that more than 50 percent of musculoskeletal injuries in athletes may be eliminated with strength-training exercises. (For more discussion, see chapter 9, *Cardiovascular Conditioning and Health,* p. 227.)

Trail horses and jumping horses depend on strength in their rear quarters, back, and abdominal muscles to drive them up a mountain or over a jump, and to help brake them on descents. Dressage horses, reining horses, roping horses, and cutting horses require muscle strength to execute maneuvers that require agility. To best develop muscle strength and joint stability, integrate a strategy of strengthening exercises within regular training rides to elicit the appropriate response for the intended work. An effective strategy for strengthening the muscles is to work a horse up hills starting first at the walk, then gradually adding trot, and finally canter as strength improves over months of graduated demands. Increasing the speed of ascent, the steepness of the grade, or duration of climb are valuable methods to increase resistance to develop strength and cardiovascular conditioning effects (see p.150). Cantering uphill synchronizes the thrust from the hindquarters and builds strong muscles in the haunches and back.

A horse's mass, the rider, and tack provide "weight" on the end of the muscular levers. The horse must push all this against gravity, and in the process, muscles build in strength, in endurance, and in cardiovascular development. As the musculoskeletal system develops, so does the development of the circulatory system within the muscles, along with efficient use of aerobic metabolism, and improvement of the heat dissipation abilities of the skin through capillary beds (see p. 356). Eventually, over a period of months, a horse tackles the work with greater ease. Other strength-training exercises that further improve a horse's skill level include cross-training use of cavalletti work, jumping grids, and more advanced levels of dressage training. It is important to vary the work and the exercises to develop many different muscle groups. A horse should be kept even and straight beneath the rider in any riding circumstance. If one side of a horse's body is stronger than another, injury could occur in the weaker links. It is equally as important to improve a horse's flexibility with stretching exercises, both mounted and unmounted (see p. 153), and by incorporating cross-training in various disciplines. Supple muscles are at less risk of strain; this is particularly true of strong, highly developed muscles.

INTERVAL TRAINING TECHNIQUES

Either speed or more intense gradients are used to elicit an *interval* training effect to improve muscular endurance (see p. 227). This strategy pushes a horse into and past the anaerobic threshold for several minutes at a time so the fast twitch muscle fibers are recruited and learn to function efficiently despite the absence of tissue oxygen. This stage of training is usually reserved for horses in their second or third season. By then the other support systems (bone, joints, ligaments, tendons, and hooves) have reached a degree of development so that injury will less likely occur as greater speed or exercise intensity is applied.

The horse evolved as a fright-and-flight animal able to escape from predators by fast bursts of speed. Studies confirm that training specifically for intense bursts of speed does not change the metabolism of glycogen. However, conditioning does improve nerve signals, coordinating muscle movement. The rate of muscle contraction and the removal of lactic acid are also improved by anaerobic conditioning of muscles.

The technique of interval training requires a horse to exercise at fast canter or gallop speeds that bring the heart rate above 160 bpm (beats per minute), and preferably above 180 bpm. The horse need only run at this speed for a couple minutes to elicit a training effect in the tissues. A similar effect is gained by climbing very steep hills at a walk, or trotting up moderate gradients. The key is to bring a horse's heart rate beyond the point of the anaerobic threshold for a short period of time. This point differs for each horse, but generally is a heart rate greater than 160 to165 bpm. Once an interval "sprint" is incorporated into the workouts, the horse should be allowed to recover by slowing the pace or intensity for at least four times as long as the period of time he had been asked to accelerate his heart rate. The fast/intense exercise is repeated for a few minutes again, followed by sufficient recovery time. As a horse gets more accustomed to this kind of work, interval training can be interspersed periodically within a workout to amplify training of the muscles and the cardiovascular system.

As with any exercise session, a horse should be warmed up sufficiently before starting intervals. Similarly, an appropriate cool down period is important (see "Warm-Up and Cool-Down Strategies," p. 153). Use of a heart rate monitor assists in achieving a level of effort within the anaerobic range, and allows accurate tracking of a horse's recoveries (see chapter 9, *Cardiovascular Conditioning and Health*, p. 222).

Muscle Exercises

RESISTANCE

As an example of the effect of resistance on muscles, consider the development of a horse's neck muscles as he is trained to accept bit contact. With the neck in a normal, relaxed position, the nuchal ligament stretching from the poll to the withers passively assumes the load of the head. The muscles along the top of the neck are not stressed when the neck is in a relaxed position. When a horse is asked to accept bit contact, his neck and head arch and activate those muscles on the top of the neck. The head acts as a "weight" to provide some resistance to the exercise. The horse then actively holds his head and neck with muscular effort rather than by passive support from the ligaments. Continual exercise of the neck muscles develops them over time and bulks up the neck.

Faster Gaits

To increase the resistance of anaerobic exercise, add a faster gait to the muscle-training period. For example, trotting up a hill places more demand on muscle tissues than walking up a hill.

Hill Work

An inclined grade or a hill challenges and strengthens body muscle. The resistance of a horse's body weight as he climbs a hill develops hind leg, forearm, and shoulder muscles. Walking or trotting a hill develops independent muscles in each hind leg.

As the horse accelerates into a canter or gallop, he propels himself forward by pushing off the ground with both hind legs at about the same time. A hill climb in a canter or gallop exercises the hind legs as a unit, with considerable strain on the rump and back muscles. These muscles strengthen accordingly.

Downhill work strengthens pectoral, shoulder, and forearm muscles, while braking strengthens the quadriceps muscles in the hind legs. Hill work has more advantages besides muscle strengthening. A horse gains as much training effect on the muscles and cardiovascular system doing a hill climb as he would covering three times the distance on flat ground. Bones and joints receive less impact stress with hill work than with flatwork, which attempts to reach the same heart rate by increasing speed.

Deep Footing

Exercise in deep footing, like sand, snow, or a spongy meadow, creates resistance in thigh and pectoral muscles. Mud is not a good medium for resistance training as it can cause tendon injuries and even bone fractures. If mud is incorporated into a training routine, restrict exercise to the walk, never trot or canter. Slow and careful conditioning accustoms a horse to deep footing, preventing tendon strain.

BENEFITS OF CROSS-TRAINING

Sprint work benefits endurance performance by improving the efficiency of the fast twitch fibers. These fibers contribute to the staying power of a horse as eventually he depletes aerobic fuel supplies and resorts to the recruitment of FT fibers.

Endurance conditioning benefits a sprint horse by improving aerobic metabolism, which reduces the horse's dependency on anaerobic energy production. Then, less lactic acid is produced. In addition, aerobic conditioning develops the capillary beds and circulation to improve efficiency of lactic acid removal. Aerobic conditioning increases muscle glycogen stores. This is beneficial to a sprint horse as he relies almost exclusively on glycogen metabolism for energy.

An abundance of equestrian disciplines provides a variety of exercises to develop and strengthen muscles. Long rides stretch and supple muscles, teach balance and rhythm, and strengthen all body systems. Negotiating obstacles such as cavalletti poles teaches precision through a gymnastic routine. The even footing of a track is excellent for speed workouts. Cross-training builds a versatile and durable athlete.

SPORT-SPECIFIC STRENGTHENING EXERCISES

Dressage

Combining *calisthenics* (developing muscular tone) with strength training improves the back, belly, and hind leg muscles in a dressage horse, enabling him to perform precision movements with ease. Work the horse on bit contact and in a dressage frame, and then allow him to relax and stretch between difficult exercises. Repetitive practice and correct execution of advanced movements of half-pass, piaffe, passage, and pirouettes strengthen associated muscles. Trotting over cavalletti teaches rhythm and balance, and teaches the horse to work with his hocks up and under his body. Cantering over 2-foot fences spaced one stride apart encourages simultaneous hind leg use, developing croup and back muscles. Downhill walking also teaches a horse to balance with his hindquarters, an important element of collected work.

Jumping

A jumping horse not only propels off the ground with strong hindquarter muscles, but the landing exerts considerable force on shoulder and neck muscles. These horses benefit especially from hill climbs at a canter, with slower downhills to rest the muscles between strengthening exercises. Cavalletti work, gymnastic grids, and dressage exercises additionally strengthen hindquarter muscles.

Reining

A reining horse executes sudden stops and rollbacks, and benefits from exercises that strengthen muscles over the croup and back. These muscles tuck the hindquarters beneath the body for abrupt changes in direction. Besides practicing sliding stops and spins, a reining horse may benefit from hill work at a canter or slow gallop to build buttock muscles. Downhill walking improves balance and coordination. Exercise in deep footing strengthens thigh muscles.

Cutting

A cutting horse relies on strength in the shoulder and chest muscles, as well as buttock and thigh muscles that enable him to move quickly in front of a calf. Hill work, both ascents and descents, exercises all these muscles, and provides a break from the mental pressure that comes from persistent cutting practice.

"Detraining" the Muscles

Once a horse has reached a peak level of tolerating a specific exercise demand, training intensity can be reduced. The objective is to maintain a horse within a required level of fitness with a minimum of conditioning time; this saves his musculoskeletal structures from too much wear and tear. For aerobic disciplines, this means exercising the horse at his skill level 2 to 3 times a week. For distance sports, this means a horse needs only be ridden twice a week, with one of those rides being a longish distance, maybe 15 to 20 miles. A third ride that week could be a shorter distance, maybe 6 to 10 miles, at a faster speed. For any athletic discipline, light exercise once or twice a week is usually sufficient to retain musculoskeletal strength. Several weeks of rest following a competition or rigorous work will not reduce muscle strength or stamina. Usually a rested horse comes back to work stronger and full of enthusiasm.

It is not uncommon for there to be a lengthy interruption in a horse's conditioning program either due to a rider's busy schedule, a musculoskeletal injury, or adverse weather conditions. Horses don't "detrain" as rapidly as people. A layup of 4 to 6 weeks shouldn't pose an obstacle for bringing a horse rapidly back to his previous level of condition, assuming he was fit to begin with. Metabolic muscle adaptations are maintained for at least 5 to 6 weeks. The enhanced oxidative enzymes achieved with conditioning won't decline to pretraining level until a horse has been idle for about 3 months. A longer layup will require rehabilitation strategies to counteract decline of muscle strength and cardiovascular conditioning. Rehabilitation of an idle horse relies on application of basic conditioning principles of long, slow distance training to bring him back to work. If plagued by a specific injury, specific physical and medical therapies are also implemented. Usually, the time necessary for recovery from a mild injury does not cause a horse much loss in ability or competitive edge. A general rule suggests that following a month's layup, a horse should receive a month's conditioning for every succeeding idle month.

Monitoring Muscular Efficiency: Tools and Tests

Thermistor

While the heart rate monitor is an essential tool to both cardiovascular and muscular conditioning, the use of a *thermistor* assists in determining internal temperature of the working muscles (see p. 362). The thermistor sensor pad is placed on the skin just beneath the front of the saddle. Skin temperature is displayed on a digital readout on a box that is attached to the saddle. As a horse begins to overheat due to excess exertional demands or extreme environmental conditions, the skin temperature will exceed 101 to 102° F (38 to 39° C) as the working muscles strive to dissipate heat through the skin with sweating. Elevation in skin temperature is a signal that it is time to back down on speed and/or intensity of the horse's exercise. Skin temperature less than 97° F (36° C) also warns of impending problems with dehydration or poor circulation to the periphery.

Blood Lactate

Measuring blood lactate levels (see p. 458) is not a specific test for a horse exercising at submaximal (aerobic) demands since levels of circulating lactic acid in the bloodstream generally occur only with anaerobic work. Distance horses, dressage horses, and pleasure horses achieve optimal locomotor efficiency when able to maintain submaximal output of aerobic exercise. Continued sweating that occurs with protracted endurance-type exercise amplifies the loss of electrolytes (particularly potassium and chloride) with the potential to develop *metabolic alkalosis*, an aberration in the acid-base status that also has adverse effects on muscle function. This is the opposite effect to lactic acid buildup during anaerobic work in other intensive athletic disciplines, such as polo, track racing, steeplechase, timber racing, or endurance races at gallop speeds.

Warm-Up and Cool-Down Strategies

The horse is naturally designed for short bursts of speed to flee from predators. In the wild, this flight response need not be sustained for more than a few moments. Today, horses are asked to perform for extended periods at a maximal level of work. Many equine sports require fast bursts of speed combined with abrupt stops and turns, or jumping over obstacles while carrying a rider. Other sports involve long hours of steady work under saddle with infrequent rest periods. Just as with human athletes, a horse needs to limber up and stretch before beginning a workout.

To prevent injury, each workout should include a routine of warm-ups and cool-downs before and after exercise. Muscles, ligaments, and tendons should be properly prepared for the demands of athletic exertion. This preparation involves at least 15 to 20 minutes of warm-up to stimulate blood circulation to the tissues, and to slightly raise body temperature a few degrees. Warmth and circulation improve the flexibility of the musculoskeletal system, improving efficiency of muscle work and reducing the risk of injury to ligaments, tendons, and joints.

Warm-Up Exercises

WALKING
Walking is a preliminary exercise to gradually increase the respiratory rate and heart rate, flushing the muscles with blood and oxygen. Walking lightly stretches tendons and ligaments to improve their elasticity as the tissues heat up from movement. Joints are also warmed and lubricated.

Walking can be done under saddle, in hand, on a longe line, or by using a hotwalker. Brisk walking for 5 to 10 minutes sufficiently prepares the musculoskeletal system for more work.

TROTTING
After walking, the horse can then be trotted for another 5 to 10 minutes to further warm the muscles, and to stretch tendons and ligaments. Urge the horse forward at a vigorous pace to improve the respiratory intake of oxygen and to accelerate the heart rate. These physiologic changes allow the musculoskeletal system to handle increased stress.

MANUAL STRETCHING EXERCISES
A light warm-up, such as walking in hand for about 5 minutes, should precede stretch exercises. Once the muscles, tendons, and ligaments are warm, manual stretching exercises add flexibility and suppleness. If a muscle is stretched 100 percent of its functional length before contraction, the strength of the muscle contraction achieves maximum efficiency. Most horses are trained at a muscle exertion of only 60 percent of maximum contraction length, leading to tight, rigid muscle with diminished range of motion. Sudden loading of a short, tight, and inelastic musculotendinous unit may tear muscle or tendon fibers. (Much like an unbraided rope, tendons are made up of fibers that are arranged in tightly packed alignment parallel to each other.) To maximize muscle and tendon elasticity, apply stretching exercises in both warm-ups and cool-downs.

During a stretch, maintain each limb in a slightly flexed position to avoid strain to the tendons and ligaments of the lower leg. Grasp the limb above the carpus (knee) or just below the hock. Each pull should be concentrated above the carpus or hock for a greater range of motion in the shoulder or hip joints and their associated muscles. Each limb is stretched with gentle traction, allowing the weight of the horse's leg to attain the stretch while the horse relaxes. Do not force the stretch. Ask the horse to passively "let go" in response to a gentle tug. A hold of 10 to 20 seconds is usually suffi-

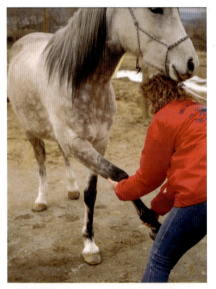

6.3 *One stretch relies on pulling the front leg forward and across the body toward the other front leg, then gently to the outside, and then backward toward the hind legs. Each stretch is held for 10 to 20 seconds, whereupon the limb is returned to the ground between each repetition or direction change.*

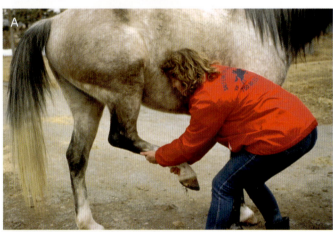

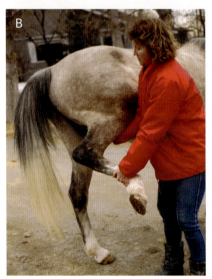

6.4 A & B *A hind limb stretch also includes gentle traction of the limb toward the horse's front legs to release extensor muscles and tendons (A), then the hip and upper leg is gently pulled to the side (B).*

cient, with repetition of the stretch 3 times, allowing for rest in between. It may take several days of practice for a horse to become accustomed to the strange feel of these stretches without resisting.

Forelegs

Pick up each front leg individually and gently pull it forward to stretch the shoulder and forearm muscles. Then ease the limb forward and across the body toward the other foreleg (photo 6.3). Also pull the leg gently to the outside, and then backward toward the hind legs.

Hind Legs

Hind leg stretches are similar to foreleg stretches. Each hind leg is first stretched directly behind the horse, then toward the opposite hind leg. The hip and upper leg are then stretched forward toward the front legs, and finally gently tugged out to the side (photos 6.4 A & B).

Neck and Back Stretches

A long, downward stretch of the head and neck can be accomplished by making the horse reach down for a carrot or other treat. This stretch loosens the back and loins, while the horse also relaxes mentally (photos 6.5 and 6.6). Sideways stretches can be achieved by offering carrots to the horse's side or flanks, with the carrot held at mouth level. Hold a carrot beneath a horse's belly at the same time you apply a *belly lift* so the horse stretches his neck while the back is raised; this prevents jamming of the lower neck region. Gentle pressure with the hands or tickling a horse along his abdominal midline encourages lifting of his back. Back massage prior to asking for belly lifts improves favorable effects. When applying stretches to rehabilitation of an injury, be careful not to overuse these techniques as they could worsen a horse's discomfort and irritate healing tissues.

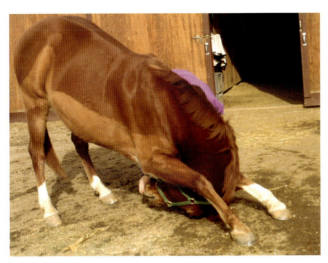
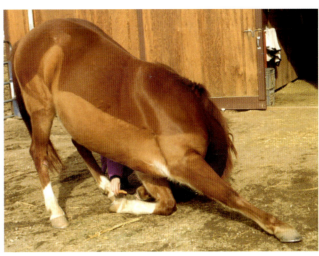

6.5 Asking a horse to reach for a carrot or treat helps to stretch his head, neck, and loins.

6.6 Reaching down and to his side for a carrot releases and stretches neck and head tissues. Remember to ask your horse to reach on both sides.

MOUNTED SUPPLING EXERCISES

While mounted, relax the horse's neck and back muscles by bending the head and neck to the side (toward the rider's leg) with a slight jiggle of the rein. This technique softens the poll and jaw as the horse gives to the rein (photo 6.7). Then, stretch him through his neck and topline by asking him to yield in the bridle, and touch his nose to his chest (photo 6.8). Asking the horse to move in circles, figure-eight patterns, and serpentine patterns requires the horse to step under the body with the inside rear leg; this stretches the back and haunches.

Lateral exercises, such as leg-yields or sidepasses supple the poll, neck, shoulders, back, and haunches (photo 6.9). The horse gradually begins to actively carry himself by using muscle groups in concert.

LONG-TERM BENEFITS

Stretching and suppling exercises have more long-term benefits than just the immediate

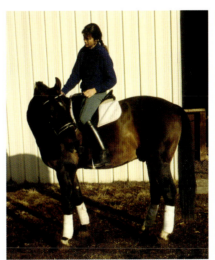
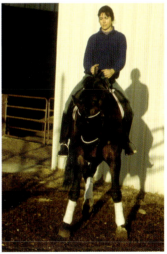

6.7 One effective mounted suppling exercise gently asks your horse to touch your boot with his nose. This bend helps relax his jaw, neck, poll, and back.

6.8 Another mounted suppling exercise asks the horse to touch his chest with his nose. This is accomplished by jiggling the reins a little, asking him to relax his jaw, and then as he gives to repeated nudges, his poll, neck, and back also stretch and relax.

improvement of tissue elasticity. Daily application of stretching exercises both before and after exercise ultimately:

- Develops a longer stride as a horse's shoulders move with greater freedom
- Improves the range of motion in both shoulder and hip muscles to facilitate lateral movements
- Improves flexibility in the upper limbs, reducing the risk of injury during stressful demands
- Minimizes fatigue because muscles and joints are pliable
- Improves circulation to all the tissues, requiring less effort during a warm-up and conserving energy for athletic exertion

SPORT-SPECIFIC WARM-UP

The entire warm-up process, exploring all varieties of stretching and suppling exercises, can take as long as 30 minutes. As the warm-up intensifies after the first 20 minutes, a jumping horse might be asked to trot cavalletti, or jump several small obstacles less than 2 feet high. A Western performance horse would be worked at intervals of jog and lope in figures using the entire arena. A trail horse could gradually begin a mild incline after 10 or 15 minutes of trotting on the level. A racehorse would be breezed at a slow canter after the initial warm-up to gradually increase cardiac output and blood flow to the muscles.

Cool-Down Exercises

After a horse has finished a workout, devote 15 to 30 minutes to cooling down at a walk or slow trot. It is best to keep a horse moving during a cool-down to dissipate heat generated by working muscles. Dissipating heat allows muscle and body temperature to decline slowly. Blood that was routed to the muscles is gradually redirected back to internal organs. Oxygen is replenished to muscles that reached an oxygen debt, and accumulated lactic acid is flushed from the muscles. Removal of lactic acid from the muscles is important for alleviating muscle soreness that can occur after exercise.

POST-EXERCISE STRETCHES

While walking, a loose rein encourages the horse to stretch his own neck and back, relieving tension on overworked muscles that might begin to tighten (photo 6.10). Once dismounted, the same manual stretches that were used during warm-up can also be used in a cool-down. Stretching reduces post-exercise muscle soreness.

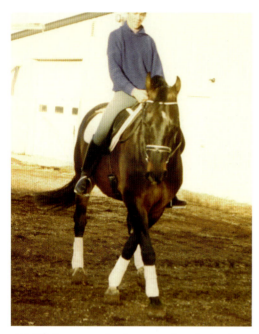

6.9 *While mounted, a horse can be asked to leg-yield or sidepass, which stretches his abductor muscles in the hindquarters, as well as muscles in his back and neck.*

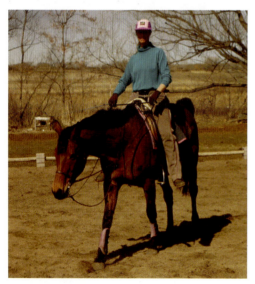

6.10 *Walking on a loose rein following a workout is good for releasing tension.*

Muscle Endurance   157

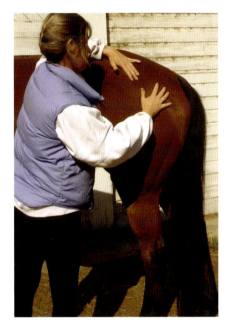

6.11 *Massage of large muscle groups is helpful to relax tension, and to improve oxygen circulation and remove heat and waste products of muscle metabolism.*

MUSCLE MASSAGE

Muscle massage relaxes tight muscles, improving oxygen circulation in the muscles, and removing toxic by-products. The large muscles over the hip, neck, back, and thighs particularly benefit from 20 to 30 minutes of massage. With firm pressure, use the heel of the hand or the fingertips to create a circular massaging motion over each muscle group (photo 6.11). The horse will relax and most likely will lean into the pressure. As a finishing touch, apply a thick rubber currycomb in a circular motion to stimulate the skin and superficial muscles, as well as to remove sweat and dirt from the coat.

FOOD AND WATER

Once the horse's chest is cool to the touch, offer hay and water. Wait about a half hour after the horse is fully cooled down before offering grain. Then blood flow is restored to the intestines, and the horse is less likely to develop gaseous colic.

WARM WEATHER COOL-DOWNS

During hot and humid weather, a horse may need additional help cooling down. Sponging the head, neck, chest, and legs helps remove body heat by improving evaporative cooling (photo 6.12). Soak the large blood vessels along the neck and legs for maximum cooling, but stay away from the large muscle groups over the back and hindquarters unless in a very hot and humid climate. In an arid, cool, or windy climate, sponging water on overheated, large muscle masses may cause muscle spasms whereas in hot, humid climates, a full body soak may be ideal for cooling (photo 6.13). After a pleasure ride that stimulates only a light sweat, a horse can be bathed following 15 to 30 minutes of cool-down.

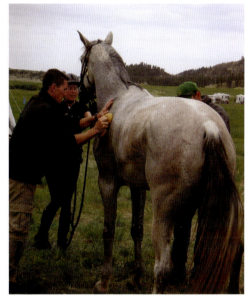

6.12 *Soaking the head, neck, chest, and legs with water assists release of heat from muscles of an exercising horse by capitalizing on the principles of evaporative cooling.*

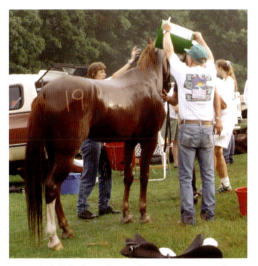

6.13 *A full body soak may be necessary in a hot, humid climate to prevent a horse from overheating.*

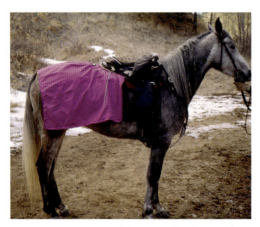

6.14 *A rump rug acts like a windbreaker to keep the large haunch muscles from being chilled by a brisk wind or from cooling too quickly when exercise stops.*

Besides soaking the neck and chest, place the horse in an area shaded from the sun. If the air is particularly still, improve heat dissipation by directing a fan on the horse to push cool air past the skin. For any horse that exercises during warm weather, it is best to maintain as lean a body weight as possible (see p. 345 and p. 360). Extra body fat delays heat dissipation from the muscles, and dramatically increases the cooling period.

COOL WEATHER COOL-DOWNS

It is important to cool down the working muscles adequately after a hard workout any time of the year, but it is essential during the cooler seasons. Working skeletal muscle generates a large amount of heat, and if insufficiently cooled down, or if exposed to cold rain or water directly after a workout, muscle tissue may begin to spasm and cramp. A rump rug is effective to protect haunch muscles from cooling too rapidly (photo 6.14).

Insulation Delays Cool-Down

Fat Insulation

Fat is an insulating layer that acts as a "cushion" against climatic elements. A thin horse has fewer fat reserves against chills than an individual with a healthy covering of flesh. On the other hand, an overweight horse has the opposite problem. Heat dissipates slowly from an overweight or underconditioned horse. An overweight horse may finish exercising with only slight dampness around the neck. Then, a couple of hours later, he may be soaked in the neck, chest, and girth areas because heat loss through the skin continues after exercise.

Hair Coat Insulation

When dry, the horse's hair coat provides insulating protection from chills and damp (photo 6.15). A dense, winter hair coat protects a horse from the elements, but its length makes it difficult to cool down a horse. Shortened daylight hours of winter stimulate hairs to grow longer due to the effect of reduced light on the brain's pineal gland. A horse with a thick, heavy coat experiences the same phenomenon as a fat horse because the hair layer insulates against cooling. Delayed sweating is a natural occurrence, yet steps must be taken to protect damp horses from drafts and chills. Horse hairs are evenly distributed on the body, rather than in clusters, as in dogs or cats. The loft in a horse's hair coat insulates him and retains body heat.

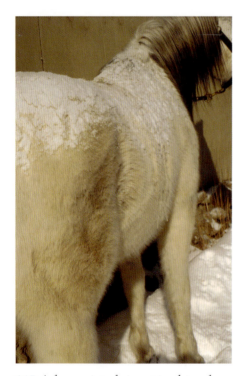

6.15 *A dense, winter hair coat insulates a horse from climatic elements. In this photo, you can see that this horse's body heat is not escaping through the thick insulating fur; snow remains unmelted on his back while he retains warmth and body heat beneath his coat.*

COOL-DOWN METHODS

An adequate cool-down permits the circulation to flush away toxic by-products and heat, and prevents tying-up syndrome (see p. 166).

Consider special cool-down procedures during winter weather such as walking, drying the hair coat, cover-ups, and body clipping.

Walking

Walking for 15 to 30 minutes cools muscles after an exertion, releasing much of the heat that contributes to sweating. Walking is the best way to cool down a horse in cold weather. Both hand walking or mechanical hotwalkers are useful. Walking maintains good circulation to the muscles, which dissipates heat. However, there is a mistaken belief that walking a horse after exercise dries a damp hair coat. Sunshine dries a wet coat as the horse walks, but a dry coat does not mean the horse is fully cool. And, although a horse has cooled down, his fur may remain wet for a while.

As muscles cool down, so do ligaments, joints, and tendons. Walking maintains flexibility in these structures, making the limbs less susceptible to injury. Bandages retain warmth and circulatory flow in the lower legs, so it may help to leave on splint boots or leg bandages during the cool-down period to cool lower limbs slowly.

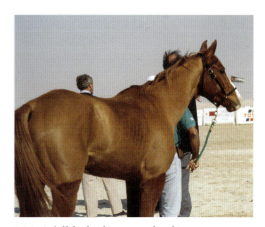

6.16 *A full body clip opens the skin to evaporative cooling with sweat by removing the insulating layer of fur.*

Drying the Hair Coat

Sweat scrapers are great for pulling extra moisture from the hair coat to regain "loft" and insulating capacities quickly. A brisk rub with a dry towel or brush also removes moisture from the coat, while exposing more hair surface to the air for faster drying. Toweling also "polishes" a dull coat. If necessary, an electric hair dryer set on low heat may speed up drying of a soaked coat.

Body Clipping

To avoid prolonged cool-downs in the wintertime, many horses are body clipped to facilitate heat loss during exercise. Shaving hair away from the chest, abdomen, neck, and shoulders exposes a large area for evaporative cooling (photo 6.16). Shaving also helps large, surface blood vessels in these areas radiate heat away from the horse. However, if a horse has been body-clipped and the insulating fur layer removed, it is important to cover the horse during resting hours.

COVER-UPS

Blanketing serves as a substitute for natural hair on clipped horses, protecting from wind chill or wet weather. Blankets may also give additional protection against the elements for horses with a full hair coat. Many varieties of horse blankets are commercially available, each appropriate for different conditions.

Blanketing a Wet Horse

Only cover a wet horse with a blanket if he will be checked periodically for drying, or else use a blanket that has a wool or polar fleece liner and a "breathable" shell material, like Gore-Tex®. When soaked with sweat, a blanket of some fabrics (cotton or Dacron or nylon) increases the rate of body cooling, creating a "refrigerator effect," resulting in a chilled and miserable animal: such a wet blanket causes moisture to evaporate from the skin faster than the body is able to warm the skin. Skin temperature decreases, and eventually chills the body as well.

OTHER OPTIONS

Enclosed Barn

Access to an enclosed barn provides greater cool-down options in cold or wet weather. A barn provides a draft-free environment with consistent temperatures. If a barn is well-insulated and warm, it may be acceptable to wash the horse after a workout. Hair that is matted with sweat, or caked with mud removes the loft and allows vital body heat to escape. It is best to avoid bathing a horse during the winter months unless a warm barn is available to allow complete drying. Repeated bathing removes natural oils from a horse's hair and skin and reduces the water repellency of the hair coat. Bathing a horse in cold weather risks accidental chilling even when using warm water. Use common sense: a dirty horse is better than a sick horse.

Management

Each horse tolerates climatic changes differently. Consider the horse's body weight, length and distribution of the hair coat, the stabling facilities, and blanketing options available. When cooling down a sweat-soaked horse, an educated approach coupled with instinct and common sense will prevent trouble. Keeping a horse current on respiratory vaccine boosters allows him to fend off chill-related respiratory viruses (see chapter 10, *Respiratory Conditioning and Health*, p. 265). Intelligent management can maintain a horse's conditioning program year-round

Dietary Manipulation of Muscle Performance

Attempts at dietary manipulation of muscle performance by using carbohydrates or fat have little impact on the content of glycogen in the muscles unless the horse previously has suffered imbalances in his nutritional plane. Glycogen stored in the muscles is called upon for energy during exercise (see "Food for Muscle Energy," p. 139). It is the adaptations induced by training that develop a horse's top performance (see "Response of Skeletal Muscle to Exercise," p. 144). In addition, it is a wise strategy to feed a high fat diet to an equine athlete, especially one that specializes in aerobic sports, in order to provide calories without depending on a high-carbohydrate source such as grain. High-fat and high-fiber diets facilitate the muscles' ability to use lipids and fatty acids as energy sources. Although this does not increase muscle glycogen content directly, it does create a noticeable glycogen-sparing effect to retain this valuable energy source in reserve.

Ergogenic Acids

As examples of other strategies of dietary manipulation, oral "nutraceutical" supplements are fed in an attempt to promote an improved ability of the muscles to work. These substances are considered *ergogenic acids*. When considering use of these products, it is important to recognize that most studies have measured the effects of these products in human sports medicine with only speculation as to their effects on equine muscle physiology. Of those products that have been examined in horses, studies have been performed on racetrack horses that compete in high-intensity anaerobic exercise for short periods. Their exercise demands are far different from those of a horse exercising at submaximal effort (distance riding, trail riding, dressage, hunter/jumpers, and show horses, as examples). Any information gained could only be extrapolated between athletic disciplines.

Many supplemental ergogenic acids probably have little value for use in aerobically exercising horses that maintain a steady level of aerobic exercise output. Lactic-acid levels do not significantly elevate in the muscles until a horse is pushed to higher speeds or intensity, or ridden past his level of fitness or ability. In these situations, lactic acidosis may develop for variable and transient periods of time, but other fatigue factors additionally interfere with continued performance. In the horse that is ridden within his aerobic capacity, lactic acidosis is not normally present; then, these supplements that are meant to reduce lactic-acid concentrations would have no application.

CARNITINE

Carnitine is an amino acid that is responsible for mitochondrial uptake of free fatty acids during submaximal exercise. It is normally found in skeletal and cardiac muscle. This substance increases with age and training and is highly correlated to the oxidative capacity of muscle fibers. Proponents of the use of nutraceuticals speculate that this product should improve muscle function by sparing glycogen use and minimizing production of lactic acid. However, as an oral supplement, it is very poorly absorbed from the gastrointestinal tract so it has a limited advantage, if any.

BRANCHED CHAIN AMINO ACIDS

Another example of supplements provided in an attempt to improve muscle metabolism in prolonged aerobic activities includes branched chain amino acids (BCAAs) such as leucine and isoleucine. BCAAs allegedly decrease the blood-lactate concentration primarily during anaerobic metabolism. Another theory suggests that BCAAs reduce the uptake of *tryptophan* by the brain, and since tryptophan is used to synthesize other chemical substances that induce sleep, less of its presence during performance may minimize an athlete's fatigue. The use of such supplements is purely speculative at this time.

GLYCINE

Glycine, which comes in the oral form of DMG (*dimethyl glycine*) is also an amino acid that supposedly reduces the production of lactate while increasing the use of oxygen in the muscles. It allegedly has beneficial effects on the immune system as well. To date, no studies have supported any evidence that feeding this material will minimize lactate production or improve a horse's performance.

BLOOD BOOSTERS

The objective to achieving stamina and staying power is to improve the oxygen-carrying capacity of the blood and hence oxygen delivery to the muscles of locomotion. One drug that has come to the attention of those involved with sport horses is a product called *erythropoietin*, or EPO. This medication is used to treat humans suffering from suppression of blood cell regeneration in the face of cancer chemotherapy or diseases affecting the bone marrow. Some have extrapolated that if it is good for people, then it must be applicable to horses.

However, the reality is considerably different. Use of this product can cause fatal anemia in horses. There are several facts to consider:

- Horses already possess a large splenic reservoir of blood cells. At the beginning of exercise, the spleen contracts and releases a large supply of red blood cells into circulation, driving up the packed-cell volume. Red blood cells are circulated through the body to deliver oxygen to the lungs and to working muscles. At rest, a horse has a packed-cell volume of around 40 percent whereas splenic contraction raises the packed-cell volume to around 60 percent. This natural physiological process in a horse's body enables it to "blood-dope" itself. Adding more red blood cells to the body by use of EPO would increase viscosity of the blood thereby slowing blood flow in the capillary beds; this would be counter-productive to oxygen delivery.
- EPO is a synthetic form of the human hormone. Giving a human product to a horse stimulates an antibody response by the horse to this foreign substance. Such an antibody response can cross-react to inactivate a horse's own EPO, leading to a severe and potentially fatal anemia. This feature of cross-reactivity is worsened by the fact that a single dose of EPO is insufficient to increase red cell production in a healthy horse so multiple doses are often used. Multiple dosing with EPO increases the likelihood of a horse developing antibodies to his own EPO with fatal consequences.

SELENIUM

Selenium deficiencies are known to be associated with muscle disease or tying-up syndrome in horses, however horses fed a high quality diet are unlikely to develop selenium deficiencies unless the soil in a geographic area is known for its lack of selenium. In those instances, consult a veterinarian about the wisdom of supplementing this micronutrient. Care should be taken to avoid indiscriminate supplementation unless there is justification. Feeding an excess of selenium when it is not needed can easily result in toxicity with associated thinning of mane and tail, horizontal cracks in the hooves, and laminitis. (See chapter 3, *The Hoof*, p. 57.)

Electrolytes

For most short-term equine athletic events, a primary problem is heat dissipation from working muscles. In athletic pursuits that require extended exercise, like endurance, competitive trail, eventing, combined driving, polo, steeplechase and timber racing, horses lose a significant amount of body salts in the sweat. Many horses begin an event already depleted from the stress of trailering a distance. Some horses don't drink or eat well when on the road due to changing routines. Studies done at endurance and competitive trail rides have shown that many horses experience the greatest loss of fluids and electrolytes within the first segments of exercise; for a distance horse these losses occur within the first 20 miles. Once a horse falls behind, it is hard to catch up in both departments. As body salts are lost, and especially sodium, the thirst drive diminishes and the horse is no longer interested in drinking even though that is the most important thing for him to do. Drinking plain water without any electrolyte supplementation exacerbates this problem by further diluting the concentration of remaining salts in the bloodstream.

A delicate balance in concentration of salts is essential for normal biochemical functions, such as muscle contraction, and normal intestinal function. Not only does extreme and prolonged sweating lead to dehydration, but also horse sweat consists of more than just water. Sweat releases important electrolytes, including:

- Sodium
- Calcium

- Chloride
- Potassium
- Magnesium

In sports that cause sweating for prolonged periods or during athletic efforts in hot, humid climates, a rider is able to help a horse replenish these salts as he is exercising. Supplementation with electrolytes is essential to maintaining sodium, potassium, and chloride levels within safe concentrations not only for efficient muscular contraction, but also for continued function of the thirst drive that keeps a horse drinking (see chapter 12, *The Digestive System: Nutritional Management*, p. 333).

EFFECTS OF ELECTROLYTE DEPLETION

Usually sports that require hours of steady exercise have the potential to create metabolic problems for a horse. However, in hot and humid climates, a horse that is trailered and/or exercised for any duration of time may undergo metabolic problems related to dehydration, electrolyte losses, and heat exhaustion.

Neuromuscular Depression

Electrolyte deficits often lead to neuromuscular depression: the muscles respond slowly or not at all to nerve signals.

Loss of Sodium

A relative loss of sodium in the bloodstream depresses neuromuscular activity, impairing muscle contraction. The horse is prone to fatigue and performance falters. Muscle cramping may occur due to interference in enzymes that control the sodium and calcium *ion pumps* within the muscles (see "Tying-up Syndrome," p. 166). Ion pumps are microscopic pores within the cell membrane that regulate the movement and exchange of electrolytes in and out of the cells.

Not only is sodium crucial to neuromuscular function, but it also helps retain body fluids so a horse does not become dehydrated. Normal sodium concentrates stimulate thirst. Sodium is not available to the horse in feed, so it must be offered as a supplement on the grain or by syringe.

Loss of Chloride

With exercise of short duration (an hour or two), chloride loss is not usually a concern. However, extended aerobic exercise stimulates the kidneys to compensate for a loss of chloride in sweat by retaining bicarbonate from the blood. Bicarbonate retention by the kidneys results in a mild *metabolic alkalosis* to increase the pH of the bloodstream (see p. 170).

Loss of Potassium

Potassium is an important electrolyte controlling the force of contraction in the muscles, both skeletal and heart. It is also responsible for dilating small arteries to improve oxygen supply to the tissue. If oxygen and blood supply to the muscles are compromised with potassium depletion, tying-up syndrome may develop. Potassium loss also results in fatigue. Hay is rich in potassium so this mineral is normally replenished when a horse stops working and eats. If exhaustion or metabolic problems depress the appetite, potassium must be replenished by supplementation.

Neuromuscular Hyperirritability

Neuromuscular *hyperirritability* develops from electrolyte imbalances of calcium and magnesium. Hyperirritable muscles twitch or spasm.

Excess Calcium or Magnesium in Muscle Cells

Muscle tissue is particularly sensitive to calcium concentrations. Increased concentration of calcium in muscle cells coupled with energy deficits contributes to hyperirritability. Each muscle fiber has a "pump," fueled by energy

6.17 *Thumps: The phrenic nerve crosses the atrium of the heart to innervate the diaphragm for breathing. With electrolyte imbalances, the phrenic nerve becomes overly irritable, such that the diaphragm contracts with every beat of the heart. This is visible or felt as a flutter or "thumping" in the flank region.*

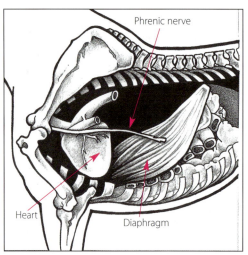

and magnesium from the bloodstream may develop multiple syndromes, including:

- Intestinal shutdown
- Colic
- Heart arrhythmias
- Tying-up syndrome
- *Synchronous diaphragmatic flutter*, also known as *thumps* (see below)

THUMPS

Thumps, or synchronous diaphragmatic flutter (SDF), is not a disease in itself, but is a distress flag indicating electrolyte imbalances. The *phrenic nerve* passes directly across the heart muscle as it runs to the diaphragm, and provides nerve impulses for contraction of the diaphragm muscle (fig. 6.17). Excess loss of calcium and magnesium through the sweat, and rising levels of lactic acid in the body sensitize the phrenic nerve. In response to electrical discharges of each heartbeat, the diaphragm contracts at the same time as the atrium of the heart contracts. This is visible as a twitching in the flank, or can be felt as a "thump" when a hand is placed against the flank. The thumping or twitching is not related to respiratory movements, but occurs simultaneous with every beat of the heart.

Dietary Cause of Thumps

Hard work and hot, humid weather promote loss of calcium and magnesium through sweat. As a horse sweats, hormones from the *parathyroid gland* remove calcium from the bones to the bloodstream, while the kidneys retain calcium to prevent its loss through urine. Such an internal regulatory system maintains calcium at precise levels in the bloodstream.

Alfalfa hay is rich in calcium. If fed a diet primarily of alfalfa hay, a horse is predisposed to thumps and tying-up syndrome: consistent, high consumption of calcium "turns off" the

(ATP) molecules, that removes calcium from the cell. With energy depletion, the pump cannot remove calcium from the cells, resulting in persistent contraction, or spasms of muscle fibers.

Accumulation of lactic acid alters muscle pH to an acid environment, which interferes with the activity of the calcium pump and energy use. Imbalances of sodium, chloride, potassium, and magnesium further impair muscle function and pump activity, resulting in fatigue and *myositis* (*tying-up syndrome*—muscle inflammation or cramping).

Lack of Calcium in the Bloodstream

Rigorous work increases the demand of calcium and magnesium for muscle contraction, and accelerates their depletion. Calcium depletion creates an insufficient availability of calcium stores in the *sarcoplasmic reticulum* to achieve proper muscle contraction. Calcium or magnesium loss from the bloodstream through the sweat can lead to stress *tetany*, which is a visible form of hyperirritability: a horse becomes nervous and jumpy, muscles twitch or spasm, or the limbs stiffen.

A horse with excessive losses of calcium

parathyroid gland so it is unable to mobilize calcium from bone stores during periods of excess calcium loss in the sweat. A horse with this tendency can be fed alfalfa hay during and after a competitive event to replenish these losses, but should not be fed excess alfalfa between events.

Encouraging Water Intake

It is always desirable for a horse to drink well. Not all horses take care of themselves in stressful situations. Some need enticement to consume water. Obvious strategies come to mind, like soaking the hay and feeding sloppy mashes. Dry hay is only 5 to 8 percent water whereas grass pasture contains water content of 50 to 90 percent; grain is only 9 percent moisture. The more dried feed offered, the more water is required for digestive processes. Hay and dry feed pull water into the intestinal tract and away from the muscles and general circulation. There is a fine line between providing ample energy and electrolytes from food during an athletic event, and interfering with water balance in the body.

Offer water at a temperature a horse prefers. Some like it tepid; some like it cool. Find the type of bucket a horse likes to drink out of, experimenting with plastic, rubber, or galvanized materials. Syringe electrolytes into a horse's mouth after he has eaten and drunk well, or offer a bucket of electrolyte-laced water along with plain water.

Muscle Injury or Disease

Muscle injury in an athletic horse comes in several forms:

- A strained or "pulled" muscle from overexertion or a slip in bad footing. Other injuries must be ruled out by a thorough exam to identify a specific muscle injury.
- Muscle fatigue
- *Tying-up syndrome* or muscle cramping (*myositis* or *exertional rhabdomyolysis*—see p. 166) due to electrolyte/fluid imbalances, heat stress, and/or problems with muscle metabolism (*equine polysaccharide storage myopathy*—see discussion on p. 172).

An area of pain may be detectable by diligent palpation and massage of each part of the large muscle groups along the hip, thigh, groin, and back. Muscle pulls or strains require rest and time, along with careful rehabilitation strategies before your horse should return to full work.

Muscle Fatigue: Losing the Peak

Muscle function is limited by the onset of fatigue. This does not occur all at once in all muscle fibers, but a horse's performance begins to suffer gradually at first, and then quickly deteriorates. When muscles fatigue, the tendons assume a greater load to compensate for reduced muscle tonus. This renders the tendons at greater risk of strain and serious injury. The objective is to recognize fatigue before it becomes hazardous to a horse. Fatigue occurs as a result of any of the following biochemical events:

- Depletion of energy stores such as glycogen
- Diminished energy production (ATP) due to muscle fiber damage or lactic acid accumulation in the muscles: under optimal conditions, ATP is effectively produced by oxidative metabolism within the mitochondria. Within the muscle cells, ATP is necessary for reuptake of calcium, for maintenance of proper gradients of sodium and potassium to enable propagation of nerve impulses, and for contraction.

6.18 *A muscle cramp is sometimes visible as an obvious spasm in a large muscle group, as seen here on this horse's haunch muscles.*

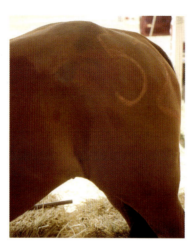

- Changes in calcium uptake and release that interfere with normal muscle contraction
- Aberrations in neuromuscular irritability due to depletion of electrolytes such as calcium, potassium, sodium, chloride, and magnesium
- Dehydration creating decreased blood flow and inadequate circulation of oxygen to maintain aerobic work
- Excess tissue temperature: muscle contraction is only 20 to 25 percent efficient, with the remaining energy of metabolism being released as heat within the muscles. Blood circulation and natural cooling mechanisms (sweating and respiration) dissipate heat from the muscles provided environmental temperature and humidity are not too extreme. A moderate increase in tissue temperature is favorable to muscle metabolism, but if temperature remains too high or is high for too long, efficiency of contraction suffers, leading to fatigue.

Intensive training and competition depletes glycogen reserves gradually, but may finally reach a threshold that is incompatible to further performance. Repletion of glycogen in the muscles is a slow process, requiring at least 72 hours to return to normal following intensive or prolonged exercise. This is important to consider when peaking a horse's performance for an event.

Tying-Up Syndrome aka Exertional Rhabdomyolysis aka Myositis

CLINICAL SIGNS

One of the primary problems experienced by athletic horses is the propensity to develop muscle cramping. Any inflammatory event in a muscle is called *myositis*, while a muscle cramp is often referred to as *tying-up syndrome*. When muscle tissue undergoes damage at the cellular level, especially related to exercise, it is referred to as *exertional rhabdomyolysis*. These terms are often interchangeable.

Clinical signs of myositis vary greatly: the muscles may be taut, or they may be flaccid. An affected horse often demonstrates poor heart rate recoveries during exercise, and may work at a higher heart rate than usual. The muscles may visibly spasm and cramp or enlarge with swelling (photo 6.18), or may simply be painful to finger pressure. The horse may have a stiff, stilted gait, or be obviously lame in a rear leg, or in a front limb if the shoulder muscles are affected. Some horses sweat as a response to pain; some refuse to move; others act as if they have colic pain.

RECURRENT EXERTIONAL RHABDOMYOLYSIS

Most cases of myositis are sporadic and do not occur on a regular basis in an individual. Yet, sometimes a horse is affected with myositis on numerable occasions. *Recurrent exertional rhabdomyolysis (RER)* is a form of myositis that occurs as repeated episodes of tying-up syndrome under various circumstances, even when a horse has had minimal exercise. Certain stressful events, like environmental changes, climatic factors, dietary changes,

Muscle Endurance

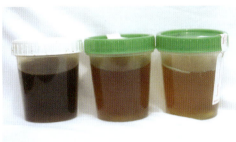

6.20 *The urine in these bottles was taken from a horse with severe myositis over the course of 12 hours. Abundant myoglobin was filtered into the urine, giving it a molasses-colored hue. The bottle on the far left is the first sample taken by bladder catheterization, and the subsequent samples show some slight clearing while the horse was on intensive intravenous fluid therapy. This degree of myoglobin filtration through the kidneys can lead to kidney failure and death.*

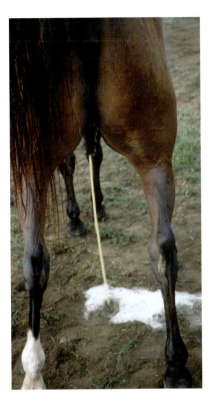

6.19 *Normal horse urine is straw-colored, thick, and viscous due to normal components such as mucus and calcium crystals.*

pain, or anxiety, may trigger RER. There may be an inherited problem with muscle contraction that is an important component to these recurrent bouts; Thoroughbreds are mostly affected, while Standardbreds and Arabians show a higher propensity than many other breeds. Some horses with seeming attacks of RER may, in fact, suffer from *equine polysaccharide storage myopathy* (*EPSSM*—see p. 172).

THE SIGNIFICANCE OF DISCOLORED URINE

Normal horse urine is straw-colored, and cloudy in appearance due to mucus and calcium oxalate crystals, which are normal components (photo 6.19). Certain feeds, like legume hays, influence the degree of cloudiness, so not all horse urine appears exactly the same. However, urine that is dark yellow or light amber in color is concentrated because of dehydration. The body responds to dehydration by conserving every drop when too much body fluid is lost in the sweat and is used by the working muscles. A horse that hardly urinates is dehydrated. Any dark discoloration to the urine is cause for concern. Urination should be monitored for:

- Frequency of urine output
- Amount of urine output
- Color of urine in all phases of the stream passed, from beginning to end

Urine that is brown or red-tinged indicates that there has been some muscle damage due to dehydration, electrolyte imbalances, acid-base disturbances, and/or too much heat buildup in the muscles. A reddish color to the urine is a result of *myoglobin* being filtered through the kidneys into the urine, referred to as *myoglobinuria* (photo 6.20). Myoglobin is a large protein molecule of muscle tissue that is released from dehydrated, injured, or cramping muscle. Via

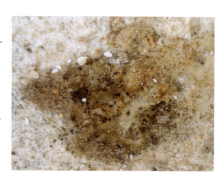

6.21 *Horse urine oxidizes to a reddish-orange color when it contacts the air, and this is highly visible in white snow. This is a normal process, and it occurs at all times but is not visible in dirt.*

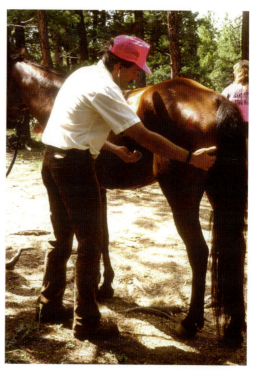

6.22 *A horse with myositis may resent pressure placed along a sore muscle. He may try to kick, put his ears back, or move away, but he makes his discomfort known. Not all horses with myositis have muscle pain, and not all tied-up muscles feel firm to touch.*

the blood circulation, myoglobin passes through the kidneys, but here is where it can cause problems. Because of their large size, myoglobin proteins block the kidney tubules, potentially leading to kidney failure. Any sign of red-tinged or brown urine is clear evidence of muscle breakdown, with myoglobin passing through into the urine.

Whether a horse is showing overt signs of muscle cramping (tying up, myositis, or exertional rhabdomyolysis) or not, discolored urine is a sure sign that some degree of muscle inflammation is occurring.

Red Discoloraton of Urine in Snow

Not all discolored urine is related to myositis. Reddish-orange spots that are visible in the snow after urination often are mistaken for a bleeding problem from a horse's urinary system (photo 6.21). When oxygen and moisture interact with horse urine, an oxidation reaction turns yellow urine to a reddish-orange hue. This is true even in summertime, but dirt and sand obscure color changes of the urine; white snow provides a dramatic and visible background.

Such "red" urine is not necessarily representative of a problem but other sources should be evaluated such as inflammation caused by urinary tract stones. If the insides of a horse's rear legs are chronically spattered with blackish stains, there could be real cause for concern. Any blockage or infection of the urinary tract, tumors, or bladder stones can result in actual blood in the urine.

Muscle Tone

Sometimes with myositis, the haunch or thigh muscles are more flaccid than normal due to electrolyte derangements; sometimes the muscles are painful to palpation (photo 6.22), or overtly spasm into a knot (photo 6.23); and sometimes there are no outward signs of muscle inflammation other than a discoloration of the urine. Not all muscle cramping leads to myoglobin release or discolored urine. If a horse continues to exercise in the face of a muscle cramp, the muscles could undergo

Muscle Endurance

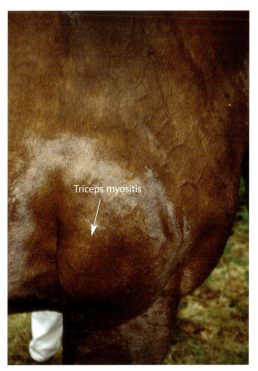

6.23 *In severe cases, more than one muscle group may develop a cramp, such as is seen in the knotted triceps muscles of this horse's shoulder.*

more and potentially significant damage. Many horses compensate quite well in the face of dehydration. Many recover quickly from a mild muscle cramp. However, it is known that in human marathons, muscle damage and pain incurred from muscle cramps persists for several weeks subsequent to the event, with the potential for scarring of muscle tissue.

THE SIGNIFICANCE OF MYOSITIS

Myositis occurs for many reasons. Key among them is persistent dehydration that reduces circulation in the muscle tissues and impairs oxygen delivery to the muscles.

Dehydration

Stiff muscles, muscular weakness, or tremors tip one off to the fact that a horse is dehydrated. In order for a horse to maintain himself in exercise, his circulatory system must have sufficient blood volume to deliver oxygen, nutrients, and energy to contracting skeletal muscles. Heat and metabolic by-products are carried away from the muscles in the bloodstream. Muscles cannot function properly when they lack oxygen from inadequate blood flow, or when too much heat or metabolic waste products accumulate, or when electrolyte imbalances develop. Affected muscles stiffen, or sometimes they weaken. There may be trembling of forearms, shoulder muscles, flanks, or hindquarter muscles. The tendency is to think the horse might be chilled because he is standing still and his sweat is drying. Muscle tremors occur not just from fatigue, but also from dehydration and electrolyte imbalances (see chapter 13, *The Skin as an Organ*, p. 359).

Electrolyte Depletion

Hand-in-hand with dehydration in the working horse are attendant electrolyte depletions and imbalances as body salts are lost in high proportion in the sweat, as discussed in "Effects of Electrolyte Depletion," p. 163. Intravenous fluid replacement may be necessary to treat dehydration and electrolyte depletion.

Elevated Muscle Temperature

Excessive muscle temperature due to prolonged exercise and/or high heat and humidity conditions interferes with the ion pumps that are important to regulating electrical polarity of sodium, potassium, calcium, magnesium, and ATP within each muscle cell. Similarly, alterations in muscle and blood pH created by electrolyte imbalances affect the membrane ion pumps. Likewise, glycogen depletion results in ATP energy deficiency to further affect their function. Due to interference with function of the ATP-driven ionic pumps, calcium concentration rises within the sarcoplasmic reticulum to adversely affect normal mitochondrial respiration so important to aerobic energy production; the cellular membranes are damaged and myofibrils disrupted. Energy depletion and insufficient ATP traps calcium in the muscle cells, causing persistent muscle contraction and cramping.

Metabolic Alkalosis

In horses with persistent sweating during lengthy bouts of exercise, depletion of potassium, chloride, calcium, and magnesium through the sweat may create *metabolic alkalosis* (pH of the blood is more alkaline due to loss of potassium in sweat). This alters the membrane potentials necessary to elicit muscle contraction; neuromuscular transmission suffers leading to muscle cramps, synchronous diaphragmatic flutter (see "Thumps," p. 164), reduction in intestinal function (see chapter 11, *The Digestive System: The Oral Cavity, Dental Care, and the Intestinal Tract*, p. 317), and occasional cardiac arrhythmias. In higher-speed endurance-racing sport events, horses are trained to gallop over a 100-mile course. This style of competition alters previously believed tenets of exercise physiology for aerobic sports; in these cases, the blood becomes more acidic, with increased levels of lactate and its attendant adverse effects on muscle function (see p. 147).

MEASURING MUSCLE DAMAGE BY ENZYME LEVELS

Once a horse has suffered a bout of myositis, if the basement membrane surrounding muscle fibers is not damaged, the muscle fibers will completely heal with no scarring or residual problems. The best means to monitor the resolution of muscle damage is by testing levels of circulating muscle enzymes in the blood. After muscle damage, the level of myoglobin reaches its highest level (peaks) in the bloodstream within 5 minutes, *creatine phosphokinase* (CPK or CK) peaks within 5 hours; both of these components clear the bloodstream within 3 to 4 days following the end of fiber disruption or damage. On the other hand, *lactate dehydrogenase* (LDH) does not elevate to its peak for 12 hours, and *aspartate aminotransferase* (AST) does not peak for 24 hours. AST requires at least 2 to 4 weeks to clear to baseline levels.

This data is important for tracking the body's ability to heal, and as a measure of when to return the horse to work. In general, once the CPK has returned to less than 1000 U (units) per liter and AST has returned to normal values (less than 500 U per liter), light exercise can be reinstated. Usually, serial blood tests are done at weekly intervals to ensure complete resolution of the muscle injury so a horse is not prematurely returned to work.

A horse that has tied-up in the past is not necessarily at greater risk of doing so again unless there is an inherent problem in that individual's muscle metabolism. In most cases, intelligent conditioning strategies and appropriate riding for the conditions on the day of a competition are critical to successful performance.

WHAT TO DO WITH A TIED-UP HORSE WHILE EXERCISING

As soon as a horse demonstrates signs of tying up, dismount, and let him rest. Allow him to graze. If water is accessible, and if the horse's skin feels hot and sweaty, cool down his neck and chest by sponging, but refrain from soaking the tied-up muscles of the rear quarters. If there is no available water, give him a bit of rest time before heading to the barn. If the horse can walk without too much distress, then walk slowly for a short bit, stop, rest, then walk a little more. Send a friend to get help when possible. Consider the nearest access for veterinary equipment and/or a trailer to reach the horse. Pull the saddle and use the saddle blanket to keep painful muscles warm. If a muscle cramp isn't too severe, light massage might help. However, too much massage compression on damaged muscle adds to the problem and causes further damage and pain. In most cases, massage and manipulation of cramped muscles should be delayed until several days following the crisis when cellular damage has halted.

PREVENTIVE THINKING

- Consider the fitness level of other horses when riding in a group. Maintain realistic expectations. An unfit or overweight horse should not be expected to keep up with a fit companion. Consider body condition of each horse to determine the appropriate exertion level for any given day. Many tie-up emergencies occur in unfit horses, or horses ridden beyond their level of conditioning. Others occur in hot and humid climates that elicit fluid and electrolyte losses from sweating. On occasion, an exercising horse that is suddenly exposed to a chill from wind or cold rain will start to cramp in the heavy haunch muscles.
- Horses that sweat heavily or those working in hot and humid climates should receive oral electrolyte supplementation and have ample opportunity to drink anytime during exercise.
- Dark urine, a stiff gait, or "colicky" signs should be addressed promptly. Seemingly transient problems can result in serious and potentially fatal consequences. A delay in treatment could prove costly. Haul the horse to the nearest medical source of help.
- Signs of "colic" such as depression, lack of appetite, lying down, and sweating may be caused by pain from an abdominal problem, although these are similar features to pain from tying-up syndrome. It is important to differentiate the source of illness. A stiff gait that is accompanied by any of these signs is often indicative of early cases of myositis, or even laminitis. Learn how to obtain a rectal temperature, heart rate, and digital pulse, and evaluate sounds for intestinal motility (see chapter 11, *The Digestive System: The Oral Cavity, Dental Care, and the Intestinal Tract*, p. 299). Gathering this information sorts out the significance and severity of an immediate crisis, and enables communication with a veterinarian.
- If traveling away from home, plan ahead and know where to find the nearest treatment facility. Ask your local veterinarian for a referral in the area you will be going, or peruse a phone book at the nearest town.

Muscle Spasms Caused by Ear Ticks

An irregular cause of muscle cramps can be attributed to an unlikely parasite particularly found in arid climates: *spinose ear ticks (Otobius megnini)*. An affected horse is in pain and acts as if he is experiencing a bout of colic. A horse will paw and sweat, and have intermittent muscle spasms and muscle tremors. The third eyelid may prolapse across the eye.

Exam of the ear canals for larvae or adult spinose ear ticks may lead to an immediate diagnosis and rapid resolution of the problem once the ear ticks are eliminated by topical (1 percent dioxathion) treatment. Spinose ear ticks elicit a waxy secretion in the ears; some horses respond adversely to the irritation by rubbing their ears or by shaking their head. (See also "Other External Parasites," p. 385 and "Headshaking," p. 515.)

Equine Polysaccharide Storage Myopathy

Equine polysaccharide storage myopathy (EPSSM) is a condition related to a defect in energy storage within muscle cells. It is most commonly seen in draft horse breeds, or draft-related breeds such as Warmbloods, Quarter Horses, Paints, and Appaloosas. Studies indicate that 50 percent of draft horses or draft crosses are affected.

WHAT CAUSES EPSSM?

EPSSM is a disorder of glycogen storage resulting in up to four times greater concentrations of glycogen and abnormal polysaccharides accumulating within muscle cells. Muscle tissue is able to metabolize glycogen, but in EPSSM horses there is an enhanced sensitivity to insulin that occurs when carbohydrates or sugars are consumed. The result is an increased rate of glucose transport into the cells with accumulation of excess muscle glycogen. Even a mild exertion may elicit an acute onset of muscle stiffness and discomfort, or colic-like symptoms.

SYMPTOMS OF EPSSM

Clinical signs of EPSSM mimic many other muscle conditions. Typical signs seen include:

- Poor muscle development, particularly of the haunches
- Muscle tremors, particularly associated with exercise
- Signs comparable to myositis (tying-up syndrome)
- Stiff gait, particularly in the rear limbs
- Suspicion of a gait disorder such as *fibrotic myopathy* (p. 173), *shivers* (p. 518), or *stringhalt* (p. 524)
- Stumbling, clumsiness, weakness, reluctance to move, difficulty in backing
- Stretched-out stance, as if to urinate
- Colic-like episode following exercise
- Low energy and/or poor performance and exercise intolerance
- Symmetrical muscle atrophy of haunches and/or topline
- Back pain and soreness
- Upward fixation of the patella (see p. 118) due to muscle dysfunction

DIAGNOSIS OF EPSSM

Diagnosis is based on breed predisposition, clinical signs, laboratory evaluation of muscle enzymes, and muscle biopsy, which is achieved by taking a sample of tissue from the *semitendinosus* or *semimembranosus* muscles of the thigh. Without a definitive diagnosis by muscle biopsy, it is common to try dietary modifications to track improvement in suspect cases.

MANAGEMENT OF EPSSM

A horse afflicted with this metabolic disorder does not seem to be able to derive energy from a diet that is high in carbohydrates or sugars, and most equine diets rely on feeding grain or pelleted horse feeds that happen to be high in these ingredients. The strategy for feeding EPSSM horses relies on substituting grain products with a high fat diet, and on maintaining the horse on a high fiber diet (see "Fat for Energy," chapter 11, *The Digestive System: The Oral Cavity, Dental Care, and the Intestinal Tract*, p. 330). Glucose in the bloodstream is markedly suppressed when fat is added to a grain meal making it useful in managing EPSSM. Incremental addition of fat to a horse's diet can reach the full component of required daily fat over a two-week period. Full adaptation of muscle function to dietary modifications may not be appreciated for 2 to 4 months.

The feeding objective is for a horse to obtain at least 20 to 25 percent of his total daily calories from fat. Good quality hay and pasture continue as mainstays of the diet, but rapidly growing, lush pasture is not recommended as forage due to its high sugar content. Elimination of all grain is important, as is supplementation with fat: 2 cups of vegetable oil a day added to alfalfa-based pellets or cubes or soaked beet pulp provides the necessary dietary fat component. A 1000-pound horse requires 1 pound, or 1 pint, of fat per day. The feeding of rice bran requires supplying 5 pounds to achieve a diet close to 20 percent fat; rice bran is not intended to be fed at such a volume so it is a less useful feed to manage an EPSSM horse. Caution must be taken to prevent obesity by limiting total daily intake while maintaining a high fat component. When feeding fat, Vitamin E should be supplemented at an amount of at least 1000 IU (international units) per day. Dietary strategies should continue through a horse's lifetime.

Consistent exercise is extremely important in managing EPSSM. Daily turnout and routine work minimize flares of clinical signs. Combining dietary changes with exercise has achieved a decrease in the severity and frequency of clinical signs.

White Muscle Disease

A diet that is deficient in selenium can create muscle problems known as white muscle disease. Foals may exhibit stiff and painful muscles and have cardiac problems, while older horses experience recurrent episodes of tying-up syndrome. Another symptom related to selenium deficiency is pain and swelling of the *masseter* (cheek) muscles of the face. Selenium deficiency occurs in certain geographic areas such as the Northwest and the northeastern United States. Caution must be taken to not supplement with too much selenium as toxicity can occur (see chapter 3, *The Hoof*, p. 57).

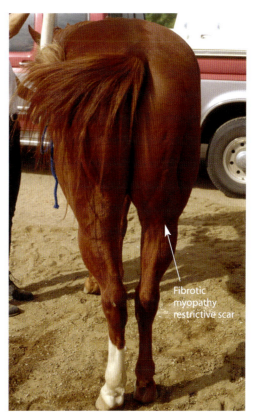

6.24 *Scar tissue that forms at the junction of the thigh muscles and attaching tendons can restrict forward extension of the limb. This tight band can be felt along the back of the thigh, and in addition, a horse with fibrotic myopathy, like this one, has a very diagnostic gait in which he doesn't lift the limb very high as he advances it, then slaps it back down—abruptly.*

Fibrotic Myopathy

Scarring that forms in muscle tissue of the thigh near the junction of the muscle and tendon may result in a lameness syndrome called *fibrotic myopathy*. Forward extension of the hind leg is reduced due to mechanical constriction by fibrous scar tissue; this creates a functional shortening of muscle and tendon stretch (photo 6.24). Usually a horse experiences no pain with this syndrome, but his gait is asymmetric and abnormal in the affected rear limb. The gait of

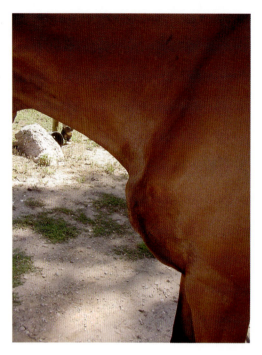

6.25 *Dryland distemper or pigeon fever is known for its propensity to develop large abscesses in the pectoral muscles, giving the appearance of a pigeon breast when viewed from the side, as seen here.*

an affected horse is characteristic: the limb is slapped down quickly before it reaches its normal forward phase of the stride, and before it reaches full forward extension. In contrast to a stringhalt gait in which the limb is elevated abnormally high toward the belly, a limb affected by fibrotic myopathy shows no excess elevation before it abruptly "catches" and the foot is slapped hard to the ground. In many cases, the restriction can be felt as a thickened band where the muscle joins the tendon at the lower portion of the back of the thigh.

Development of fibrotic myopathy is often attributed to sudden sprint activities. A racehorse may tear muscle tissue as he bolts from the start gate. A cutting, roping, reining, or gymkhana horse that abruptly slams on the "brakes," setting his hind legs far under him, can pull or tear a thigh muscle in the process. This syndrome may also develop from a kick injury, from catching a limb in a fence or halter, or from an infection in the thigh muscles. Injured or infected tissue repairs with scar tissue to varying degrees. There is no medical treatment for this condition. Minimal improvement has been reported with surgical cutting of the affected muscle and/or tendon, with more than one-third developing recurrence of fibrotic myopathy post-surgery.

Dryland Distemper aka Pigeon Fever

During a drought year, particularly in the western United States, it is not uncommon to have epidemics of *dryland distemper*, also known as *pigeon breast* or *pigeon fever* (photo 6.25). Although occurring mostly in the fall months, it can show up as early as springtime or summer. Dryland distemper is caused by a bacterial infection of *Corynebacterium pseudotuberculosis*, which localizes in deep abscesses in the breast (pectoral) muscles, along the abdomen, and/or in the groin (sheath or udder) region. It is called "pigeon breast" because, in profile, the swelling on the chest resembles the appearance of a pigeon's breast. At first glance, it might seem the horse had been kicked in the chest, but in fact the horse may be growing an infection.

These abscesses can take weeks to months to grow to the point where they can be lanced and drained. Some horses will spike a fever for a day or many days. Most continue to eat. Most become lame due to the swelling, which usually gets worse before it gets better. Often swelling migrates around the abscess and between the legs or along the belly. The udder or sheath may enlarge greatly due to localized edema secondary to tissue inflammation.

INCIDENCE AND FORMS OF INFECTION

Corynebacteria organisms live in the soil and become most pathogenic during drought conditions. Dryland distemper is thought to be transmitted through some abrasion or break in the skin, or through mucous membranes. Most probably, flies serve as vectors, particularly horn flies, houseflies, and stable flies (see p. 377 and p. 380). Just because a horse on a property has contracted pigeon breast does not mean all or any other of the other horses there will develop this disease. The presence or extent of infection may depend upon an individual horse's immune system, and how well he can respond to exposure of this organism. Even when fly season has abated with freezing temperatures, it is still possible for an infection to show up due to lengthy incubation time. A horse with a seemingly cured infection may relapse with occurrence of another abscess, even months later.

Although not common, it is possible for the infection to travel to internal areas, creating weight loss, fever, depressed appetite, lethargy, colic, and a variety of other symptoms dependent on where in the body the abscess has landed. A veterinarian should examine any horse that displays these symptoms or stops eating or drinking in the face of this illness. Any swelling in the groin or difficulty in using one or both rear legs should also receive prompt veterinary attention. If infection lodges in the rear limbs, it can cause a chronic syndrome known as *ulcerative lymphangitis* that can be difficult to resolve. This is usually restricted to one rear limb, which may swell to gargantuan proportions. Once lodged in the lymphatic system in that limb, some degree of limb swelling may remain indefinitely, and signs of systemic illness and limb swelling may recur intermittently over many years.

TREATMENT

When an abscess on the chest finally "points" and matures, and eventually feels soft to the touch, it can be opened and drained by a vet. Abscesses located along the belly may open and drain on their own because there is less tissue to break through; since these belly abscesses are pointing downward, gravity brings them to the surface more quickly.

In an effort to wall-off an infection, the body builds a thick capsule around the abscess to contain it. Pectoral abscesses develop within a thick, fibrous capsule that extends deep into the breast muscles. This necessitates local anesthetic and a scalpel incision to make an opening through the skin and the capsule. An ultrasound exam is helpful in locating the abscess pocket. These capsules are loaded with thick, creamy pus, as much as a quart at a time, which flows freely through the incision. The abscess pocket is irrigated with a dilute povidone-iodine solution made by mixing 10 ml povidone-iodine in 1 liter of saline.

The use of antibiotics is controversial: unless there are extenuating circumstances such as an internal abscess or ulcerative lymphangitis, it is recommended to not put a horse affected by external or pectoral abscesses on any antibiotics. If a horse is placed on antibiotics prematurely, in most cases, the infection will simply simmer along, only to resurface when the antibiotics are discontinued. Supportive care includes:

- Hot packing of the swollen area.
- Administration of a low dose of nonsteroidal anti-inflammatory (NSAIDs) medications (phenylbutazone or flunixin meglumine) once a day if swelling or lameness is extreme or if the horse feels so poorly that he is not taking care of himself by eating and drinking. Only administer such anti-inflammatory medications under advisement of your veterinarian.

Recovery can take as little as 2 weeks or as long as 2 to 3 months. Even after a horse receives medical attention and an abscess is lanced and drained, it is possible that one or more abscesses will form near the original swelling. Usually these are of lesser consequence and some abate spontaneously.

CONTROL
Since the bacterial organisms persist in the environment in the soil, the primary means of control is through management practices since it is impossible to eliminate the bacteria completely. Ideally, strategies reduce the possibility of exposure, and if a horse is exposed, then techniques are applied to minimize the risk of infection. The best means of prevention and control rely on common hygienic practices:

- Affected horses should be isolated, particularly if an abscess is actively draining.
- Purulent material from an opened abscess should be collected into a container as best as possible and disposed of properly.
- Contaminated stalls, bedding, blankets, tack, tools, and equipment should be disinfected.
- People should be aware that they, too, can serve as vectors to transmit infectious material from horse to horse. Sick horses should be handled or fed only after well horses have been attended. Hands should be washed after handling sick horses. Care should be taken to change clothing and shoes that have been contaminated with pus or that have contacted a sick horse.
- Rakes, shovels, and manure carts should not be transferred from areas containing sick horses.
- Insect vectors should be controlled with ample use of fly spray, and the use of protective fly sheets and fly face masks.

The bacteria that are present in the pus of draining abscesses can remain infective for almost 2 months in manure, hay, straw, and shavings. On surfaces of stalls, floors, and equipment, infective material is present for at least a week, and may persist longer in cold environmental temperatures.

A similar strain of Corynebacteria occurs in small ruminants, for which there is a vaccine. Current research efforts are focused on development of an equine vaccine but to date, there is no reliable vaccine for horses for this disease.

Hyperkalemic Periodic Paralysis
Hyperkalemic periodic paralysis (HYPP) is a condition of skeletal muscle weakness that has been genetically linked to a certain line of Quarter Horses, specifically of the Impressive line. Usually an affected horse begins to show signs of this genetic defect between the ages of 2 and 4 years.

CLINICAL SIGNS
Early in an HYPP episode, an affected horse experiences persistent muscle twitching over the trunk, hindquarters, flanks, neck, and/or shoulders. Facial muscles also spasm, the nostrils flare, and lips become taut and drawn. The third eyelid often drops over the eye as muscles spasm around the orbit. The horse might sway or stagger from muscle weakness. He may buckle at the carpal joints (knees), sag in his hocks, or be unable to raise his head and neck. If an episode progresses, further weakening of the skeletal muscles causes a horse to collapse to the ground, or to assume a dog-sitting pose on his haunches. During an HYPP crisis, the horse remains alert, although slightly depressed, and is in no pain. The relaxed attitude of a horse during an attack helps distinguish HYPP from similar appearing syndromes of colic or myositis. Episodes vary in intensity, and are unpredictable. Most episodes are non-fatal, lasting 15 to 90 minutes. Between episodes of HYPP, a horse appears completely normal.

THE CAUSE OF HYPP

HYPP occurs due to a genetic defect in the transport system that regulates the movement of potassium and sodium across cell membranes. Horses afflicted with HYPP have less potassium content in the muscles than normal individuals, due to increased permeability of the muscle membrane that causes potassium to accumulate in the bloodstream. This causes leakage of sodium across the cells, resulting in a hyper-excitable muscle membrane and muscle twitching and spasms. As muscle contractions persist, potassium further exits the cells to add to elevated blood potassium levels. After several minutes, muscle membranes can no longer fire; muscles become paralyzed, and the horse weakens and collapses.

HYPP is potentially fatal due to the adverse effects of high blood potassium levels on the heart and the potential for diaphragm muscles to become paralyzed. An attack is elicited by excess potassium in the diet, as occurs with alfalfa hay. Sudden dietary changes, irregular feeding schedules, withholding food or stress from training or transport can precipitate an attack.

GENETIC TEST

A genetic test (University of California, School of Veterinary Medicine, Davis, California) detects if a horse is at risk of developing HYPP by evaluating mane and tail hairs for a specific gene in the DNA. Not all horses of the affected lineage have the HYPP gene. If only one parent has the mutant gene, a foal has a 50 percent chance of being afflicted. If both parents possess the gene, there is a 75 percent chance of a horse developing HYPP. A horse that tests negative for the mutant gene may be confidently used as breeding stock as it cannot pass the syndrome to future generations.

PREVENTING HYPP EPISODES

Prevention relies predominantly on feeding strategies: the recommended diet should contain no more than 1 percent potassium; alfalfa hay, rich spring pasture, molasses, and sweet feed that contains molasses should all be avoided. If grain is fed, it should restricted to small amounts offered 2 to 3 times daily using oats, barley, and corn, which contain less than ½ percent potassium. Water-soaked beet pulp can supplement grass hay to meet normal roughage needs while minimizing potassium intake. Have hay analyzed as some grass hays contain as much as 2½ percent potassium. Affected horses should not be supplemented with potassium-containing electrolytes. Labels on protein, and vitamin and mineral supplements should be checked for inclusion of potassium. A salt block should be available at all times.

Horses with HYPP should be turned into paddocks for self-exercise rather than being confined to stalls. Preventive medical management of HYPP includes a diuretic (*acetazolamide*) that stimulates potassium excretion through the urine.

TREATMENT

At beginning signs of an attack, walking or longeing the horse stimulates circulation of adrenaline, which drives potassium back into the muscle cells. In addition, feeding a small amount of oats or Karo® syrup stimulates the release of insulin, which also drives potassium back into the muscle cells. Severe attacks require immediate veterinary attention.

Therapy for Muscle Injury and Pain

Cold Therapy

Muscle tissues require application of cold compresses for 30 to 50 minutes to achieve the desired effect. Initially, muscle temperature rises due to a reflex that increases circulation. Then, the temperature begins to decline in deep muscle layers, and continues to drop up to 10 minutes after cold application has been discontinued. If no activity follows therapy, the muscle tissue may not warm up to normal temperature for 4 hours. Confinement of the horse ensures prolonged cold-therapy effects. Deep muscle massage also loosens muscle spasms.

Therapeutic Ultrasound

Once the initial muscle inflammation has settled down after a few days, therapeutic ultrasound is useful for deep tissue "heating" to stimulate metabolic activity and blood flow through an injured area (see p. 197). Caution must be taken to avoid overheating deep tissue or injuring bone. Use of this therapeutic modality should be restricted only to a person trained in its use.

Acupuncture

Acupuncture stimulates specific nerve fibers with needle penetration. Acupuncture points may also be stimulated with heat application to the points or by acu-injection of drugs or saline to prolong stimulation of the nerves.

ACUPRESSURE

Acupressure, as a variation of acupuncture, seeks to stimulate the same points as acupuncture, but without penetrating the skin. One means to apply acupressure on the horse is by massage therapy.

Electrical Therapies

TRANSCUTANEOUS ELECTRICAL NERVE STIMULATION

One method of electrically stimulating acupuncture points to reduce pain is *transcutaneous electrical nerve stimulation*, known as TENS. Conventional TENS therapy provides a voltage of electrical pulses high enough to stimulate the acupuncture points, but low enough to avoid sustained muscle contractions. Impulses are passed to the nervous system using a padded electrode placed over the skin. These electrodes send impulses to nerve receptors in the skin and in the superficial tissues. Sensory information is relayed to the central nervous system by specific pain receptors (*nociceptors*) located in areas of motor and trigger acupuncture points. A *motor point* excites muscle tissue and causes it to contract. *Trigger points* define hypersensitive areas afflicted with inflammation and tenderness.

Relieving Pain

Many acupuncture points are located in the superficial skin layers, where nerves and nociceptors transmit impulses from both the internal and external environments to the central nervous system. Stimulation of these nerve fibers and pain receptors by TENS results in the production and release of *endorphins* and *enkephalins* from the brain. Although the half-life of enkephalins is as brief as 1 minute, endorphins have a half-life of 2 to 3 hours, providing opiate-like pain relief.

TENS provides pain relief based on a *"gate theory."* Repeated, non-painful stimulation of sensory nerve fibers fatigues nerve endings, limiting transmission of pain sensation to the brain. Such an overload of stimulation elicits release of serotonin, a chemical that blocks pain impulses and reception by the brain, and, in effect, "closes a gate." Then, the brain "ignores" the less intense stimulus from an injury.

TENS as a Diagnostic Tool

TENS may be a valuable diagnostic tool to direct appropriate therapy to a specific site of injury, particularly if used in conjunction with *infrared thermography*. Infrared thermography visually identifies heat gradients that are related to inflammatory conditions with increased circulation. Because pain reflexes already stimulate an inflamed area, less voltage is required from TENS to "fire" a trigger-point nerve: TENS locates sensitized nerve tracts. This technique corroborates information attained from an infrared thermograph about the presence of acute inflammation. In structurally sound areas with no inflammation or reduced circulation, infrared thermography shows "cold" patterns.

ELECTROANALGESIA

Another type of electrical stimulation, *electroanalgesia*, is similar to TENS therapy, but uses different frequencies than TENS. Unlike conventional TENS, electroanalgesia amplifies electrical output mildly to produce visible muscle twitches.

Low Frequency Electroanalgesia

Low frequency electroanalgesia (LFEA) may provide pain relief for 1 to 3 days. LFEA is helpful for chronic pain of degenerative joint disease; it stimulates large nerve fibers in the joint to elicit a central pain-suppressing effect.

High Frequency Electroanalgesia

At a higher frequency than used for TENS, electroanalgesia also provides pain relief by the gate theory, and by releasing endorphins. *High frequency electroanalgesia* (HFEA) relieves pain more quickly than LFEA, but pain relief is sustained for shorter periods than LFEA.

ELECTRICAL MUSCLE STIMULATION

Electrical muscle stimulators (EMS) are useful to stimulate contraction of muscle that has atrophied or weakened from long-term disuse. Initiation of electrical activity and passive contraction within muscles improves tone, and nutrient and oxygen circulation. Muscle tissue is strengthened through this process via "retraining" of biochemical and enzymatic reactions essential to muscle contraction. An injured limb that needs rest for bone, joint, ligament, or tendon repair may be "exercised" by EMS without weight-bearing or stress while healing. The pumping action of electrically produced muscle contractions indirectly improves circulation to the area. Improved blood flow enhances the healing process while removing waste products, including lessening of edema formed by stagnant circulation.

PULSING ELECTROMAGNETIC FIELDS

The application of *pulsing electromagnetic fields* (PEMF) allegedly improves oxygen supply and increases temperature within the tissues (particularly bone) by improving dilation of blood vessels and circulation. This, in turn, promotes healing. PEMF has been applied to bone injuries, especially of long bones, such as bucked shins or splints.

Two electromagnetic coils are placed on opposite sides of the injured area, with each coil "capturing" the electromagnetic field of the other to align it into a uniform field. In theory, this uniform field produces a uniform electric current within the tissues. Normally, bone has an electrical polarity. The pulsing field generated on the coils mimics normal electrical potentials of long bone to stimulate faster healing. Theoretically, varying wave patterns and pulse rates determine the biological response of bone. There is still no evidence as to which specific pulses and waves affect what or how. It is speculated that magnetic fields increase oxygen levels in tissue and improve energy production to fuel healing processes. Improvement in circulation and oxygen supply to the tissues has the potential to limit pain created by lack of oxygen.

A similar principle attempts to use bio-magnetic, flexible, rubber or plastic pads surrounding a foil. The foil contains a magnetized iron compound, producing alternating magnetic fields. Such magnets come in commercial form as boots and blankets, with the expectation that when applied over areas of large blood vessels, circulation will increase to that area. In theory, the principle of PEMF seems sound, but controlled research projects comparing different electromagnetic devices show no improvement in the healing rates of bone, tendon, or muscle

Strong Tendons and Ligaments 7

As you picture a horse at a strong working trot suspended in the air for but a brief moment, you can see the nostrils flared, the muscles working, sinews taut and defined. With each stride, there is a coordinated movement between muscles and sinewy parts, each one relying on the other. The complex interrelationship of bones, muscles, tendons, and ligaments enables the musculoskeletal system to perform with precision (fig. 7.1).

The Difference between Tendons and Ligaments

Tendons connect muscles to bones. Like a system of levers and pulleys, muscles contract, transmitting their force through the tendons to the bones. With each muscular movement, connecting tendons move the bones to propel a horse along the ground. In design, tendons withstand loading of a horse's mass on his skeletal system by dissipating concussion and strain. Tendons must be strong yet retain sufficient elasticity to deform and return to their resting shape and length. An example of a major tendon in the lower leg is the *superficial digital flexor tendon* (SDFT) that runs along the very back of the cannon bone, con-

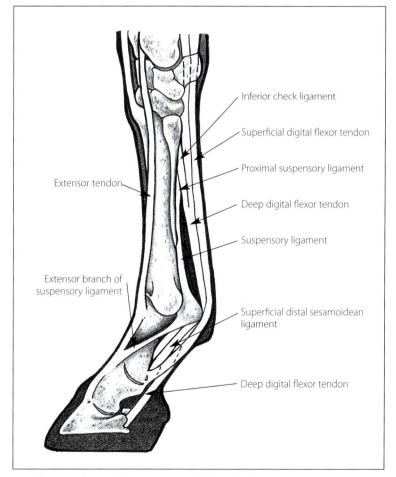

7.1 *Main tendons and ligaments in the lower limb.*

necting the superficial flexor muscle of the forearm to the bones of the pastern.

Ligaments, while of similar fibrous composition as tendons, are less elastic. Their function is to attach bones to each other across a joint. Ligaments stabilize the joints from overstretching, overflexing, or twisting. An important ligament to an athletic horse is the *suspensory ligament,* which originates just below the bottom of the carpal joint (knee) or the hock. It runs as a pair down each side of the cannon bone to the back of the *sesamoid bones* of the fetlock joint where it then branches out along each side of the pastern. The suspensory ligaments take a considerable amount of punishment during downhill travel, over jumps, and during sudden stops and turns. Other important ligaments, the *collateral ligaments*, are located alongside joints, helping to hold them in place by limiting side to side movement. Collateral ligaments may be injured by abnormal rotation of a joint from a misstep.

Prevention of Soft Tissue Injury

Conditioning

Both tendons and ligaments have the job of resisting "high-tensile" loads, i.e. those that place tension on soft-tissue components and stretch the fibers. The more inactive these structures are, the less organized the fibrous components within the ligament or tendon. Subsequently, a confined or inactive horse has weaker soft tissues that are less tolerant of withstanding the stress of exercise. This is a critical feature when considering the level of activity a horse is asked to undertake, or when considering returning a horse to work after a lengthy layup period. As exercise is renewed, the soft tissues will strengthen, but they do so slowly. An appropriate conditioning strategy should be applied when training an unfit horse or when rehabilitating an injured horse. Months of slow miles of training (*long slow distance* or LSD) should be the basis of any conditioning foundation. A stall-confined horse needs a more strategic approach to riding than a horse that is turned out and allowed to exercise at free will.

Conditioning tendons and ligaments to the stress of exercise is a lengthy project, requiring years to develop them to peak strength. Conditioning techniques as described for developing the cardiovascular system, muscles, and bone also apply to tendons and ligaments. The main means of prevention of injury is to develop a horse's muscle strength and endurance. Strong muscles developed by a foundation of strategic conditioning enable a horse to do his job with minimal fatigue. In this way, the muscles assume some of the load-dampening effect for the tendons so the tendons are not overly strained. A horse must be prepared for a specific athletic endeavor with months and years of training and fitness targeted to that particular athletic effort. Common sense suggests that a rider should not exceed the pace or the duration for which a horse has been prepared.

Other Strategies

Institute a methodical warm-up and cool-down *before* and *after* exercise. A warm-up period of 15 to 20 minutes raises tissue temperature. This improves elasticity of the soft tissues, allowing them to stretch with minimal strain when a horse is put to work. A cool-down period allows heat to dissipate from the tendons, muscles, and joints before the horse is brought to a standstill (see "Warm-Up and Cool-Down Strategies," p. 153).

Icing the legs after a rigorous workout checks a mild inflammatory process. Commercial ice boots make this half-hour job easy, or a plastic bag of frozen peas can be wrapped around the leg and bandaged into place, changing as often as necessary to retain cold over the 30-minute period. Hosing the lower legs with cold water is another means of cooling the tissues. Monitor the limbs for abnormal swellings before and at the end of each ride.

Attention to proper shoeing on a regular schedule (every 5 to 7 weeks) is critical to prevention of soft-tissue injuries. The hoof and pastern should run parallel to each other in alignment and not have a broken-back axis (see chapter 3, *The Hoof,* p. 50). The toes should not be too long, and the heels should not be too high or too low. It is helpful to allow a horse to go barefoot for a few months to see how he crafts his feet if left to his own devices.

Predisposing Factors to Soft Tissue Injury

Most tendon or ligament injuries occur during exercise involving an intense activity and/or as a horse performs a movement with a leg not quite square beneath him. Each time a horse sets his foot down, tendons are loaded and stretched. This is normal, as they stretch and rebound to their original configuration. If soft tissues are asked to perform beyond their developed strength during a particularly rigorous exercise, or if a horse's muscles are fatigued, failure can result.

A tendon is comprised of many fibers arranged parallel to one another. Like a rubber band that is stretched too far, a tendon and its fibers may similarly overstretch and fail to return to original length. Or, tendon fibers may tear or rupture. (This results in a *bowed* tendon.) Ligament doesn't have nearly the elastic stretch of a tendon, and is more easily stretched and torn. A sudden twisting force on a joint may result in ligamentous injury. Injury to a tendon is called *tendinitis*, while to a ligament it is referred to as *desmitis*.

A traumatic blow from an opposite foot, a kick, or contact with a stationary object like a rock or tree also creates soft-tissue injury that must be treated as a stress-related failure. A wound or laceration can irritate tissues surrounding tendons or may disrupt tendon fibers. Constriction of soft tissues and surrounding circulation by an incorrectly applied bandage also has the potential to create significant tendon or ligamentous injury.

Not all soft-tissue injuries occur during a single event. Sometimes damage results from cumulative overuse, ultimately leading to failure. Repeated stretching of a tendon with each footfall may damage surrounding tissues that supply nutrients to the tendon tissues. With intensive exercise, such as galloping, the interior portions of the tendons heat up and may be subject to thermal injury. In either case, with time, progressive degeneration may transform a simmering problem into a recognizable injury.

A previously injured tendon or ligament is more at risk for reinjury since these soft tissue structures "heal" with scar tissue instead of normal fiber architecture. Sometimes the tissues thicken and occasionally may calcify. Elasticity is less than optimal so fibers are more prone to disruption from stretching.

Other predisposing factors exist that increase a horse's risk of developing a tendon or ligament injury.

Conformation

Conformation plays an important role in whether or not soft-tissue structures are at risk of injury. Long, sloping pasterns increase the risk of injury to the SDFT because long pasterns permit more fetlock drop than is desirable. This places more tension and stretch on the SDFT. A long toe and low heel (LTLH) amplify tendon strain in a horse with poor conformation while artificially creating excess fetlock drop in a more desirably conformed horse. In addition, a LTLH foot configuration delays breakover of the foot so that the fetlock joint overextends while loaded. This particular syndrome is easily rectified with excellent farrier technique, squaring back the toes, and the application of shoes with ample heel support.

An upright pastern, with or without a low heel places a horse at risk of tearing the *distal sesamoidean ligaments* along the back of the pastern. This injury is usually accompanied by swelling and lameness, however, not always. It is common to discover past evidence of its occurrence as an incidental finding on radiographs (X-ray films).

Poorly Conditioned for the Task

A horse that is overridden for his level of fitness often experiences muscle fatigue. This is significant because the muscles play a dampening role in how much stress is transmitted across the tendons. Tired muscles lose their supporting role, thus allowing tendons to stretch beyond their normal limits. Contraction of fatigued muscles is delayed or weakened so the limb isn't moved off the ground as quickly as normal. The foot "sticks" and then the fetlock drops too far (*dorsiflexion*—see figs. 5.27 A & B, p. 124). The result can be minor strain, or the more severe injury, a bowed tendon.

Difficult Terrain

Slippery, or uneven terrain creates hazards that can cause a horse to take an uncoordinated step. As long as he isn't fully supporting his weight on a misplaced leg, he'll probably be able to recover his footing. However, if his full body mass is moving forward over a limb placed crookedly beneath him, injury can occur from overstretching or twisting of soft tissues. Similarly, deep mud or shoe caulks can cause a leg to "stick" longer than it should while the horse continues forward (see photo 3.45, p. 63). This places excessive strain on tendons, and may result in soft tissue injury.

Quick Turns

Quick turns may overload a limb, placing too much downward force too quickly on soft tissue structures. A similar phenomenon occurs when a horse comes off a jump, or a steep hill or ledge. And, an overweight horse potentially overloads the limbs, particularly if he is muscle weary.

Concussion Injury

Vibrations occur within soft-tissue structures from the concussion of movement. Over-training may create microdamage within a tendon or ligament, or to surrounding tissues and blood supply. Over time the soft tissues degenerate and ultimately fail. This is particularly true of injury to the suspensory ligament, which results from cumulative stress. Speed work on downhill inclines imposes great strain on the suspensory ligaments that support the fetlock joints from over-extension. Persistent exercise of this nature places a horse at risk of incurring suspensory desmitis.

Injury-Prone Areas

There are a multitude of tendons and ligaments throughout a horse's body, but discussed on the following pages are those that most commonly incur injury in an athletic horse.

Strong Tendons and Ligaments

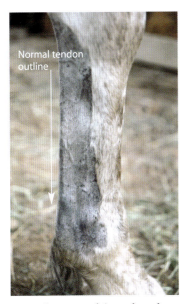

7.2 When viewed from the side, a normal tendon profile has a straight, regular appearance with no enlargements or thickenings.

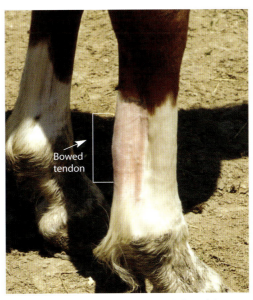

7.3 This acutely bowed superficial digital flexor tendon shows a bulge from swelling and inflammation.

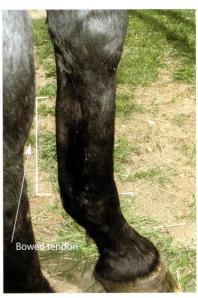

7.4 An acute injury to the flexor tendons created lameness and swelling in this limb, visible as a distinct bow.

Cannon Bone Region

SUPERFICIAL DIGITAL FLEXOR TENDON

One of the most commonly injured soft tissue structures of the athletic horse is the *superficial digital flexor tendon* or SDFT (photo 7.2 and see fig. 7.1, p. 181). As said earlier, significant strain to this tendon results in a bowed appearance, giving it the name *bowed* tendon (photos 7.3, 7.4, and 7.5). Injury occurs when the SDFT is placed under excess tension, especially as the fetlock is at its maximum drop just before a horse's foot leaves the ground. The danger of injury increases if a foot "sticks" and cannot lift off the ground, yet the horse's body continues to propel forward. The SDFT is at greatest risk of strain because its point of rotation is farthest from the fetlock joint than other tendinous structures. Many SDFT injuries occur at the point where the superficial digital flexor tendon has the smallest cross-sectional area, which is in

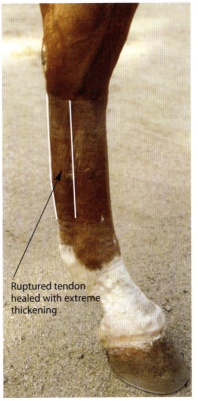

7.5 This horse fell off a mountainside, and ruptured her superficial digital flexor tendon. At eight months of healing, the tendon has scarred in and thickened to a large degree. The horse remains lame and her athletic career is finished due to massive and irreparable damage.

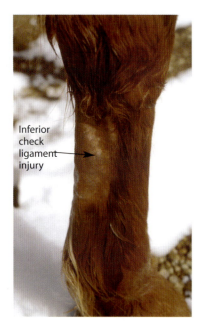

7.6 *An injury to the inferior check ligament elicits swelling in the middle of the tendons along the cannon bone.*

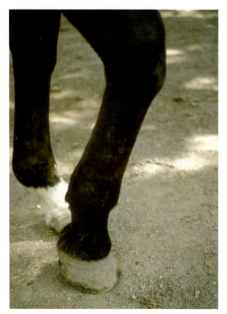

7.7 *A horse with tendon pain in the lower part of the limb often stands with his ankle flexed to relieve weight off the back portion of the leg.*

the middle of the cannon bone area. As the tendon's cross-sectional area decreases, it becomes stiffer and less elastic. In addition, there is an increased force per unit area on this narrower segment of the tendon.

INFERIOR CHECK LIGAMENT

The accessory ligament of the deep digital flexor tendon is also referred to as the *inferior check ligament*, or IFCL (see fig. 7.1, p. 181). Injury to this ligament usually occurs in older horses as a result of athletic strain, most often developing on a front limb. In an acute injury, there is pain and swelling just above the midpoint of the cannon bone (photo 7.6). A horse in pain may tip his heel off the ground and stand with the fetlock slightly flexed (photo 7.7). An ultrasound exam defines the extent of injury, and examines surrounding structures, like the superficial and deep digital flexor tendons, that might also be affected.

This is a difficult injury to resolve, with successful return to athletic function noted in only 43 to 75 percent of those treated with 3 months of box-stall rest, anti-inflammatory medications, and controlled walking rehabilitation over another 3 month period. Recurrence is likely with this injury. One recommendation that has been made for chronic or recurrent cases is to cut the IFCL by a surgery referred to as an *inferior check desmotomy*. A more guarded outlook must be taken when there is concurrent injury to the superficial and/or deep flexor tendons, as well.

PROXIMAL SUSPENSORY LIGAMENT

Injury to the uppermost third of the suspensory ligament (see fig. 7.1, p. 181) is known as *proximal suspensory desmitis*, and can develop on a front or rear limb. Horses with straight hocks, or those engaged in activities that require hyperextension of the fetlock (jumping, cutting, reining, calf roping, polo, or trail events with downhill trot or canter) are most at risk. Use of the longe line is incriminated in creating proximal suspensory injury as well as fostering reoccurrence. Heel wedges also increase the risk of this injury, as does a long-toe low-heel (LTLH) hoof configuration (see chapter 3, *The Hoof*, p. 51).

Initially, when a horse suffers a front limb suspensory injury, he may demonstrate discomfort by shortening the stride. This can be an insidious lameness that starts out as a seemingly mild problem and responds to rest and confinement, only to reoccur following any exercise.

In a rear limb, lameness is worse when the affected hind is on the outside of a circle, or when a horse is exercised on a soft or deep surface. When a rear limb is affected, the lameness doesn't usually respond to rest, and instead continues to worsen. Some horses demonstrate discomfort by reluctance to go forward when asked; there is often a noticeable reduction in hind limb impulsion. Lameness also worsens when a rider "sits" on the weight-bearing diagonal of the affected limb.

Digital pressure over an injured proximal suspensory ligament does not always elicit a pain reaction from a horse. The normally sharp margins to a ligament may feel rounded along with a stiffer feel to an affected ligament. Radiographic exam is necessary to identify if there is a concurrent fracture of the outermost portion of the cannon bone or an *avulsion* (tearing away) fracture that sometimes accompany a suspensory injury. Definitive diagnosis depends upon a diagnostic nerve block to infuse anesthetic locally in the area of concern, coupled with a thorough ultrasound exam.

Proximal suspensory desmitis is a difficult problem to manage. Affected forelimbs reoccur 20 percent of the time, while hind leg proximal suspensory desmitis reoccurs 65 percent of the time. Application of *extracorporeal shock wave therapy* (ESWT—p. 106) along with conventional anti-inflammatory therapy and controlled exercise has yielded a greater success rate for continued return to athletic function. ESWT returned 41 percent of hind limb cases to their previous level of work by 6 months following treatment. In all cases of proximal suspensory desmitis, rest is paramount for resolution of the injury. At least 1 to 4 months is required for a front leg, whereas a hind leg requires 4 to 6 months minimum. Assessment of improvement is based on progressive ultrasound exams.

CURB

Curb refers to inflammation or tearing of the *plantar tarsal ligament* at the back outside aspect of the hock. It is easily confused with an overly developed splint bone (photo 7.8). Also, inflammation of a rear limb superficial flexor tendon is sometimes confused with a curb because of close proximity of the tendon to the plantar tarsal ligament. Sickle-hocked conformation increases the propensity to develop inflammation of the plantar tarsal ligament. It may also occur as a result of a horse's rear limb slipping as he pushes up a steep hill or as a result of rapid sprint acceleration.

Fetlock Region

LOW BOW

If the *deep digital flexor tendon* (DDFT) is injured, a *low bow* results (photo 7.9). Tendon injuries in the fetlock area or below have a poorer prognosis than injuries higher on the limb. Because of the digital sheath over the tendon in this area, more connective tissue develops beneath the skin (subcutaneous) in the healing process (photo 7.10). This tissue restricts gliding of the tendon through the sheath.

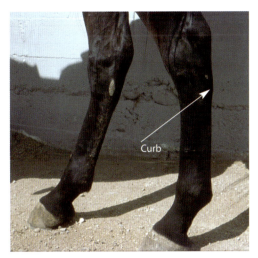

7.8 *Curb is an inflammatory condition of the plantar tarsal ligament at the rear of the hock on the outside, as seen here.*

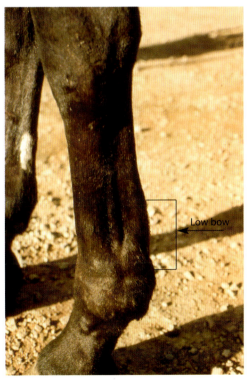

7.9 *Injury to a flexor tendon along the lower part of the back of the cannon bone is referred to as a low bow.*

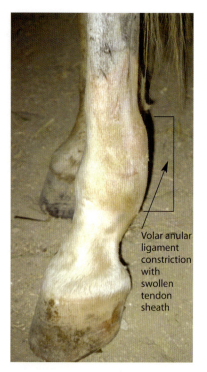

7.10 *The deep digital flexor tendon sheath runs along the back of the leg from just above the fetlock all the way into the lower pastern area. Injuries to this tendon sheath form a windpuff swelling with varying degrees of lameness. With chronic inflammation, adhesions can form within the tendon sheath, leading to constriction of the volar anular ligament. This is usually accompanied by significant swelling of the tendon sheath, as seen here.*

VOLAR ANULAR LIGAMENT INJURY

The *volar anular ligament* (VAL), a non-elastic band of dense connective tissue, runs horizontally across the back of the fetlock, and may be involved in a low bow. The volar anular ligament does not stretch as the deep digital flexor tendon swells; then the ligament binds down the inflamed tendon. This unrelenting pressure reduces blood flow to the tendon over time. Fiber death, reduction in gliding motion, and development of adhesions bind the two structures together as a result of reduced blood flow. The ligament constricts, resulting in a visible depression over the back of the fetlock, with a pronounced bulge above and/or below, near the digital tendon sheath (photo 7.11).

Immediate surgical intervention to release the constricting ligament allows a more favorable prognosis for a horse to return to function. If adhesions are allowed to progress too long before surgery, they "glue" the structures together, permanently restricting the tendon and causing a mechanical lameness.

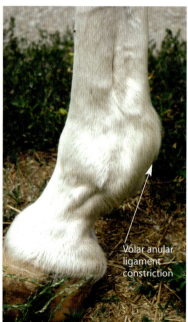

7.11 *This horse is experiencing constriction of the volar anular ligament. Such a constriction may create lameness due to pain and mechanical restriction of the gait.*

DEGENERATIVE SUSPENSORY DESMITIS

Some horse breeds, such as Peruvian Pasos, Paso Finos, and Andalusians, experience notable degeneration of the branches of the suspensory apparatus for reasons unrelated to trauma or injury (photo 7.12). A high degree of breed-related incidence implicates a possible genetic component. Older horses of any breed, especially broodmares, may suffer the same condition. Previous injury to a suspensory ligament increases the chance of ligament degeneration. The problem typically appears in the hind limbs. The fetlocks sink as suspensory support progressively declines (photo 7.13). There is often associated stiffness or lameness related to suspensory and/or fetlock pain. Nothing can be done other than to keep a horse comfortable on soft ground or bedding to prevent abrasions of the fetlock. Attempts can be made to support the fetlock and pastern joints by extending the heel branches of the shoes, or using elongated egg bar shoes.

Strong Tendons and Ligaments

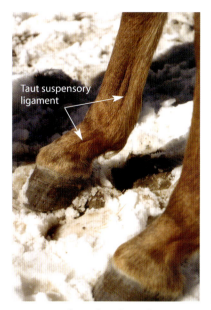

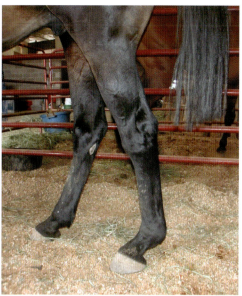

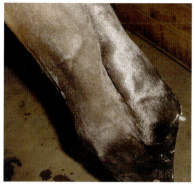

7.14 *Injury to the Achilles tendon along the back of the hock is accompanied by swelling and lameness. The best way to identify the extent of this particular injury is with diagnostic ultrasound (see p. 190).*

7.12 *Some horse breeds, such as Peruvian Pasos and Paso Finos, are prone to suspensory ligament degeneration as seen here. Note the bulge and tautness visible along the overstretched suspensory ligament in this photo.*

7.13 *Degeneration of the suspensory ligaments allows excessive dropping of the fetlock, as seen here in this aged horse. Such hyperextension of the fetlocks leads to joint and soft tissue injury, with pain and lameness.*

Signs of Injury: Diagnostic Aids

Pain, Heat, and Swelling

Both before and after exercise, it is important to monitor the legs for abnormal signs. Regular monitoring compares tendons on a daily basis to alert one to change. If caught early, many injuries may be treated with excellent results. When tendons or ligaments are injured, a horse often experiences pain and swelling, but not always (photo 7.14). Sometimes, the only notable indication may be that a horse's stride has shortened, he is unwilling to move forward, or he seems to move with a stiff gait. Swelling may be present due to serum or blood filling within or around the tendon or ligament. An inflammatory response by the body increases blood flow to the area, so in some cases, the tissues may feel warm. Distention of the tissues and inflammatory chemicals released by the body generate pain for the horse. A horse may feel pain when the injured tendon is squeezed between your fingers, called *palpation* (photo 7.15).

7.15 *To identify pain in a tendon along the back of the cannon bone, it is best to lift the limb off the ground, then to gently palpate along the extent of the tendons, one structure at a time. Compare the suspect leg with the opposite normal leg to determine if a horse reacts by pulling his leg away because he is overly sensitive to touch or because there is true pain.*

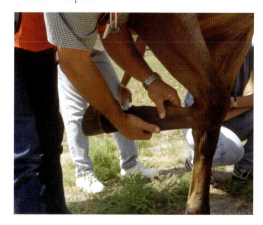

7.16 A & B *Ultrasound is the best diagnostic tool to evaluate integrity of the tendon fibers and structure. This longitudinal view of a normal tendon shows a compact, parallel arrangement of the fibers of each tendon (A). In comparison, it is easy to see the ruptured area of tendon fibers, visible as dark areas in the longitudinal view (B). This is a serious disruption to the tendon, requiring a lengthy healing time and possibly limited return to athletic work.*

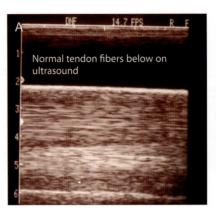
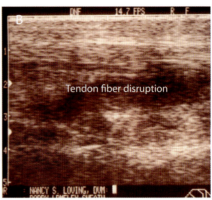

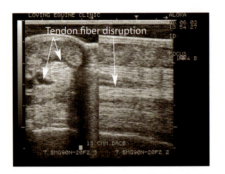

7.17 *Here are two images placed side by side. The one on the left is the tendon structure viewed in cross-section, while the one on the right is the same location of that tendon but in longitudinal view. There is evidence of tearing and fiber disruption in both orientations.*

The presence or absence of overt clinical signs (such as pain, heat, swelling, or lameness) correlate poorly with the severity of a tendon injury. The only accurate method of assessment is with diagnostic ultrasound.

Diagnostic Ultrasound

A *diagnostic ultrasound* exam provides a noninvasive method of "imaging" the internal fibers of a tendon or ligament (photos 7.16 A & B and 7.17). It is possible, then, to accurately "see" which structures are damaged, the exact degree of injury, and to measure the size of a lesion. This gives an understanding of how long a horse must be rested, and when he can return to work with the least chance of recurrence. To track healing progress, ultrasound exams are repeated at 2 to 3 month intervals. Ultrasound information gives a baseline to which to compare future serial exams.

It is valuable to ultrasound the opposite limb as a means of comparison. The cross-sectional measurement of tendons compared between the two limbs should have less than a 5 percent difference. It is possible for a tendon injury to occur in both limbs, and this can confuse analysis of the measurements.

Tendon and Ligament Repair

The principles of healing and treatment are the same for tendons and ligaments, however ligament injuries are much more difficult to resolve. Ligaments tear away from bone and although the area of bone attachment may heal, an injured ligament may never regain its original strength or structure. Many ligamentous injuries alter the athletic career of a horse to lesser demands, whereas tendon injuries have a better chance of returning to function, if given time and therapy. Microscopic tears in the orderly arrangement of tendon fibers may expand to a larger tear.

Accompanying inflammation produces clinical symptoms of pain, heat, or swelling. Edema and bleeding interrupt a tendon's fiber patterns that are normally arranged in tight, longitudinally-oriented and parallel bundles. A tendon is weakest at 5 to 7 days following injury, with the acute inflammatory stage lasting up to 14 days.

Fibrin and Granulation Tissue Repair Process

Fibrin is a blood component that binds together torn tendon collagen. In the initial weeks following injury, fibrin forms a "callus" around an injured tendon that connects wounded structures, in effect hardening the fibrin cells into a scaffold for repair. Then, like a skin wound (see chapter 14, *Equine First Aid, Medication, and Restraint*, p. 407), the body repairs a tendon injury with granulation tissue that organizes into fibrous tissue. Over following months, a tendon repair "matures." Collagen fibers redevelop to a normal, longitudinal orientation. Usually, by 6 weeks following injury, collagen formation exceeds collagen breakdown within a tendon. By 3 months, collagen fibers begin to form discrete bundles that approximate normal tendon fibers by 4 to 6 months. The inflammatory process has the potential to permanently thicken a tendon with scar tissue, giving the visual impression of a bow where previously there had been a straight structure (photos 7.18 and 7.19).

Blood supply within a tendon only nourishes 25 percent of the tendon volume. Because inflammation limits internal blood flow, healing components must come from tissue around (*peritendinous*) the tendon. The more actively peritendinous cells contribute to healing, the greater the development of adhesions and scar tissue. Adhesions restrict normal gliding of a tendon through its sheath, and scar tissue limits its elasticity. Excellent tendon repair depends on limiting the inflammatory response throughout the healing phase.

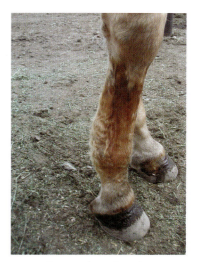

7.18 *The term bowed tendon describes the obvious appearance of an injured healing tendon—it thickens with scar tissue giving it the appearance of a bow rather than a straight structure.*

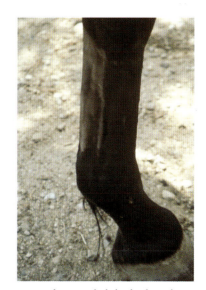

7.19 *This is a slightly thickened tendon bow due to a mild injury. With time, this injury will remodel so that finger palpation may identify a slight thickening, but the tendon will visibly appear relatively straight and normal.*

Exercises That Promote Healing

During the repair process, controlled passive motion exercises realign collagen fibers longitudinally by placing mild tension on the tendon. Slow, range-of-motion exercises include manual flexion and extension of the limb for 10 to 15 minutes, 2 or 3 times a day. After the acute inflammatory stage, light hand walking can begin. Progressively increase these exercises over the months. It is not known how much passive physical therapy is appropriate; therefore it is wise not to overdo this practice. Aggressive physical activity interferes with repair, and reinjury can occur. Attempts to forcibly break down adhesions are counterproductive, whereas gentle lengthening and stretching of scar tissue gives better results.

Healing Time

Time required for tendon healing varies, depending on the extent of the injury. A minimum recovery period for slight tendon injury may require only a month. More severe injuries require at least 10 months for a tendon to heal to its best. In some cases, recovery times as long as 1½ years may be necessary to achieve optimal repair. Veterinary recommendations should be followed so a long enough recuperative period is given to prevent a relapse. Indications of "healing" can be misleading. Many horses at 10 weeks after injury may not be sensitive to finger pressure over the tendon. They may also have no heat or swelling in the area. However, there are still areas of tendon damage that are in the earlier healing stages and require a longer rest period than other areas of the same tendon.

Successful Outcome versus Recurrence

RECURRENCE OF TENDON INJURY

Recurrence of a tendon injury is possible if the tendon is prematurely stressed while an injury is visible on ultrasound. Not all healed tendon injuries are immune to further damage. Prior tendinitis does not result in loss of strength in the tendon, but does result in reduced elasticity. A previously injured tendon, bowed or not, may be unable to withstand stresses placed on it by exercise.

Transition Zone

Subsequent tendon damage does not necessarily occur at the site of the original injury. It often occurs just above or below the point where tendon structure least resembles normal structure. These areas are called *transition zones*. Adhesions in a transition zone may prevent the fibers from orientating longitudinally as they heal. Instead, they orient abnormally and may tear prematurely before they reorganize in a longitudinal pattern. Fibers with a loosely structured and random pattern are a weak link in the collagen chain. Adhesions are unyielding, causing the inelastic tendon tissue above or below the original injury to "super stretch." Continued microtrauma in this area enlarges the traumatized area, and causes lameness due to chronic inflammation.

Tendon and Ligament Therapy

There are many approaches to therapy for tendinitis or a bowed tendon. The ultimate goal is to restore elasticity and gliding function to the tendon. Lameness, heat, sensitivity, and swelling of the tendons are unreliable indicators; diagnostic ultrasound is the tool of choice in assessing progress. Once symptoms appear, emergency measures minimize damage.

Controlling Swelling and Inflammation

THERMAL TREATMENT

Local swelling and hemorrhage further damage tendon and ligament fibers. Therefore, control of swelling is essential if the tendon is to heal well and with limited adhesions. Ice and heat therapy are well-respected treatments for a myriad of injuries and lameness conditions in the horse. Horse owners have effectively treated sore legs with cold, followed by hot packs, for centuries.

Cold Today and Hot Tomorrow

Cold therapy is typically applied in the first 24 to 48 hours of injury, and heat therapy 72 hours following injury. (A jingle helps to remind you which order to apply therapy: "cold today and hot tamale.") But, depending on the extent of an injury, the acute inflammatory stage may last from 2 days to 2 weeks, and cold therapy is best applied throughout the course of the acute phase of injury.

Ice-water immersion reaches desired therapeutic tissue temperature levels in the skin and subcutaneous tissues, but not in the deeper tissues. However, one main effect of either hot or cold therapy is its modification on enzyme actions and on tissue metabolism. It is known that cell activity, enzyme reactions, and metabolic rates of the tissues will change up to threefold for every 18° F (10° C) change in tissue temperature. Cold water/ice immersion reduces temperatures by as much as a 14° F (8° C) range. Warm water hosing changes temperatures by as much range as 13° F (8° C). Based on these values, there should be an accompanying change in metabolic rates of the tissues when subjected to hot or cold therapy. Appropriate treatment methods have beneficial effects to a tissue depth of 2 cm, especially when applied for at least 20 to 30 minutes.

COLD THERAPY

Examples of injuries that benefit from cold therapy are:

- Strained tendons or ligaments
- Splints
- Muscle injury
- Joint injury
- Kick trauma
- Interference trauma (striking one leg with another)

Apply cold for the first 48 to 72 hours after an injury occurs. Water immersion (with ice in buckets, boots, or the cold of a running stream) is the best form of cold therapy (photo 7.20). If water immersion is not used, wrap ice in a towel to prevent freezing the superficial skin layers. The therapeutic threshold for cold therapy is considered to be at a temperature below 66° F (19° C); this is accomplished best by using ice or ice water.

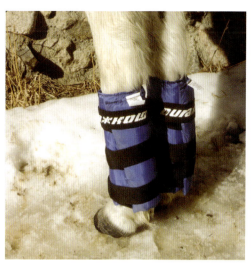

7.20 Commercial ice boots are helpful in applying cold therapy to limb injuries. Soak the skin in water first, then apply the boots. Body warmth will melt the ice packs, so it is best to change to a freshly frozen boot after 15 to 20 minutes if longer therapy is necessary.

Effects of Cold Therapy

Decreasing Inflammation

Cold therapy arrests the inflammatory process by decreasing blood flow to the area as capillaries constrict from the cold. Slowing of bleeding and hematoma formation controls fluid leakage into the injury site. Hemorrhage and edema disrupt tendon or ligament fibers. The initial use of cold treatment and a compression bandage minimizes scar tissue thickening in the tendon.

Pain Relief

Cold provides pain relief (*analgesia*) because nerve signals are limited at temperatures of 50 to 59° F (10 to 15° C). Analgesia lessens muscle and tendon spasms. By "cooling" a tendon or ligament, pain and lameness subside and give a false impression of a "cure." But cold therapy also increases the stiffness of the collagen in tendon or ligament fibers, reducing

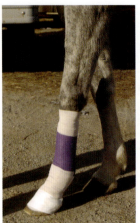
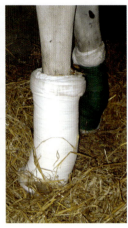

7.22 *A Robert Jones bandage is an excellent means of providing tendon compression without danger of blood flow constriction. Such a bandage is created by wrapping the limb with multiple layers of roll cotton to make thick padding, then applying a polo wrap or bandaging tape around the cotton.*

7.21 *Compression bandaging from the carpus (knee) to the hoof helps to limit limb swelling.*

the elasticity of these structures. Although a horse may not be visibly lame, premature or strenuous exercise is detrimental and may result in additional injury. Rest is the time-honored therapy for treatment of most tendon strains.

BANDAGING

After cooling down a strained tendon, a splint, or injured muscle or joint, it is advantageous to bandage the limb when possible. The benefits of bandaging include:

- Reduced swelling encourages tissues to heal with limited scar tissue
- "Support" of soft tissues in proximity to damaged structures
- Prevents the spread of swelling to other areas of the leg

Gravity encourages swelling of structures below an injury site. If an injury occurs above the fetlock, it is best to bandage from just below the carpus (knee) or hock to the hoof (photo 7.21). A full limb bandage is less likely to slip into a position where it hinders blood flow.

Monitor for excess bandage constriction. Signs include swelling above the bandage, or signs of discomfort with a horse chewing at the bandage or stamping his foot. Cotton padding prevents inadvertent tightening of bandage materials that could hinder circulation or compress tendons (photo 7.22). Apply bandages uniformly with no bumps or wrinkles.

HEAT THERAPY

Heat therapy can be applied after the initial inflammatory phase has passed following injury: this could be 2 days to 2 weeks (see p. 191). Heat therapy works by warming the tissues around an injury site. This warming stimulates the body to "cool" the area by dilating vessels and increasing blood flow. Oxygen supply improves, and blood components such as white blood cells, antibodies, and nutrients are delivered to the tissues. The lymphatic vessels remove waste products and excess edema fluid. Elasticity and stretch improves in tendons and ligaments with warmth. Pain decreases, and healing is enhanced. Light bandaging after heat therapy is advantageous to limit mild tissue edema.

Hair and the thick layer of horsehide serve as an insulating barrier to heat, and more time is required to warm deeper structures than surface structures. Application of heat to a limb for 20 minutes is usually adequate. Problems that benefit from heat therapy include:

- Contusions (bruising)
- Mild sprains
- Strains
- Muscle or nerve inflammation
- Joint arthritis

Water immersion or hot water bottles are more effective than dry heat as produced with an electric heating pad. A towel placed between the skin and a hot pack prevents burning and insulates the pack. Any temperature that you can tolerate on your own skin is safe to apply to a horse's skin. For heat treatment, tissue temperature should reach at least 106° F (41° C). A horse will not tolerate heat above 113° F (45° C).

If you apply heat in the acute phase of an injury, you increase circulation and tissue metabolism, furthering damage and swelling. But in most cases, 2 or 3 days later, microscopic bleeding has ceased, and the healing process has begun. At this time, heat therapy decreases spasms in the area to provide pain relief, while promoting cellular cleanup of the injury.

Sweat Bandages

Use of a leg "sweat" is another one-step method of heat therapy. An effective leg sweat is prepared by combining DMSO and a nitrofurazone preparation. "Sweat" bandages work by increasing heat and circulation to an area to remove swelling. A plastic wrap placed under a standing wrap traps sweat produced by the leg, creating a fluid barrier and retaining heat by preventing evaporative cooling. To prevent skin rash, a sweat bandage should not be left on for more than 48 hours.

Epsom Salt Soaks

The benefits of wet heat therapy can be improved by adding Epsom salts (magnesium sulfate). A solution is prepared by dissolving 2 cups Epsom salts per gallon of warm water. The limb is soaked in this solution for 20 minutes.

Poultices

A commercial poultice preparation "pulls" swelling from an inflamed area as do Epsom salts. A poultice compound is applied beneath a layer of absorbent material, such as roll cotton. Swelling is pulled away from the tissues in the presence of a warm, moist environment. A light pressure wrap over the cotton holds the preparation in place and supports soft tissue. Gelocast®, zinc oxide-impregnated bandages, and Animalintex® pads serve as excellent, ready-made poulticing materials, and need only be covered with an elastic, adhesive bandage, such as Elastikon®.

Liniments and Balms

Many old-time horse liniments and leg balms also elicit heat and increase circulation by chemical action and by mild irritation of the skin. Human and equine athletes use these balms to advantage, but most should not be applied beneath a bandage, as there is a possibility of "burning" the skin. Follow manufacturer's recommendations.

OTHER BENEFICIAL THERAPIES

DMSO

When applied in the same manner as a poultice, DMSO is an effective anti-inflammatory agent (see p. 127). It occasionally irritates the skin, and may result in mild hair loss. Do not apply it to any raw or deep wound surfaces. Wear protective gloves when applying DMSO as it easily penetrates human skin.

Massage and Hydrotherapy

Deep massage is beneficial to an injured muscle or tendon along with cold and heat therapy. It increases circulation and breaks down adhesions formed by scar tissue. Massage can be done by hand, or by hosing the limb with a forceful spray of water (hydrotherapy). Whirlpool boots are a commercially available option. A whirlpool can be made by reversing a vacuum cleaner to convert the sucking air into blowing air. Inserting the vacuum hose into water achieves a turbulator effect, but exercise extreme caution when using electrical cords and water in close proximity.

Physical Therapy

Soft tissue injury responds well to controlled mobilization of the lower limb. This is achieved by passive flexion and extension of the joints below the carpus (knee) or hock. The advantages gained from passively stretching the tissues include:

- Increase in localized circulation to improve oxygen delivery for tissue repair
- Activation of lymphatic and venous drainage to decrease swelling
- Prevention of adhesions that limit movement
- Maintenance of muscle tone and suppleness

Following a period of applied exercises of controlled physical therapy, a horse can then be started back to controlled exercise.

Controlled Exercise

Controlled exercise enhances circulation to a limb and reduces the buildup of fibrous scar tissue adhesions in tendon or ligament injuries. Light exercise, such as handwalking, can begin after the acute inflammatory stage has subsided. *"Stocking up"* from confinement, or swelling created by pregnancy responds quickly to light exercise.

"Support" Bandages

After a layoff for a tendon injury, support wraps are often applied during reintroduction to work in an attempt to delay the onset of fatigue in an injured leg. It is speculated that a bandage limits dorsiflexion of the fetlock when a limb is fatigued. A leg bandaged with the Equisport® (3-M) bandage may absorb up to 39 percent more energy of dorsiflexion of the fetlock than an unbandaged leg (see figs. 5.27 A & B, p. 124). In theory, the bandage assumes the elastic function of the tendons as the fetlock sinks with weight-bearing, reducing strain on the tendons. Studies with these bandages focus mainly on racetrack application; in this situation the bandage only needs to aid limb support for 2 to 5 minutes. Materials that absorb the most energy also tend to wear out fastest. Bandage support of a limb declines rapidly with an increasing number of fetlock dorsiflexions. This limitation makes "support bandaging" impractical for most other equine athletic pursuits like dressage, trail, jumping, reining, cutting, and roping.

Bandages may be more of a hindrance than a help if they are applied too tightly and impair local circulation, or if they partially restrict the range of motion of the fetlock joint. The supportive capabilities of a bandage depend on the tension with which it is applied, and the bandage configuration. The tighter a bandage is applied, the greater is its energy-absorption capacity. The most versatile method of applying a bandage is at half-stretch tension in a low figure eight, starting just below the carpus (knee) and spiraling down with a two to three layer figure eight over the fetlock, and the bandage spiraled up again to the carpus (knee). Applied in this manner, the bandage does not inhibit fetlock mobility, and at half-stretch tension it should not impair local circulation or constrict the tendons.

Drug Therapy

Drug therapy is used in conjunction with hydrotherapy and rest of an injured leg. Commonly used drugs are the nonsteroidal anti-inflammatory drugs (NSAIDs), such as phenylbutazone or flunixin meglumine. NSAIDs limit the inflammatory process before it begins, and limit edema, swelling, and pain. However, NSAIDs may mask a severe problem that requires professional attention. A horse might further inflict injury subsequent to lessening of a protective pain response by NSAIDs.

Surgery

For superficial digital flexor injuries, one surgical technique, called a *superior check desmotomy*, involves cutting the superior check ligament to release tension on the scarred tendon. The superior check ligament is an extension of the superficial digital flexor muscle and is located just above and toward the rear of the carpus (knee). When performed during the initial repair stage, there may be reduced scarring in the tendon. The superior check ligament lengthens as it heals, reducing tension on the injured tendon. Its transitional zone is not subjected to much stress because both the muscle and tendon above the carpus actively assume some of the load of weight-bearing.

THERAPEUTIC ULTRASOUND

Ultrasound is a therapeutic tool because it "heats" musculoskeletal components that may be too deep, too large, or too dense to benefit from hot soaking. The penetrating warmth of ultrasound therapy reduces spasms in muscles or tendons, particularly in the large muscles over the back, buttocks, and shoulders. It is especially difficult to use conventional heat therapy in these areas because only superficial warming would result.

Mechanics of Ultrasound

Ultrasound's therapeutic advantage comes from its mechanical effects. As sound waves enter the tissues, the tissue molecules "vibrate." Energy created by the friction of sound waves entering the tissue generates heat. Ultrasound energy is barely absorbed by skin, but is well-absorbed in tissues with a high protein and low fluid content, such as muscles, tendons, and ligaments. Muscle absorbs two-and-a-half times as much of this energy as fat; bone absorbs 10 times as much energy as muscle.

Types of Therapeutic Ultrasound

Continuous Wave

Ultrasound is used as either a continuous wave, or as a pulse at regular intervals. Continuous wave ultrasound provides deep heat, improving elasticity and pliability of tight, thickened, and scarred tissues. Horses involved in sports that require collection, pushing from behind, or stretching the back can form scar tissue in their backs. These sports include endurance, eventing, jumping, and dressage. Or, scar tissue can form as fibrotic myopathy within the thigh muscles (see p. 173).

Problems with Continuous Wave

If ultrasonic waves are generated continuously, excessive heat builds in the shallow tissues. Ultrasound can raise tissue temperature by 7 to 8° F (8 to 12° C) at 2 inches below the skin surface if applied continuously over one spot or for too long. Too much heat in the tissues is counterproductive, resulting in permanent damage to bone and surrounding tissue. The appropriate amount of time the ultrasound is applied depends on the type of tissue and the injury involved.

Bones are very dense, and the sound waves cannot pass all the way through them. The energy reflects back to the source, overheating the bone and surrounding tissue. Ultrasound treatment of fractured, inflamed, or growing bone results in excessive blood circulation to the bone, with resultant demineralization and thinning of the affected area. Excessively heating bone and surrounding tissues destroys the blood supply, causing part of the bone to die and separate from the healthy bone.

Pulsing Wave

Pulsated waves can be compared to waves crashing on a beach. Unlike the ocean, however, medical pulsing waves can be adjusted to penetrate the exact distance desired into the tissues, thereby limiting overheating. Greater intensity of ultrasonic waves increases the tissue absorption of the waves. Not only can the ultrasonic waves be adjusted to limit penetration, but the interval between pulses also allows heat dissipation from the tissues.

Applications of Ultrasound

Reducing Swelling

A useful application of ultrasound for tendon and ligament injuries is to combine it with cold therapy. An ice pack or cold water is applied for 20 minutes; then ultrasound is pulsed at 25 percent frequency (every fourth wave) for 20 minutes. A massaging effect known as "microstreaming" or "acoustical streaming" encourages moving molecules to go from areas of high concentration to areas of low concentration. Applying ultrasound in this way improves circulation, limits edema and pulses the swelling out of the limb.

A "sweat" bandage (see p. 195) can be applied to the limb for 24 hours after using a combination of cold and ultrasound therapy. Then, therapeutic ultrasound can be applied over topical medication (*phonophoresis*). Therapeutic ultrasound encourages small, molecular-weight molecules, such as topical corticosteroids, to penetrate up to 2 inches. It should not be used over open and contaminated wounds where it could drive bacteria deep into the tissues, spreading infection.

Relieving Pain and Promoting Healing

Deep heating of ultrasound relieves pain by changing the rate at which the nerves react and by limiting tissue spasms. Warmth restores the pliability of collagen fibers and relieves joint stiffness. Deep heat enhances circulation and metabolism that accelerate the healing process.

EXTRACORPOREAL SHOCK WAVE THERAPY

Extracorporeal shock wave therapy (ESWT—see p. 106) has been found to be useful particularly in treatment of chronic *proximal suspensory desmitis*. Historically, this form of suspensory ligament disease has been a fairly unrewarding syndrome to manage. Conventional treatment methods have met with a low success rate in diminishing lameness as well as a high rate of recurrence. Now, using the ESWT strategy, 40 percent of horses with proximal suspensory lameness duration of greater than 6 months returned to work as compared to none of the control horses treated by conventional methods that did not include ESWT. The treatment protocol included 3 treatments, each applied at 2 to 4 week intervals.

Tendon Disease: Flexural Contracture

A *flexural contracture* describes an inability of an affected joint(s) to be fully extended due to tension within the tendons. The limb is flexed to varying degrees, and in extreme cases in a foal may be folded past 90 degrees. Acquired cases of contracture may begin in a subtle fashion. Many contractures develop when a horse is young, but may persist into an athletic age if not corrected early on. Any degree of flexural contracture has consequences to the athletic potential of a horse so rapid recognition and intervention is important.

Congenital Flexural Contracture

Congenital flexural contractures may occur due to malposition of the foal in utero. A congenital condition also arises from ingestion of *teratogens* (an agent that is toxic to fetal growth) or toxic weeds like locoweed or Sudan grass (see *Appendix C*, p. 571). Most cases of congenital flexural contractures involve the carpal (knee) or fetlock joints (photo 7.23). In some cases, a foal may not be able to stand due to pronounced restriction of joint movement. Milder forms involve the lower limb joints.

Acquired Flexural Contracture

Acquired conditions develop due to pain reflexes that cause a foal to resist full stretch of the limb. Limb pain may be caused by trauma, infection, rapid growth, or overuse. Flexural contracture of the pastern or coffin joints is often precipitated by rapid growth associated with overfeeding and under-exercised foals, as is commonly seen with halter horses. Many cases of acquired lower limb contractures visibly develop over a 3 to 5 day period. The foal ends up walking on his toes within the week (photos 7.24 and 7.25 A & B).

Acquired flexural contractures are graded as mild, moderate, or severe. With a mild case, the hoof-ground angle is increased from its normal, but is less than 90 degrees. In these cases, a broken hoof-pastern axis is obvious. A moderate case has a hoof-ground angle increased past 90 degrees, while a severely affected foal bears weight on the dorsal (front) surface of the hoof wall.

Acquired fetlock flexural contractures generally occur in rapidly growing youngsters between 10 to 18 months of age. Usually both fetlocks of the front limbs are affected at the same time. Grading of the degree of contraction in the fetlock joints describes the degree of deformity. A foal with a mild grade fetlock contracture has fetlocks that are relatively straight. A moderate grade contracture describes fetlock joints that appear buckled forward when at

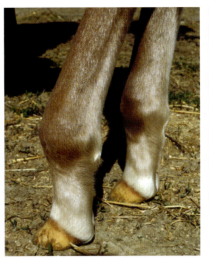

7.23 *Flexural deformity of the fetlock joint creates a buckling of the ankle due to contraction of the superficial digital flexor tendon. This is referred to as contracted tendons.*

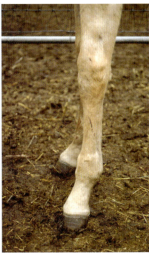

7.24 *This horse is afflicted by various elements of developmental orthopedic disease. He has epiphysitis of the carpi (knees) and fetlocks (see p. 132), as well as a flexural deformity or contraction of the left front hoof.*

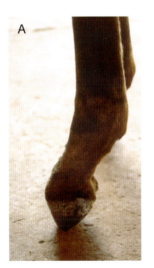
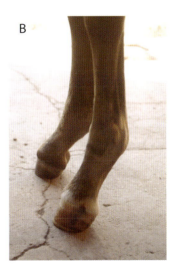

7.25 A & B *Contracture of the deep digital flexor tendon causes lifting of the heel off the ground (A), although it does not necessarily lift the heel all the way from contact with the ground (B).*

rest. If the joint flexes to an angle of more than 180 degrees (135 degree flexion is normal), the extensor tendons become taut and visibly pronounced. In a severe grade contracture, the fetlocks are knuckled over.

Club Foot

A more slowly developing process of *distal interphalangeal joint* (coffin joint) deformity occurs in which the heel stays in contact with the ground but tends to overgrow. There is a noticeable bulging of the coronary band, and the foot appears boxy; this condition is known as a club foot (photo 7.26, and see p. 52). Over time, internal changes of the coffin bone within the hoof capsule result in a hoof wall that grows out with a dish, much like a laminitis horse.

Treatment of Flexural Contracture

In a newborn foal with a congenital mild to moderate flexural contracture of the lower joints, the initial treatment of choice is the use of intravenous *oxytetracycline*, which is in fact an antibiotic. In this case, it is not used for its antibiotic properties. It is theorized that oxytetracycline binds calcium in such a way as to prevent calcium influx into the muscle fibers of the deep digital flexor tendon and its associated structures, thereby stimulating tendon laxity. Beneficial effects of this treatment often only last a few days so may need to be repeated again. The most successful results are seen when oxytetracycline is given within the first few days of life. Kidney function should be monitored with the use of oxytetracycline in a neonate, especially one that may already be sick.

Nonsteroidal anti-inflammatory (NSAIDs) medications (flunixin meglumine or phenylbutazone) are used in neonates, but with extreme caution because of the likelihood of development of gastric ulcers. These drugs help reduce pain reflexes while improving the foal's use of his limbs but should be administered with care and in conjunction with anti-ulcer medications.

If a foal cannot stand due to severe congenital flexural deformities, more aggressive procedures must be implemented in addition to splinting the affected limb(s). A foal with carpal contracture may require surgery of the *superior check ligament*. Cutting this check ligament (located just above the carpus) away from the tendon facilitates release of soft tissues for correction. Severe congenital flexion abnormalities often involve the carpus, fetlock, or multiple joints. Due to contraction and *fibrosis* (scarring) of the joint capsule and associated ligaments, severe congenital cases rarely respond to treatment and result in euthanasia.

In addition to use of oxytetracycline, multiple therapies are applied to mild to moderate lower limb flexural contractures. If the foot sits flat on the ground, then the foal may benefit from splinting and corrective shoeing with toe extensions. Toe extensions are glued on to the hoof to increase stretch of the tendons. The heels are also rasped down with a file to facilitate tendon stretch. Splints and bandages induce ligament laxity and may help the tissues to stretch. Another technique is to apply physical therapy with controlled manual stretching of the limb 2 or 3 times throughout the day. Gentle and repeated extension exercises lengthen and stretch the soft tissues. Restriction of the foal to controlled exercise (hand-walking) with no turn out protects the limbs from overuse. If these treatments are not successful within 10 days, then surgical release of the *inferior digital check ligament* (located in the cannon region) is recommended. Radiographs of the coffin bone and lower joints are important for monitoring health of these structures

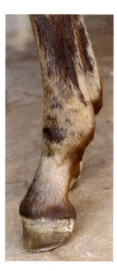

7.26 *A club foot is caused by flexural deformity at an early age. As seen here, the foot appears boxy and upright, and there is a noticeable bulge at the coronary band at the coffin joint.*

and are particularly helpful in guiding proper trimming of a club foot.

In all cases, it is important to balance the foal's nutritional plane with attention to minimizing excess energy intake. When possible, a foal with a flexural deformity should be pulled off a heavily nursing mare as well.

Weak Flexor Tendons

Some foals are born with relaxed and weak flexor tendons that may be severe enough that the fetlock contacts the ground. Such cases usually correct within a few days given controlled exercise and protection from ground abrasion. Bandaging is not recommended as bandages further relax tendon support.

Systemic Illness as Cause of Limb Swelling

In some cases, a horse is suffering from something besides a tendon injury that causes a lower limb to swell. This limb edema can occur from simple stocking-up from sluggish circulation caused by standing idle in a stall or small pen. Advanced pregnancy often slows circulation in the tissues, resulting in swollen, stocked-up legs. However, complete swelling of more than one leg may signal a systemic illness (photo 7.27). These diseases include:

- Heart disease
- Tumor or abscess or infection that blocks the lymph system
- Dietary protein deficiency
- Protein loss due to intestinal parasitism, or liver, kidney, or intestinal disease
- Viral infections, such as equine influenza or *equine viral arteritis*
- Vaccination reactions
- An allergic form of *strangles* (*Streptococcus*

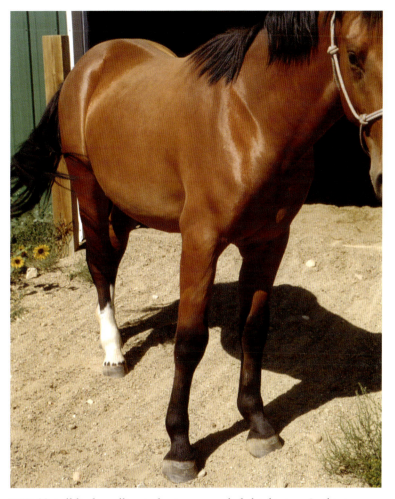

7.27 *Not all limb swelling is due to a musculoskeletal injury. In this image, the swelling of all the legs is caused by systemic illness related to strangles infection.*

  equi) called *purpura hemorrhagica*, which causes blood vessels to leak (*vasculitis*—see p. 277)
- *Ehrlichia equi* infection, also called *Anaplasma phagocytophila*
- *Ulcerative lymphangitis* (see p. 175)

A single limb may swell for causes unrelated to tendons. Examples include a hoof abscess, edema from a musculoskeletal injury, or an infected puncture wound.

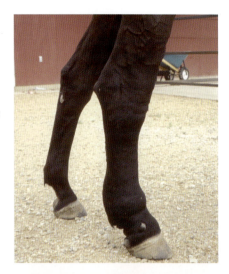

7.28 *Inflammation of the lymphatic vessels of the limb may become a permanent swelling due to scar tissue replacement of normal tissue. The limb remains swollen and enlarged as seen in this horse's right rear lower limb.*

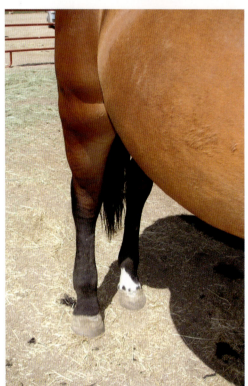

7.29 *In an acute case of lymphangitis, as seen in this horse's right rear limb, the entire limb may be swollen from stifle to hoof, and the horse shows signs of systemic illness.*

Lymphangitis

Lymphangitis is an inflammation of the lymphatic vessels that are responsible for moving fluids in and out of the cells in the body, and particularly in the legs (photos 7.28 and 7.29). When there is a lengthy duration of this problem, scar tissue in the leg deters adequate lymphatic drainage. In these cases, the leg swelling may never reduce in size. Exercise is the best method to improve circulation in the limb, assuming it is not painful to the horse to use it. Support bandages on the leg can be helpful to limit the amount of limb swelling, but once the bandages are removed for a short time, the swelling often reappears.

The Horse's Back

8

Considering that the horse evolved to be fleet of foot to outrun predators and did not evolve to support the weight of a rider, it is a wonder that horses don't suffer back problems more frequently than they do. Yet, there are often subtle problems that make themselves apparent to an astute observer. Low-grade back pain can elicit a variety of performance issues.

Conditioning a horse's back to withstand the stress of exercise encompasses the variety of techniques important to building strong muscles, ligaments, tendons, bones, and joints. Application of strengthening strategies is important, but so also is the ability to recognize if a horse is having a back problem. A sore back has put many a talented horse out of commission for a time. The trick is to identify subtle beginning symptoms and to track them down and find solutions to the problems. Performance and behavioral changes often warn of back discomfort.

Horse Communication of Back Pain

A horse's behavior and posture speak volumes about how he is feeling (photos 8.1 and 8.2). Good horsemanship skills allow one to know how to listen, and what to listen for. When being groomed, a horse may have much to say if he is experiencing pain. He may be more irritable than usual when the brush is run across his back. Muscles tighten beneath the brush. Displeasure is expressed with flattened ears, or wrinkling of the lips in a grimace. When approached with a saddle, the horse moves away instead of standing still. Girthing him up elicits a more belligerent attitude, his neck snaking around in warning.

Such displays of "emotion" may be shrugged off as thinking that a normally placid horse is having a bad day. A horse may communicate his distress more vigorously when mounted, as he humps his back or bucks. As a rider settles into the saddle, a sore-backed horse might sink down low, crumpling through the back and haunches.

Once under way, the horse may seem to require more effort than usual to "warm" him up. Energy and impulsion are lacking as he moves with a short, choppy stride, particularly behind. When asked for lateral movements and bending, he resists, proclaiming his unhappiness with a wring of the tail. When asked for more extension, the response is an upward jerk of the head, an elevation of the

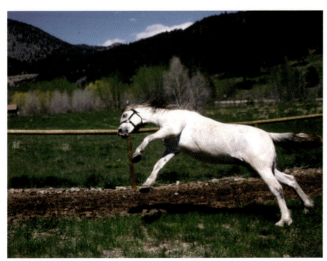

8.1 *A horse that is feeling good has little hesitation about bucking and romping in the field to blow off steam. This horse is both twisting and elevating his back, not postures he would make if in pain.*

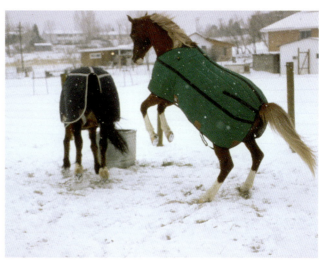

8.2 *A horse that is willing to rear in play is not suffering from back pain. This posture causes the back to flex and contract, and a horse with spinal or muscular back pain would be reluctant to assume this stance, even briefly.*

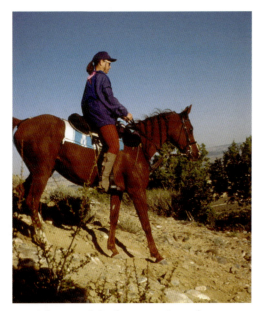

8.3 *A horse with back pain is often reluctant to negotiate a downhill incline, taking tentative steps and bracing his back as he creeps down the hill. This type of mincing gait is also typical of a horse protecting himself from other forms of musculoskeletal pain, such as problems in the hooves or joints.*

neck carriage, and a quickening of movement, resulting in faster, but not longer, steps. The back is braced and rigid beneath the rider, with no connection between front and rear limbs. The horse refuses to pick up canter leads immediately when asked. He isn't very interested in lowering and extending his head and neck when asked to go long and low. Attempts at collected work do not give a normal quality of movement. In a rein back, the horse braces against the bit, and does a pretty poor job of it as he raises his head, arches his back, and drags his front toes with each backward step. Instead of a nice fluid motion, the exercise is performed with an erratic and sticky movement. The more that is asked, the less he gives. If asked to move along on a downhill grade, he acts as if he wants to put on the brakes, and balks at going forward (photo 8.3). His back remains stiff and hollow no matter how many exercises he is asked to do in an attempt to limber him up. Demands for more speed and extension are only met with more mental resistance.

A jumping horse with back pain may refuse or rush a jump, jump too flat, or twist his hind legs when clearing a jump. An event horse may demonstrate similar problems: the horse's speed may slow, and his enthusiasm may wane as he fatigues sooner than normal.

A back-sore horse may have displayed behavioral changes for a while with a more subdued disposition, some grumpiness, gnashing of the teeth, or wringing of the tail. A farrier may have commented that the horse has resented having one of his hind legs picked up for shoeing.

The horse hasn't been seen playing in the field, or rolling to scratch itches along his back. Overall, his enthusiasm for life and work is deflated.

Identification of Back Pain

Besides non-specific performance inconsistencies that a horse displays, what else can be monitored to identify the presence of back pain? A veterinarian can give a horse a thorough exam as part of the information-gathering process.

THE HORSE AT REST

When thinking about normal behavioral characteristics of a horse that may be displaying subtle signs of a problem, consider whether the horse lies down, or if he rolls to scratch in the field or stall. Consider how well he cleans up his food, and the preferred posture of eating. How good is his body condition? Also, examine his personality and behavior for other subtle clues.

THE STANDING HORSE

One important feature of an exam includes observing a horse in his stall, when he is at ease and not expecting any touch or manipulation. Does he stand comfortably? What does his posture display?

As he is led out of the stall, how does he negotiate the curve between the stall and the aisle? Square him up on a level surface and look for asymmetry between the hipbones or top of the hips. Are the gluteal muscles of his rump of similar dimensions? If not, there may be some muscle atrophy on one side relating to disuse. Or, if a muscle of the back or haunches is in spasm it may appear larger than surrounding tissues. It is helpful to stand on a chair or rail at a safe distance above a horse to evaluate straightness of the spine and symmetry of the muscles.

Palpation of the back with the flat of the hand and the fingers is important to localize the area of pain (photo 8.4). It is normal for a horse to arch and dip his spine slightly when the loins are pinched. A horse that drops his back in an exaggerated fashion to slight pressure may be displaying true pain. A horse that holds himself very rigid when squeezed in this area may feel sufficient back pain that he prefers to brace the muscles rather than move his back.

THE HORSE IN MOTION

Next, the horse should be watched in motion. A firm, level surface is

8.4 *Palpation of the back is best achieved initially by using the flat of the hand. Then, as in this photo, a gentle squeeze using flexed fingers identifies pain in deeper muscles of the back.*

helpful to tell if the horse is tracking straight. Watch for pelvic rotation, shoulder swing, and movement of the back, all of which are normal features of equine locomotion in a comfortable horse. Does the horse easily make transitions from trot to canter and canter to trot indicating a willingness to step his hind legs beneath him? Does he pick up the correct lead when asked? Or, does the horse swish his tail, gnash his teeth, or brace his head and neck when asked for precision movements?

In addition, the horse should be examined in motion on an inclined surface and again in deeper footing as sometimes stifle and hock problems become more evident on less even footing.

A practical and inexpensive method of detecting subtle pain is to ride a horse consistently with a heart rate monitor. After many readings of the normal heart rate response to a given exertion, it may be possible to identify beginning signs of discomfort. Heart rate may elevate during exercise that elicits pain as compared to the response seen when the horse was previously comfortable.

FLEXION TESTS

A horse with chronic back pain often demonstrates poor results with hock-flexion tests. (See "Flexion Tests" in chapter 5, *Joints*, p. 115.) Frequently, the front part of one or both rear hooves is worn away due to toe dragging since stepping well under himself requires a horse to activate the back muscles, which he isn't likely to do if his back is sore. Some horses with low-grade back pain tend to *plait* behind (one foot swings inward and is placed almost in front of the opposite hind foot), with the rear feet practically stepping in each other's tracks. More moderate back pain elicits a wide, straddling type of rear-limb gait. Many affected horses have difficulty in making tight turns.

ENSURING PROPER SADDLE FIT

To assess fit of a saddle, square the horse on a level surface. Being careful not to place the saddle so far forward that it restricts movement through the the shoulder blades, the saddle is placed on a horse's back without any padding or girth. The pommel and cantle should be positioned such that a rider's seat is centered between them, with the cantle slightly higher than the pommel. The pommel should clear the withers by at least 2½ to 3 fingers width. Then, place a hand beneath the center of the saddle's seat, and push downward on the seat with the other hand. There should be no rocking in any direction. There should be no pressure points, or areas with large gaps (bridging) in the contact of the saddle with the back. The saddle should not extend beyond the horse's last rib. Viewing the saddle from behind, there should be adequate space the entire length of the gullet so the saddle panels do not place pressure on the spine. With a rider mounted, the saddle will make closer contact with the back, so it is important that the spine is free and clear of any pressure.

Just because a saddle looks as if it fits when a horse is standing still on a level surface does not mean it fits when the horse is in motion. A saddle may create pressure points on the back of a horse in motion, especially when asked to negotiate uneven terrain or jumps. Computerized saddle-pressure measuring equipment, such as a mechanical pressure-sensor pad, can display specific pressure points to identify potential problem spots when a horse is mounted and during locomotion. Another means of saddle assessment relies on *thermography*: the horse is saddled with a cotton pad, longed til warm, usually 20 minutes or so, and then thermography is applied to the panels of the saddle to evaluate symmetry of all areas in contact with the horse's back. It is best to do this unmounted as a rider may sit slightly off center and so skew the results. Another technique for assessing saddle fit uses a saddle pad that contains a gel-like substance that will squish around to accommodate pressure points of saddle contact.

It is helpful to engage the services of a professional saddle maker to fit an individual horse with a saddle that is appropriate for the intended athletic task and skills of the rider. A custom saddle can be designed from a plaster cast built to the exact shape of a horse's back. Saddle pads also come in many styles and materials, but one that has been ancillary in reducing pressure points from mild saddle-fitting concerns is the Supracor® pad. A Supracor® pad is made of a flexible honeycomb material that ventilates and is shock absorbing. It has been used in medical applications as for wheelchairs and hospital mattresses to ease pressure points in injured and sick patients.

Misleading Signs of Back Pain

Palpation of the back muscles can cause horses to flinch away from finger pressure. Sometimes this is true pain within the soft tissues, but it is also possible that unknowingly the horse was pinched over specific acupuncture points that relate to problems within a channel or meridian (see *Appendix D*, p. 574). There are many diagnostic acupuncture points on the back alongside the spine that refer to pain in other areas of the body; pain from back palpation must be interpreted appropriately.

Not all horses that drop their backs when mounted are showing true back pain. Sometimes, a horse is hypersensitive to the weight of a saddle and/or rider, and will become stiff or dip his spine when mounted. A so-called "cold-backed" horse usually moves off just fine once a rider is in position; there is no interference with performance.

A horse with muscle problems in any part of the body quickly stiffens and tires with exertion, leading to poor performance. Tying-up syndrome (myositis or exertional rhabdomyolysis) can cause a horse to stop work because of severe pain (see chapter 6, *Muscle Endurance*, p. 166). A mare with a painful ovary at the time of ovulation may exhibit signs of back pain, or she may appear to have signs of colic. This can be identified by rectal palpation and ultrasound exam of the ovaries.

A horse with chronic arthritis often experiences days when the pain is aggravating enough that performance suffers. In an effort to protect painful feet or joints, his stride shortens, and muscles are restricted and tight, including those of the back.

Considering the Cause of Back Pain

Usually, all back-related "problems" are not seen simultaneously, but each single issue is a common complaint by an owner of a horse with back soreness. Probably the most consistent findings are a change in temperament and a decline in performance. Subtle signs develop slowly over time until a sore-backed horse just can't do the job asked.

Trauma

Many reasons are at the root of back pain. Pain might be related to a traumatic incident such as a fall or a slip, or too much speed in unconditioned muscles. Another traumatic situation occurs with trailer loading when a rebellious horse rears, backs up rapidly, or spins away from the trailer door. The *thoracolumbar* or *sacroiliac* areas may be injured when a leg slips out behind while a horse is pushing off with it, as with an uphill gallop or a leap out of a start gate.

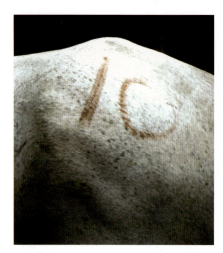

8.5 *Enlargement related to injury of the sacroiliac joint and/or ligaments at the top of the croup is referred to as a hunter's bump.*

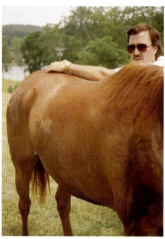

8.6 *Palpation at varying depths along the top of the croup is helpful to identify sacroiliac or lumbosacral pain.*

SOFT TISSUE TRAUMA

The Epaxial Muscles

The *epaxial* muscles (*longissimus dorsi* mm.) of the back that run along the spine are prone to injury when a horse slips or falls, or launches poorly over a jump. These muscles extend the back and control stiffness of the back. The epaxial muscles most commonly are injured in the lumbar region, sometimes with evident swelling and pain. Performance suffers, as does quality of movement. To brace against the pain, a horse with lower back pain will become restrictive in the swing of the pelvis and in length of stride of the rear limbs. The hind legs are placed wider than normal, and the limbs become disunited at canter, with a horse cross-firing behind or falling out of a canter lead.

Sacroiliac Strain

The pelvis is connected to the spine by slinging *sacroiliac ligaments* that support and stabilize the *sacroiliac joint*. These ligaments and the joint itself are often strained during equine athletic demands. This may be visually appreciated as a *"hunter's bump"* at the top of the croup, but not always (photo 8.5 and see chapter 2, *Conformation for Performance*, p. 30). If actively inflamed, a horse reacts adversely to finger pressure placed over the swelling (photo 8.6). Some more obscure signs of injury in this location may be related to:

- Poor performance
- Unwillingness to work
- Reduced hindlimb impulsion and stride, or obvious hindlimb lameness
- A stiff back and rigid spine particularly evident during exercise
- Difficulty performing lateral movements, going on the bit, changing canter leads, or jumping
- Asymmetry or weak development of the back muscles and hindquarters.

The horse may drag his toes, or may plait, particularly noticeable at a slow trot. An affected horse may also stand with a roached appearance to the top of the loins, or may hold his tail to the side during locomotion. Many horses affected with sacroiliac pain are reluctant to stand with weight on one hindlimb, and may refuse to pick up one hindlimb at all.

A rider may feel a limited push from the hind end in a dressage horse, and at higher levels, a horse with sacroiliac pain may have difficulty performing collected movements like piaffe. A jumping horse may continue to tackle his regular jump height, but a rider on a horse with sacroiliac pain may notice that the horse loses scope over the jumps. The horse may move in a disjointed way that tends to throw a rider out of the saddle. He might display behavioral changes, such as bucking or kicking out when ridden, as if striking at something painful behind him.

REPETITIVE STRESS

High speed is often incriminated as a cause of musculoskeletal trauma, but low speed concussion experienced over time is ultimately as destructive to a performance horse. Repetitive motions, such as a horse executes in distance trail riding, or in arena training pursuits like dressage, show equitation, or reining lead to stiffening of the soft tissues throughout the body, and particularly the back. Use of restrictive devices, such as side-reins or draw-reins, or anything that forces a headset, further tightens the torso and back with time.

Horses that are asked for continuous efforts of collection and engagement of the hindquarters, like in the discipline of dressage, may incur repetitive injury to soft tissues of the back.

POOR SADDLE FIT

Poor saddle fit is a common cause of back pain in a working horse. Young horses have a relatively straight back that drops slightly as the horse reaches maturity at 5 to 6 years (photos 8.7 A–C). The saddle that fits a two- or three-year-old needs to be altered to accommodate change in body contours. Increased muscular development from maturity and conditioning also requires that saddles be refitted periodically in keeping with a horse's changes in physique. It is impractical to try to compensate for a poor-fitting saddle by bulking it up with extra saddle pads. The more padding placed on the horse's back, the narrower that makes the gullet, which further impinges on the withers. A heavily padded saddle shifts and moves, adding to increased friction and pinching to elicit more pain and soft-tissue damage.

The back should be examined for areas of muscle atrophy or areas with asymmetric overdevelopment or spasm. Examine the coat for indication of white hairs on a dark horse (photo 8.8) or black hairs on a light horse that might indicate improperly fitting tack. After a

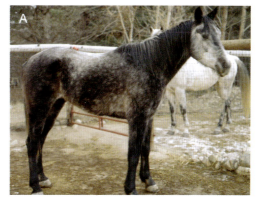

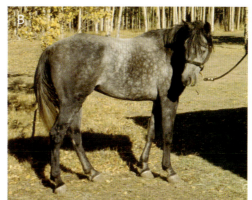

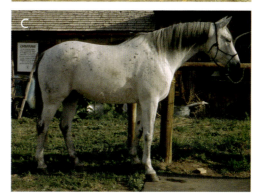

8.7 A–C *A thin horse, as seen here at age 4, has a relatively straight back with little padding to accommodate good saddle fit (A). This is the same horse as in (A) at age 6 (B). He has more flesh on his frame and his back, but is still a little too undeveloped to allow for a permanent saddle fit. The same horse, now at age 11, fit and strongly muscled (C). His physique matured by age 8 to allow for a custom saddle fit that fits well into his teen years.*

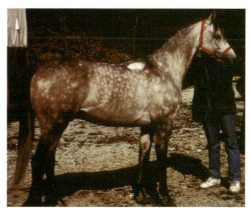

8.8 *The bright, white hairs behind the withers on this horse indicate chronic saddle irritation that has cause permanent damage to the hair follicles.*

8.9 A & B *A tense horse and tense rider exacerbate stress on a horse's back, each compounding the other's problem. The horse is restricted in his movement, and the rider braces to combat the horse's tension. This unrelenting cycle makes it difficult to achieve good performance from either team member (A). In contrast, the horse and rider in this picture demonstrate harmonious relaxation in the task of backing up. The horse is yielding well to the rein-back through his head, neck, poll, and back. The rider is light in her hands in the asking of the task as seen with a relatively relaxed rein (B).*

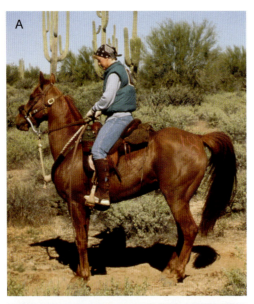

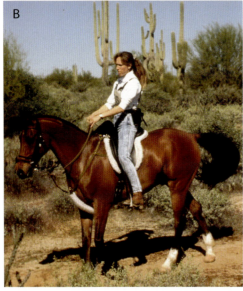

horse has been ridden, look for dry spots beneath the saddle pad, for ruffled hairs, areas denuded or with broken hairs, or swellings and lumps; any of these signs indicate poor saddle fit (see "Saddle Sores and Girth Galls," chapter 13, *The Skin as an Organ*, p. 364). A saddle that is too high in front rocks back and forth, similar to what would be felt with a flat pebble under the heel of a human foot while hiking. First it is uncomfortable to the surface tissues; then it damages deeper tissues of the heel, requiring a long recuperation time to heal the bruising. Poor saddle fit causes a horse to experience similar problems.

RIDER ABILITY

A rider's abilities affect whether or not a horse will experience back pain. A saddle may fit perfectly, but a rider who is stiff or tense in the saddle restricts a horse's back, shoulder, and pelvic swing (photos 8.9 A & B). An unbalanced or inexperienced rider creates problems for a horse's back. Leg position and seat position of a rider are important for achieving proper and consistent balance. Uneven stirrups are one cause of tilting of a rider in the saddle. A tilted rider places more weight on one side of the back, while the horse needs to adjust his posture to compensate for an imbalanced person perched on his back. This is especially a problem when a rider becomes fatigued after hard or long exertion in the saddle. This leads to overuse of one side of a horse's body, setting up conditions for muscle or joint strain. Similarly, horses that are not ridden straight between hand and leg aids do not use their muscles evenly. Twisting of the horse's head, neck, hips, or back can lead to muscle strain of the back.

POOR DENTAL CARE

Poor dental care may create sufficient soreness in a horse's mouth to cause him to carry himself with a constrained head carriage that makes the back rigid and fixed. Such an abnormal position of bracing through the neck and back elicits stiffness of the torso over time.

RIDER'S WEIGHT

A heavy rider in relationship to the size of the horse can also generate trauma to a horse's back. Most horses can carry up to 20 percent of their body weight without too much trouble, meaning a 1000-pound horse should be able to carry 200 pounds that includes rider *and* tack. Excessive time spent at sitting trot, particularly by an inexperienced rider, or poor posting technique can lead to back trauma. A horse that is overridden for his level of fitness can experience muscle fatigue and trauma of all his muscles, including soft tissues of the back. Couple the exercise of repetitive movements with a horse that is overfed and under-conditioned, and back injury is inevitable.

HORSE NOT FIT FOR THE TASK

Inconsistent training schedules potentially create strain of muscles and ligaments of the back. This is particularly true for aged horses that are inherently less flexible in their spines and have reduced muscle tone and strength than when they were of a younger age. Joint degeneration is also more of a concern in an older horse or in a horse that has campaigned hard through his athletic career. In effect, accumulated microtrauma to the back for any of the above-mentioned reasons might lead to back injury and pain over time.

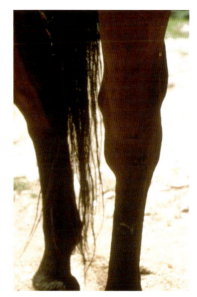

8.10 *Degenerative arthritis of the hock (bone spavin) as apparent here is one reason for persistent back pain. Lameness related to hock pain causes a horse to alter his way of going, to brace his back, thereby creating muscle soreness in his back. Stifle lameness is also known to create chronic back soreness.*

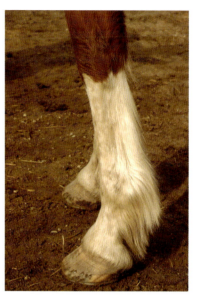

8.11 *Poor shoeing techniques are responsible for altering a horse's gait enough to elicit back pain. This horse has long toes, low heels, and a broken-back hoof-pastern axis, all of which may cause him to stumble more, to shorten his stride, and brace his back, particularly if these hoof configuration problems are found in the rear feet.*

Lameness

One of the main reasons for back pain to develop is as a compensatory response to lower limb lameness, particularly related to problems in the hocks or stifles (photo 8.10 and see chapter 5, *Joints*, p. 117). A horse with leg pain may not stride forward fully, may stab rear legs with each step instead of pushing off efficiently from behind; in so doing, this horse fixes the upper body to compensate for lower-leg discomfort. Over time, this leads to bracing and tightness of the soft tissues and muscles of the back. Similarly, front-leg lameness may force a horse to shift his weight to the rear quarters; this causes strain to the back muscles and joints of the spine.

SHOEING ISSUES

Shoeing issues also can generate pain in a horse's back. Long toes and low heels of the rear feet cause as many problems with the hind end and back as they do with the front limbs (photo 8.11). Low heels alter the mechanical advantage of hind limb thrust, and a horse may strain his back in an effort to drive his legs forward. Deep or muddy footing creates a similar stress on the back. Toe grabs and heel caulks cause a foot to stick when what is desired is for the foot to slide to prevent back muscles from experiencing a sharp and sudden stretch (see chapter 3, *The Hoof*, p. 62).

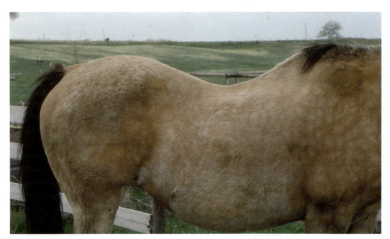

8.12 *A horse may be born with a sway back or it can develop with age or overuse by a heavy rider that causes ligament and spinal damage.*

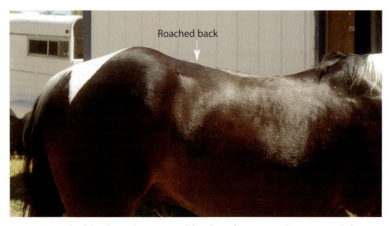

8.13 *A roached back is often created by the inherent conformation of the horse, but a spinal injury can create this feature, as well. Atrophy of the lumbar muscles may make a horse appear to have a roach back, when, in fact, his spinal vertebrae are normal.*

CONFORMATIONAL FAULTS

Horses with conformational flaws are more at risk for developing back problems. A horse with a long back is predisposed to muscle and ligament strain, while a horse with a short back may have reduced spinal flexibility that creates lesions within the bony vertebrae. Poor conformation in the form of a long back exaggerates other factors that contribute to back injury. Horses with a large frame and relatively weak quarters are predisposed to injury of the sacroiliac joint. The spine is always at risk of injury when carrying a load (a rider) through irregular or mountainous terrain, particularly if the footing is slippery and/or quite steep. Similarly, execution of precision motions like jumping, spinning, or rapid turns puts a marked strain on the spine and back.

Vertebral Problems

VERTEBRAL MALFORMATION

On occasion, a horse will be born with a congenital malformation, varying in severity. Some horses with vertebral deformities are able to be ridden for a time, but suffer secondary soft-tissue trauma as a result. The most common examples of vertebral malformations include:

- *Scoliosis* (lateral curvature of the spine)
- *Lordosis,* or dipped or swayed back (photo 8.12)
- *Kyphosis,* or roached back (photo 8.13)

IMPINGEMENT OF THE DORSAL SPINOUS PROCESSES

The dorsal spinous processes are the areas of the vertebrae that stick upward where muscles attach. The spinous processes of the thoracic spine are most commonly involved in a condition referred to as *overriding* or "*kissing spines.*" With this condition, not only are the vertebral

The Horse's Back

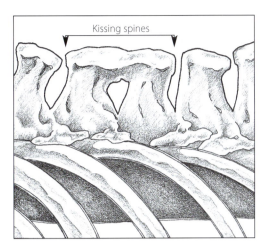

Fig 8.14 *Injury or impingement of the spinous processes of the thoracic vertebrae can elicit new bone formation such that two or more spinous processes touch and/or override one another. This condition, called kissing spines, can create pain in the vertebrae as well as in surrounding soft tissue structures.*

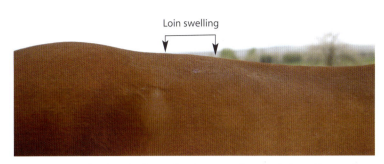

8.15 *Injury to this horse's thoracolumbar spine has created swelling and inflammation over the loins, as often occurs with "kissing spines."*

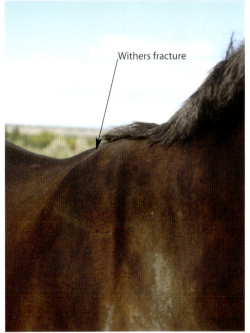

8.16 *A common injury when a horse flips over is to fracture the dorsal spinous processes of the withers. These usually heal well although create a cosmetic defect that make it difficult to fit a saddle.*

spines painful, but surrounding soft tissue structures like the epaxial muscles and interconnecting spinous ligaments are also inflamed (fig. 8.14 and photo 8.15).

Jumping horses and dressage horses are particularly affected. A rider may complain that a horse will not maintain impulsion, or will not be able to maintain collected work. A horse may resist small circle work, rapid changes in direction, or rapid and consistent lead changes of upper-level dressage demands. Another complaint is that the horse gallops flat, or that his back feels braced.

FRACTURE

One of the most common areas of a horse's spine to be fractured is one or more of the *dorsal spinous processes* of the withers (photo 8.16). Usually this occurs following trauma incurred by a horse rearing up and falling over backward. The highest point of the back is the withers so this area is most likely to be smashed. Initially, the area is swollen and the horse is not willing to elevate his head and neck. Most cases heal within 6 months and do not have any lingering effects on performance.

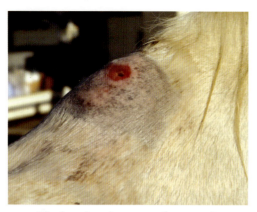

8.17 *This horse's withers injury began with a saddle sore. If such an infection extended into the supraspinous bursa beneath the withers, it could lead to a chronic infection called fistulous withers.*

Other fractures may occur anywhere else along the spine. (For more discussion, see "The Fallen Horse" in chapter 17, *The Neurologic System in Health and Disease*, p. 520.) Nuclear scintigraphy is able to localize an area of a fracture lesion, and more detailed investigation is possible using radiography.

OSTEOARTHRITIS

Osteoarthritis of the vertebrae can occur just as with any other joint in the body. Over time, excess bone that develops around an arthritic vertebral joint may cause impingement of other vertebrae creating pain or may contact the spinal cord causing neurologic signs. Horses with degenerative disease of one or more vertebra will display many of the symptoms of back pain listed earlier. An affected horse moves with a rigid spine, resents circling or performing any motion that requires back movement: performance declines and behavioral problems surface.

SPINAL INFECTION

Fistulous Withers

Chronic inflammation and infection may occur in the region of the *supraspinous bursa* and associated soft tissue structures of the withers. This condition is known as *fistulous withers*. Infection is introduced by a wound over the withers region, or by pressure necrosis created by saddle damage (photo 8.17). Infection is usually contained in the soft tissues but can invade deeper to infect the thoracic vertebral processes.

Therapy and Solutions for Managing Back Pain

Rest

A key element to resolving back pain is to implement rest from forced exercise or riding. This may require at least 3 and up to 8 months rest along with other supportive therapies.

It is critical to identify the primary source of pain prior to initiating therapy. Otherwise, a horse may receive rest and treatment for back pain, only to suffer a recurrence of the problem since an inciting cause such as a hock or stifle ailment has not been managed concurrently.

Massage, Therapeutic Ultrasound, and Electrostimulation

There are many ways to manage back pain. Initially, gentle massage improves tissue circulation as do warm-water soaks with towels or a hose (weather depending). Therapeutic ultrasound and electrostimulation are also means of breaking the pain cycle created by muscle spasms. (For further discussion, refer to "Electrical Therapies" in chapter 6, *Muscle Endurance*, p. 178.)

Acupuncture

Acupuncture is an excellent adjunctive therapy to quiet the pain reflex and to stimulate circulation (photo 8.18 and see discussion in chapter 5, *Joints*, p. 129, and chapter 6, *Muscle Endurance*, p. 178). Acupuncture performed once or twice weekly has returned 70 percent of sore-backed horses to maximum improvement between the fifth and eighth week of therapy.

Anti-Inflammatory Medication

Traditional treatment for back pain includes the use of system nonsteroidal anti-inflammatory medications (NSAIDs), like phenylbutazone, flunixin meglumine, or ketoprofen. In some cases, local injection of corticosteroids, extract from the pitcher plant (*Sarapin*), local anesthetic, or internal blisters assists the healing process (see *Appendix B,* p. 568).

Studies have shown that 39 percent of horses with back pain experience injury to the soft tissues of the back. Soft-tissue injury includes:

- The muscles along the spine
- The ligament that runs down the back of each dorsal spinous process
- The sacroiliac ligament

Manipulative Therapy

Although it is tempting to rush out and employ a chiropractor to "fix" a horse's back, this is contraindicated during the acute stages of soft-tissue injury. Chiropractics may have its place to restore normal joint movement and to release a muscle spasm during the healing phase, but at all times chiropractor work should be performed only under direct supervision of a veterinarian. No matter the therapy, frequent re-evaluation by a veterinarian is important to track healing and to make appropriate changes in management according to the response of each individual horse.

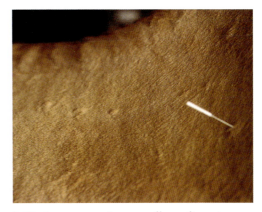

8.18 *Acupuncture is an excellent adjunctive therapy to quiet pain and stimulate circulation. This horse is demonstrating a desirable response by the small wheals (hives) local to the acupuncture needles.*

Joint Therapy

Many horses with back pain have hock discomfort as the primary cause, and so may need to have their hocks injected with anti-inflammatory medications. This therapy can aid as a diagnostic tool to get to the root cause of back pain. This is a legitimate treatment strategy that helps to rule out an underlying cause.

Intra-articular injection of anti-inflammatory medications into the sacroiliac joint is an appropriate therapy for back issues related to pain in this joint.

Exercise

In most cases turnout is superior to long-term confinement. Turnout maintains tone and strength in all muscle groups. Also, the physical act of grazing stretches neck and back muscles to maintain flexibility. Unless a horse is very severe in his presentation of pain, it is

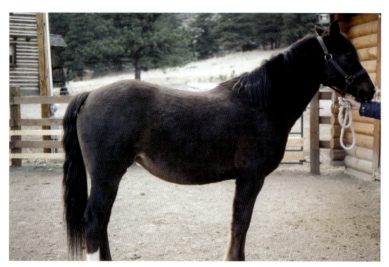

8.19 *An unconditioned horse will have weak abdominal and back muscles, as seen here in this horse with a flaccid belly and back.*

best to continue him in some form of controlled exercise. This is especially true for an older horse since it is difficult to restore condition on an aged horse if let down for too long.

Ponying a horse on a loose rein beside another is a means of legging-up a horse that has been rested for a time without adding weight to his back. Or, light riding (hacking) on level and firm terrain is helpful to restart exercise during the rehabilitation process of a horse with back pain. During convalescence, work in deep sand or mud should be avoided, as should hill work. Longeing is useful for light exercise if used only for a short period, while longeing for extended periods can cause back strain, particularly if a horse's posture is restricted with draw-reins, side-reins, or other restraining devices.

Stretching

Stretching of the back muscles prior to and following exercise is beneficial to both prevention and treatment of back problems. (For a discussion of stretching exercises, see chapter 6, *Muscle Endurance*, p. 153.)

Long-Term Strategies to Manage Back Injury

STRENGTH TRAINING

A key strategy to strengthening the back and preventing injury is to develop a horse's abdominal muscles. If a horse's torso is considered to be a bow and string, then the spine is the bow and the breastbone and abdominal muscles are the string. *Back flexion* (arching) is achieved by contraction of the abdominal muscles along with retraction of the forelimbs and protraction of the hind limbs. *Back extension* (dipping) is accomplished by contraction of the long back muscles that sit alongside the spine as well as protraction of the forelimbs and retraction of the hind limbs. Just as it is critical for humans to build abdominal strength to avoid injury to the back, so too a horse must activate his abdominal muscles to properly engage the back muscles (photo 8.19). Haunch and quadriceps muscles also need to be developed to prevent back injury.

Strength-training exercises to build abdominal muscles and the haunch and hip muscles include:

- Walking under saddle with neck stretched long and low
- Trot work over cavalletti
- Working in proper collection with engagement of the hindquarters
- Lateral movements
- Backing in hand and under saddle
- Use of backing in collected posture for one or two steps between gait transitions into trot or canter
- Counter-canter using a figure-eight pattern
- Hill climbs

While a horse is recuperating from a back injury, most of these strength-training exercises would be contraindicated, but such riding approaches are important to prevent injury or reinjury.

ATTENTION TO ALL DETAILS

Effort should be made to minimize a horse's anxiety and stress as body tension is propagated into all the back muscles. A tense horse that carries himself with a hollowed back and inverted neck ends up worsening back problems. A relaxed mental state is conducive to relaxation of the back, jaw, and neck muscles (figs. 8.20 A & B).

All other elements of horsemanship should be evaluated and fine-tuned to achieve success in preventing or managing chronic back pain. Saddle fit should be accurate; dental care and bitting should be explored; equitation skills should be honed; shoeing should be supportive and advantageous to the intended sport; and conditioning techniques should be implemented to guard against fatigue.

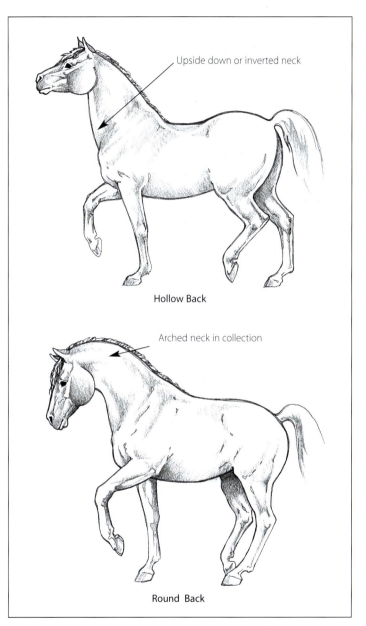

8.20 A & B *A horse that is tense or unwilling to take bit contact often carries himself with a hollowed back and upside down (inverted) neck that implies tension in the back and makes an uncomfortable ride for the rider (A). A horse that uses his abdominal muscles to lift his back is better able to achieve collection, agility, and energy-efficient gaits (B).*

Cardiovascular Conditioning and Health 9

The marvel of a horse's athletic ability depends on adequate preparation and conditioning of one of the more malleable systems in the horse's body: the cardiovascular system, which encompasses the heart and blood circulation. In contrast to years of lengthy preparation required by the skeletal system and bone, the cardiovascular system most quickly responds and adapts to training. With an intelligent conditioning strategy, the cardiovascular system can be brought to peak within 4 to 6 months.

The Cardiovascular System

The Heart
Accomplished equine athletes are said to have a lot of "heart," and a lot of heart they have. Since the heart is the central organ comprising the cardiovascular system, a horse's performance depends on his heart being an effective pump to move blood and oxygen to the tissues. This is particularly important for protracted exercise related to sports where a horse is undergoing lengthy aerobic exercise, such as distance riding, eventing, and steeplechase. A strong heart is also important to propel a horse through intense speed efforts. Features that dictate a horse's staying power and stamina include:

- The efficiency by which oxygen is delivered to the working muscles
- The effectiveness of heat dissipation from the core of the body

Blood Vessels
The heart moves blood through an intricate network of arteries, veins, and capillaries. Like branching limbs of a tree, the blood vessels diminish in size yet logarithmically increase in number the farther away they are from the heart. Through this *vascular* network, nutrients are transported to all tissues in the body while metabolic waste products are removed. Necessary nutrients and biochemical substances needed by the tissues include oxygen, water, electrolytes, and fuel for energy derived from digestive processes.

The Spleen
A unique feature of the horse that enables him to achieve athletic superiority in the animal kingdom is his large *spleen*. This organ is a holding reservoir of blood cells, which are

delivered to the circulation when the spleen contracts with exercise. The additional supply of oxygen-rich blood cells dumped into the system improves the *aerobic capacity* of the horse to imbue him with endurance.

Definitions of Exercise Efforts

Submaximal Exercise (Endurance)

Most horse sport activities involve work at *aerobic* levels of heart rates less than 150 beats per minute (bpm). Such exercise is called *submaximal*, or aerobic exercise. Examples of this level of activity include pleasure riding, competitive trail events, endurance racing, show hunters, dressage, team penning, and Western pleasure riding. At or below this heart rate, lactic acid does not accumulate in the muscles. Any small amount of lactic acid that forms is flushed from the muscles by the circulation or undergoes aerobic metabolism.

Maximal Exercise (Sprint or Gallop)

Sprint sports require *maximal* exercise, which in most horses occurs at heart rates above 180 to 200 bpm. These sports depend almost exclusively on *anaerobic* energy metabolism. Quarter Horse racing, barrel racing, roping, steeplechase, and timber racing are examples of such athletic efforts.

Combination Exercise

Examples of activities that depend on both *aerobic* and *anaerobic* metabolism are Thoroughbred and Standardbred racing, jumping, polo, cutting, reining, combined driving, and eventing.

Functional Cardiovascular Adaptations

Heart Rate

As a horse begins an athletic effort, the heart rate accelerates rapidly in the first 2 to 3 minutes of exertion. Several minutes of animated walk or slow trot warms up the system so the circulation gears up to meet oxygen demands of the muscles. Once the system is "turned on," the heart rate levels off to a steady state with the heart rate changing directly in relationship to the horse's speed or the intensity of the exercise. Faster speeds, greater difficulty in terrain (footing or slope), or a heavier rider create more demands on the system with insistence on more rapid conversion of fuel sources to energy in working muscles. In order for this to proceed in the most metabolically efficient manner, the muscle cells need a steady supply of oxygen. The role of the cardiovascular system is to supply blood, and thereby oxygen, to the demanding tissues of locomotion. The heart beats faster to fulfill these demands. Training elicits specific adaptations by the cardiovascular system to rally in time of need.

Cardiovascular Adaptations at Exercise

HEART EFFICIENCY

Many changes occur in the cardiovascular system and other body systems during exercise to accommodate the increased metabolic demands necessary to fuel locomotion. For starters, a horse's heart rate increases to more quickly push blood to the periphery. The amount of blood pushed with each pumping action of the heart (*cardiac output*) increases. Heart muscle (*myocardium*) responds to signals from the central nervous system to more completely empty the ventricles with each pumping action. More blood flows through the lungs to be saturated with oxygen as the pulmonary capillaries and *alveoli* open in response to exercise. Similarly, the respiratory rate increases favorably, changing the pressures within the thoracic cavity so that more blood returns to the heart with each beat.

Studies done at an elite 100-mile endurance competition (Purina *Race of Champions,* 1985) compared the differences in heart parameters between 53 elite-caliber competitive endurance horses and 34 non-conditioned horses that had done little more than walk around a small pasture for a year. Heart parameters were measured using *echocardiography*. Aerobic conditioning experienced by endurance horses revealed the following results:

- The dimension of the left ventricle slightly increases during its relaxation and filling stage (*diastole*) to increase the amount of blood delivered with each heartbeat.
- The thickness of the posterior wall of the left ventricle increases to improve muscular contraction to deliver more blood under high pressure; the thicker wall decreases tension on the heart muscle while increasing contractility of each beat; these features are critical to the heart's ability to function as an efficient pump.
- The left ventricle increases in mass as a result of conditioning.

Studies using electrocardiograms on racetrack horses indicate that heart mass may increase during the immediate few months following the start of training, but then the heart does not seem to enlarge any further.

SIZE AND DISTRIBUTION OF BLOOD VESSELS

The coronary vessels increase in size in response to greater metabolic demands by the heart muscle for oxygen and blood. Blood is effectively redistributed to the skeletal muscles in trade for reduced circulation to the intestinal organs. And, blood flow to the skin increases to assist in improved heat dissipation out of the core. With conditioning, the number and size of capillaries in the skin increase over 4 to 6 months to improve the efficiency of heat dispersal from working muscles. Movement by muscles during locomotion further improves circulation to quickly return blood to the heart so it can be fed through the lungs, be saturated with oxygen, and pushed to the muscles once again.

INCREASED RED BLOOD CELLS

During intense exercise, a horse increases his oxygen consumption thirty-six-fold. Red blood cells contain hemoglobin that binds oxygen and carries it through the bloodstream to the organs and tissues. To accommodate the huge demand for oxygen, the bloodstream is flooded with a reserve of red blood cells. These cells are stored in the spleen for occasions when more oxygen is required in the muscle tissues. With conditioning, the number of hemoglobin molecules in the body increases up to 50 percent. At high altitudes, a horse's body similarly compensates for reduced oxygen by manufacturing more hemoglobin, and this increases the oxygen-carrying capacity of the blood. More oxygen in the blood means more oxygen available in the muscles for aerobic metabolism.

PERFUSION OF DIFFERENT ORGANS

Skeletal muscle of a resting horse receives only about 13 percent of the body's overall circulation but during exercise more than 80 percent of the blood flow is diverted to working muscles. This is done at the expense of other organ systems, and particularly the gastrointestinal (GI) tract. At rest, the GI tract receives 26 percent of the body's circulation, and in the face of exercise this is reduced dramatically. Under

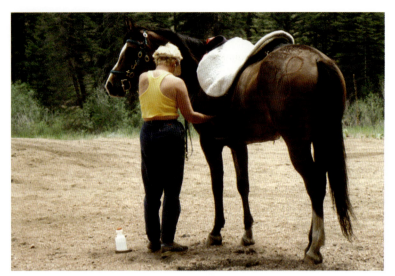

9.1 *Taking the heart rate from the ground with a stethoscope is not an accurate measure because by the time a rider stops, jumps off the horse, and counts for 15 seconds, the heart rate can drop by half the working rate.*

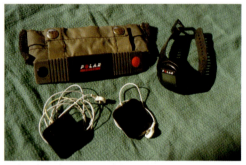

9.2 *A cardiotachometer (heart rate monitor) provides an accurate measure of a horse's working heart rate while being ridden. The kit uses a digital watch to give a heart rate reading. The heart rate is sent to the receiver watch by electrode pads that are attached with small wires to a transmitter contained in this small pouch that is affixed to the breastplate. One electrode pad is placed beneath the girth at the level of the elbow, and the other is placed beneath the saddle and pad alongside the withers on the opposite side.*

normal circumstances during submaximal (aerobic) exercise, the central nervous system, the kidneys, and the heart still maintain ample circulation.

Invaluable Equipment

The Cardiotachometer

An most useful tool for a rider to use to continually evaluate a horse's performance is an onboard *heart rate monitor*, also referred to as a *cardiotachometer*. This device enables immediate reading of a horse's working heart rate while exercising. There is no other means to appropriately track a horse's working heart rate since the heart rate will drop by almost half by the time a rider pulls a horse to a stop, jumps off, and counts the heart rate or pulse for 15 seconds (photo 9.1). A heart rate monitor has particular value for horses training for distance sports, like endurance riding, competitive trail, eventing, and combined driving (photo 9.2). It is also invaluable to use for training in racing sports, like Thoroughbred and Standardbred track racing, steeplechase, and timber racing. In addition, benefits can be gained in using a heart rate monitor to measure effort expended in dressage work to track conditioning progress.

A heart rate monitor consists of two rubber electrode pads, electrode wires that connect these pads to a transmitter that is clipped to the saddle or breast collar, and a receiver in the form of a digital wristwatch. One electrode pad is affixed to the girth to contact an area near the heart. A second pad is placed to the side of the horse's withers under the saddle pommel to act as a ground. Electrode gel is smeared on the electrode pads to facilitate good contact with the horse's skin. Wetting the skin with a saltwater solution or clipping away the coat beneath an electrode pad will further improve contact. Activity from the heart is averaged every 2 seconds with a number continuously appearing on the digital readout of the wristwatch display. The heart rate continually changes to correspond with varying exercise intensities as you ride. If the monitor gives erratic readings, check the contact of the electrode pads against the horse's skin.

More sophisticated units with computer memory chips are available for slightly more expense. Information can be stored within these units for up to an hour's worth of work, and then downloaded into a computer to develop comparison graphs of a horse's working ability.

USE OF A HEART RATE MONITOR TO IMPROVE CONDITION

This device is invaluable for assisting in conditioning a horse. Almost instant feedback is obtained on how much effort a horse is asked to do. A horse's heart rate is directly related to the work effort undertaken. This effort is determined by level of fitness, the intensity of the terrain, the type of footing encountered, the climatic conditions of the day, and the combined weight of the rider and tack. The monitor allows a rider to maintain a horse within a specified target working heart rate. Aerobic working heart rates range at rates less than 140 to 150 beats per minutes (bpm). An aerobic training effect can be achieved by riding at heart rates of 135 to 150 bpm during conditioning rides. But, a heart rate monitor should not be used like a tachometer in cases of difficult terrain; pushing a horse to run over rocks just to drive the heart rate up would be impractical. On good trails, a solid working trot should initiate some training, and hill climbs can be used to advantage to elevate the working heart rate.

A heart rate monitor enables a rider to gradually increase distance at a specified heart rate, incrementally and safely stressing the cardiovascular and musculoskeletal systems. Each progressive level of challenge created by an increase in speed or distance stimulates the body's adaptive response. A heart rate monitor is also useful to note heart rate recoveries: a horse that is fit for the level of exercise demand being asked for the conditions of the day will show a rapid drop in heart rate within a couple of minutes. With this information at hand, a more scientific approach can be made to determine when it is time to expand each step of the conditioning program.

Monitoring a Horse

To maximize an interval-training strategy once a horse has developed a solid long, slow distance (LSD) base, the horse should be reaching heart rates of 170 to 180 bpm for several minutes at a time. This is accomplished with fast canter work, sprints, and/or steep hill climbs. Increasing the heart rate bumps a horse into his anaerobic threshold, the place where muscles convert to the use of anaerobic metabolism with a by-product of that work being lactic acid. By exposing a horse's muscles to small amounts of lactic acid while in training, his aerobic capacity develops to improve the efficiency of how muscle fuel substrates are used for locomotion. Then, a conditioned horse develops greater endurance for aerobic efforts while fatiguing less quickly than an unfit horse.

The working heart rate for a given work intensity will decrease as a horse's muscles become stronger and the aerobic capacity improves. This is appreciated with use of an onboard heart rate monitor: the horse won't have to work as hard for the same effort as he did in earlier training.

Identifying Problems with a Cardiotachometer

A heart rate monitor should be used consistently in training in order to learn each horse's "normal" working and recovery rates. It can be used also to monitor for musculoskeletal problems, although it is not reliable in this application. Start looking for a problem if the working heart rate runs 10 to 20 bpm higher than usual for a given exercise effort. It is possible that an obscure lameness issue is bothersome enough to accelerate heart rate. Early recognition may identify a problem before it becomes too serious. Check the heart rate while posting on both diagonals and on both canter leads. Try the horse on different surfaces such as a hard-packed and a soft surface and note if the heart rate changes. A pressure point from an ill-fitting saddle can drive the heart rate up. A horse with a back or soft-tissue problem may show a higher heart rate on a softer surface if pain is elicited, and a horse with foot or joint problems may show an elevated heart rate on the hard-packed surface. In many cases of musculoskeletal injury, an overt problem may not show up until days later but the heart monitor may detect a problem earlier on. This is not to say that all mechanical problems will be reflected by an elevated heart rate, but this does have value for monitoring. Some horses are stoic in their discomfort; some don't feel pain in the face of adrenalin while working, especially if competing or buddying with another horse.

The greatest value of a heart rate monitor is the information gleaned about a horse's level of metabolic efficiency during exercise. A low-grade fever, a respiratory problem, and colic are examples of metabolic situations that cause a heart rate to elevate. Dehydration and electrolyte imbalances drive a heart rate up, and maintain it at a high rate for longer periods of time. Exercise in hot and humid climates exacerbates the heat load in the muscles, as well as fluid and electrolyte losses through sweat. Don't rely entirely on the heart rate monitor to detect a brewing problem. Use intuition and good "horse sense."

The Thermistor

A thermistor is used to measure skin temperature as a reflection of core temperature. The thermistor is an excellent monitoring device to evaluate the efficiency of blood flow to pull heat from the working muscles. (For more information, refer to chapter 6, *Muscle Endurance,* p. 152 and chapter 13, *The Skin as an Organ,* p. 362.)

Conditioning Techniques

Ultimately, each athlete is trained for a specific task. However, any performance horse must have a strong foundation on which to build for each phase of the conditioning process. A strategically planned conditioning program means a commitment to pursue it for months and years. Consistency of workouts is an important ingredient to increasing cardiovascular and biomechanical strength. "Progressive training" methods include a recovery period for the body to adapt to training and stress. In this way, a horse continues to build strength with less risk of strain or fatigue while developing into a fit athlete.

Humans typically require about 10 weeks to increase muscular strength by 50 percent because neuromuscular coordination is required for "neural learning" and control. Similar biophysical processes occur in horses, and all body tissues must respond to incremental challenges. Tissue with a generous blood supply responds most quickly: muscle tissue is the fastest (about 3 to 6 months), ligaments and tendons take longer to condition (6 to 12 months), and bone takes the longest time to fully condition (2 years). To advance a horse to absolute peak condition may require a couple of years (fig. 9.3).

Specific Tasks

VALUE OF REPETITION

Progressive increases in speed or distance over time (*conditioning*) enhance strength and durability. Once a conditioning program is begun, commitment is required for success. For a horse to achieve fitness, he must be repeatedly and consistently stressed before the tissues have a chance to fully recover from a prior workout. This method promotes adaptation and strengthening of body structures to build a solid foundation. Bone, cartilage, ligaments, and tendons must be slowly trained over time to meet the demands of added exertion. Although muscle responds rapidly to training, sudden speed bursts on unconditioned support structures in the limbs can overload the components that take longer to develop, resulting in damage and lameness. Progressively applied stresses, however, challenge the tissues and result in strength training of muscles, ligaments, and bone along with cardiovascular improvements.

VALUE OF WALKING

Walking improves condition by slowly stimulating ligaments, tendons, and muscles to accept a slight increase in load. Walking loads a horse's ankle with two-and-a-half times his weight. The stifle and hip are loaded with one-and-a-half times the horse's weight. Walking increases the heart rate to 90 bpm. Blood vessels dilate and become more elastic, allowing blood to flow with less resistance. An adequate warm-up of 10 minutes of walking enhances delivery of blood and oxygen to working muscles. However, only a small percentage of muscle fibers are recruited at a walk, primarily the slow twitch (ST) and a few of the fast twitch high oxidative (FTH) muscle fibers (see chapter 6, *Muscle Endurance*, p. 143). These muscle tissues learn to improve oxygen delivery

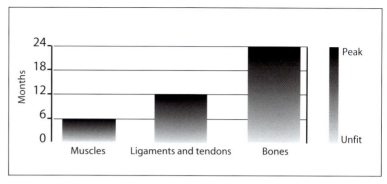

9.3 *Conditioning Levels of Various Body Structures: Tissue with a generous blood supply responds most quickly: muscle tissue is the fastest (about 3 to 6 months), ligaments and tendons take longer to condition (6 to 12 months), and bone takes the longest time (2 years).*

and removal of toxic by-products. Walking alone does not adequately stress the tissues to train them to higher levels of effort. But, it is an excellent starting point to build on, and is useful for a relaxed exercise.

VALUE OF SWIMMING

When available, swimming can be added to a routine conditioning program of flat and hill work to provide cardiovascular and respiratory conditioning without concussive stress on the limbs (photo 9.4). It is also a useful form of training that can be applied to a young horse or while rehabilitating an injured horse. Swimming strengthens the cardiovascular system without straining growing bone, and develops joints, tendons, and ligaments. The exercise of swimming maintains cardiovascular and respiratory fitness of an injured horse without loading an injured limb. Movement of the limbs through the water passively stretches healing joints and tendons, while water massages the tissue to improve circulation.

However, using swimming as the sole means of exercise while rehabilitating a horse will not provide cyclic loading stress on bones,

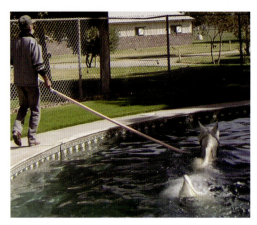

9.4 *Swimming is valuable exercise for maintaining cardiovascular and respiratory fitness without loading the musculoskeletal system. In addition, it's an effective tool to maintaining condition in a horse with a healing leg injury. Not all horses swim well; a horse that swims with his head and neck held high and back arched risks straining his back muscles. The horse in this photo is comfortable in the pool and doesn't mind getting his face and muzzle wet as he swims horizontally in the water. Photo: Carolyn Hock.*

joints, tendons, ligaments, and hooves that is part of a normal conditioning process. A horse requires the weight-bearing stresses of adequate land preparation before beginning or returning to competitive athletics. In addition, swimming forces a horse to invert his back, with a potential to elicit back spasms.

Long Slow Distance Training

The essence of developing the cardiovascular system depends on long slow distance conditioning, also referred to as LSD training (see p. 148). LSD is used to build a foundation for further training for any equine sport. This is the foundation for aerobic athletics of low to moderate intensity such as a horse experiences in distance riding, or dressage, or show equitation. To accomplish this end, a horse is exercised at the walk, trot, and slow canter. Slow gaits like these maximize the use of *aerobic metabolism*, which depends upon the use of carbohydrates and fats to generate energy in the presence of oxygen that is delivered to the muscles by an ample blood supply. Consistently applied cardiovascular conditioning improves a horse's *aerobic capacity*, which is the intensity of exercise a horse can sustain using aerobic metabolism to fuel muscular contractions.

In the beginning stages of LSD training, the optimal frequency of riding is every other day, 3 to 4 times per week, moving up to 5 to 6 days per week as a horse gets stronger. In all cases, it is important to start each exercise period with a good warm-up for 5 to 10 minutes, or longer in cold weather. The warm-up literally warms the tissues by increasing circulation and by activating enzyme systems within the muscles to convert chemical fuel to mechanical energy. In addition, the elastic stretch of tendons and ligaments is improved, which not only adds to the efficiency of a horse's gait, but also minimizes the risk of injury to musculoskeletal components (see p. 153).

TARGET HEART RATES

In LSD conditioning, the heart rate is maintained below 150 bpm, and preferably below 130 to 140 bpm. In general, this keeps a horse working within aerobic limits. Usually, the most basic cardiovascular adaptations are achieved within 2 to 3 months. The goal during this time is to improve a horse's fitness sufficiently that he can exercise for an hour or two at an average speed of 4 to 10 mph using gaits of walk, trot, and slow canter. If a horse is destined for recreational trail use, dressage, or equitation, then this level of fitness can easily be maintained by riding 2 to 3 times a week at the same light to moderate intensity.

INCREASING INTENSITY

For the competitive long-distance trail horse, event horse, jumper, polo horse, or working ranch horse, this level of LSD fitness provides a foundation to build upon to develop more endurance for longer periods and at greater exercise demands. As the next step is addressed in developing a horse's cardiovascular system, the duration of exercise periods is reduced, with substitution of greater intensity either in speed or difficulty. Increased intensity relies on incorporation of fast trots or gallops into workouts or by increasingly rigorous hill climbs to elevate a horse's heart rate. Deep footing, like sand, will increase the heart rate by 50 percent as compared to a conventional firm surface. The objective is to drive a horse's heart rate into the 140 to 150 bpm range for longer periods while staying within the aerobic limit. The overall result of this training is improved oxygen delivery to the tissues during exercise. Eventually, more time can be added back on each exercise period once a horse adjusts to the greater intensity.

As more rigorous exercise demands are applied to workouts, a horse need only be ridden a couple times a week. This gives him an opportunity to recover from the training effect and to improve in cardiovascular fitness from the intensity of the workouts, while minimizing the risk of cumulative musculoskeletal injury that occurs with overtraining. A third day of light hacking or arena work can be incorporated each week to work on training skills such as lead changes, balance, rhythm, and sport-specific proficiency.

Strength Training

As the foundation of LSD training develops, strength-training exercises should be added into the program (see p. 148). Not only is strength training a muscular response to cardiovascular conditioning, but a horse reaps other benefits as well, including reduction in the risk of musculoskeletal injuries, along with overall improvements in performance. As muscular endurance (the ability to sustain work for prolonged periods) improves, a horse should be able to perform repeated submaximal muscular contractions for longer periods without fatigue. This is accomplished through repetition of low to moderate intensity work such as climbing hills, trotting gymnastic jumping grids or cavalletti, practicing dressage skills, or cautiously working in footing that is deeper than usual. Even if the intended sport does not involve trail riding or jumping, use of hills and grids help develop a more versatile athlete. Integration of a variety of strengthening strategies prevents a horse from incurring repetitive stress and overuse on specific areas of the body that might be used in competitive skills. Ideally, some form of strength training should be incorporated three times a week, and then reduced to twice a week when workouts increase in intensity.

Interval Training

After a horse is accommodating more intense demands easily and with rapid heart rate recoveries, interval training (IT) techniques can be implemented (see p. 149). IT relies on the use of short bursts of speed or difficult hill climbs to elicit a cardiovascular response within the anaerobic range of metabolism. Interval training teaches a horse's body to tolerate the anaerobic state, and it develops a horse's inborn potential for speed. These goals are accomplished by performing repeated bouts of high intensity exercise for a set distance or time, followed by a walk or trot recovery period between each high intensity effort. This technique conditions horses for maximal exertions up to 3 minutes without risking structural damage. Usually IT is not introduced until a horse's second riding season since musculoskeletal structures need to be prepared to withstand the stresses incurred by speed or intensity of athletics.

SPEED PLAY

Brief sprints, called *fartleks*, teach a horse's muscles and metabolism to bump against the anaerobic threshold. These bouts of speed play are meant to bring his working heart rate to 160 to 170 bpm by speeding up his trot, or cantering or galloping at a moderate pace, then quickly dropping him back to an aerobic heart rate for rapid recovery. To develop more anaerobic tolerance, interval training pushes a horse to work at higher heart rates for longer periods.

WORK IN THE ANAEROBIC RANGE

Ever more challenging workouts drive the heart rate near to or into the anaerobic range between 160 to 180 bpm, and keep the heart rate elevated in that range for several minutes. Anaerobic workouts teach the tissues to respond to utilizing energy fuels (specifically carbohydrates) in the absence of oxygen, and to effectively metabolize waste products such as lactic acid in order to delay the onset of muscular fatigue. Anaerobic metabolism is a relatively inefficient mechanism for locomotion as compared to muscle contractions generated by aerobic metabolism. A horse working within the anaerobic range can generate rapid bursts of muscular contraction that can be sustained for only several minutes until lactic acid builds to excessive levels within the bloodstream. As an example of the time to fatigue at different maximal heart rates, a horse working at 170 to 180 bpm can maintain the pace for about 24 minutes, while a horse galloping at 208 bpm will fatigue in about 4 minutes.

Anaerobic metabolism is appropriate to fuel quick sprints or strenuous mountain climbs, but cannot be sustained for any distance. Yet, the fitter a horse becomes, the higher his heart rate must be to reach the anaerobic threshold. It is important for a horse to be developed to also withstand bursts of anaerobic output, necessary in sport pursuits that require sustained exercise or speed efforts.

Interval training capitalizes on the principle that a horse's body responds to a short but intense workout without the risks incurred from fatigue that is associated with sustained periods of strenuous activity. An ideal regimen incorporates periods of IT within longer periods of slower work. For example, a horse is galloped for a couple of minutes, then allowed ample recovery time at the trot or walk for a period of 2 to 4 times as long as he performed the speed work. Then another "interval" of speed or difficulty is repeated followed by sufficient recovery time. With this technique, a horse's tissues and muscle enzymes recognize the metabolic change and respond accordingly, ultimately giving him greater ability and endurance in the face of a competitive challenge.

TRAINING EFFECTS

Cardiovascular effects of interval training (IT) include:

- Strengthening of the heart, with increased blood pumped with each contraction
- Expansion of blood vessels
- Increased blood-vessel elasticity to improve blood flow

OPTIMIZING OXYGEN USE

With interval training, fast twitch high oxidative (FTH) muscle cells increase numbers of mitochondria (see chapter 6, *Muscle Endurance*, p. 146). More mitochondria increase the use of available oxygen and produce more energy. Interval training also encourages the spleen to increase its storage capacity for red blood cells. These red cells should enter the circulation twice a week by sprinting the horse about ¼ mile. If this does not occur, aged red blood cells distort and lose their oxygen-carrying capacity while the spleen destroys other inactive red blood cells.

Long Fast Distance Training

Long fast distance training methods often lead to failure. Prolonged speed creates breakdown injuries or exhaustion. This training method does not allow the body to repair, much less strengthen, between efforts. The horse continually disintegrates and cannot improve past a certain performance level.

Evaluating Cardiovascular Conditioning

Fitness Indicators

Training often concentrates on skills essential to an intended discipline. Yet, another training ingredient is essential to the success and well-being of any athletic horse: fitness of the cardiovascular system. As the muscles train to better efficiency, less work is needed to achieve a desired level of athleticism, with less heat generated by the body. Competition places critical physiological demands on a horse at every moment. A horse's level of fitness is not the only influence on his ability to perform well. Also consider the horse's metabolic condition and body weight, his age, the weight of the rider relative to the horse's size, the terrain or footing, and the weather.

Specific criteria determine how well a horse is holding up to stress, and his ability to continue a performance. One general fitness indicator is a horse's attitude. The look in his eyes, the degree of alertness, the impulsion of stride, and the posture of body and ears indicate his overall well-being.

HEART RATE RECOVERY

The most effective means to monitor fitness depends on measuring a horse's *heart rate recovery* during and following a performance effort. During exercise, the heart rate may increase as much as six to seven times the resting rate, increasing blood flow and oxygen to working muscles. For example, if a horse's resting rate (HR) is 30 beats per minute (bpm), his heart rate at maximal exertion could be 180 to 210 bpm. (Normal resting heart rate varies between individual horses, ranging between 24 to 40 bpm, with 36 bpm being average.)

One of the best indications that a horse tolerates the effort asked is how quickly his heart rate drops when the demand is lightened. Recovery rate depends on fitness, environmental temperature, and the type of athletic exertion. Typically, the heart rate decreases rapidly in the first minute once exercise ceases, and then it steadily and gradually declines toward the resting heart rate value over the next several minutes. As an example, as a horse crests a steep climb and starts down the other side, the heart rate should drop quickly to less than 100 bpm. When a horse is stopped for a rest break in the arena or along a course, his heart rate should drop to less than 60 to 64 bpm within 5 to 10 minutes. Measuring heart rate recovery of a horse that relies on bursts of speed for performance is also useful for evaluating conditioning training. For a sprint horse, the heart rate should drop to 150 to 180 bpm after 30 seconds, and 100 to 140 bpm after 1 minute. After a gallop near 200 bpm, the heart rate should recover to less than 120 bpm within 2 minutes, and to less than 80 bpm within 10 minutes. Within 30 minutes, the heart rate should be below 60 bpm following any kind of exertion. A heart rate monitor belt placed around the girth is helpful to continue to assess heart rate recovery (photo 9.5).

Below 120 bpm, the heart rate is affected to some degree by psychogenic factors like fear, anxiety, anticipation, pain, or other external stimuli. When a buddy horse leaves the immediate area; anxiety and herdbound behavior often delay slowing of the heart rate,

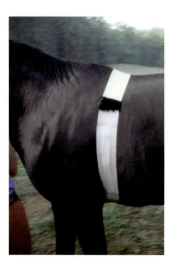

9.5 *A heart rate monitor belt is useful for continual monitoring of a horse's heart rate recovery. The belt has self-contained electrodes and a transmitter, which send digital information to the same watch used with the heart rate monitor kit in photo 9.2, p. 222.*

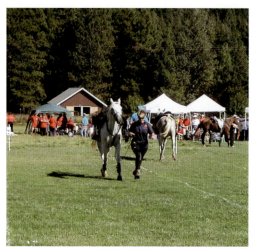

9.6 *The cardiac recovery index is a useful tool to evaluate how well a horse is coping with the stress of exercise. Count the horse's resting heart rate over 15 seconds. Then trot the horse out 250 feet. At the moment the horse starts the trot, mark the time on a stopwatch. At exactly one minute, take the heart rate again over 15 seconds. The recovery rate should return to the same or less number of beats than the starting resting rate.*

but this is a brief response. Some horses react adversely to handling by strangers or to other odd environmental stimuli. However, if the heart rate remains elevated for an extended time past expected return to normal values, then it could indicate significant adverse events for the horse:

- Consequences of dehydration and electrolyte depletion
- Musculoskeletal pain

A horse's inherent resting heart rate does not lower with conditioning, unlike the effect seen in humans. This aspect of the equine constitution coupled with rapidly changing mental responses to the world around him makes a horse's resting heart rate an unreliable indicator of fitness.

CARDIAC RECOVERY INDEX

Once a horse's heart rate returns to less than 60 to 64 bpm, a *cardiac recovery index* (CRI) is helpful in discovering subtle problems before they become serious. The resting heart rate is counted over a 15 second period. Then, the horse is trotted out a total of 250 feet (125 feet out and 125 feet back). A stopwatch is started at the precise moment the horse begins his 250-foot trot (photo 9.6). At exactly 1 minute, the heart rate is counted again over 15 seconds. It only takes 20 to 30 seconds to trot the measured distance, so the horse is standing still at the time of both comparison counts. The heart rate of a fit horse or a horse that is coping well with the stress of exercise returns to the initial "resting" rate or 4 beats below. As an example, if the resting rate is 56 bpm, then the reading at the minute, after the trot-out, should be 52 or 56, although 60 bpm could be considered in an acceptable range.

A CRI heart rate that is 4 or more bpm above the resting rate may indicate exhaustion or pain. At endurance or eventing competitions, the CRI is one parameter used to determine if a horse should be held at the check for a longer rest period or taken out of the competition. A count of 4 bpm higher is commonly seen with no untoward problems, but an elevation of 8 bpm or more may imply impending metabolic problems or a musculoskeletal injury. Questionable horses (such as 52/60) are re-evaluated 10 to 15 minutes later to monitor for progressive recovery. Under all circumstances, multiple metabolic parameters obtained during a veterinary physical exam are reviewed in conjunction with the CRI to determine fitness to continue in competition. A CRI check can also be implemented during training rides to evaluate appropriateness of the intensity of riding related to a horse's ability to cope.

OTHER METABOLIC PARAMETERS TO ASSESS CARDIOVASCULAR FITNESS

Capillary Refill Time

Gums should be a healthy pink color, and if blanched (pressed) with a fingertip, they should be come pink again in approximately 2 seconds (photo 9.7). This evaluation tests that the circulatory system is in good shape, pumping blood to all parts of the body. The time required for this response is called the *capillary refill time* (CRT).

Jugular Refill Time

Another method to evaluate circulatory efficiency and hydration is achieved by pressing a finger into the jugular furrow (groove) and watching how long the jugular vein takes to fill with blood (photo 9.8). Each horse's exact jugular refill time will vary; however, the jugular vein typically fills to pencil-size within 2 seconds. Checking the jugular refill time at the beginning of an athletic endeavor helps the rider monitor dehydration during the event. If the refill time lengthens throughout an event, this is a sign of lower circulating blood volume related to dehydration.

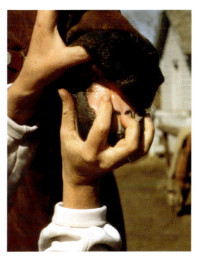

9.7 *Capillary refill time (CRT) is measured by blanching the gums with a finger and seeing how rapidly they become pink again when refilling with blood. Normal CRT is less than 2 seconds.*

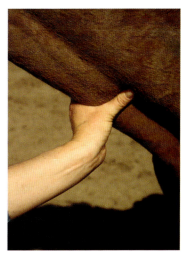

9.8 *Holding off the jugular vein in the neck gives a measure of how quickly the vein fills with blood. Typically, a normal horse's jugular refill takes less than 2 seconds. A very fit horse may have a slower refill time, as will a dehydrated horse. It is best to compare a reading to a horse's normal reaction taken when he is not working in rigorous athletics.*

Gut Sounds and Intestinal Activity

Intestinal activity and associated gut sounds heard on both sides of the flanks are important indicators of normal physiological function. An exercising horse may have fewer gut sounds because a large percentage of blood is diverted to the muscles. Less blood reaching the intestines slows intestinal activity. However, the intestinal tract should not be silent. Also, a horse's appetite should be active, preferably greedy, at rest stops or after a performance. (For more discussion, refer to chapter 11, *The Digestive System: The Oral Cavity, Dental Care, and the Intestinal Tract*, p. 316.)

If a horse is exercised at anaerobic levels, he can be watered and fed hay after he is cool to the touch on the chest. After 30 to 60 minutes, a horse may be fed grain with less risk of colic.

If a horse is working at aerobic, submaximal exercise, it is safe at any time to allow him to drink water and eat hay or grass. A small amount (no more than a pound or two) of grain may be offered once a horse has achieved heart rate recovery of 60 to 64 bpm.

Veterinary Evaluation

When available at equine sport events, a veterinarian can play a crucial role in achieving safe and successful competitions. In addition to evaluating a horse's metabolic condition, a veterinarian also assesses swelling in the limbs, or an obvious lameness that might prevent a horse from competing. Nicks, scrapes, minor injuries, and sores from improperly fitted tack are also pointed out in case a rider may have overlooked these. Such a veterinary resource can be invaluable so communicate with the veterinarian, ask questions, and discuss inconsistencies in a horse's performance.

Standard Exercise Test

Besides using recovery rates to monitor fitness, relative changes of the working heart rates can be tracked using a *standardized exercise test* (SET). A SET exercises the horse over a specified distance at a specified speed and evaluates the working heart rate. This value can be checked every 2 weeks and compared to previous performance by graphing heart rates over time.

As a horse's fitness improves and strength develops, his heart rate during a workout will decrease relative to the starting rate of previous months. As an example, trotting down a level road a horse may work at 136 bpm, but a few months later, a trot along that same road at the same speed elicits a heart rate of only 117 bpm. The work is easier because the muscles are stronger and the body has learned to maximize its systems of oxygen delivery to the tissues and heat transport from the muscles.

The lower the working heart rate, the less oxygen will be consumed by the heart muscle. Overall, the heart has to work less hard to accomplish the same objective of moving the horse along a course.

In most cases, training may only elicit drops in heart rates of 10 to 20 bpm for a particular task. Because of this small increment of change, it can be difficult to use working heart rates as a consistently reliable measure of fitness. Maximal heart rates achieved at gallop speeds or very intense hill climbs do not change much with improved fitness.

FIELD FITNESS TEST

Another variation on the SET is to use a heart rate monitor to perform a *field fitness test* to evaluate a horse's aerobic capacity. This test measures the velocity (mph) at 200 bpm (V_{200}) after a warm-up period. To perform the field test, measure and mark off a set distance of ¾ to 1 mile, and then record the time it takes for a horse to cover that distance with the heart rate maintained as close to 200 bpm as possible. The fitter the horse, the faster he must go to achieve a heart rate of 200 bpm, and the greater his aerobic capacity. V_{200} can be compared every month, determining improvements in fitness. However, heart rate measurements only evaluate aerobic capacity, not structural strength.

For most athletic pursuits, it is only necessary to evaluate the horse at 160 bpm (V_{160}). This is the heart rate at which lactic acid accumulates faster than it can be metabolized. The speed a horse can go at this heart rate while lactic acid is being formed defines the horse's aerobic capacity. V_{160} is not an accurate indicator of fitness because pain or excitement can artificially drive the heart rate up to 160 bpm without muscular work being performed. However, it is a useful rate to start with for a horse re-entering training after a long layoff, or for an old or young horse at risk of musculoskeletal injury at fast speeds.

CARDIOVASCULAR DRIFT

In some instances of persistent, strenuous submaximal exercise, despite a constant exertion the heart rate may elevate slowly in a phenomenon known as *cardiovascular drift*. As an example of this situation, the working heart rate may start at 154 bpm and by 30 to 90 minutes of strenuous endurance exercise may elevate to 173 bpm, despite the fact that the work effort seemingly remains the same. Such a rise in heart rate may be a combined result of ongoing fluid and electrolyte depletion, muscular fatigue, and environmental factors like heat and humidity that tax the system; then what started out as a moderate-intensity effort now is amplified due to metabolic changes within the horse. This change in working heart rate is a warning flag to lessen the speed or intensity.

Maintaining Peak Form

An issue a rider must face is how to maintain a horse's strong level of fitness during a competitive season. It is tempting to continue training between competitions, but there is a calculated risk that a horse may be overridden. As relates to the cardiovascular system, it is not necessary to present continual exercise pressure on a fit horse. When a horse is rested for a time, referred to as *detraining*, there are only minimal decreases in the cardiopulmonary system and blood-lactate responses to aerobic exercise over a two- to six-month period (see chapter 6, *Muscle Endurance*, p. 151). One month of layup time has little to no effect on a horse's cardiovascular abilities. Some changes do occur during detraining, such as a slight reduction in oxidative enzyme systems that generate energy through aerobic metabolism. At 6 weeks of detraining, a horse's ability to dissipate heat is slightly less efficient.

However, once a solid cardiovascular base has been achieved, a horse responds rapidly to reconditioning whether he has two weeks off or a winter season of light work. During the competitive season, resist the urge to keep the level of intensity of riding as high as what was applied for "conditioning" and developing the system. Sufficient recovery and rest time (days to weeks) should be allowed following a demanding event. During the weeks between competitions, cardiovascular conditioning can be maintained by riding the horse lightly once a week with a more intense ride another day each week.

Exercise Intolerance and Poor Performance

Not all horses have the ability to be a premier athlete. It is sometimes puzzling when a horse that has everything in his favor is unable to meet an expected level of performance, especially when compared to similarly endowed horses. Sometimes a horse does not have the combination of attributes to drive him to a pinnacle of excellence. At times a horse's genetic capabilities are not properly suited to the assigned career. In other instances there is a physiologic reason for failure to perform to expectations. Examples of system failure leading to exercise intolerance include:

- Musculoskeletal pain (see chapters 3–8)
- Respiratory illness (see chapter 10, *Respiratory Conditioning and Health*)
- Cardiac disease (see this chapter, *Cardiovascular Conditioning and Health*)
- Anemia or vascular disease (see this chapter, *Cardiovascular Conditioning and Health*)

- Gastrointestinal problems (see chapter 11, *The Digestive System: The Oral Cavity, Dental Health, and the Intestinal Tract*)
- Dental problems (see chapter 11, *The Digestive System: The Oral Cavity, Dental Health, and the Intestinal Tract*)
- Mental stress and anxiety (see chapter 15, *Preventive and Mental Horse Health*)
- Dehydration (see p. 235)

Overtraining

An equine athlete must be able to summon all his resources to maximize performance. Some days everything clicks into place, and a horse performs flawlessly. But occasionally a horse reaches a period of crisis where performance begins to wane, imperceptibly at first, and then more consistently with each workout. Due to cumulative physical and psychological stress, a horse may reach a state of crisis.

A common reason for poor performance is a phenomenon known as *overtraining*: a horse is ridden too often at too high a level of demand without sufficient recovery periods. Muscles exhaust their energy supplies during strenuous exercise, and they need time to restore energy and enzymes to drive biochemical reactions. Usually complete recovery only takes 12 to 24 hours. After extreme exertion, such as a competition or hours of rigorous work, several days of rest may be necessary to replenish energy stores. If a horse is continually pushed past the body's limit, all his reserves are depleted. A horse cannot compensate for the lack of muscle fuel needed to drive performance and fatigue results.

Without rest and replenishment of energy, depleted muscle cells of a horse will consume each other in an attempt to metabolize protein into glycogen. The horse will lose weight or fail to gain condition, and the bright bursts of brilliant performance typical of that individual fail to appear.

INITIAL INDICATIONS

Initial indications that a horse is stressed from an excessively intense training schedule include:

- Elevated resting pulse
- Elevated working pulse
- Abnormal sweating
- Poor heart rate recovery
- Muscle tremors
- Diarrhea

SYMPTOMS OF OVERTRAINING

An overtrained horse is recognized by:

- Failure to gain weight
- Weight loss
- Stiff and sore muscles
- Dull eyes
- Less alert stance
- Nervousness
- Behavioral changes
- Poor appetite and picking at food
- Poor immune system

REST AND RELAXATION

If a horse starts to fail in performance, try backing off to an every other day training schedule rather than a daily workout, or consider walking for an hour on one of the days scheduled for a rigorous training period. Once a horse's fatigued body begins to recuperate, appetite will improve. A horse facilitates his own rehabilitation by consuming needed nutrients and energy. Often, attempts are made to supplement a horse with food additives and vitamins to restore luster, when what is really needed is rest and relaxation. To determine whether a horse is suffering from muscle damage or nutritional deficiencies, blood chemistry profiles can be analyzed before and after exercise.

Dehydration

Dehydration has adverse effects on health and performance.

BODY WATER, WHAT IS IT?

Think of a horse as a walking vat of saltwater with four legs. Body water is distributed within several main locations:

- In blood vessels and between the cells (referred to as *extracellular fluid* or ECF)
- Within the cells (referred to as *intracellular fluid* or ICF)
- Within a reservoir of about 18 to 21 gallons in the intestinal tract

As water is depleted from the bloodstream through losses in sweat, fluid shifts from the ICF to the ECF. This enables the cardiovascular system and heart pump to continue to function well, and circulation is maintained to the skin to dissipate heat from the body core and muscles. In the meantime, tissues are rapidly dehydrating as fluid shifts out of the cells into the ECF. (The ECF volume is maintained at the expense of the ICF.)

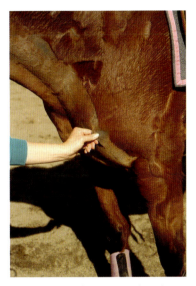

9.9 *The best place to test skin elasticity is by pinching the skin over the point of the shoulder. The rapidity with which it snaps back to normal reflects hydration of the tissues.*

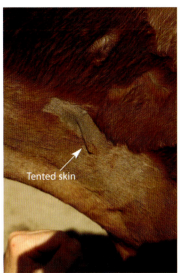

9.10 *Pinching the skin on the side of the neck is not always an accurate measure for determining hydration. Due to less subcutaneous fat in that area, the skin may remain in a "tented" position (a sign of body dehydration) in normally hydrated horses that are fit, thin, or old. Wet or sweaty horses also may show less skin elasticity.*

WATER LOSS

Sweating usually begins within 10 minutes of exercise, immediately pulling water out of the ECF. For aerobic rides of any distance in a hot climate, by 15 miles there could be 1 to 4 gallons of water loss. Along with this water loss, electrolytes also are significantly diminished. As water is depleted from the bloodstream, as much as 10 percent of the total body stores of electrolytes will be lost along with it. With depleted body water, the horse experiences reduced blood volume with less available blood to bathe the tissues, especially those of the muscles, skin, and intestines.

HYDRATION ASSESSMENT

There are many levels of dehydration, and there are variable indications of it. Pinching a fold of skin on the point of the shoulder or the eyelid provides a rough estimate of dehydration (photo 9.9). The speed at which it snaps back into position denotes tissue hydration. A horse that is not dehydrated experiences normal blood flow to the skin so the skin rebounds immediately. Pinched skin that remains "tented" and does not return to normal indicates a moderate to dangerous level of dehydration (photo 9.10).

A skin pinch test may have a poor correlation with degree of hydration; in general there is often not much change in the skin until a horse is at least 5 percent dehydrated. By this time, a horse is experiencing a significant degree of body fluid loss. Also, if fluid losses happen rapidly, the skin pinch test lags behind so a more accurate assessment is not identifiable immediately. And, the elasticity of the skin depends a lot on age of the horse and breed. Thin horses and those breeds with thin skin (many Arabians and Thoroughbreds) tend to have less elastic tissue because there is less fat in the skin layers. These animals often show a delayed skin pinch, as does skin that has been soaked with water used for cooling.

On a hot day, it is possible for a 1000-pound horse exercising for protracted periods to lose 2 to 3 gallons (7.6 to 11.4 liters) of fluid each hour of exercise, or 6 to 12 gallons (22.7 to 45.5 liters) during a workout. A racehorse may lose as much as half a gallon (2 liters) of body water during a mile race. Such extensive fluid loss may lead to severe dehydration of 7 to 10 percent, resulting in circulatory collapse and exhaustion.

On a hot, humid day, even mild dehydration of 2 to 3 percent loss of body fluid adversely affects performance, whereas severe dehydration of 7 to 10 percent body fluid loss places a horse in life-threatening danger. A horse with mild dehydration (2 to 3 percent) may demonstrate a prolonged capillary refill time (see photo 9.7, p. 231), a dry mouth, or dry mucous membranes. Other signs of dehydration include depressed intestinal activity, and slow heart rate recovery (see p. 239). At moderate dehydration of 5 percent:

- The eye sockets appear sunken.
- Skin elasticity is markedly reduced.
- The horse is weak, and appears dull.

The flanks in a moderately dehydrated horse often appear tucked up in a wasp-waisted, gaunt way (photos 9.11 A & B). Scanty or absent manure, dry feces, or manure covered with mucus also point to a horse suffering from dehydration (photo 9.12). Minimal urine output is another means for a horse to conserve body water. Urine that is concentrated in appearance (dark yellow) and of small volume speaks of dehydration. With muscle damage from dehydration, urine often turns brown or red-tinged (see chapter 6, *Muscle Endurance*, p. 163).

THIRST REFLEX

Progressive dehydration and excess loss of electrolytes such as sodium, chloride, and potassium, eliminates the stimulus to trigger thirst. By not drinking, a horse worsens his dehydration problem. Just because a horse won't drink does not mean he is not in need of fluids. He may be suffering a marked electrolyte imbalance, requiring immediate intravenous fluid and electrolyte therapy.

What Is Normal Water Intake?

An idle horse needs about 5 to 7 gallons of water a day just to maintain normal physiologic function. With the work of protracted exercise, a horse needs to drink at least 20 gallons of water each day to keep abreast of the losses. Performance suffers with just 3 percent dehydration at any time, which is equivalent to a loss of 4 gallons of body "water."

Doctoring Drinking Water

Some horses do not like the taste of strange water and will refuse to drink. If a horse is finicky about strange water, begin to "doctor" the drinking water at home with a small amount of cider vinegar or sugar about a month before competition. Vinegar or sugar disguises a strange water source so a horse may continue to drink well. As an alternative, carry water from home when you travel.

Cardiovascular Conditioning and Health

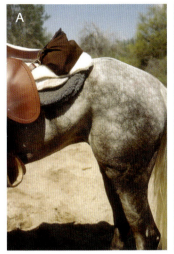
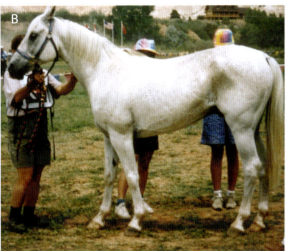
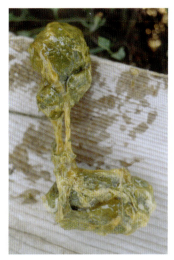

9.11 A & B *Both these horses demonstrate overall body dehydration by the tucked-up and splinted appearance of the flanks. The darker grey horse experienced dehydration through the course of a competitive event, while the white horse arrived at an event after a day in the trailer traveling through extremely high summer temperatures. Although the presence of splinted muscles is sometimes associated with a pain response, these two horses are suffering only from dehydration. Were this allowed to persist in the course of continued exercise, such horses could develop signs of exhausted horse syndrome and/or impaction colic.*

9.12 *When intestinal contents are dehydrated, the body attempts to lubricate the feces with a mucoid coating to facilitate passage of manure through the bowel.*

PREVENTING DEHYDRATION

Conditioning helps prevent dehydration. The more fit the horse, the less demand exercise has on his body so exercising muscles produce less heat. Indirectly then, conditioning reduces fluid loss from sweat. By sweating less, the body conserves vital electrolytes and body fluid.

A horse should be allowed to drink at every opportunity. A hot horse can be allowed to drink as long as he continues to move afterward. Otherwise, cool out slowly and offer small amounts of water at frequent intervals.

If an overheated horse abruptly stops work, blood pools in the muscles. Less blood is available to the circulation, contributing to a horse's relative dehydration. An exhausted horse that refuses to move may benefit from massage of major muscle groups in a rhythm with the heartbeat to circulate blood through the muscles.

BODY TEMPERATURE

Working muscles expend at least 20 times the energy of their resting metabolic rate, with the natural by-product being heat. A thermoregulatory center in the horse's brain sets the normal temperature and maintains it within a very narrow range. Rectal temperature provides another valuable parameter to monitor a horse's well-being and is a reasonable indicator of internal temperature. Normal rectal temperature for a horse ranges between 97 to 101° F (36 to 38° C). An exercising horse typically works within a rectal temperature range of 101 to 103° F (38 to 39° C). Should rectal temper-

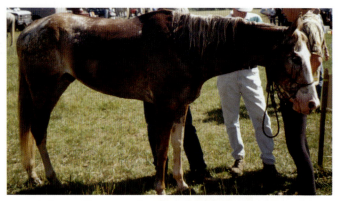

9.13 *A fatigued horse stands with a deflated body posture, ears turned back, head drooping, with an anxious expression.*

ature surpass 103.5° F (40° C), a horse is showing signs of overheating. Once a horse has been pulled up to rest, rectal temperature should decline steadily over 20 minutes. External cooling strategies hasten the return of internal temperature toward normal.

Rectal temperature exceeding 105° F (40.5° C) is abnormal in any horse and poses a dangerous situation; rapid cooling measures should be initiated at once. An overheated horse may experience weakness and incoordination. Loss of muscle control and strength can lead to serious accidents. An exhausted horse may stumble and fall or he may not safely clear an obstacle, placing both horse and rider in jeopardy. The higher the internal temperature, the more metabolic demands are placed on the system; this metabolism needs to be fueled by oxygen. If body temperature exceeds 106° F (41° C), the body's demand for oxygen may surpass the amount that can be supplied by the respiratory system. Oxygen deficit in the tissues (*hypoxia*) potentially leads to kidney, liver, and brain damage. At temperatures greater than 107° F (42° C), a horse in severe heat stress may go into convulsions or coma, and die.

SUBTLE SIGNS OF DEHYDRATION

Many times, the clues are present to a rider who is tuned-in to his horse. A horse owner intuitively knows when his horse is normal, and when he is not. Be cognizant of very subtle changes in your horse's demeanor and attitude; you need only "listen" and pay attention. This doesn't always apply if a horse is influenced by herd adrenalin and commotion, or in stoic, highly competitive animals that don't know something is wrong.

But, in the best situation, subtle signs may be evident. Often, a horse will communicate flagging energy in subtle ways long before a crisis develops. Such clues are abundant in the way a horse stands, moves, and relates to his rider and the world around him. Many seemingly obscure signs may be obvious behavioral clues to an observant rider. An unhappy horse is reluctant to move out, maybe wrings his tail, pins his ears, or tosses his head when asked to pick up speed or agility. A horse that leans increasingly onto the forehand, stumbles, or continually slows is communicating fatigue. A horse that stretches his head and neck downward while asked to move out is telling of muscle fatigue, or he may be seeking more air to accommodate the effort asked.

At rest, a droopy, "deflated" body posture signals fatigue (photo 9.13). Odd positions, such as a camped-out stance, or a shifting of weight from foot to foot are a horse's way of seeking a more comfortable position. This implies that something is bothering him, either fatigue or pain. When a tired horse is asked to lead forward, his head and neck follow, but he moves his body as little as possible. Wrinkling of the muzzle around the nostrils is often an expression of discomfort (photo 9.14). Other signals of dehydration and fatigue include a sunken appearance to the eyes, or dull eyes.

A horse that plays in the water rather than drinking is one to watch carefully. A picky appetite or slow chewing signal distress. A horse that doesn't want to eat at all should be monitored very closely and may need veterinary attention. Lack of interest in surroundings or lack of normal response to insect irritation indicates that a horse is sick or overly tired.

Stress Indicators

OBVIOUS WARNING SIGNS OF FATIGUE

A horse that is experiencing fatigue and/or heat buildup will demonstrate various signs, some subtle, some quite obvious. A knowledgeable rider will continually monitor for any of these signs:

- Slow heart rate recovery
- Elevated heart rate following exercise
- High respiratory rate, often shallow and inefficient
- Deep, gulping breaths that persist for over 1 minute
- High rectal temperature (greater than 103.5° F or 39.7° C) for longer than 20 minutes
- Dehydration with dry or pale mucous membranes, prolonged capillary refill time and jugular refill time, lack of intestinal sounds, and/or lack of skin elasticity
- Depression
- Disinterest in surroundings or environmental stimulation
- Lack of appetite or thirst
- Muscle tremors or twitching
- Muscle cramping
- Thumps, or synchronous diaphragmatic flutter (see "Thumps," chapter 6, *Muscle Endurance*, p. 164)

Poor Recovery

Outward signs of a persistent heat load in the muscles and body core are evident as a horse's

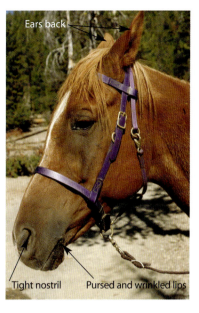

9.14 *Discomfort is often expressed by wrinkling of the muzzle around the corners of the mouth and the nostril, as seen here in this fatigued horse.*

respiratory rate increases or he pants, and heart rates stay elevated for longer times. An overheated and/or dehydrated horse demonstrates poor recoveries and/or has elevated cardiac recovery indexes. Rectal temperature often remains elevated above 103° F (39° C) with heat stress, and the use of a thermometer is one useful means to monitor recovery.

The effects of prolonged sweating result in loss of body fluids and loss of necessary electrolytes involved in muscle contraction, intestinal function, and blood perfusion to the skin. Each organ affects the other in its activity; one cannot function efficiently without the full and efficient functioning of the other. Dehydration is an athletic horse's greatest enemy as all body systems are adversely affected, leading to potentially serious metabolic problems.

Persistent Heart Rate Elevation

Persistent elevation of heart rate may indicate an impending metabolic collapse. As mentioned, heart rate remains high due to fatigue or exhaustion. Pain also elevates heart rate. If other metabolic signs such as attitude, gut sounds, level of fatigue, level of dehydration, and body temperature seem normal, seek out a source of pain, particularly in the limbs or muscles.

Respiratory Rate
The respiratory rate should decrease along with heart rate recovery. Preferably, the respiratory rate will drop below the heart rate within 10 minutes. However, environmental conditions, hair coat, obesity, and level of fitness influence the rate of this drop. In hot and humid climates, horses may pant in rapid, shallow respirations. A high respiratory rate is also associated with high body temperatures. If rectal temperature is greater than 103° F (39° C), it would be prudent to stop exercise.

Inversion
When the respiratory rate remains faster than the heart rate, it is called an *inversion*. As a horse's flanks move rapidly in and out with each breath, there is an impression that he is "panting." Panting respiration is shallow and rapid, and nostrils are flared.

If the heart rate recovers within 10 minutes, but the respiratory rate remains high, the horse is not necessarily in trouble; he may need help in ridding his body of extra heat. After extended exercise, a few extra minutes spent slowly walking the horse enables flushing of heat and lactic acid from the muscles by the circulation. Head and neck soaks with water further speed cooling (see chapter 13, *The Skin as an Organ*, p. 358).

Heart Irregularities
Heart disease is uncommon in horses, but heart murmurs or irregularities in heart rate (*arrhythmias*) do occur. Evaluation of the heart can be achieved with ultrasound and an ECG (electrocardiogram). *Degenerative myocardial disease* is unusual, but does occur. Chronic respiratory disease places strain on the heart, and may create an arrhythmia. Viral, bacterial, or protozoan infections can injure heart valves. Electrolyte imbalances in an exercising horse have profound effects on heart contraction and cardiac output. Any condition that creates anemia or interferes with blood flow to the heart muscle also compromises the heart's effectiveness as a pump to supply blood and oxygen to the tissues.

Certain drugs, toxins, or electrolyte imbalances can mimic heart disease symptoms, including:

- Rapid heart rate
- Irregular heart rate
- Poor recovery rate
- Acute fatigue
- Fainting or *syncope*

ATRIAL FIBRILLATION
One of the most commonly encountered heart arrhythmias in the horse is *atrial fibrillation*. It is usually identified upon examination of a complaint of poor performance and/or exercise intolerance. The heart rhythm is irregular and lacks a standard "lub-dub" heartbeat; this irregularity persists even during exercise. Atrial fibrillation may occur following chronic heart failure, ventricular failure, or infections by *Streptococcus equi*, influenza virus, or pharyngitis (inflammation in the back of the throat). It may occur subsequent to migration of *Strongyle* endoparasites, snake bite, pulmonary disease, or abdominal surgery. In sports requiring prolonged endurance exercise, potassium depletion through sweat may create transient atrial fibrillation.

Anemia

PACKED CELL VOLUME

The *packed cell volume* (PCV) measures the percentage of circulating red blood cells in the bloodstream. Normally a horse has a PCV of around 40 percent. A highly fit individual may store up to one-third of his red blood cells (RBCs) in the spleen, so a fit horse may show a PCV of about 30 percent. A horse with a PCV of less than 30 percent is considered anemic, and efforts should be made to identify the source of the loss of RBCs or lack of production of RBCs.

CAUSES OF ANEMIA

RBCs contain hemoglobin, which carries oxygen to the tissues as the blood circulates through the body. Losses of red blood cells or hemoglobin reduce oxygenation of the tissues. Any condition that results in blood loss, destruction of red blood cells, or failure of the body to manufacture red blood cells leads to anemia. Some examples:

- An intestinal parasite load may consume blood.
- A chronic infection or inflammatory condition consumes both white and red blood cells resulting in a loss of RBCs.
- Gastrointestinal ulcers may bleed, slowly leaking away red blood cells.
- Nutrient deficiencies of iron, copper, protein, and B vitamins impair the body's ability to manufacture sufficient RBCs.
- Hemorrhage may cause acute blood loss.
- Toxic plants, like red maple leaves or onions, destroy RBCs (see *Appendix C*, p. 571).
- A blood sample provides information whether a horse is anemic and if he is capable of producing more red blood cells.

Red Maple Toxicity

Wilted or dried leaves of the red maple tree cause a serious and potentially fatal hemolytic anemia when ingested. Red maple leaves cause oxidant damage and destruction of red blood cells. Intake of 1½ pounds of leaves causes toxicity and consumption of 3 pounds is fatal. Fatality occurs in about 30 percent of cases.

EQUINE INFECTIOUS ANEMIA

Equine Infectious Anemia (EIA) has been present in the United States for over 100 years, called *equine relapsing fever*, or *swamp fever* because of its distribution along wet areas. EIA is a viral disease resulting from infection by a *retrovirus* similar to the HIV virus of humans.

A horse with an acute infection with the EIA virus (EIAV) may exhibit clinical signs within 1 to 3 weeks after exposure. Illness appears suddenly with a high fever, depression, small hemorrhages (*petechiations*) on the mucous membranes, and dependent edema of the limbs, abdomen, and sheath. An overwhelming infection may result in death within four weeks.

Once infected with EIAV, a surviving horse remains infected for life, and may suffer through episodes of intermittent fever, progressive weight loss, and anemia. Stress from management, hard exercise, or transport can precipitate a crisis. A horse that recovers from an acute episode becomes a chronic carrier to infect normal horses. The most worrisome form of EIA is that of the *inapparent carrier,* which is a horse that has shown no clinical signs of the disease yet carries sufficient virus in his system to be a potential source of infection to others (see "Carrier Horses," p. 242).

Transmission of EIA

Insect vectors, particularly the horsefly (*Tabanus* spp.) and the deer fly (*Chrysops* spp.) are the primary means by which infected blood or serum is transferred mechanically from a sick horse to a well one. These large flies are able to transfer large enough amounts of blood and virus to be infective. The bites of these flies are painful so feeding is often interrupted as a horse dislodges the fly. Then, the fly retires to another horse to complete a blood meal, carrying freshly contaminated blood on its mouthparts, and virus is injected into a new host. The fly itself does not become infected, but the virus remains infective in the fly's blood meal for up to 4 hours. Mosquitoes do not transmit the disease for several reasons: not only do their secretions contain inhibitors that inactivate EIA virus within 30 minutes, but also it is not likely that a mosquito will be interrupted from a blood meal feeding to transfer contaminated blood to another host.

Small amounts of blood can also be transmitted from horse to horse by contaminated syringes, needles, and surgical instruments, or through abrasions or mucous membranes from tack that has been contaminated with blood or serum secretions.

An EIA-infected stallion can transmit the virus to a mare via his semen, despite being asymptomatic. Also, the virus can cross the placental membranes in a mare to infect a growing fetus. If the fetus survives and is not aborted, it will be infected serologically with EIAV, and the foal will probably die within a few months. A foal can also be infected by virus passage through the colostrum (first milk).

Carrier Horses

Not all horses develop obvious clinical manifestations of EIA. Besides the acute and chronic forms of the disease, there exist *inapparent* cases. These horses are infected, but are not sick. The likelihood of mechanical transmission of virus from inapparent carriers is much less than from a horse suffering an acute attack with high fever and virus rampant in the bloodstream. However, studies have proven that inapparent carriers harbor enough virus to be considered a threat to normal horses. The United States Department of Agriculture (USDA) states statistical probabilities as follows:

- One-fifth of a teaspoon (1 milliliter) of blood of a horse infected with *acute* illness contains enough virus to infect one million horses.
- One-fifth of a teaspoon of blood of a horse infected with *chronic* illness during a feverish episode contains enough virus to infect 10,000 horses.
- Only one horsefly out of 6 million is likely to obtain and transmit EIAV from an *inapparent carrier*.

Transmission probabilities are dependent on the density of horses, the incidence of insect vectors, the season, and the environment that determines insect habitats.

Regulation of Horses

In much the same way as the AIDS virus in man is incurable, once infected with EIAV, a horse possesses the disease for life. Because of the threat of unidentified carrier horses to the safety of equine health in the population at large, necessary regulatory measures have been instituted across the United States. A lab test (called a *Coggins test*, see p. 457) screens for the presence of EIA in a horse's blood.

The USDA prohibits interstate movement of any horse that tests positive to the Coggins test, or of any horse that is clinically sick. A horse that tests positive to an official Coggins test can move interstate only if he returns to the farm of origin, to an immediate slaughter facility, or to a specified diagnostic or research facility. Not all states follow the same regulatory procedures as to timing requirements of a negative Coggins test so each state must be consulted about its specific entry requirements. Some states require a negative test within 6 months, while others require only a yearly test.

If a horse is pronounced a positive reactor to the test, the options are few and brutal. Either the horse must be euthanized, or branded or tattooed with a special number or letter and quarantined for life. Quarantine requires isolation of the horse within a 200-yard buffer zone separation from other horses. The 200-yard rule works because 99 percent of the time horseflies return to the original host to finish feeding from an interrupted meal if another horse is more than 160 feet away.

Adherence to these stringent control regulations over the last several decades has reduced the incidence of EIA in a large proportion of the United States. The predominant areas of concern remain mostly in the southeastern states. In these warm, humid states, high insect vector populations persist through many seasons, thus increasing the opportunities and risk for transmission.

Control Recommendations to Limit Spread of EIA

- All horses should be tested at least annually for EIA, and horses that travel to high-risk areas should be tested twice a year.
- A negative Coggins test certificate should accompany any new horse to his new premises.
- It is recommended to test all horses for EIA prior to purchase, and in some states this is mandatory.
- Any horse involved in events, trail rides, races, assemblies, or gatherings where he will comingle with other horses must have a current negative Coggins certificate.
- New horses to a premise should be quarantined for 45 days or until a negative Coggins test has been confirmed before allowing comingling with the resident horses.
- Fly control strategies are important to minimize risk of exposure: cleaning stalls and paddocks regularly, composting manure, and minimizing poor sanitation on a farm as well as using pesticide sprays.
- Specify individual equipment and tack for each horse and minimize sharing.
- Sterilize equipment such as dental and surgical instruments that may be used in common with other horses, and discard needles, syringes, or blood-contaminated supplies once they are used on a horse.

Respiratory Conditioning and Health 10

When we paint an image in our minds of a galloping horse, we see nostrils flared, the horse straining with neck extended, his flanks heaving with the effort. It is fitting that horses are oft referred to as "drinkers of the wind." What makes an equine athlete so capable of sustained performance is the ability to use oxygen for as long as possible to fuel muscle locomotion. The better able a horse is to assimilate oxygen from his lungs to the bloodstream to be carried to the muscles, the more stamina and more mental willingness the horse will display.

The Respiratory System

The respiratory tract includes two parts (fig. 10.1):

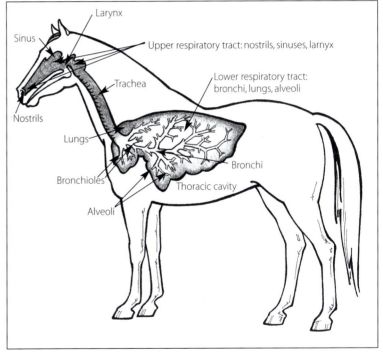

10.1 *The upper and lower respiratory tracts.*

- The upper respiratory tract: the nostrils, sinus passages within the head, the larynx
- The lower respiratory tract: trachea (windpipe), bronchi, bronchioles, lungs, and diaphragm (see fig. 10.3, p. 248).

The respiratory system does not directly adapt to conditioning. However, as other body systems (such as the circulatory system) become stronger, the respiratory system must maintain its efficiency of oxygen intake to fuel performance. The lungs provide oxygen to fuel the musculoskeletal tissues, heart, liver, kidneys, and intestinal tract. Each of these parts is dependent on the others for fueling and maintaining optimal performance.

The Upper Respiratory Tract

In its most simplistic form, we can think of the upper respiratory tract as the head region with a series of tubes through which air flows. As the horse inhales, air enters the nostrils and travels through the long sinus passages within the head to the back of the throat. Horses are incapable of breathing by mouth, and all air must pass through the nostrils. The shape and function of the tissues in the nasal passages, sinuses, and larynx contribute directly to resistance of airflow through the "pipes." (See p. 247 for more on size and shape of airways.)

Even the conformation of the head is important for ensuring maximum air intake. An exaggerated Arabian "dish" to the face may limit the width of the nostrils and sinus passages and thereby restrict air intake. Any dysfunction within the pharynx or larynx in the back of the throat makes it hard for a horse to get enough air to the lungs to fuel locomotion; performance suffers accordingly (see "Recurrent Larnygeal Neuropathy aka Roaring," p. 258). Air restriction is particularly a problem during the high demands associated with speed and can be a problem with the high demands for oxygen created by aerobic exercise.

STREAMLINED SYSTEM

Under normal circumstances, the upper respiratory tract is streamlined to minimize the resistance of flow of air in a healthy horse. As an example, the flaring of the nostrils and constriction of abundant blood vessels within erectile tissue in the nose all serve to functionally widen the nasal passages (photo 10.2). Once air has passed through the head region, it goes through the larynx at the back of the throat into the trachea. The *vocal folds* around the larynx pull backward to reduce airway resistance. Also, the elastic mucosa lining the top and bottom walls of the nasopharynx and larynx is stretched, pro-

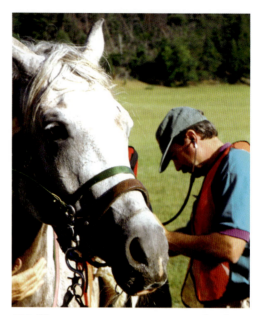

10.2 *The upper respiratory tract is streamlined to allow smooth passage of air flow. The nostrils flare and blood vessels constrict to functionally widen the nasal passages for lessened resistance to air flow.*

viding a smoother surface and reducing airflow resistance. Small muscles hold the soft palate down and "raise" the roof of the nasopharynx, but these muscles need head and neck extension to prevent fatigue during strenuous exertion. As the larynx outwardly expands and opens, the air passages leading into the trachea become smooth to limit resistance. As the horse extends his head and neck, the airway is straightened, eliminating bends and turbulence. During exercise, a normal larynx expands its cross-sectional area three times wider than at rest, allowing ease of passage of air through minimal air resistance by the tissues.

Many special adaptations in the system best accommodate flow of air. Air is a mixture of gases, the most important of which is oxygen. As a horse inhales, his rib cage and thorax expand to create a negative pressure, or vacuum, within the thorax. Air then flows into the nostrils, along the nasal passages, over the soft palate and through the pharynx, through the larynx, down the trachea, and into the lungs, sucked-in to fill this void. Due to differences between the relatively positive atmospheric pressure outside and negative pressure inside the thorax, twice the energy is required for the horse to inhale as to exhale. With any suction force, structures surrounding the airway would tend to collapse. Yet, the equine respiratory tract is protected from such dynamic collapse in many ways:

- The nasal cavity is supported largely by bone.
- Special dilating muscles in the nostrils, the nasopharynx above the soft palate, and the larynx help to overcome the suction force of inhalation.
- The larynx is suspended from the base of the skull by a rigid bony scaffold called the *hyoid apparatus*.
- The trachea is kept spread and open by reinforcement with rings of cartilage.
- A strap muscle (*sternothyrohyoideus*) extends from under the sternum (the breastbone), up the chest and along the underside of the neck to attach onto the hyoid apparatus. Contractions of this muscle bundle keep the trachea and larynx open under athletic demand. This muscle group is visible as a bulging strap along the underside of the neck in a horse that travels with head his up and back hollowed.
- Contractions of the diaphragm (a dome-shaped muscle behind and beneath the lungs) additionally enlarge the airways and keep the trachea open.

SIZE AND SHAPE OF THE AIRWAYS

The size of the air passages directly influences the efficiency of airflow. According to the laws of physics, air flows best down a straight tube with smooth, rigid, and preferably parallel walls. Resistance to airflow is affected by the diameter of the tube. For example, flow of air through a tube that is opened to a diameter of twice its normal size is improved sixteen-fold in efficiency. Consequently, airways that are as straight and smooth as possible, with minimal bends or obstructions, result in optimal air and oxygen intake to enhance performance.

For a normal horse that does not suffer from respiratory disease or mechanical obstructions of the airways, the upper airway is still responsible for more than half of the total air resistance. Any situation that functionally reduces the diameter of the airways further increases resistance of airflow. Such situations include:

- Inflammation of the airways with swelling or mucus
- A mechanical obstruction such as created by laryngeal hemiplegia (roaring), displacement of the soft palate, chronic pharyngitis, soft palate hypertrophy (enlargement), or nasal polyps
- Any bend in the airway such as head flexion

Flexion at the Poll and Neck

The mechanics of breathing in the exercising horse are quite different from the resting horse because more oxygen is needed to metabolically support the body in exertion. The anatomy of the pharynx, larynx, and trachea require the exercising horse to stretch out his neck and head; this streamlines the airway to minimize resistance.

Partial flexion of the head and neck, required by many athletic pursuits such as show jumping and dressage, interferes with streamlining by creating a bend in the airway. When a horse is asked to flex at the poll and neck to improve his balance and impulsion, it is not unusual for a horse to react with mental resistance and evasion as he struggles to opti-

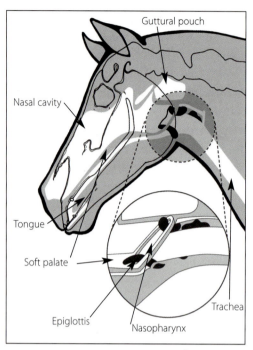

10.3 *Soft tissue structures within the cavity of the mouth have functional effects on how efficiently a horse breathes. This sheet of soft tissue, called the soft palate, arises from the hard palate and covers the nasopharynx. The larynx (inset) is made up of cartilages called the epiglottis, and it is these that should fit like a "button in a buttonhole" to create an airtight fit to minimize turbulence in the throat region as a horse breathes.*

MEETING THE AIR DEMAND

Because the horse is strictly a nose-breathing animal, physical adaptations accommodate the demand for air at faster speeds. In the back of the mouth, a sheet of tissue arises from the bottom of the hard palate and extends backward and up across the nasopharynx. This sheet of tissue is called the *soft palate*, and an opening at the back of it provides a "buttonhole" through which the larynx fits. For normal respiration, there must be a perfect, airtight fit between the soft palate and the larynx so the "button" larynx fits snugly against the "buttonhole" (fig. 10.3). Because the tongue is connected to the larynx, when one moves the other must move such as occurs with swallowing, hanging the tongue out of the mouth, or pulling the tongue behind the bit. Movement of the larynx or soft palate breaks the seal between them (referred to as *laryngo-palatal dislocation*), then creating an obstruction with partial closure of the airway. Because swallowing requires complete disconnection of the larynx from the opening in the soft palate, the airway closes so food and/or saliva are not drawn into the lungs.

Bit Evasion

A horse may evade a bit in the mouth by moving his tongue around, and in so doing, the larynx slides backward to separate from its snug fit with the soft palate. Generally, swallowing returns a misplaced tongue to its normal position.

Other bit evasion tactics include opening the mouth. This action breaks the airtight seal of the lips. Air entering the mouth causes the soft palate to vibrate or rise; laryngo-palatal dislocation may result. Use of a dropped noseband, a flash, or figure-eight noseband keeps the mouth shut and deters these evasion tactics. The noseband should not be clamped down so tightly as to pinch the nostrils.

A bit that is fitted properly and is comfortable encourages a horse to accept it. A goal in

mize air intake. In an attempt to improve breathing, the horse might carry himself "upside down" in a position that arches the neck toward the ground and hollows the back. This upside-down carriage allows him to extend the head and neck, opening the airways.

When a horse is trained to go "on the bit," he loses some of his airway freedom. The upper and lower walls of the nasopharynx are relaxed and flaccid. In this position, air might vibrate in the pharynx and create noise. If the head is maintained in this flexed position during faster and more difficult demands, performance could falter.

riding a horse "on the bit" is to achieve jaw flexibility and softness with a minimum of hardware or accessories. Bit acceptance is often accompanied by salivation, which may stimulate swallowing with a brief laryngo-palatal dislocation.

The Lower Respiratory Tract

BRANCHING AIRWAYS

At the bottom of the rigid trachea, the tubes branch into a series of *bronchi*, which subsequently expand into a web of smaller *bronchioles* and on into the *alveoli*. As the airways branch, like the branches of a tree they decrease in size the further into the lungs they reach, but the overall cross-sectional area increases exponentially (see fig. 10.1, p. 245). The huge expanse of surface area of the lower airways makes for a minimum of airway resistance in healthy lungs. You can think of alveoli as clumps of "grapes"—tiny air sacs juxtaposed next to a vast network of tiny blood capillaries. It is at this *alveolar-capillary interface* that air gases are exchanged to and from the blood by the process of diffusion.

THE LUNGS

Although the lungs only constitute about 1 percent of a horse's weight since they are mostly comprised of air and blood vessels rather than dense tissue, the lungs are an incredibly large organ relative to the size of the horse. The large surface area of the equine lungs facilitates diffusion of gases across the tissues. Pulmonary arteries bring oxygen-deficient blood into the lungs to the alveolar-capillary interface. There, carbon dioxide (a normal by-product of tissue aerobic metabolism) is transferred from the blood (returning from deep body tissues) to the alveoli to be expired into the air. At the same time, oxygen enters the capillaries from the freshly air-filled alveoli during this gaseous exchange. As oxygen passes the alveolar-capillary barrier, it goes into solution within the blood plasma or it reversibly binds to hemoglobin molecules (a protein attached to RBCs) of the red blood cells. Once the capillaries along the alveoli are saturated with oxygen, this blood is taken by way of the pulmonary veins to the left chambers of the heart where it is pumped to the rest of the tissues of the body.

The main route by which oxygen reaches the tissues is by hemoglobin carrying it through the blood stream. Once in the deeper tissues, oxygen unbinds from the hemoglobin and enters the tissue cells where it is utilized by aerobic *mitochondria* (cellular machinery to generate energy in the presence of oxygen) to generate energy for muscle contraction (see p. 140). The continuous exchange of oxygen and carbon dioxide to and from the tissues maintains the acid-base status of blood within a normal range during moderate exercise. This is critical to superior metabolic function of the athletic horse.

MUSCLES OF BREATHING

The muscles of breathing are important to the overall picture of what happens as air travels through the nostrils to the lungs and then to the tissues. Hyperextension of the neck during fast exercise maintains stiffness and opening of the trachea to decrease airway resistance so air can easily reach the lungs. The chest walls and the diaphragm create a triangular-shaped "housing" for the lungs; this housing is referred to as the *thoracic cavity* (see fig. 10.1, p. 245). Air is pulled into the lungs by the muscles of inspiration, the diaphragm being the main inspiratory muscle. Other muscles connecting the head to the sternum or ribs also assist in enlarging the thoracic cavity on inspiration. As they contract, these muscles pull the sternum and ribs forward, "expanding" the thorax and lungs. Unique

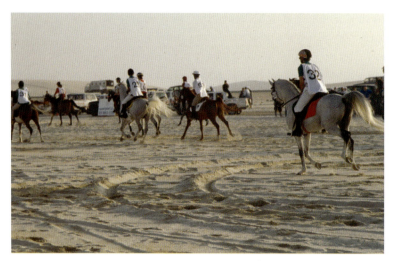

10.4 *At canter speeds, horses tend to synchronize the breathing rate with stride frequency.*

to the horse, a portion of the expiratory cycle is an active process facilitated by the abdominal muscles. As these muscles contract, abdominal pressure increases as the momentarily relaxed diaphragm is forced forward to reduce the size of the thoracic volume. With expiration, unused gases in the lungs and carbon dioxide are expelled into the environment.

Coupling of Breathing with Gait

At rest, a horse's respiratory rate normally ranges from 12 to 20 breaths per minute, depending on the ambient temperature. At the walk and the trot, a horse's respiratory frequency has little relationship to the timing of each stride, whereas at canter and gallop speeds, fit horses tend to synchronize the respiratory rate with the stride frequency (photo 10.4). Horses may possibly select a gait or speed that corresponds with minimal oxygen consumption. However, as speed increases, oxygen consumption proportionately increases. At a gallop, the respiratory rate may be as high as 128 bpm (breaths per minute), which requires increased blood flow to, and more work effort by the muscles of breathing. Muscles that work the respiratory system (the diaphragm, abdominal, and thoracic muscles) become stronger with conditioning. The advantage gained by this locomotor-respiration coupling is a result of movement of the chest wall with the limbs that spares the work effort by the breathing muscles.

Consider the respiratory system in a mechanical analogy: think of the head and neck as a pendulum and the intestines as a piston. Then, consider the movement of a horse at speed. As the forelimbs swing forward, the horse's head and neck swing upward, pulling forward the muscles connecting the head and neck to the breastbone and lower thorax. This pulls the rib cage forward and out. During this propulsive "leap" at the canter or gallop, the hind limbs push to drive the horse forward. When this happens, the torso accelerates forward while at the same time, the intestines shift to the rear. This further opens up space in the thorax as the horse inhales, and so air rushes in.

As the forelimbs land and support the horse's mass, the head and neck drop, the rapid deceleration of the thorax causes the intestines to move forward, and the rib cage is compressed as it absorbs some of the concussive force of landing. As a fast-moving horse decelerates slightly, like a piston, the internal organs slide forward to squeeze air from the lungs. This abrupt abdominal/thoracic compression facilitates exhalation.

Measurements done on Arabian horses indicate that at rest, an adult horse inspires and expires about 6 liters of air with each breath. At the gallop, the volume of each breath more than doubles to 14 liters and the respiratory rate increases to 128 bpm (breaths per minute). Improvement in ventilation is achieved mostly by increased respiratory frequency and only slightly from an increase in volume of air inspired. (In contrast, humans rely more on increasing volume inspired with only a small increase in respiratory rate.) At the gallop, stride and respiratory rate are coupled such that the greater the stride frequency, the greater the respiratory rate. Despite an attempt to keep up, ventilation of the airways becomes less efficient at speed. Horses cannot pull in sufficient oxygen despite more rapid respiratory rates so they depend greatly on improved cardiac output (see p. 220) to compensate for large oxygen demands of working muscles at high intensity exercise.

Functional Adaptations of the Respiratory System

Conditioning the respiratory system is linked closely with cardiovascular conditioning. The respiratory and cardiovascular systems work in harmony to supply working muscles with ample oxygen. With exercise, a horse's oxygen consumption increases by thirty-fold compared to that of a horse at rest. The body accommodates this increased demand for oxygen by the following adaptations:

- Ventilation increases up to twenty-three-fold, accomplished by an increase in respiratory rate and/or an increase in the volume of inspired air, called the *tidal volume*.
- Cardiac output and blood flow increase five- to eight-fold to bathe the tissues in oxygen.
- Improved capillary development occurs in all the tissues, including the lungs, the alveolar-capillary interface, the working muscles, and the skin to facilitate exchange of gases (oxygen and carbon dioxide) within the tissues, along with dissipation of heat from the exercising body.
- Hemoglobin in the blood increases by 50 percent due to contraction of the spleen to discharge red blood cells (RBCs) into the bloodstream; hemoglobin has an affinity to bind oxygen molecules to transport them through the blood to the tissues.
- Hemoglobin increases its affinity for oxygen such that a fit horse has to breathe less air to achieve enhanced oxygen uptake.
- With exercise, oxygen extraction from the blood is enhanced at the tissue level where it is favorable for oxygen to unload from the hemoglobin molecules. Tissue "warmth" from increased circulation and acid-base changes within exercising muscle beds encourages release of oxygen from hemoglobin. When hemoglobin is completely saturated with oxygen, 100 ml of blood holds about 20 ml of oxygen. Exercise encourages the release of oxygen from hemoglobin within the working muscles.

CARDIOVASCULAR ADAPTATIONS TO SUPPORT RESPIRATORY EFFICIENCY

A horse accommodates the need for aerobic energy transfer by additional cardiovascular adaptations, which include increased heart size/contractility, increased number of hemoglobin molecules, increased development of capillary beds within the muscle and skin, and increased numbers of mitochondria within muscle cells. At rest, hemoglobin concentration is about 15 percent, while with exercise, hemoglobin concentration approaches 40 percent. This is due to contraction of the large equine spleen, which serves as a blood reservoir to be called upon in time of need. As increasing cardiovascular fitness improves blood supply within working muscles, more oxygen can be extracted from the blood during aerobic exercise. In addition, cardiac output and blood flow are selectively routed to exercising muscles in a fit horse. An adult Arabian horse delivers 1 liter of blood with each heartbeat, whether at rest or during exercise. An increase in heart rate facilitates greater output of blood from the heart, with the cardiac output increasing five- to six-fold during high intensity (maximal) exercise. As an example, a resting rate of 32 bpm can increase to at least 160 to 184 bpm with exercise. At sub-maximal aerobic exercise, cardiac output is three times its resting value (see chapter 9, *Cardiovascular Conditioning and Health*, p. 220).

RESPIRATORY ADAPTATIONS FOR EFFICIENCY

Improvements in Breathing Muscles

The cardiovascular adaptations result in a reduction of energy demands by the ventilatory muscles, making more oxygen available to the working skeletal muscles. In addition, improved efficiency of breathing spares the respiratory muscles so they are not likely to fatigue quickly.

It has been suggested that with submaximal prolonged exercise, horses do get a "second wind." This occurs as the muscles of breathing compensate for an increased oxygen demand with persistent exercise. This is accomplished by the following: the diaphragm improves its contraction force, the release of *catecholamines* (like adrenalin) improves the contractility of the diaphragm muscle, and more blood flow is supplied to the diaphragm.

Heat Dissipation by Panting

In addition, the respiratory tract is an important means to relieve internal heat buildup as occurs with sustained exercise, especially in hot and humid conditions. During prolonged exercise, respiratory frequency may increase to assist in thermoregulation as another means of dissipating the heat load created by persistently working skeletal muscle (see p. 357). Once the horse stops exercising, he will continue to "pant" to blow off heat. Cooling strategies are important to relieve the internal heat load that is forcing the respiratory tract to work harder.

It should be noted, however, that respiratory limitations on performance are more an issue for performance at high-speed, middle-distance work, as seen with Thoroughbreds, harness racing, eventing, and timber racing and not as significant to sprint or long-distance exercise. Nonetheless, an excellent and unending oxygen supply to fulfill the demand by working muscles is paramount to performance in any task.

Ventilatory improvements occur rapidly with conditioning similar to the rapid changes associated with conditioning of the cardiovascular system. However, ventilatory improvements "detrain" and return to baseline after just a three-week layoff time.

Situations That Overtax or Compromise the System

Good "wind" is essential for continued aerobic performance. Without efficient lung function, an exercising horse may not acquire sufficient oxygen to maintain aerobic metabolism throughout an exercise effort. Then, an increasingly greater reliance on anaerobic metabolism more quickly elicits poor performance and fatigue. Any strategies that encourage maintenance of respiratory health will provide a performance advantage.

EFFECT ON LUNG FUNCTION BY RESPIRATORY VIRUSES AND ALLERGENS

Respiratory viruses should be avoided by judicious use of viral vaccines. To minimize risk of respiratory allergies, quality hay free of dust or mold should be fed. Damage to the lower airways and alveoli from viruses or allergens cause sections of alveoli to remain collapsed and not filled with air. This dramatically reduces the amount of cross-sectional lung tissue available for transfer of oxygen to the blood.

ANEMIA

Anemia creates a decrease in the number of available red blood cells and hemoglobin so the blood has less oxygen-carrying capacity no matter how excellent the lung function (see chapter 9, *Cardiovascular Conditioning and Health,* p. 241). Anemia may be caused by intestinal parasitism, a chronic infection, inadequate nutrition, or bleeding, gastrointestinal ulcers. A comprehensive and aggressive deworming program eradicates an internal parasite load. Careful monitoring of a horse's enthusiasm for work, working heart rates, and recovery rates can alert to a horse being slightly "off" in his performance. Periodic or annual blood screens monitor for anemia. Once or twice yearly complete blood counts may detect a chronic infection or anemia; blood tests at the very least establish a baseline to compare to at a later date should problems arise (see p. 457).

BITTING

How a horse is ridden in the bridle also affects how much air he takes in as he works. As mentioned earlier, a horse that is kept coiled in the rider's hands necessarily moves with chin and head tucked under in tight flexion. This configuration puts a bend in the upper airways of the throat and may restrict air intake. However, a horse does not need to run with head high or outstretched without any bit contact for him to achieve efficient breathing; some slight flexion still allows good air intake and rider control. The horse should be encouraged to push from behind through his back and poll to engage his hindquarters. A relaxed horse in a relaxed frame allows ease in breathing. The mildest bit possible also keeps his mouth soft, his muscles supple, and permits him to swing his limbs with a big, easy stride. Too much hardware or the use of nosebands cramps mobility; tie-downs or martingales create unnatural flexion of the head and neck. In some cases these "aids" may be necessary for rider control and safety, but in most cases, less is better.

TRAILER TRANSPORT

Transport (see "Transport Stress," chapter 15, *Preventive and Mental Horse Health,* p. 478) exerts adverse influences on the equine respiratory tract, as well. Long-distance hauling with a horse's head maintained in an upward position limits the normal physiologic clearance mechanisms to remove dirt and debris from the airways. Mucus collects in the airways while at the same time the mucociliary clearance process is hampered. Then, the airways may be less permeable to gas exchange and more susceptible to invasion by viruses and bacteria. It is a good strategy to off-load a horse periodically during long transport so he can drop his head and neck to clear mucus and debris as well as have an opportunity to walk around to loosen his muscles.

HEAT AND HUMIDITY

Environment plays a role in limiting the efficiency of the respiratory tract to supply oxygen to the tissues. In hot, humid conditions, more blood flow is diverted from the working muscles to the skin to dissipate heat, so less oxygen is carried to the muscles. The skin competes with the muscles for cardiac output during exercise. With ongoing dehydration and persistent sweating, this can have serious consequences when neither skin nor muscles receive sufficient blood or oxygen flow. The horse not only overheats, but also the limitation on oxygen delivery to the muscles causes a greater reliance on anaerobic metabolism with rapid development of muscular fatigue. Recovery will suffer, with the heart and respiratory rates remaining elevated.

For the equine athlete exercising in any climatic conditions, dehydration has the most profound repercussions on ventilatory performance. With ongoing dehydration, circulatory efficiency is impaired throughout the tissues, including at the alveolar level where gaseous exchange occurs. As the horse undergoes sustained exercise, dehydration increases while oxygen consumption and demand concurrently increase. Ventilation may not be able to keep up with the tissue need for oxygen so the horse must bump more into the anaerobic threshold to maintain the current level of performance. Anaerobic metabolism can only be sustained for a short period before performance declines. When a horse can't accommodate oxygen demands by the muscles, he slows down and demonstrates other indications of fatigue. These signs may be as subtle as deflated body posture, diminished impulsion, or reluctance to move. Or, more overt signs of fatigue appear such as poor heart rate recovery, decreased gut activity and intestinal sounds, and/or a lack of interest in eating and drinking. Subtle signs occur early on; an attuned horseman often appreciates these demeanor changes before a crisis develops.

FRIGID AIR

Human joggers find that rapid intake of cold air during a sub-zero workout stimulates reflex constriction in the airways. Horses working at moderate or slow speeds are not as prone to injury of their throats, sinuses, or lungs during cold weather exercise as are people. The long shape of a horse's head provides a "tunnel" between the nostrils and throat. Copious blood vessels course through the roof of this tunnel to warm and moisten air as it enters the nasal passages. By the time outside air reaches the back portion of the nasal passages and throat, it approximates body temperature, preventing cold shock to the tissue. As air is warmed along its extended passage through a horse's head, condensation of moisture alleviates abrasive effects of cold and/or dry air on delicate tissue in the upper respiratory passages. Respiratory rates of moderately exercising horses are also lower during cold spells because a horse needs to dissipate less body heat.

Because respiration is synchronized with the stride at high speeds, a galloping horse must hyperventilate to keep pace with locomotion. Air that enters rapidly without warming or humidification in the passages of the head is called *unconditioned* air. Research studies have shown that cold (unconditioned) air that is breathed during gallop exercise does cause injury to the mucosal lining of the peripheral airways. Such cooling and dessication of the respiratory lining may contribute to airway inflammatory disease in the equine athlete.

Respiratory Health and Illness

Just as good quality nutrition provides a horse with resources to build healthy tissue, so does air quality determine the health of the respiratory system. Management greatly influences a horse's respiratory health. During winter, many horses are confined inside a stable, which may contain irritants to the respiratory tract. Evaluation of the barn atmosphere includes noting:

- Noxious fumes, such as ammonia
- Dust particles floating in the air
- Musty odors
- Coughing horses

The result of poor management is a heavily polluted environment. A stabled horse breathes this environment around the clock with adverse effects on his respiratory tract.

Defense against Foreign Particles

UPPER AIRWAYS

Nasal Passages

A horse's airways filter a large percentage of particles in the air during inhalation, with the nasal passages filtering the largest particles. Humidity in the air increases a particle's size and density as water condenses on it. Such large particles are easily trapped by the nasal passages, preventing entry to the respiratory tree. However, some large particles are so heavy that they fall out of the nasal filtration trap and are inhaled into the upper airways.

Mucociliary Apparatus

An invaluable clearance mechanism in the upper airways is referred to as the *mucociliary apparatus* (MCA). Particles deposited in the upper airways are cleared away from the lungs by a one-way flow of mucus that lies on top of *epithelial cells* lining the airways. Epithelial cells cover all surfaces of the body, but in the airways, they are specialized with beating *cilia* (tiny hair-like structures protruding from the cells that trap debris.) The cilia propel the mucous layer, with attached particles, outward toward the throat, where debris is swallowed or coughed away.

Epithelial cells may be damaged by infectious agents, noxious gases such as ammonia or carbon monoxide, or by extremes in temperature or humidity. Interference in their function reduces the efficiency of the MCA. Poor barn ventilation creates inadequate air exchange, and promotes a buildup of humidity, irritants (dust, allergens, and gases), and an increase in numbers of airborne, disease-causing agents (*pathogens*) in the environment. Ammonia fumes degenerate ciliated epithelial cells, in essence paralyzing them, as well as decreasing secretion of the protective mucous layer.

Ammonia suppresses the ability of *macrophages* (large blood cells that ingest and destroy foreign particles—see "Lower Airways" below) to kill bacteria. If you can smell ammonia fumes, the levels are too high.

High humidity enables formation of aerosolized *droplet nuclei*, which enclose bacteria or viruses, protecting them from the lethal effects of drying or temperature extremes. Dust not only irritates the respiratory lining, but it also provides a vehicle for particles, increasing the dose of pathogens introduced into the airways.

Coughing

Another airway clearance mechanism is coughing. Specific nerves in the upper airways respond to dust, ammonia, and other irritants by eliciting a cough reflex. Coughing forcefully expels mucus and particles from the airways.

Excessive inflammation caused by irritants stimulates reflex constriction of the bronchioles in the lungs. Constricted diameter of air passages diminishes the efficiency of the coughing clearance mechanism.

LOWER AIRWAYS

In conjunction with an effective mucociliary apparatus, specialized white blood cells, called *alveolar macrophages,* provide a primary line of defense against infection of the lower respiratory tract. An alveolar macrophage binds microorganisms, such as bacteria and viruses, to its cell membrane, and internalizes and inactivates the foreign material.

Smaller particles and droplets of water that contain bacteria and viruses (droplet nuclei) may remain suspended in the inhaled air, not falling out until they reach the bottom of the lungs. Normally, any particles that descend past the mucociliary apparatus are removed from the lungs by a fluid layer that slowly moves outward until it reaches the MCA. Or, the particles may penetrate through the mucous layer to be consumed and destroyed by alveolar macrophages, or they are circulated with the alveolar macrophages to the MCA. Nerve endings in the smaller airways do not elicit coughing, but they will stimulate airway constriction. Interference in any of these events results in inadequate control of infection. Both the macrophage and the MCA are adversely affected by poor air quality.

Factors Affecting Air Quality

HAY AND BEDDING DUST
Many barns place hay storage areas overhead; this management technique can compromise a horse's respiratory system. As hay is thrown from the loft above, quantities of dust and mold spores are cast out to sift down through the atmosphere. It may take several hours for small fungal spores to settle out of the air. Horses moving in their stalls kick up bedding and dust. Dust concentrations in the air of a barn may increase up to three-fold, further irritating the respiratory tract.

FUNGAL SPORES
Damp, decomposing bedding generates ammonia fumes, and promotes development of fungal spores. Warm temperatures, coupled with high relative humidity caused by inadequate ventilation, encourage fungal growth. Fungal growth is greater in straw than in wood shavings. Horses lying in straw and moldy bedding are subjected to massive numbers of mold spores even in a well-ventilated stable.

Hay "dust," fungal spores, and other irritants initiate a degenerative process in the airways by causing a hypersensitivity reaction similar to allergies in people. Horses continually exposed to these air contaminants may develop *recurrent airway obstruction* (RAO) or *heaves* (see p. 259). Feed and bedding are the main sources of stable dust.

RIDING ARENA DUST
Many exercise and riding arenas connect to the stabling area, providing a warm enclosed space to ride during bad weather. Unfortunately, this practice complicates the problem of confinement in the barn. As horses and people move around these arenas, stirred dust mixes with still air inside the barn. Not only are working horses exposed to this polluted air, but stalled horses are, as well.

Attempts to water the arena to hold down the dust further increase humidity in the barn. Oil droplets that result from "moistening" an arena with an oil mixture also exert toxic effects on the equine respiratory tract.

HUMIDITY
High humidity levels contribute to respiratory infection. Adequate and effective floor drainage of water or urine is essential to limit humidity in the barn, and to remove moisture from bedding.

CARBON MONOXIDE
Machinery, such as tractors, driven in and out of barns to assist with stall cleaning or raking of an arena contributes to buildup of carbon monoxide fumes within the stable. Appropriate ventilation is important especially when this equipment is in operation.

Maintaining Air Quality

BENEFITS OF VENTILATION
An increase in numbers of circulating pathogens in the air presents an increased dose to a horse's respiratory tract. Under normal circumstances, the immune system may be able to inactivate a low-dose level, whereas a greater dose can overwhelm and infect a horse with disease. Most infections are dose-dependent, meaning that exposure to a small quantity of a pathogen results in a milder disease or one that passes unrecog-

nized. Frequent and rapid air turnover by a good ventilation system reduces the concentration of particles in the air (and dose).

NATURAL VENTILATION

Cross-Ventilation

A natural ventilation system is achieved by holes in the walls and/or under the eaves of the roof, or by cross-ventilation created by doors open at opposite ends of the barn. Wind and currents force air through a building, but if openings are inappropriately placed, drafts may be created. Effective ventilation is achieved in stalls with openings of the following dimensions: 2 by 2 feet in the walls, and 1 by 1 foot near the roof. Larger wall openings allow a horse to put his head outside, giving him fresh air, and relieving mental boredom.

Convection

If the air is still, or the holes are baffled to prevent drafts, the only means for air movement is by natural convection. Convection results from a temperature difference between warmer stable air (generated by the horses) and cooler outside air. Hot air rises to exit from the upper holes, while cool, fresh air enters lower holes.

Effective insulation of a building increases temperature differences between the inside and outside of the barn, maximizing natural convection. Roof insulation reduces radiant heat loss during cold winter nights, decreasing condensation (and resultant humidity) in the building.

In a large horse barn (twenty or more horses), it is difficult to maintain precise mixing of the air masses. Barns that are shut up tightly in the winter, with all doors and windows closed, have still air with inadequate ventilation. Auxiliary ventilation openings along the roof allow entry of air into and out of the building, or specialized airflow systems should be installed.

MECHANICAL AIRFLOW SYSTEMS

Mechanical airflow systems should exhaust the air rather than recirculate it, with a minimum air exchange of four times every hour. Anything less than two air exchanges per hour results in a dangerous buildup of mold spores. Exhaust units should be placed at a sufficient distance from the air inlets for adequate air turnover.

IDEAL MANAGEMENT PRACTICES

Optimal air quality in a barn to promote respiratory health depends on specific measures:

- Institute an ideal ventilation system in the barn to bring in fresh air, and to exhaust stale air.
- Separate riding and exercise areas from the stabling section.
- Hay should be stored in a separate building from where horses are housed to reduce air pollutants and decrease the fire hazard. Hay stored under cover from the weather develops less mold.
- Use good quality, dust-free bedding.
- Ensure adequate drainage for water and urine.
- Clean stalls frequently to reduce ammonia levels, and apply 1 to 2 pounds of hydrated lime or *clinoptilolite* (Sweet PDZ® or Stall Freshly®) to the stall floors and sawdust bedding after cleaning to reduce ammonia levels.

Not only will the air quality and health of the horses improve, but also humans directly benefit from these management procedures. Air quality will be healthful, and the horse will feel better, look better, and perform better.

Stress Factors

TRAINING AND EXERCISE

Stress increases the risk of respiratory infection. Routine training and strenuous exercise are frequent stresses to a horse. Stress results in increased *cortisol* secretion by the body, coupled with exercise-related inflammation of the lung tissue. Cortisol is a steroid hormone that inhibits immune function of the alveolar macrophages and other white blood cells. Cortisol depletes the number of *immunoglobulins* in respiratory secretions. Immunoglobulins are specialized proteins that decrease the ability of bacteria and viruses to attach to and infect epithelial cells. They also coat the organisms with a substance to enhance uptake by white blood cells. Immunoglobulins chemically attract other white blood cells to the area to help clean up infection.

TRANSPORTATION

Transportation over long distances is a stressful condition that increases a horse's susceptibility to viral or bacterial infection, particularly one week following a trip. Horses subjected to stresses such as hard training, competition and travel benefit from optimal air quality. (For more on this, refer to chapter 15, *Preventive and Horse Mental Health*, p.478.)

RAPID TEMPERATURE CHANGES

It is preferable to maintain a constant temperature within a barn rather than having extreme fluctuations between hot and cold. Many stalled horses are blanketed and often are body clipped. The only insulating layer of protection against cold for a clipped horse is the blanket. If a horse is blanketed at the beginning of the winter season, or clipped to prevent growing a winter hair coat, it is necessary to consistently blanket him throughout the cold season (see p. 159). If the horse has a fur coat and is not used to being blanketed, be careful of overheating him by blanketing on a sporadic basis. Chills and drafts, or improper cooling out of an overheated horse can further compromise the immune response.

Upper Respiratory Problems

RECURRENT LARYNGEAL NEUROPATHY AKA ROARING

As an example of how finely tuned the system must be for air to flow through the "tubes," let's consider a common syndrome described as "roaring." This syndrome, also termed *recurrent laryngeal neuropathy* (RLN) or *laryngeal hemiplegia*, is created by a problem with the nerve supply to an arytenoid cartilage within the larynx. Under normal circumstances, an increase in the cross-sectional area of the larynx during exercise is created by the opening of the two *arytenoid cartilages* located on either side of the larynx. The *recurrent laryngeal nerve*, a branch of the vagus nerve, regulates opening of each arytenoid cartilage. Damage to one or both of these nerves or loss of their function results in laryngeal hemiplegia with paralysis generally occurring on the left side of the larynx. Partial paralysis of the cartilage causes it to hang flaccid within the larynx rather than contracting flush against the side with breathing. The relaxed arytenoid cartilage creates a mechanical obstruction that limits the amount of air passing through the larynx while also generating a lot of turbulence that does get through to the trachea. The turbulence creates a "roaring" noise with breathing.

Racehorses, steeplechasers, eventers, jumpers, and polo ponies are often asked to perform at peak speeds, and the tiniest impairment to respiratory ability can quickly turn a potential winner into a loser. At least 5 percent of Thoroughbred racehorses suffer from RLN. A horse with this condition is unable to breathe enough oxygen to fuel the demanding muscles; therefore speed and performance are compromised. A severely affected horse is subject to "choking down" or suffocation, followed by abrupt halt of exercise.

A narrow jaw width has been linked (Dr. W. Robert Cook) with RLN. The average Thoroughbred has a normal jaw width equivalent to at least four fingers (2.8 inches or 7.2 centimeters). To measure the jaw width, fold the fingers at the joint below the knuckles with the back of the hand resting against the underside of the horse's neck. The fingers are placed between the lower jawbones, at the level of the throatlatch. The narrower this measurement, the greater the likelihood the horse will be afflicted with some degree of RLN.

RLN is diagnosed by passing an *endoscope* into the horse's nose to the back of the throat. To determine the extent of laryngeal paralysis, it is sometimes necessary to examine the horse while he is working on a treadmill. Surgery is moderately successful in returning affected horses to top performance. The most common surgical procedure is the *tie-back* procedure, in which the cartilage is actually tied into an open position.

Not all roaring and gurgling sounds are caused by laryngeal paralysis. Some horses just like the noise that resonates in the nostrils and purposefully allow them to flap with inhalation.

OTHER THROAT PROBLEMS

Other throat problems may cause a diminished opening of the larynx and subsequent airway obstruction. These may be identified with an endoscope. Such problems include:

- *Dorsal displacement of the soft palate* (DDSP)
- *Epiglottic entrapment*
- *Pharyngeal lymphoid hyperplasia*
- *Arytenoid chondritis*

The first two syndromes interfere with the seal created by the soft palate and the larynx that maintains air pressure in the airways. The other two syndromes involve inflammation and distortion of the back of the throat that may obstruct normal airflow.

Lower Respiratory Problems

The lower respiratory organs include the branches of the trachea, bronchi, and the left and right lungs (see p. 245). Problems relating to the lower respiratory system usually result from viral or bacterial infection, or allergic reactions. Viral respiratory infections can predispose to:

- Bacterial pneumonia or pleuropneumonia
- Lung abscesses
- *Inflammatory airway disease* (IAD)
- Recurrent airway obstruction (heaves)

These problems may produce lasting conditions that permanently interfere with a horse's respiratory capacity and performance. On rare occasions, cancer in the thorax may slowly compromise a horse's lung capacity.

INFLAMMATORY AIRWAY DISEASE

Inflammatory airway disease (IAD) is a condition of the lower airways related to irritation from infectious (viral or bacterial) or non-infectious problems such as environmental allergens that do not include mold exposure. Respiratory viruses or chronic respiratory infections create inflammation within the airways, leading to spasms and *bronchoconstriction.* Injured ciliated epithelia that line the respiratory tract regenerate with thickened or altered cells; in many cases, an excess of mucus is produced. Many horses with IAD experience a chronic cough that occurs particularly with exercise due to accumulations of mucus in the lower air pas-

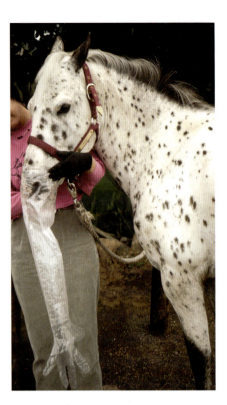

10.5 *One means of evaluating lung sounds with a stethoscope is to hold off a horse's air for a minute or two, forcing him to take deep breaths. In this case, a plastic rectal sleeve serves as a simple re-breathing bag placed over the horse's nostrils to restrict air intake.*

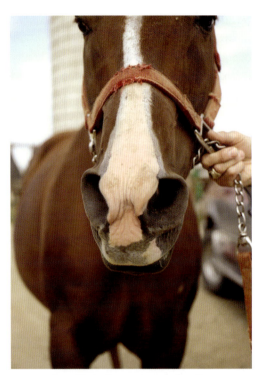

10.6 *Labored breathing associated with airway inflammatory disease is evident in this horse that is taking hard breaths through flared nostrils. The fact that he is not exerting himself and standing at rest demonstrates the difficulty he is having acquiring oxygen in the lungs.*

sages. Exercise intolerance, early fatigue, lessened stamina, and poor exercise recoveries are common findings in a horse affected by IAD.

RECURRENT AIRWAY OBSTRUCTION AKA HEAVES

Heaves, or *recurrent airway obstruction* (RAO) is a recurring respiratory condition that is triggered by moldy hay or by an overwhelming concentration of organic dust allergens (including molds and mold spores) in the environment. Historically, heaves has been referred to as *chronic obstructive pulmonary disease* (COPD) or "broken wind" because of a similar, but less treatable condition of humans called COPD (emphysema), but the correct terminology is RAO. Stabled horses are particularly afflicted, while some are reactive to alfalfa hay because of the abundance of mold and spores that proliferate in legume hay.

Symptoms of Heaves

Hyper-reactivity of the small airways results in constriction and spasm, or bronchoconstriction. Mucus accumulates as part of the allergic response. Narrowing of the air passages from constriction and debris accumulation leads to mechanical obstruction. An affected horse has difficulty exhaling or properly ventilating the lungs (photo 10.6). He stands depressed, with nostrils flared and with an increased respiratory rate greater than 20 to 24 breaths per minute. A white, mucous nasal discharge is often present. Wheezing may be audible. An increased effort is obvious with each exhalation. Over time, abdominal muscles become overdeveloped as they labor to push air out of the lungs. This is visible as a *heave line* between the flank and the thorax. A horse with severe RAO loses his appetite, loses weight, and appears unthrifty. Chronic coughing is a key symptom of this disease, particularly if a cough persists for several weeks yet the horse seems otherwise normal.

The Disease Process of Airway Inflammation

The sequence of events that stimulates heaves begins with an inhaled allergen, such as mold. If hay is baled with high moisture content, heat generated in the bale encourages the growth of mold. Symptoms may develop within 1 to 10 hours following exposure. An allergic response proceeds rapidly, calling inflammatory cells to the lungs.

Mast cells release substances, such as *histamines*, that cause spasms and constriction of the smooth muscles of the airways, along with an increase in mucus production. A type of white blood cell, *neutrophil,* releases substances that further constrict the airways and enhance mucus production. Normal airflow is interrupted by all these changes:

- Thickening of epithelial cells lining the airways
- Bronchoconstriction
- Excess mucous congestion
- Inflammatory cell infiltration

The inflammatory process impairs the mucociliary-apparatus-clearance mechanism. Inflammation in the lower airways triggers spasms and constriction of the bronchioles and bronchi (see fig. 10.1, p. 245). As the diameter of these air tubes closes down, resistance increases to airflow through them. Irritated lung tissue is coated in mucus and fibrin in response to the inflammation. Eventually, adhesions and scar tissue "glue" together localized areas of the tiny saccules of alveoli so they no longer expand to fill with air nor are they able to completely empty of residual air. For all these reasons, the extent of air capacity in the lungs is limited. Nerve receptors in the lungs are stimulated to elicit a cough reflex. What may start as an intermittent and infrequent cough may become persistent as more lung tissue is affected and the lower airways become more sensitive to the effects of mold and dust.

Any damage to the lower airways and alveoli reduces the amount of cross-sectional lung tissue available for transfer of oxygen to the blood. The result is that the horse's tolerance for exercise diminishes and performance suffers.

MANAGING IAD AND HEAVES

The goal for managing lower airway inflammation is to reduce irritant or allergen levels below a threshold that causes clinical disease. It is not possible to remove all allergens from the environment. Each horse responds differently to inhaled particles, just as do people. What may be below threshold level for one horse may still cause reaction in another. To successfully manage a horse with compromised respiratory health requires diligent attention to detail. Management of airway disease depends upon the same strategies as used for prevention: unpolluted open air, and clean living. (For more discussion, refer to "Maintaining Air Quality," p. 256.)

Housing

When possible, horses should be housed in open air and out of the barn area. Bedding should be restricted to wood shavings, peat moss, or shredded paper, but not straw, which is abundant in mold and mold spores. Horses should be located at least 50 yards upwind of any hay supply. A horse afflicted with heaves or IAD should be kept in as dust-free an environment as possible.

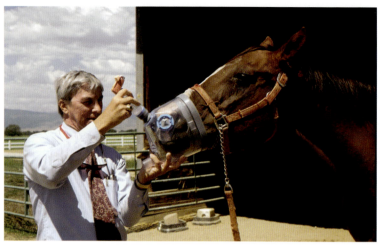

10.7 *This horse is being given respiratory relief by dosing with a metered dose inhaler (MDI) squirted into an Aeromask held over his face. The MDI bronchodilating medication circulates through the mask and is inhaled with each breath.*

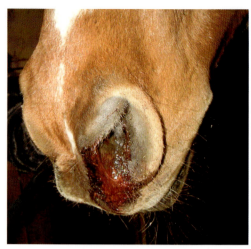

10.8 *A horse with exercise-induced pulmonary hemorrhage (EIPH) is also referred to as a bleeder. During or following intense exercise, a bleeder will have a bloody nose unless the blood from the airways is swallowed before it passes through the head.*

Feeding

Horses should be fed off the ground, not out of racks or raised feeders. Head down feeding enables a horse to eject particles from the nasal passages by blowing his nose repeatedly as he eats. Moldy hay should never be fed. Alfalfa hay should be removed from the diet if a horse seems at all sensitive to it.

A cubed or pelleted diet is preferable, or in the very least, grass hay should be soaked well before feeding. Even good quality grass hay contains a large amount of fungal spores. Wetting the hay may not completely prevent allergic effects due to continued mold and dust exposure from the local environment. A pasture situation is ideal, particularly if plants are not in bloom. Tree and grass pollen have been implicated as allergens, as are straw mites.

Vaccinations

A viral respiratory infection weakens a horse's resistance to other disease, and renders a horse more susceptible to IAD. Once a horse has developed IAD, his respiratory immune system is weakened against further viral and bacterial insult.

Drugs

Many pharmacological drugs are available to deal with IAD or heaves, but have temporary effects unless management and environment are altered. Systemic drugs include *prednisolone* (a corticosteroid) to control inflammation and the allergic response, and *clenbuterol* (a bronchodilator with ability to loosen secretions) to open the airways. Aerosolized forms of respiratory medications elicit improved effects with longer duration (photo 10.7).

EXERCISE-INDUCED PULMONARY HEMORRHAGE

Exercise-induced pulmonary hemorrhage (EIPH) is primarily a condition seen in racehorses or horses engaging in strenuous speed events. Affected animals are called *"bleeders."* Blood accumulates in the airways, and occasionally flows from the nose, a condition known as *epistaxis* (photo 10.8). It is not always easy to diagnose a horse affected by EIPH. Sometimes the horse coughs, or swallows excessively. A bleeder may exhibit exercise intolerance due to reduced lung function. The best way to identify a bleeder is to examine a suspect horse with an endoscope after 20 minutes and within 2 hours of exercise. In conjunction with endoscopy, a *bronchoalveolar lavage* is also useful for detecting the presence of blood in small airways.

Lung Damage

One theory of how EIPH occurs blames airway inflammation on creating fragility within lung capillaries. With maximal exertion, the lungs are inflated to full capacity at rates greater than 120 breaths per minute. If a previously damaged region of the lung fails to inflate, the adjacent good lung tissue that has inflated may distort the diseased area. Altered pressure differences develop between the good and bad lung tissue. Pressure changes and tissue tearing may rupture fragile capillary walls in the diseased lung area, causing bleeding.

Less inflatable areas of diseased lung may result from:

- Previous infection or inflammation that has healed with scar tissue
- Mucus or debris in the airways following an attack of influenza or pneumonia, which reduces the opening of the airway, creating uneven pressure in the lungs
- Allergies that cause bronchoconstriction and mucus within the airways, functionally reducing their size

Cardiac output is maximally increased in horses exercising in strenuous exertions. This creates hypertension within pulmonary capillaries with subsequent rupture of the tiny vessels. Repeated episodes of bleeding result in scarring of the lung tissue, and the cycle continues. An alternative explanation for the presence of EIPH suggests that pressure waves occur across the lungs by expansion and compression of the rib cage during galloping. These pressure waves cause rupture of the capillaries and hemorrhage by shearing stresses on the lungs.

Predisposition to EIPH

In summary, a horse may be predisposed to EIPH because of any of the following conditions:

- Inflammation increases blood flow in the walls of small airways, making them susceptible to rupture.
- Lung tissue is damaged by inflammation from viral, bacterial, parasitic infection, or allergic reactions.
- Blood pressure increases due to tremendous heart pumping during strenuous exertion.
- Genetics predispose the horse to weak blood vessels lining the lungs.
- Recurrent laryngeal neuropathy (RLN) may create abnormal pressure changes in the lungs.

Chronic bleeding permanently alters lung tissue with an adverse effect on performance and a propensity to continue to bleed.

Treatment Options for EIPH

Furosemide (Lasix®)

The impact of isolated incidents of EIPH on performance is not very well understood. Pre-exercise prevention using a diuretic called *furosemide* has improved racing times and performance in horses afflicted with EIPH. As a diuretic, furosemide causes urination within minutes; it is given 4 hours prior to an event. Furosemide appears to reduce pressures in the pulmonary vessels, thereby limiting capillary failure and reducing the severity of bleeding episodes. Furosemide lessens bleeding by 80 percent in EIPH horses.

External Nasal Strips (Flair®)

Up to 50 percent of airway resistance is attributable to the nasal passages in a horse. About 30 percent of airway resistance relates to the remainder of the upper airways, while 20 percent of resistance comes from the lower airways within the thorax. Since horses are obligate nose breathers, any strategy to minimize resistance of the nasal passages may improve performance. One technique is the application of Flair® nasal strips to reduce collapse of unsupported nasal passages during exercise. The nasal strip is meant to support the nasal passages between the incisor and nasal bones. These strips do not have any action on the opening of the nostrils. Bleeding has been reported to decrease by 44 to 74 percent when Flair strips are used on a horse with EIPH. In addition, by decreasing a horse's breathing, these strips also reduce oxygen consumption during exercise.

Nitric Oxide and Nitrovasodilators

Nitric oxide (NO) relaxes the smooth muscle lining of blood vessels to achieve vasodilation. Attempts to generate NO from metabolism of nitroglycerin by infusing nitroglycerin to exercising horses have not yielded any beneficial effects. Nitric oxide is created by the action of an NO enzyme on L-arginine. In an attempt to generate more NO, other nitrovasodilators have been tried to increase levels of L-arginine in the system. L-arginine can be found in several pharmaceutical products, specifically ketoprofen and some immune stimulant products. These therapeutic methods also do not reduce EIPH in the exercising horse.

Prevention of EIPH

Any management strategies implemented to minimize disease of the small airways help prevent EIPH. These techniques include:

- Improved ventilation in barns
- Dust-free bedding
- High quality, dust-free, and mold-free hay
- Ample recovery time (3 weeks) for respiratory infections
- A viral vaccination program against influenza and rhinopneumonitis of 2 to 4 times per year
- Deworming every 6 to 8 weeks to minimize damage from worms migrating through the lungs
- Screening for RLN via endoscopic exam and measurement of jaw width

RESPIRATORY VIRUSES

Urbanized living congregates horses together in big barns and stables, increasing the opportunity for viral respiratory illness. More horses are housed under one roof and are stressed by training and competition. A viral respiratory outbreak can easily grab hold and maintain itself in a concentrated equine population. Transcontinental and intercontinental transport of competition and breeding horses increases possibilities for spreading viruses on a global scale.

Spread of infectious respiratory viruses occurs by droplet nuclei in the air, or directly from nose-to-nose contact. Viruses are also spread by indirect contact with tack, equipment, and/or stable personnel, in trailer transport, or in a contaminated grooming or wash stall common to all horse traffic.

Replication of a Virus

Unlike bacteria, viruses cannot duplicate themselves without inserting themselves into a host cell. There, they command the cell's replication mechanisms to reproduce the virus.

Eventually, the cell is so full of new viral particles that it bursts. The cell is killed and viral particles are released to infect other cells. The horse's immune system recognizes viral proteins as foreign, and begins to produce antibodies. Specifically, antibodies recognize *hemagglutinin (HA) spikes* on the surface of viral particles. They attach to the virus and neutralize it. Each HA spike is made of a specific sequence of amino acids (components of proteins). Recognition of these specific amino acids on the spike is essential for the antibody to attach to it, with subsequent neutralization of the virus. In this way, antibodies disrupt viral replication by preventing the virus from entering host cells.

Effects of Vaccination

On the Immune System

Vaccines train a horse's immune system to respond to viral proteins. The initial vaccination, called *primary immunization,* primes the cells that produce antibodies. Subsequent boosters stimulate actual antibody production. A booster vaccine stimulates a rapid immune response, and the antibodies rise to high levels due to antibody "memory," or *anamnestic response.* To invoke this response, it is necessary to wait 3 to 6 weeks to give the second injection in the primary series in accordance with manufacturer recommendations.

Vaccination stimulates the immune system to produce specialized antibodies against a specific strain of virus, such as influenza or rhinopneumonitis. Vaccine may also stimulate cross-protective antibodies against variations of a viral strain. Antibodies developed against a specific strain are better at neutralizing that particular virus than are cross-protective antibodies. Yet, cross-protective antibodies rally when a horse is exposed to a similar, but unfamiliar virus.

When antibodies prevent the virus from invading respiratory cells, an immunized horse does not develop clinical symptoms of disease. Vaccinations are not completely protective, but they reduce the risk of contracting disease, while minimizing symptoms. Both illness time and recovery time are shortened significantly in a vaccinated horse.

On Herd Health

Vaccination of a herd or a large population of horses reduces the number of susceptible horses. With antibody levels present in the entire group, there is a better chance that a viral infection won't create an epidemic. Assume, for example, that only 10 percent of a herd has been vaccinated. During an outbreak, virus carried by the other 90 percent presents an overwhelming challenge to the immune systems of the vaccinated horses. In this case, vaccination may be insufficient to protect the vaccinated 10 percent against an overwhelming viral assault. In spite of vaccination, clinical disease may occur in epidemic proportions.

To prevent serious epidemics, at least 70 percent of a population should be vaccinated. When an outbreak occurs, as yet unaffected individuals should be vaccinated to limit spread of disease. Vaccinated horses develop a high-level immune response that "blocks" further transmission of virus from horse to horse. There is no point in vaccinating already sick animals.

Factors Affecting a Vaccination Program

Aggressive immunization programs ensure respiratory health. However, the most aggressive vaccination program will not entirely eliminate disease if horses are stressed, overcrowded, or faced with poor stable hygiene, inadequate nutrition, or parasitism.

Age of the Horse

Each horse's immune system is unique in its ability to respond to vaccines. The age of a horse determines how frequently he should receive boosters. Young horses under 2 years old are most susceptible to respiratory viruses. Because a youngster has not encountered a full spectrum of viruses or bacteria, his immune system is not fully competent to ward off all infections.

Occupation

The occupation of a horse is critical in determining a vaccination schedule. A highly competitive and mobile horse is frequently exposed to respiratory viruses, and may require vaccination every 2 to 3 months. Although a horse may not be clinically ill, he can carry a virus home and spread it to others. Horses in boarding stables, or in barns with these transient individual share a high risk of exposure.

A horse that rarely socializes with strange horses may only need boosters twice a year. This may be sufficient to maintain a protective antibody level. In 6 months, antibodies do not decline so low as to prevent an anamnestic response to a booster vaccine.

Timing of Vaccination

Ideally, your competition horse should receive vaccine boosters at least 2 to 4 weeks prior to travel, competition, or a known risk of exposure. This gives him an opportunity to develop good antibody protection against worrisome disease, while also giving him a chance to recover from transient muscle soreness or fever should an intramuscular vaccine induce such adverse reactions. In the face of an outbreak, it is worthwhile to vaccinate non-sick horses. The immune system of horses with a previous vaccination history should respond with protective antibodies within 4 to 7 days.

Vaccine Types

The type of vaccine used determines booster frequency. *Inactivated* or *"killed"* injectable vaccines protect for at most 3 months, whereas a *modified live* vaccine protects for 4 to 6 months, depending on the product. Some killed vaccines use carrier agents, called *adjuvants* that affect how well immunity is stimulated. A "depot" adjuvant enhances both the level and duration of antibody response by slowly releasing the vaccine over several weeks. As the foreign protein is presented to the immune system over a prolonged period, it continually stimulates antibody production. Intranasal vaccines used against respiratory disease stimulate a more long-lived immunity, up to 6 months in many instances.

Respiratory Virus Modification

Viruses can modify themselves so they are no longer recognized by the immune system. There are various strains or subtypes of viruses, and it is necessary to immunize against those that are currently prevalent, and not outdated. Effective immunization is best achieved by using vaccines that contain current reference viruses that are known to be present in specific geographic locations.

Viral Shift

Viruses modify themselves in two ways. The first, called *viral shift,* is the appearance of an entirely new strain of virus due to a combination of two different strains. For example, the last major shift of equine influenza virus in the United States occurred in 1963 with the outbreak of the Miami/63 strain. In the past few years, new subtypes of equine influenza virus have appeared in Europe and China. Intercontinental movement of horses increases the possibility for exposure to new subtypes that a horse's immune system is unable to combat.

Antigenic Drift

The second method by which a virus alters itself is *antigenic drift*. An *antigen* is any foreign protein presented to the immune system to stimulate antibody production. Drift is a minor change in the viral antigenic structure and makeup. If viral proteins are altered in a process of *mutation,* antigenic drift results and a horse's immune system cannot defend against it. Neutralization by antibodies is prevented, and viral infection and clinical disease develop.

Viral Duplication

Whenever a virus successfully infects a horse and begins to duplicate itself, there is an opportunity for drift and mutation. The rate of drift is relative to the number of passages through horses, so the more horses infected in a population, the greater likelihood of antigenic drift. Antibodies are less effective at neutralizing the "different-looking" viruses created by antigenic drift. Disease produced by a viral mutant is not necessarily more severe, but a horse's immune system is less able to defeat a mutant virus. Unvaccinated horses and those that have never before been exposed to certain viruses (*immunologically naïve*) are susceptible to illness. Sick horses are reservoirs for disease.

It is important to report outbreaks of respiratory disease in a horse or herd to a veterinarian; this enables tracking of epidemics, shifts in viral subtypes, and antibody response to various vaccines. This practice ensures that vaccines are kept up-to-date with the current reference viruses. Advising others about the need and frequency of immunizations against respiratory viruses benefits the entire horse population. Limiting the number of susceptible animals that could carry viral respiratory disease promotes health within a population. Staying current with an aggressive immunization program prevents loss of valuable training, conditioning, and competition time.

Influenza Virus

Equine influenza can strike a horse regardless of time of year. Competitive horses that attend events where other horses are congregated and horses that live in large boarding barns are particularly at risk. Strenuous or prolonged exercise has been proven to significantly suppress the immune response of an otherwise normal horse, making him more susceptible to challenge by the influenza virus. Not all horses that contract a viral infection will display overt clinical signs, but a horse with such a *subclinical infection* may be a carrier capable of infecting those with a less hearty immune system. In this way, a horse that has never even left the property could become infected. Any age horse, and particularly the young or the old, may not be sufficiently capable of fighting off an infection. Any respiratory inflammation incurred sets up the potential for that horse to develop *inflammatory airway disease* (IAD) or *heaves* (see p. 259). Moldy hay is one means of starting heaves, but damage from respiratory viruses is another common inciting cause of airway disability.

The National Animal Health Monitoring System (NAHMS) Equine Study (1998) identified respiratory problems as the third leading cause of the greatest number of days of lost work in the horse population. In general, prevention is the key to good airway health, but even in the best of circumstances, horses do develop respiratory infections.

Clinical Signs

The "flu" can strike rapidly and unexpectedly, usually requiring an incubation time of only 1 to 5 days. An affected horse is lethargic, depressed, and often is disinterested in food. Rectal temperature may reach 103 to 106° F (39.5 to 41° C). The respiratory rate increases to as many as 60 breaths per minute. (See *Appendix A*, p. 567, for normal health parameters.) A sick horse moves with deliberate concentration, indicating an aching head or muscles (*myalgia*). Often, a watery, nasal discharge is observed, and a dry hacking cough is heard in about 40 percent of affected horses.

Coughing is a principal means of spreading the virus from horse to horse. Respiratory secretions ejected from a coughing horse into the air contain infective doses of viral particles. If viral particles are coughed into a moist environment, such as a damp barn or shipping van, the influenza virus remains alive and infective for several days. Infectious secretions are also passed by direct nose-to-nose contact, and from contaminated housing, food, water, and *fomites* (substances capable of transferring disease) such as human hands, clothing, rakes, and buckets.

The First Line of Defense
Secretory antibodies in the nasal passages are the first line of defense against influenza virus. Secretory antibodies respond to influenza virus only if previously "trained" to do so either by a prior infection or by vaccination. If the virus is inhaled and not neutralized by secretory antibodies, it colonizes the mucous membrane lining of the upper respiratory tissues and trachea.

Circulating Antibodies
If the flu virus penetrates the first line of defense, antibodies circulating throughout the body limit the infection. Circulating antibodies also develop in response to prior infection or vaccination.

Damage to Airways
The flu virus invades and kills the ciliated epithelial cells lining the respiratory tract. By 4 days following successful invasion by an influenza virus, these cells undergo significant degeneration. By 6 days post-infection, the cells of the mucociliary apparatus are almost entirely denuded of cilia, and the respiratory tract

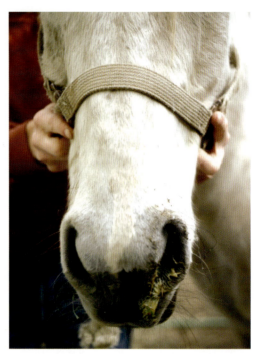

10.9 Nasal discharge that is creamy and/or yellow, as seen here, is typical of a bacterial infection.

cannot adequately clear debris, dust, viruses, or bacteria from the lungs. Depending on severity of an infection, the mucociliary apparatus needs 3 to 6 weeks to repair once the virus is defeated and healing begins. Even in an uncomplicated case of influenza, a minimum of 3 weeks is necessary for functional recovery of the respiratory epithelium.

Because the denuded respiratory tract epithelium cannot respond to further insult, opportunistic bacterial infections can develop, possibly leading to pneumonia, long-term damage to the lungs, or death. An opaque, white discharge often indicates mucus and is related to inflammation in the airways, sometimes associated with an allergic condition. A colored discharge (creamy, yellow, green) is usually suspicious of bacterial infection (photo 10.9).

Accurate Diagnosis

An exact diagnosis is not determined in all cases of respiratory infection in a horse. A general diagnosis of "the flu" is often applied to any coughing horse with a fever and nasal discharge. However, this includes a litany of equine respiratory illnesses such as infection with the respiratory form of *equine herpesvirus,* or *rhinopneumonitis* (p. 270), *rhinovirus* (p. 272), *adenovirus, equine viral arteritis virus* (p. 556), Streptococcal spp. (*S. equi, S. zooepidemicus, S. pneumoniae*—p. 273), as well as equine influenza. Historically, testing has not been done to confirm an exact respiratory disease diagnosis because treatment would likely not change, and a virus generally runs its course within a couple of weeks. To accurately identify what is causing the problem, it is necessary to run *paired serology* on blood samples taken 2 weeks apart. Due to the slow turnaround time on these diagnostic tests, they do not lend themselves well to common use. In the past, owners have opted for testing only if a horse's illness is non-responsive to treatment. But now, a stall-side virus isolation test is available to analyze nasal swabs prior to administering any treatment. Results from this stall-side test only take 30 minutes to confirm or rule out equine influenza virus as the problem. If there is a large population of horses at risk, it may be best to identify the source of the illness early on so a strategy can be planned to minimize sickness throughout a barn.

Isolation and Control

A sick or coughing horse, or a horse with a fever should be isolated from others in the event the problem is induced by a viral or infectious bacterial infection (see p. 458). Your vet can advise you of appropriate therapy and course of action as each case is individual in how it should be handled. Incubation of respiratory viral infections means that it generally takes 3 to 7 days for a horse to start showing clinical signs once exposed. An infected horse will shed (give off) virus for at least 7 days (although studies have indicated that horses that have been regularly vaccinated may only shed for a day). It is possible that if a horse was exposed or vaccinated within the previous 5 days, he may not show clinical signs but may still shed virus for up to 5 days. This poses a risk to a susceptible population and hence an epidemic outbreak may occur. It may be prudent to implement 2 to 3 weeks of quarantine on healthy horses returning after interaction with a large outside population of horses.

Efforts should be made to minimize communal use of buckets, rakes, and shared tack and equipment. These items serve as vectors for transmission of viral particles. The person tending to sick horses should care for them last in the chain of chores, and then clothing should be changed and careful hygiene measures followed. Treatment consists of supportive care to control fever and to keep horses feeling well enough to continue eating and drinking while the virus runs its course.

Clean air is a definite part of the recipe for tending to a horse with respiratory problems as well as maintaining good airway health. When possible, it is best for a horse to be housed outside where the air is fresh, rather than indoors. Hay should be fed off the ground rather than in chest-high feeders. Head-down eating enables a horse to clear dirt and dust from his nostrils and airways rather than inhaling irritating particulate matter into the lungs. Shake flakes of hay and if at all dusty, soak each thoroughly with water before feeding to hold down dust and mold spore irritants.

Resuming Exercise

Exercise can resume 7 to 10 days after body temperature returns to normal and coughing stops altogether. Once clinical symptoms such as these have abated, a horse is still infectious to others for 3 to 6 days. If exercise causes coughing, wait another 4 or 5 days before resuming a training program. A horse with a respiratory infection should be allowed at least 3 weeks for healing before being put back to full work. This enables the airways to regain full, healthful function without suffering a relapse.

Recovery Period

Having a horse removed from training and competition for a month or more for full recovery is an emotional and economic cost to a horse owner. However, if a horse is prematurely returned to work, a relapse is possible. In rare instances, the heart is affected by the influenza virus and may develop an arrhythmia (see p. 240).

An adult horse receiving adequate supportive care, rest, and protection from secondary complications usually recovers uneventfully with no permanent problems. Careful monitoring during both sickness and recovery are essential to success. In general, the mortality rate from an influenza infection is remarkably low in uncomplicated cases.

Prevention

It is best to avoid equine influenza viral infection if possible. The protective antibody response to an influenza virus infection is rapid, but short-lived. By 100 days, circulating antibodies have diminished and a horse is again susceptible to illness. (Human influenza antibody response lasts for 6 months to years.)

New arrivals to a herd or barn should be quarantined for 2 to 3 weeks. This practice isolates horses that are incubating disease or are shedding viral particles. An active performance horse is frequently exposed to respiratory viruses and can carry these viruses home to other animals. Such horses should be vaccinated often, preferably every 3 to 4 months.

Immunization Strategies

Athletic horses depend on a huge lung capacity to fuel the muscles with oxygen to maintain exercise. To protect against the flu, a *minimum* program of twice annual boosters of equine influenza ensures some good antibody protection, and may be given 2 to 4 times a year. Frequency depends on risk of exposure. In highly trafficked barns and for horses that experience travel and stress associated with competition, the vaccination plan should be more frequent. These vaccines don't guarantee that your horse won't get sick from the flu or contract other respiratory viruses, but a high antibody titer (concentration) in the bloodstream minimizes the degree of illness your horse experiences if he is exposed. Influenza vaccine imparts relatively cheap protection against the sniffles and coughs that can pull your horse out of work for weeks at a time. Any viral infection of the respiratory tract makes a horse susceptible to bronchopneumonia or to developing the allergic syndrome of inflammatory airway disease (IAD). Such secondary problems may have repercussions affecting performance far into a horse's athletic future.

Influenza vaccinations are available in an intranasal form that doesn't cause adverse reactions. The intranasal format affords a high level of protective immunity by blocking viruses or bacteria at their site of entry, the lining of the respiratory tract. Intramuscular influenza vaccinations are not thought to be as effective in protecting against influenza infection, but they do have a good track record of suppressing the degree of infection and the development of clinical signs.

Horses at greatest risk to developing influenza are those less than 3 years old. In an outbreak, about 75 percent of these youngsters get sick. Older horses may have developed some natural immunity over the years. Current recommendations for implementation of the initial vaccine series are to begin a series of three monthly immunizations starting no earlier than 9 months of age. The primary series is then followed with boosters every 2 to 4 months.

Equine Herpesvirus, Respiratory Form

Another respiratory virus for which a vaccine is available is the equine herpesvirus (EHV), or *rhinopneumonitis*. Often referred to as "rhino," the virus has different subtypes. EHV-1 is the most prevalent concern in horse populations not only because its respiratory disease is more virulent than EHV-4, but also because it is incriminated in causing viral abortion (see p. 536) or neurologic disease (myeloencephalopathy—see p. 508). Most cases of herpesvirus infection occur from weaning age to 12 months, and it is speculated that 80 to 90 percent of young horses will have been infected with EHV-1 by 2 years of age. Abortion occurs from 14 to 120 days after exposure to the virus. A mare may show no signs of disease, yet virus may invade the placenta and fetus. Most EHV-1 abortions occur in the last half of pregnancy, particularly the last trimester.

EHV-4 must replicate before clinical signs appear. It has a longer incubation time than the influenza virus, taking as long as three weeks. An infection may not be as severe as that seen with the flu because the horse's defense mechanisms begin to respond to EHV during the incubation period.

Symptoms

Initially, infection with herpesvirus (EHV-1) produces mild respiratory signs of watery, nasal discharge, fever (as high as 106° F or 41° C), and cough. There may be pinpoint hemorrhages (*petechiations*) on the mucous membranes. Some horses may also develop edema, swelling of the limbs or abdomen. After several days, the clear nasal discharge turns progressively thicker leaving a crust around the nostrils. Less than a week into the illness, this turns into an obvious yellowish, snotty discharge due to bacterial invasion of damaged cells lining the respiratory tract (photo 10.10).

The viremic phase lasts from 7 to 21 days, and during this time virus-infected cells have the potential to spread to other organs, such as a pregnant uterus and fetus to elicit abortion, the central nervous system to elicit myeloencephalitis, or the eye to elicit ocular disease like *chorioretinitis*. Typically, a horse that develops viral abortion or viral neurologic disease will have mild respiratory disease and/or fever in the two weeks preceding clinical evidence of reproductive or neurologic disease, albeit the signs may be so subtle as to be unnoticed. Once the infection moves to the lymph nodes in those first few days, it potentially reaches a pregnant uterus or the central nervous system through the blood circulation. Direct damage to the lining of the blood vessels adversely affects these organs. Abortion results from malnourishment of the fetus related to blood vessel damage within the uterus.

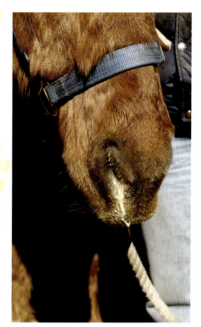

10.10 *Mucopurulent nasal discharge can be associated with herpesvirus infection, as well as strangles, bacterial respiratory infection, an infected tooth, or a sinus infection.*

Latent Infection

What makes herpesvirus unique is its ability to persist in a latent state, reappearing at intervals through an animal's life. Herpesvirus may be present in as many as 50 percent of adult horses, maintaining its presence in its hideout place within the trigeminal nerve of the face or within specialized white blood cells of the lymphatic system. It is clever in its ability to evade a host's immune recognition: the virus rests in a dormant state within latently infected cells, it does not turn on its machinery to replicate itself; instead, it lurks and waits. During this period while it is not expressing antigenic proteins that might alert the host to its presence, it is "silent" to the immune system, effectively escaping detection and destruction by the horse. During stressful periods associated with training, competition, transport, management changes, or illness, high levels of circulating corticosteroids suppress a host's normal defense mechanisms. Poor nutrition, a heavy parasite load, overcrowding, and rigorous climatic events are other stressors that adversely affect a horse's immune defenses. It is during stress periods that latent virus is reactivated and shed into the nasal secretions. A horse may appear clinically normal yet he serves as a silent shedder. This increases the potential to spread virus within a herd to individuals whose immune systems have not been previously challenged by herpesvirus.

Transmission maintains itself within a horse population in several ways:

- Passage from a latently-infected mare to her foal
- Persistence of infection in a latently-infected youngster into adult life
- Reactivation of latent virus to pass from horse to horse of any age

Of key importance in transmission of this virus is exposure by carrier horses that are incubating disease and not yet showing clinical signs, or from those horses that silently shed virus when a latent infection is reactivated by stress or illness.

Vaccination Schedule

The objective in stimulating immunity is to eliminate virus before it can enter the cells of the respiratory tract or restrict the spread of virus thereafter. Currently, the most effective control of respiratory infection lies at its site of entry, the upper respiratory lining. Based on this strategy, intranasal inoculation is particularly beneficial to limit viral respiratory disease. Immunity provided by intranasal vaccine lasts from 3 to 6 months.

The best immunization strategy is based on vaccination of young horses. Up until 3 to 5 months of age, a foal is unlikely to respond to vaccination due to blockage from maternally-derived antibodies of passive transfer that came from a mare's colostrum, particularly if she had been vaccinated prior to foaling. Vaccination titers are highest when a foal receives his first immunization at 5 months of age or older. A series of three immunizations should be administered to start a young horse on a herpesvirus vaccine program. For the best effect, all horses (young and old), within a herd should be properly immunized. Most available herpesvirus vaccines target both EHV-1 and the less worrisome strain of EHV-4. An adult horse should receive boosters every 3 to 6 months, the frequency dependent on the risk of exposure and the risk of stress-related travel and competition. The vaccine may not entirely eliminate disease, but it may attenuate clinical signs, and it may reduce viral shedding. EHV may not be a problem in some areas, but horses that travel may contact it. Although a horse may show no outward clinical signs, he might bring it home to infect high-risk individuals so those horses left on the farm should be immunized routinely, as well.

To protect against viral abortion, pregnant mares should receive EHV-1 vaccines prior to breeding and at 5, 7, and 9 months of pregnancy, using rhinopneumonitis vaccine specifically labeled for pregnant mares.

No vaccine protects against latent infection because the virus does not present itself to the horse's immune system when it persists in this silent form. Because one specific arm of the immune system, *cell mediated immunity* (CMI), is necessary to clear equine herpesvirus, inactivated injectable vaccine may not stimulate an appropriate immune response to minimize infection. Currently, no vaccine is available to protect against the neurologic form of EHV.

Rhinovirus

The rhinopneumonitis herpesvirus (EHV) should not be confused with the rhinovirus (ERV), for which there is no vaccine. ERV is associated with a fever lasting 1 to 2 days, swelling of the pharyngeal lymph nodes accompanied by a sore throat, and a watery-to-gray-green nasal discharge due to inflammation of the trachea and lower airways, or *tracheobronchitis*. Frequently, horses are infected without producing clinical signs, and serve as carriers to other, less durable individuals.

BACTERIAL INFECTION

Secondary Bacterial Infection

During a viral infection, bacteria that normally inhabit the upper airways may colonize, infect, and inflame the lower airways. Normally, the mucociliary apparatus (MCA) and macrophage systems clear bacteria, but viruses destroy the ciliated epithelial cells of the MCA, and reduce the ability of macrophages to attach to, digest, and kill bacteria.

Pleuropneumonia

Bacterial infection of the lower respiratory tract can lead to pleuropneumonia. Horses that are stressed by transport (*shipping fever*), inclement weather, or viral infections are at risk, and a horse suffering from choke may develop *inhalational pneumonia*. A horse with pleuropneumonia is lethargic, off feed, and typically has a fever. Sometimes there is a cough or nasal discharge, but not always. Blood tests, chest examination with a stethoscope, ultrasound, and radiographs (X rays) provide the best diagnosis of this serious illness.

Strangles

Strangles is a nickname given to an infection caused by a bacterial organism known as *Streptococcus equi*. These bacteria invade the respiratory tract and cause swelling of the lymph nodes around the head and neck. In some cases, swelling around the pharynx in the back of the throat becomes so severe that the horse's airway is obstructed and he sounds (and feels) like he is "strangling," or suffocating, hence the name "strangles." This disease is also referred to as *equine distemper*, but should not be confused with *dryland distemper* caused by a different bacterial infection (see p. 174). A milder form of a similar-appearing respiratory infection can develop due to *Streptococcus zooepidemicus* bacteria that are regularly present in the environment but sometimes create disease. The two strains of streptococcal bacteria can be discriminated from each other by laboratory testing.

Fortunately, most cases of strangles do not take a strangulating form. Most commonly, an affected horse stands listlessly in the paddock and is not interested in eating. He may have a fever and he may move stiffly as if his muscles ache. Most horses that are sick with this disease eventually develop a mucopurulent nasal discharge (see photo 10.10) and/or a cough. This may be all that develops, but in most cases the lymph nodes under the jaw (*submandibular lymph nodes*—photo 10.11) or alongside the throatlatch area (*retropharyngeal lymph nodes*—photos 10.12 A & B) become swollen. There may be edema around the face, and breathing may be slightly labored. At the onset, the lymph nodes feel firm and painful to touch long before they soften and break open to drain thick, creamy pus.

Typically, lymph node abscesses rupture within a couple of weeks after the horse shows

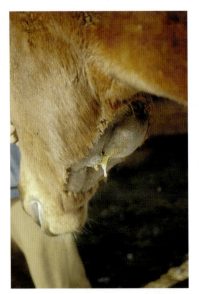

10.11 *Strangles infection of the submandibular lymph nodes causes swelling of the nodes beneath the jaw.*

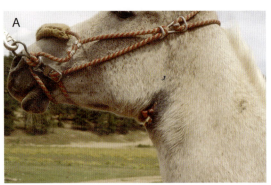

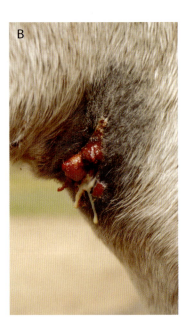

10.12 A & B *Strangles infection of the retropharyngeal lymph nodes causes swelling of the nodes beneath the jaw. When these abscesses break open, they drain a creamy, yellow discharge.*

the first clinical signs he is sick. Draining lymph nodes culture positive for the *Streptococcus equi* organism only half the time. Identification of the disease is based on clinical signs, bacterial culture of the nasopharyngeal area and/or the guttural pouch (see p. 277), and/or blood testing for strep proteins.

Who Is at Risk?

Any age horse can be affected, but it is the very young and the very old that usually suffer the worst. Most susceptible are the weanling through yearling ages; young horses may have not yet developed sufficient immunity through natural exposure in their short lives. Incubation takes 3 to 14 days once a horse has been exposed until he shows clinical signs of infection. Not all infected horses develop obvious symptoms of disease yet asymptomatic individuals may serve as carriers and shed the organism through their respiratory secretions and saliva to spread it to other susceptible horses. Older horses may show nothing more than nasal discharge, but may be more likely to harbor *Streptococcus equi* infection in the guttural pouches. The immune system of a geriatric horse may be working at less than optimal function due to age-related decline, and there may be age-related scar tissue around the openings to the guttural pouches, which could inhibit drainage.

Strangles is a highly contagious disease, particularly in conditions of stress. This includes situations where horses are housed in crowded areas, with poor hygiene, or with inadequate nutrition. Flies help spread the disease, as do fomites such as contaminated feed buckets, rakes, and human hands and clothing (see p. 458). The organism can survive for 3 to 4 weeks in water in tanks contaminated by discharges. Once established on a property, another outbreak may occur on that farm a year or two later. A strangles infection may keep cycling through a herd to become a persistent and frustrating management issue. Once a horse has been infected with strangles, he may continue to shed the organism intermittently for months through nasal secretions. In a small percentage of horses, the bacteria remain resident in the guttural pouch for prolonged periods, with the potential to carry the infection to others despite appearing fully recovered. Most horses stop shedding within about 3 weeks.

In suspected carriers, nasal washes or culture swabs of nasopharyngeal or guttural pouch contents help identify inapparent shedders of *Streptococcus equi* organisms. Reports from one study found that the average period of shedding from carriers was 9.2 months, with one horse shedding for as long as 42 months. Shedding persists in 68 percent of horses for at least 4 weeks following resolution of clinical signs. Once recovered from strangles infection, 75 percent of horses develop a long-lived immunity of at least 2 years and possibly as long as 5 years.

Treatment

This disease is labor intensive, requiring supportive nursing care. The disease must run its course, but hot packs applied to the swollen gland help point an abscess for drainage. Surgical lancing of affected lymph nodes hastens drainage and speeds a horse on his way to recovery. An opened abscess should be irrigated daily with an antiseptic solution made by mixing 10 to 30 ml of povidone iodine per liter of salt water. Supportive care is essential: the horse should be encouraged to eat by providing pelleted gruels, and food and water should be accessible in a way that he can reach comfortably.

Nonsteroidal anti-inflammatory (NSAIDs) medications make the horse more comfortable, control swelling, control fever, and encourage eating and drinking. Antibiotics may, in fact, be counter-productive by suppressing bacteria for a time, but infection may flare up when the antibiotics are discontinued. Treated horses may become reinfected because they did not develop protective immunity. Antibiotics don't penetrate into a lymph node abscess to reach the bacteria, so when antibiotics are withdrawn, there is recrudescence of disease. Antibiotic therapy may be indicated in certain instances when an affected horse remains off feed and is depressed despite other supportive care, or if the fever remains elevated (greater than 104° F or 40° C), or if the airway is obstructed by lymph node swelling, contributing to difficulty in breathing. In these cases, bacterial culture and antibiotic sensitivity can be determined in the lab to assist choice of antimicrobial therapy.

Control and Prevention

Once a horse is recognized with a strangles infection, an ideal means of containment is to isolate any sick or suspect individuals for about 6 weeks. Excellent sanitation and good common sense are important to controlling the disease from spreading through a herd. Helpful strategies include:

- Control flies.
- Use separate halters, water and feed buckets, cleaning utensils, wheelbarrows, and brushes for sick horses.
- Handle the sick horses after taking care of the healthy horses.
- Change clothes after being in contact with any sick horses, wash hands with antiseptic soaps, and wear boots that can be immersed in a footbath to decontaminate the soles.
- Scrub fences, stall walls, and anything that may have been contaminated by respiratory secretions with disinfectants known to kill the organism (phenolic products, iodophors, chlorhexidine, or glutaraldehyde).
- Reduce moisture in the environment, as *Streptococcal* spp. bacteria survive longer when protected by moisture.

- Clean and disinfect water tanks daily.
- Compost contaminated bedding beneath a layer of plastic so flies cannot access the bedding.

In the face of an outbreak, it has been demonstrated that vaccinating non-sick animals can decrease the *morbidity* (number of animals that get sick) by half. The only setback to this strategy in horses that have never been vaccinated against strangles is that to ensure the maximum effect, the non-sick horses need to receive the full protocol of 2 vaccines spaced 3 weeks apart. This may be too long a time for the horses to develop sufficient protective immunity, so they may develop the disease before the second vaccine is given. Horses that have been on a previous strangles vaccine program can be "boosted" with one dose of vaccine; this should elicit some immunity to limit the severity of infection if a horse does contract the disease. Horses that have existing high antibody titers from a previous infection or vaccination need not be immunized again. Pregnant mares should be vaccinated with approved products about a month prior to foaling so the newborn foal will receive protective antibodies in the colostrum (see "Strangles Vaccination," p. 278).

Any new horses that have entered the farm should be isolated for 2 to 3 weeks in case they are carrying a bacterial infection or virus to which the resident horses have not previously been exposed. This allows the new horses to incubate and break with disease before they've had a chance to comingle and infect all the others on the farm. Then, sickness can be identified and controlled before too much damage is done. This is especially important where foals, weanlings, and yearlings are involved. Rectal temperatures of new arrivals should be checked twice daily since shedding of the organism does not begin until 24 to 48 hours following onset of a fever, thereby giving time to separate sick horses from well ones. It is also a good idea to have a veterinarian do a health exam on new horses entering your premise.

If *Streptococcus equi* is suspected or is a concern based on a horse's past history or exposure, bacterial culture of nasopharyngeal washes or guttural pouch swabs is considered the gold standard to identify a sick or carrier horse. Ideally, a horse is considered not to be a carrier if he has three negative nasopharyngeal swabs for *Streptococcus equi* over a two-to three-week period. Nasopharyngeal bacterial cultures detect 60 percent of carrier horses. Combining this test with PCR (*polymerase chain reaction*) blood testing increases detection of carriers to 90 percent. The PCR test detects DNA from both living and dead *Streptococcus equi* bacteria and is as much as three times more sensitive than bacterial culture. Active infection should be confirmed by bacterial culture of the swab. If either test shows a positive result, endoscopic exam of the guttural pouches may be used to screen for carriers. Samples taken from the guttural pouches can be tested with PCR and culture for final confirmation.

Complications

Besides the illness associated with acute disease, strangles is not without its set of complications that arise subsequent to infection. About 20 percent of horses infected with strangles develop problems other than the basic upper respiratory signs. Some of the complications may be life-threatening, so careful monitoring is advisable following the first clinical signs.

Bastard Strangles

A difficult complication to identify is called *bastard strangles* or *metastatic strangles abscessation*. In this case, the organism spreads to other internal lymph nodes (particularly those of the gastrointestinal tract) or to other organs (like the spleen, liver, kidney, lungs, or even the brain). A horse with bastard strangles may appear relatively normal until infection wears him down. His hair coat appears dull and ragged, he may continue to lose weight in the presence of ample food and good dental care, his performance may suffer, and his listless demeanor suggests an underlying problem that cannot be explained by an obvious cause. Lab results of a complete blood count and fibrinogen level may identify a systemic infection. A rectal exam or abdominal ultrasound exam or an abdominal tap may identify the location of the internal abscess. These are hard cases to treat, requiring very long-term antibiotic therapy.

Guttural Pouch Infection

Another complication that may not become apparent for a long time is an infection of the guttural pouch (a cavity within the head that is an enlargement of the eustachian tube), referred to as *empyema* (accumulation of pus) or *chondroids* (hardened concretions of pus). This could be a life-threatening problem if the infection erodes through large blood vessels that course through the guttural pouch.

Major nerve branches may also be affected in this area creating neurologic problems referable to the cranial nerves within the head. Pus debris that accumulates within the laden guttural pouch is often swallowed as it drains into the pharynx, but is sometimes visible as a nasal discharge from one or both nostrils. An endoscopic exam and radiographs (X rays) of the head are useful to detect problems in the guttural pouches. Most asymptomatic carrier horses harbor *Streptococcus equi* within their guttural pouches.

Purpura Hemorrhagica

Streptococcal bacteria can create an immune-

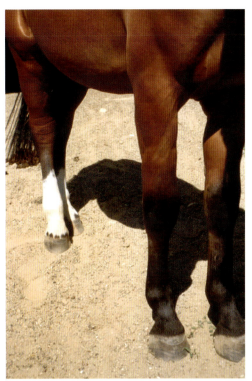

10.13 *Strangles infection can cause vasculitis with resulting limb edema and swelling as seen in this horse. Following strangles infection, a small percentage of horses may develop a hypersensitivity response called purpura hemorrhagica that causes the limbs and abdomen to swell like this.*

mediated syndrome known *purpura hemorrhagica* that leads to abdominal edema, limb edema, head edema, scrotal edema, and hives. Protein antigens of the bacterial organism combine with antibodies to elicit an allergic response in the horse, causing damage to the blood vessels. This occurs in less than 1 percent of infected horses. At least half of those horses that develop purpura have been immunized with an injectable extract vaccine. The horse may seem to be well on the mend, only to suffer a severe setback about 2 to 4 weeks following a strangles infection. Gravity dependent areas swell, like the legs, belly, and head (photo 10.13). The horse is depressed, off feed, and small blood spots (petechiations) are visible on the mucous membranes of the gums, conjunctiva, and nasal lining due to leaky blood vessels. Pronounced limb edema often elicits serum leakage and skin sloughing from swollen limbs.

If a similar event occurs in internal organs, the horse may demonstrate colic, respiratory disease, or muscle problems. Since this syndrome arises due to an immune-mediated complex stimulated by components of the bacteria, the horse needs to be treated with both corticosteroids and antibiotics for a lengthy period of time. Myositis (muscle inflammation) is another potentially fatal complication of infection that may involve an immune-mediated process (see p. 166).

Strangles Vaccination

Because the site of entry of this organism is through contamination of the upper respiratory tract, the most ideal method of stimulating immunity is by eliciting a secretory antibody response in the local respiratory tissues. An intranasal vaccine takes advantage of this means of protective immunity.

Previously, all vaccination strategies against strangles have relied on intramuscular injections (extract vaccines) that elicit a systemic immune response. Such vaccines have had limited efficacy, only curtailing disease in 60 to 70 percent of those cases challenged by the organism. They do not prevent infection. In addition, Streptococcal intramuscular injections often create sore muscles, malaise, and are accompanied by fever lasting as long as a week. Although such complications occur in only a small percentage of horses, these adverse reactions were concerning to horse owners until the advent of the intranasal vaccine.

The intranasal strangles vaccine is given as a series of 2 doses spaced 3 weeks apart. After an initial series of 2 immunizations, a horse should receive a booster annually. The material is an *avirulent* (not capable of producing disease) *Streptococcus equi* organism that is freeze-dried and then reconstituted with sterile water just prior to administration. The 2 ml dose is squirted through a nasal canula into a nostril to reach the upper nasal cavity. Here, it provides the best protective response since it stimulates local production of antibody at the site of invasion in the upper respiratory tract. The objective is to prevent attachment of wild *Streptococcus equi* to tonsil receptors, and thereby prevent invasion.

Reduction of clinical disease has been observed in horses vaccinated with intranasal product. However, despite "protection" derived from the intranasal vaccine, 40 percent of horses challenged with the organism did still develop clinical signs of disease as opposed to 60 percent of unvaccinated horses that were challenged with *Streptococcus equi*. Extent of illness is decreased, and of those that do get sick, clinical signs are reduced by 65 percent as compared to unvaccinated horses. Just as with the intramuscular vaccines, no horse can receive complete protection from the strangles organism when challenged.

There is some concern that giving a modified live organism via the nasal passages could result in shedding from the vaccinated individuals to those who were not. The safety studies performed indicate that any slight shedding that may occur does so only during the first day and the organism is not shed to any significant degree.

Pregnant mares should be vaccinated with approved products about a month prior to foaling so a newborn foal will receive protective antibodies in the colostrum.

It is recommended that the intranasal strangles vaccine be administered with care after immunizing with other intramuscular products during routine inoculations. Contamination of the site of a needle stick or a wound has been known to develop "sterile" abscesses growing the vaccine strain. An inoculated horse could wipe his face or blow the product onto a recent intramuscular injection site or on a wound, and the vaccine strain could grow. Ideally, it should not be administered on the same day as other injections or should be done with care. This strategy helps prevent inadvertent contamination of intramuscular inoculation sites with the live vaccine. It would be prudent to discuss with a veterinarian the risks and benefits of using the intranasal form of immunization against strangles relative to the immediate risk of disease in a local community.

PREVENTING RESPIRATORY ILLNESS

Maintaining excellent hygiene and minimizing stress are key elements in preventing respiratory illness. To significantly reduce shedding of bacteria and viruses in the environment, aggressive respiratory vaccine programs should be implemented. A virally infected, coughing horse sprays millions of viral particles into the air. Horses protected by vaccines are less likely to develop clinical viral disease or associated bacterial infections; subsequently, they are less likely to shed these organisms in epidemic or infectious doses. Accurate records and a calendar help implement an effective vaccine schedule to avoid respiratory illness. Respiratory vaccines are cost-effective insurance to enable a horse to train and deliver an optimal athletic performance.

The Digestive System: The Oral Cavity, Dental Care, and the Intestinal Tract 11

The horse evolved as a grazing animal, moving with the herd in search of available forage. The intestinal system was accustomed to small and frequent meals. Horses ate plants moist with dew and containing natural water. Grasses were cropped as they grew, slowly adapting microflora in the horse's intestinal tract to changes in the nutrient value of plants as they responded to season and climate. When available food sources dwindled, the horse moved on, not stopping long enough to contaminate his feed with droppings that might reinfect him with parasite eggs. In this idyllic state, the horse moved about, maintaining muscle tone and good circulation.

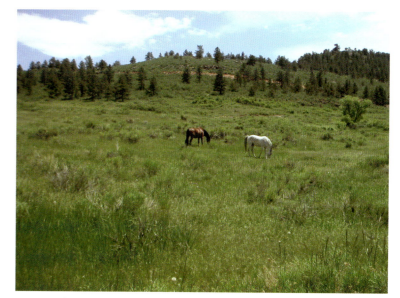

11.1 *Dryland pasture, i.e. non-irrigated, is a healthy source of roughage.*

Today, horses live quite differently. Urban development and time constraints compel us to confine horses for convenience. Horses in a natural state graze intermittently but throughout the day; by providing meals designed by humans we drastically alter how the intestinal tract handles food. People are now faced with management of an animal not naturally equipped to deal with imposed diets, feed schedules, and exercise restrictions. An understanding of how equine intestines function most efficiently enables horse owners to make appropriate management decisions. (For more on equine eating habits, see part two of the *Digestive System*, chapter 12, p. 325.)

The Importance of Dental and Oral Cavity Health

More than just about anything, horses like to spend their time eating, and an active sport horse needs to devote a lot of time to this pursuit (photo 11.1). Fortunately, it is what horses

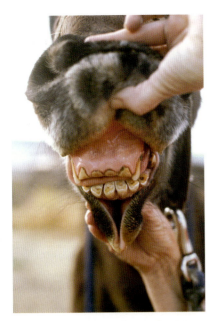

11.2 *Worn incisors and poor dentition make it difficult for a horse to get nutrition through pasture grazing, so other supplementation must be made available.*

do best, besides being a necessary function to support a large body structure on an herbivore diet. Horse teeth, with their long crowns and short roots (*hypsodont teeth*), are well adapted to grinding grass forage. A horse's large head and sinus cavities house long tooth crowns for the better part of a horse's life. As the tooth enamel of the crowns is continuously ground away by abrasive silicates embedded in forage, the molar teeth continually erupt from the sinuses into the mouth. This process maintains the upper and lower cheek teeth in contact with each other. With good care, this eruption process continues well into a horse's mid-twenties and occasionally into his thirties.

A horse's jaw grinds feed in an elliptical motion, which contributes to wear of the teeth. It is important for the molars to make even contact with each other so each tooth wears evenly and at a similar rate. Even tooth wear ensures proper chewing and grinding of the feed so it is available to the digestive tract for efficient digestion and nutrient absorption. If tooth wear differs in various parts of the mouth, then overall health and condition of a horse may suffer if nutritional demands are not met. And, pain in the mouth that develops from uneven tooth wear can lead to performance problems.

Nutritional Demands

Not only is an adequate supply of food necessary to maintain a horse's body condition, but the teeth must also be able to properly grind the feed to make full use of the diet (photo 11.2).

Horses with poor teeth place a greater demand on the wallet since they often need extra food to obtain sufficient calories to maintain body weight. Herd competition poses additional problems on horses with poor dentition. Horses with poor teeth often require longer periods to chew food, so in a herd the food may vanish before the least thrifty individuals have time to eat what they need. Broodmares in the last trimester of gestation or during lactation have intense energy demands and need to make efficient use of their feed. And, athletic horses particularly require energy to sustain performance, and they especially need to make their calories count.

Horses that receive routine dental care starting in the first few years of life tend to have good, strong teeth to take them into their geriatric years. Most severe dental problems are seen in older horses that have received minimal dental attention throughout their lives. These problems often reach the point of requiring that such horses are fed pelleted gruels or mashes to maintain body condition (see chapter 12, *The Digestive System: Nutritional Management*, p. 328). This is time-consuming as well as more costly. And, many of these problems are preventable. There are strong financial incentives to have a horse's teeth checked frequently, at least every 6 months, so preventive measures can be taken to avoid dental problems.

Problems Related to the Oral Cavity

EXCESSIVE SALIVATION

A fungus (*Rhizoctonia leguminicola*) produces a toxin known as *slaframine* that induces hypersalivation within an hour following ingestion of contaminated hay. This is often found as a contaminant of red clover hay. Other clinical signs include excessive tear production, more than usual urination and bowel movements, and some horses may develop diarrhea. Clinical symptoms usually abate within 4 days.

VESICULAR STOMATITIS

Vesicular stomatitis (VSV) is a reportable viral disease that affects horses and other livestock. Sporadic outbreaks occur in the United States during warm months, particularly in the southwestern states, Texas, and Colorado. Transmission occurs by direct contact with infected lesions or saliva from sick animals, or by contact with infective material on fomites such as water buckets, rakes, hay, hands, brushes, etc. Transmission of VSV also is linked to bites by insect vectors, such as black flies and sand flies. Shedding of the virus from an open, infected sore lasts for about a week. Incubation takes 1 to 3 days until clinical signs appear.

Early on in an infection, a horse may have a fever. Painful blisters and ulcers develop on the tongue and gums, as well as the external genitalia, the udder or prepuce (photos 11.3 A–C). Painful ulcers in the mouth discourage appetite; a horse's unwillingness to swallow due to pain results in heavy salivation. In some instances, the coronary bands may be affected, the horse demonstrating a gait suggestive of laminitis. A rare, serious case may slough the hoof, but most develop transient hoof-wall deformities related to inflammation of the coronary bands.

The disease usually runs its course within 2 weeks, the only treatment required being supportive care to keep a horse comfortable and eating and drinking.

Prevention relies on stabling management particularly during periods of high insect activity. Horses should be removed from proximity to wetlands, irrigation ditches, and other water sources, and judicious use should be made of fly repellents. In the environment, the virus is readily inactivated by common disinfectants and by steam cleaning.

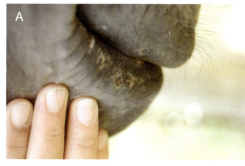
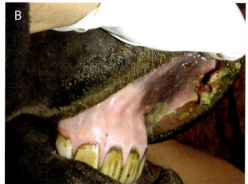
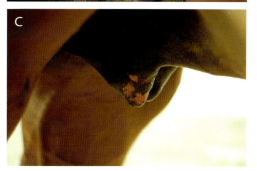

11.3 A – C *Vesicular stomatitis lesions in the mouth may only be apparent as swelling of the muzzle (A). Pain and swelling cause the horse to go off feed. Often, the lesions cause blisters, with sloughing of sensitive tissue of the mucous membranes of the mouth (B), teats, sheath (C), and at times, the coronary bands.*

AVOCADO TOXICITY

Horses that graze near avocado plants may develop an acute allergic condition that results in swelling of the head, throatlatch, tongue, lips, and cheek muscles, and swelling along the lower belly. The swollen muscles are painful to touch. Discomfort causes an affected horse to stop eating and drinking. Some display depression or colic symptoms. Toxic principles of the avocado plant usually reside in the green leaves,

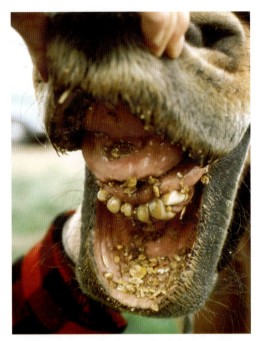

11.4 *Inadequate grinding of food due to poor teeth prevents a horse from obtaining the most from dietary nutrients. Poorly ground feed presents a large surface area to intestinal flora, which limits digestion and can lead to gastrointestinal irritation and diarrhea.*

not in the fruit or in the dried leaves. Treatment approach is to remove the horse from access to the plant, and to provide symptomatic relief (see *Appendix C*, p. 571).

Signs of Dental Problems

Health Signs

There are many signs of dental problems and inadequate grinding. Some general health issues that might be observed in a horse with bad teeth include:

- A horse may show persistent weight loss despite availability of an adequate quantity and quality of food. Improperly ground feed presents a large surface area to intestinal flora, and so may not be adequately digested (photo 11.4).
- A horse with a painful mouth may salivate excessively and drool.
- A horse may "quid," that is, wads of partially chewed hay are spit out on the ground or impacted in the cheeks.
- Whole grains or large pieces of roughage (greater than ¼ inch pieces) are often visible in the feces of a horse that has problems grinding his food.
- Intermittent or chronic diarrhea may develop due to irritation of the bowel lining by inadequately ground feed.
- A horse with dental problems may take extended time to eat a meal.
- A horse may exhibit odd head, neck, or jaw movements when eating, in an effort to relieve discomfort.
- There may be bad breath due to a rotten tooth or impacted food matter that decays within the teeth or gums.
- A unilateral nasal discharge may develop if a sinus becomes infected from a bad tooth.
- On rare occasions, mouth disease that has been present for a long time may lead to visible asymmetry of the chewing muscles of the jaw.
- A horse resents finger pressure on the outside of his cheeks when he has sharp hooks or points that dig into his cheeks.
- Horses with dental problems are prone to chronic choke (*esophageal obstruction*) from swallowing inadequately ground feed that may lodge in the esophagus (see p. 295).
- A horse may exhibit chronic colic, particularly gaseous or impaction colic, due to irritation of the bowel lining or obstruction of the intestines with feed material.
- Dental problems may make a horse difficult to bridle, or he may exhibit resistant behavior in the bridle.

Performance Signs

Horses with teeth problems also exhibit performance issues that range from subtle to very obvious. When ridden, these include:

- Abnormal head carriage
- Headshaking, head tossing, or tail wringing
- Bracing against the bit
- Refusal to stop or turn
- Unwillingness to perform collection
- Reluctance to perform the intended job

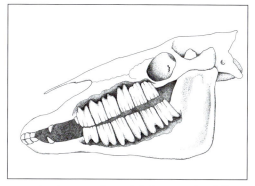

11.5 *A side view of an adult horse with a full complement of teeth.*

Besides lack of training, there are other reasons why a horse may lean on the bit, hollow his back, or move in an inefficient manner. Dental issues not only create performance problems, but may also generate habits that become so ingrained that they are difficult to change even once a source of the problem has been addressed. Any pain in the mouth will cause a horse to seek the most comfortable place for the bit. This usually means raising the head and neck to escape pain from a bit that hits tender teeth or puts pressure on oral ulcers created by sharp points on the cheek teeth. Raising the head and neck hollows the back, forcing the rear legs to trail behind rather than pushing the horse in a more collected gait. Quality of gait and performance suffer as a consequence.

Some horses cock their heads to relieve mouth pain. This twists the cervical vertebrae, throwing the horse more onto one side of his body than the other. This might hasten the onset of fatigue, with potential for over-compensation injury.

Eruption Patterns

A normal horse has a "full mouth" by 5 years of age (fig 11.5). This means all adult teeth are in place, including incisors, canines (not present in all), premolars, and molars. Once a horse is past the age of 5, it is not always simple to definitively age him based on his teeth-wear patterns. This is because abrasiveness of different soils and forages may accelerate tooth wear over expected levels.

Pastured horses are at an advantage in maintaining dental health. They are able to use their grinding teeth in the manner the teeth and jaws evolved to function most efficiently. They crop off grasses with their incisors, and then grind their jaws in an elliptical pattern with full range-of-motion. Pastured horses still are in need of dental attention, but not usually as intensively as horses that are confined or stalled. Confined horses fed a diet of dried hay and grains do not use their incisors to shear plants. Over time this may lead to overgrowth of the incisors, which then decreases contact between the upper and lower cheek teeth. This makes grinding less efficient, and also sets up conditions for such tooth issues as the development of sharp enamel points, hooks, ramps, and wave mouths (see p. 286). Similarly, pelleted diets limit a horse's normal jaw excursion so sharp points are likely to develop along the outside upper cheek teeth and the inside of the lower cheek teeth.

A range horse eats for sessions ranging from half an hour up to 3 hours for a total duration of 10 to 12 hours each day, depending on the nutritional value of the forage. Confined horses may eat dirt, manure, or fencing in an effort to satisfy the need to chew. Besides the impact that confinement has on dental health, this can lead to other health issues such as sand colic (see p. 310), parasitism (see p. 459), or *cribbing stereotypy*, which is a repetitive behavior (see p. 288).

Tooth and Mouth Issues

Wolf Teeth

Wolf teeth are vestigial premolars located at the front of the molars in the upper jaw. A wolf tooth should not be confused with a *canine* tooth. Most male horses grow canine teeth that sit in front of the bit, about halfway between the incisors and the molars. Some mares also grow canines, but not as commonly as male horses.

A wolf tooth is often very small, but its location coincides with the place a bit rests in a horse's mouth. Horses with tooth problems from either large hooks or wolf teeth resist the bridle, and many throw their heads to avoid painful bumping of the bit on the offending tooth. Wolf teeth can create other bad habits such as bridle resistance or inflexibility of the jaw. Also, the presence of wolf teeth in older horses makes it difficult to create a *bit seat* on the second premolar (see p. 290), and hooks may develop on adjacent teeth that cause future problems.

Prior to introducing a horse to the bit at age 2 or 3, the wolf teeth (first premolars) should be removed if present (photo 11.6). Not all horses erupt wolf teeth, and some only have a single one. It is rare to see wolf teeth on the lower jaw; most occur in the upper jaw sitting directly in front of the upper premolars.

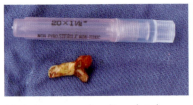

11.6 *An extracted wolf tooth is less than an inch long, but if left in the mouth, it could interfere with performance due to pressure on it from the bit.*

Retained Caps

Young horses may have *retained caps* that are remnants of deciduous molars that have not shed out entirely. This is common in two-and-a-half- to four-year-olds. Such caps may cause sufficient discomfort that a horse goes off feed or exhibits performance problems in accepting the bit. An equine dentist can locate these caps and remove them.

It is normal to see enlargements or bumps along the lower jaw or just in front of the facial crest on the upper jaw of two-and-a-half- to four-year-olds. These non-painful swellings are caused by inflammation related to the eruption of some adult teeth. With time these will subside in a young horse but such swellings would be considered abnormal in an older horse and cause for concern.

Abnormalities of Wear

SHARP POINTS ON CHEEK TEETH

Because of the elliptical grinding pattern of chewing, not all portions of each tooth are ground down evenly as teeth continue to erupt from the sinus cavities: the outside edges of the upper cheek teeth and the inner edges of the lower cheek teeth will tend to develop sharp points. These sharp enamel points can create sores and ulcers on the inside of the cheeks, causing discomfort, and they may interfere with efficient grinding of feed. The process of *floating* uses specialized files or motorized equipment to smooth these sharp points.

INCISOR OVERGROWTH

As horses age, it is important to monitor the incisor length and bite, so they don't overgrow and prevent even contact (*occlusion*) of the molars (photo 11.7).

A "grinning" appearance to the front incisors suggests that they may be too long for the

The Digestive System: The Oral Cavity, Dental Care, and the Intestinal Tract

good of the mouth (photo 11.8). Sliding the lower jaw sideways while holding the upper jaw is a way to check for incisor overgrowth (photos 11.9 A & B). If the lower jaw excursion exceeds the distance of one incisor tooth, then the incisors need to be shortened by a dentist (photo 11.10). A horse with a genetic overbite cannot help but overgrow the incisors so frequent dental procedures should be applied to reduce their length (photo 11.11 and see "Parrot Mouth," p. 12).

WAVE MOUTH

Without even contact of incisors or molars, the molars may overgrow to develop a *wave mouth* (an undulating variation in the height of adjacent cheek teeth), which is commonly seen in aged horses. A wave mouth also occurs when a tooth is missing, thereby allowing the opposite tooth to continue to grow into the mouth without opposing wear.

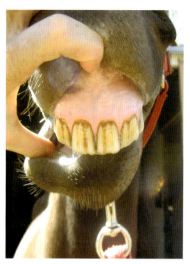

11.7 *A horse with normal length and wear on the incisor teeth; the teeth are of almost equal length with only the slightest curve in the alignment. Compare this mouth to the more aged one in photo 11.8.*

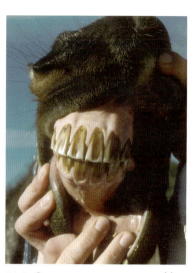

11.8 *Overgrown incisors in an older horse's mouth give the appearance of a grin with an obvious semicircular curvature in alignment. Long incisors preclude normal apposition of the cheek teeth for efficient chewing.*

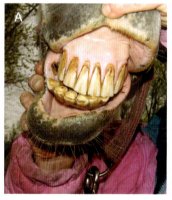 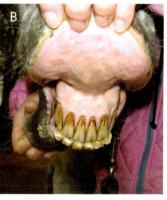

11.9 A & B *Overgrown incisors in an aged mouth showing pronounced excursion of the jaw to the side. Such overgrown incisors do not allow the cheek teeth to meet for adequate grinding of food (A). Overgrown incisors at rest without lateral jaw movement show the abnormal grin. Note the overshot lower jaw that contributed to overgrowth of these incisors (B).*

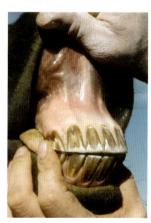

11.10 *This is how the horse in photo 11.8 appeared after dental correction to remove excess incisor growth.*

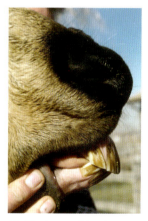

11.11 *An overbite due to an excessively long upper mandible is referred to as a parrot mouth. The incisors of this mouth configuration require regular dental care to limit overgrowth.*

11.12 *Power tools are helpful when reducing the length of overly grown incisors and removing protruding hooks on molars.*

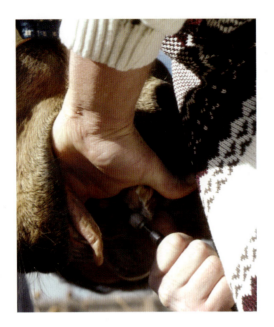

HOOKS

With time, projecting *hooks* on the upper cheek teeth may reduce the functional chewing surface by more than 50 percent of normal excursion. Poor jaw excursion or imperfect molar occlusion may cause feed to impact within the teeth; with fermentation of impacted food, *caries* (cavities) may develop as in people, leading to a rotten and painful tooth. Projecting hooks are removed with molar cutters or with power grinders (photo 11.12). A horse with hooks on the lower cheek teeth may be unable to slide his lower jaw forward particularly if his mouth is held closed with a noseband. This makes it impossible for a horse to flex at the poll no matter how hard he tries. Such resistance limits a rider's "contact" and fine control. Subsequently, it becomes difficult to engage a horse's hindquarters by developing a connection between the haunches, the back, the poll, and the horse's mouth.

RAMPS

An uneven slope angle of a tooth, with one end of a tooth being longer than the other, creates a "ramp" effect so that as a horse chews, his lower jaw is forced backward, throwing the *temporomandibular joint* (TMJ—see p. 289) out of position. Over time, this leads to degenerative arthritis of the TMJ. This may have huge performance effects in a younger horse, and may lead to eating problems and weight problems in a horse's later years due to pain and limited range of motion of the jaw.

Cribbing

Cribbing or crib-biting is a repetitive behavior that is a liability for a horse (see p. 474). A horse that cribs grabs onto a firm object like a fence rail or post, a water tank, or a stall door. The horse then flexes his neck and pulls back on the object, making an audible grunting sound. Not only does a cribbing horse turn away from eating and drinking to nurture his addictive habit, but he is also at risk of developing colic. It is hard to keep weight on a "cribber," and performance suffers. This stereotypy also causes management problems: a cribbing horse's teeth whittle down fencing, stalls, and doors, and other horses are likely to pick up the habit. There is speculation that gastric ulcers may contribute to cribbing behavior (see p. 318). In those cases, anti-ulcer medication and elimination of grain are helpful strategies to calm gastric irritation and pain.

Examination of the incisors for abnormal wear identifies a cribbing horse (photos 11.13 A & B). The incisors will be excessively worn and rounded. A cribbing collar limits the behavior by causing discomfort as the horse pulls back and flexes his throat and upper neck. The collar bites into his flesh, making cribbing physically uncomfortable.

A surgical option is available but it has limited success of less than 60 percent. The surgery involves cutting the nerve supply to the muscles under the neck that enable a horse to crib.

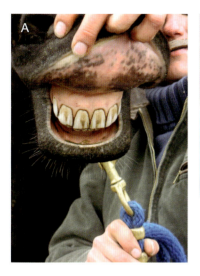
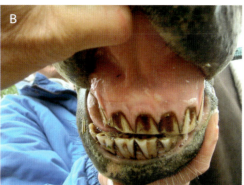

11.13 A & B *Normal incisors have a smooth lower margin with no signs of wear* (A). *A horse that cribs has worn incisors that are easily identified on visual examination. The incisors in* (B) *are excessively worn with the margins slanted in an asymmetrical fashion where the horse's teeth have repeatedly grabbed onto a smooth surface to crib. Compare the three worn upper incisor teeth on the left of this photo with the length of the more normal corner incisor on the upper right.*

Temporomandibular Joint

Comfort of the *temporomandibular joint* (TMJ) is important for the cyclical movements of chewing and grinding. "Wear and tear" injury may occur to the TMJ, particularly with dental misalignment from abnormal teeth. Trauma is another source of TMJ pain: a horse might be kicked in the face, or he might jam his head in a confined area and in a frenzied attempt to get free, injure his jaw. Ultrasound exam is useful to evaluate this joint. Correction of dental irregularities is important to manage TMJ disease. Offering a mashed or soft diet is also helpful to minimize joint pain associated with chewing. In cases of osteoarthritis of the TMJ, anti-inflammatory medications may be injected directly into the joint.

Equine Dentistry

Who Is an Equine Dentist?

Veterinarians have earned a degree in veterinary medicine, surgery, *and* dentistry, and pass state tests for a license to practice. Many vets are versed in state-of-the art dental procedures and are excited to provide these services to horses. Although it is illegal in most states for a non-veterinarian to perform dental procedures on horses, it is not uncommon for equine dentists to exist outside the veterinary profession. Many such persons work in collaboration with a local veterinarian, thus enabling the use of sedatives and anesthetics when necessary. If a horse is insured for mortality, major medical, or surgery, and any procedure that has not been performed by or under the auspices of a licensed veterinarian goes wrong, the insurance company is fully within its rights to deny coverage. Check with the state's veterinary association regarding the legalities of equine dentistry in a local area, and obtain recommendations naming veterinarians who are equipped and willing to perform elaborate dental procedures.

What an Equine Dentist Can Do

The most routine dental procedure performed on a horse every 6 to 12 months is called *floating* (photo 11.14). This technique involves the filing away of sharp enamel points on the

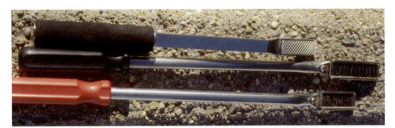

11.14 Hand tools, such as dental floats (files), are instrumental in smoothing sharp points on the cheek teeth. Power floats are also available to do this work.

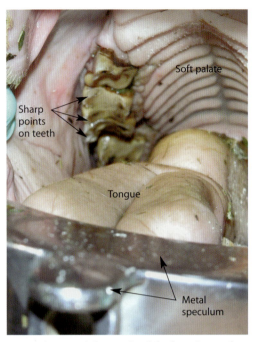

11.15 A view of the inside of the horse's mouth illustrates how sharp cheek teeth points and hooks can become. Their presence can create ulcers and pain along the sides of the cheeks, thereby limiting how well a horse grinds his food.

outer edges of the upper cheek teeth and the inner edges of the lower cheek teeth (photo 11.15). The arcades are leveled so that optimal contact is made between cheek teeth when chewing. The forward most upper premolar can be beveled or rounded to provide a comfortable *bit seat*. If hooks are present that result from a partial lack of occlusion of the cheek teeth, these hooks are also removed. They most commonly occur on the second premolar, rear upper molar, and on the rear aspect of the lower molars.

Many horses tolerate this floating procedure fairly well as it involves no pain, only an odd vibrating sensation within the mouth (photo 11.16). For an extremely thorough examination to be done on the oral cavity, a veterinarian should sedate the horse. This allows study of each tooth, and steadies the horse sufficiently so careful attention can be paid when sculpting the teeth, with minimal danger to the handler and the vet.

Prevention Is the Best Medicine

These are examples of some of the things that can go on inside a horse's warm, fuzzy muzzle. It is easy to put aside attention to those things that are out of sight, and therefore out of mind. Just because you can't "see" the inside of your horse's mouth doesn't mean that it is incapable of change. Just because a horse received

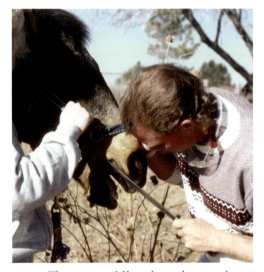

11.16 The process of filing down sharp tooth edges with hand floats is usually well tolerated by most horses, especially with the use of a light sedative to relax the horse.

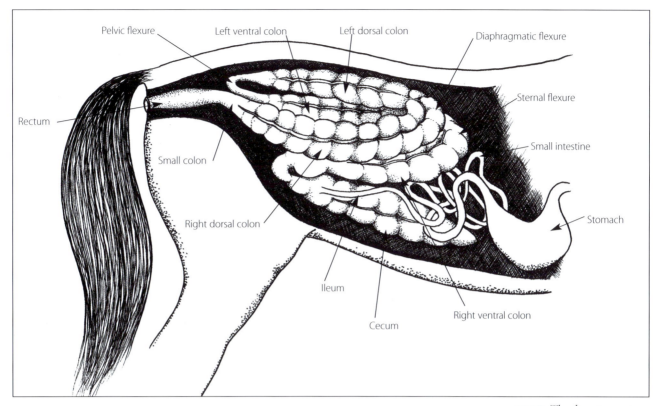

11.17 *The digestive system.*

dental work a couple years ago doesn't mean that all is well within his mouth today. Incorporate routine dental health and maintenance in a horse's preventive health program at least twice a year. It will be money well spent in keeping a horse healthy into his geriatric years and will improve his feed efficiency significantly. And, a horse with a happy mouth is better able to give his best performance.

Intestinal Anatomy: Structure and Function

Normal bowel activity creates intestinal noise that is audible on both sides of the flanks, and under the belly just behind the girth. A horse's *gastrointestinal* (GI) *tract* (fig. 11.17) can be divided into three main parts:

1. The stomach
2. The small intestines (SI)
3. The large intestines (LI)

Feed is processed differently in these three portions of the bowel, with the bulk of the active digestive process occurring in the large intestines. When empty, the total intestinal tract accounts for 5 percent of a horse's body weight. Yet, when fed and full, the digestive tract contains at least 50 gallons of fluid.

The Stomach

The stomach of a horse is quite small: a 1000-pound horse has a stomach that approximates the size of the stomach of a large man. A horse's stomach accounts for just 7 percent of the weight of the digestive tract, and its capacity approximates 4 gallons. Unlike dogs, cats, or people, horses are unable to vomit or burp to relieve building pressure in the stomach. The top half of the esophagus of a horse is skeletal muscle, capable of expulsive contractions, while the bottom half is smooth muscle. Yet an anatomical anomaly prevents regurgitation: at the point where the esophagus joins the stomach, an effective one-way valve, or sphincter, has enough tone to prevent regurgitation of material out of the stomach back up the esophagus.

The Small Intestines

Being long and large in size and volume, the small intestines of a 1000-pound horse extend about 70 feet in length and account for one-third of the weight of the digestive system. The small intestine regulates passage of *ingesta* (food material) into the cecum and prevents backflow of gas from the cecum. Feed moves rapidly (as compared to the rest of the digestive process) through the small intestines, taking only 3 to 4 hours to be admitted into the cecum's fermentation chamber. Two-thirds of all protein digestion and absorption occurs in the small intestines. It is also here that many electrolytes (potassium and chloride especially) are reabsorbed into the bloodstream. The small intestines mostly secrete water rather than absorb it. And, as will be discussed, grain is digested in the small intestines in a less efficient process than the digestion of roughage in the large intestines.

The Large Intestines

The bulk of digestive action important to the horse occurs in the large intestines (*hindgut*) that consist of four compartments that loop throughout the horse's abdominal cavity: the cecum, the dorsal colon, the ventral colon, and the small colon. The cecum and colon comprise two-thirds of the empty weight of the equine digestive tract.

A horse's intestinal tract is like a fermentation vat, capable of processing fiber and cellulose due to the bacteria and protozoa within it. In the horse, fermentation occurs behind the small intestine in portions of the large intestine, namely the cecum and large colon. Bacteria process proteins, carbohydrates, and cellulose into nutrients that are absorbed along with fluids. Microbes that live in the large colon are responsible for digesting soluble carbohydrates that come from roughage, as well as insoluble carbohydrates that are broken down from cellulose of plant material. More than 50 percent of the soluble carbohydrates in a horse's ration are digested within the large intestines.

Horses generate about 100 to 150 gallons of carbon dioxide and methane per day in this fermentation process. Cellulose breakdown by bacteria produces large volumes of gas that have no escape through the esophagus, and must travel hundreds of feet through the intestinal loops to the rectum. Gas expulsion through the rectum is a normal and expected consequence of normally functioning intestines. Any situation that inhibits intestinal motility may create excessive gas accumulation in the large intestines.

Within the large intestine near the *pelvic flexure,* is a regulator that coordinates muscle movement of the intestines and the progression of ingesta (food material) through the various loops of bowel. Large particles may be delayed for up to 72 hours to allow bacterial digestion to degrade fiber into fuels. At the same time, more easily digested foodstuffs and gases are propelled toward the rectum for elimination.

Most of the digestion of both soluble and insoluble carbohydrates in the LI generates *volatile fatty acids* (VFAs) that are important energy sources for the horse (see p. 140), especially when engaged in exercise of long duration. Volatile fatty acids accommodate as much as a third of a horse's energy needs. What is especially notable about the large intestines is the ability to reabsorb fluids, with as much as 40 percent of a horse's body weight reabsorbed from the LI every 24 hours. Also, large amounts of electrolytes are absorbed through this portion of the bowel. Under normal feeding conditions, the large intestines work at 95 percent efficiency to reabsorb fluids and electrolytes present in the bowel.

THE LARGE AND SMALL COLON

The large colon has five segments. At several junction points where the segments anatomically blend into one another, the diameter of the bowel abruptly decreases. It is at these points of stricture that ingesta or foreign bodies can cause an obstruction, and prevent normal outflow of gas and materials. The small colon has a similar function to the large colon, but it is smaller. Within the small colon, the ingesta become smaller as the feces are prepared to pass from the body.

All segments of the intestine are interrelated by allowing normal function of the other parts to continue. Consistent waves of contractions (*peristalsis*) and a healthy blood supply to and from the intestines are vital to a horse's overall intestinal well-being. Interruptions in either of these features can set off a series of events that result in digestive disorders.

Intestinal Transit

Feed material is retained in the large intestines for longer periods than occurs in the stomach or small intestines. The stomach empties quite rapidly, within a few hours, sending its macerated contents to the small intestines. Consumed roughage moves quickly from the stomach to the SI, while concentrated feed (grain, pellets) remains in the stomach for longer. Small intestinal transit takes from 3 to 20 hours. Large intestinal transit requires 50 hours. So in effect, the roughage a horse eats today will be passed as manure in about three days.

One of the most potent stimulators of intestinal motility is the act of feeding. Contrary to logic, the greater the intestinal motility, the slower the movement of ingesta down the intestinal tubes. About 75 percent of intestinal contractions within the LI resist movement of food through the colon. Intestinal contractions promote mixing and increased resistance to flow; this enables maximum absorptive efficiency in the large colon. Because of this, *auscultation* (listening with a stethoscope) of the abdomen can be misleading and does not correlate exactly with progressive movement of ingesta. However, lack of intestinal sounds is associated with abnormal motility, which can promote overgrowth of bacterial flora and a change in the pH of the bowel to a more acid environment. This elicits dying off of Gram-negative bacteria that have a cell wall composed of *endotoxin*. Too much endotoxin release through a sluggish bowel causes its absorption into the circulation to result in poisoning of the body with endotoxin. (Adverse effects of endotoxin are discussed on p. 317.)

Digestive Tract Disease

Diarrhea

Inflammatory conditions of the large intestine can lead to diarrhea, as can poor dentition (see photo 11.4, p. 284). The performance of an equine athlete suffers from diarrhea because of loss of valuable electrolytes and fluids in the feces. Persistent diarrhea also leads to weight loss or colic. With careful management practices, many cases of diarrhea in the mature horse can be quickly resolved.

Most diarrhea situations are a result of malfunction of the large intestines. Increased intestinal motility slows movement of ingesta through the tract, which is desirable to some degree so fluids, electrolytes, protein, and energy can be adequately absorbed. Diarrhea is associated with a flaccid colon, allowing more volume and fluid of contents to move quickly through the "open pipe." Inflammation of the lining of the large intestines contributes to diarrhea by interference with the absorptive capabilities of the LI and by stimulating over-secretion from inflammatory mediators. And, endotoxin circulation also elicits diarrhea by its inflammatory effects.

CAUSES OF DIARRHEA

Poor Dental Care
Poor tooth care is a common case of diarrhea, especially in older horses. If feed is not properly ground, it irritates and inflames the intestine. (For more information refer to "The Importance of Dental Health," p. 281.)

Bowel Fermentation
A horse that is fed an abnormally high grain ration or moldy food may develop diarrhea due to excess fermentation of bacteria in the bowel. Bacterial endotoxin or fungi from the food can inflame the bowel. An inflamed bowel cannot absorb nutrients, water, and electrolytes, so they are lost through the feces. Feeding at least half of the ration as roughage facilitates normal intestinal function. Discard all spoiled feed (see "Botulism," p. 525, and "Moldy Corn Poisoning," p. 527, chapter 17, *The Neurologic System in Health and Disease*).

Nervousness
A nervous horse, or a horse verging on exhaustion may have temporary diarrhea due to changes in intestinal activity. These horses may benefit from electrolyte supplements during transport or competition. It is equally important that they have frequent access to fresh water to restore fluid losses.

Parasites
Infectious organisms also contribute to diarrhea in horses. Parasite infestation of the intestines creates inflammation in the intestinal lining, the intestinal blood vessels, and the abdominal cavity. A heavily parasitized horse often has loose stools along with an unthrifty appearance and a loss of performance. (For more discussion, see "Internal Parasites and Control" in chapter 15, *Preventive and Mental Horse Health*, p. 459.)

Other Causes
Coarse food or chronic sand ingestion creates irritation that lead to diarrhea. Regular tooth care, premium hay quality, and keeping feed off sandy soil are ways to eliminate these sources.

Intestinal bacterial (*Salmonella* spp., *Clostridium dificile*, *E. coli*, as examples) and viral organisms infrequently infect adult horses and lead to diarrhea. Often there is a concurrent problem such as disease or stress that allows overgrowth of intestinal bacteria. A veterinarian should evaluate such ailments so effective treatment targets the source of an illness.

Liver disease, intestinal cancer, heart failure, and poisoning by medications, plants, or heavy metals are rare causes of diarrhea.

Potomac Horse Fever
A potentially fatal diarrhea disease that is a concern to horses is *Potomac Horse Fever* caused by *Ehrlichia risticii*. Its mode of transmission is still being defined. Previously, it was thought that the vector for Potomac Horse Fever could be a biting insect, possibly a tick. Current thinking is that the organism respon-

sible for transmitting this disease is an infected fluke worm that develops in freshwater snails found near lakes and standing water. The fluke is a transporter for the infectious agent into insect larvae of the caddis fly, mayfly, and various flying insects. Horses accidentally ingest the flies that land in water or feed; then, the organism is able to directly infect a horse's digestive tract. Bats also have a mature phase of a fluke life cycle; the bat discharges fluke eggs while flying across water, and then the eggs enter the snail to complete the life cycle. Horses that live near water sources, such as a pond, river, or stream, are most at risk for contracting Potomac Horse Fever. However, the flies can travel, contaminating feed or grain. Then they are able to infect horses that are not located where there is a direct source of water. The disease does not seem to be transmitted directly between horses. Most cases occur in late spring, summer, and early fall.

Horses infected with this disease rapidly develop severe diarrhea, accompanied by fever and depression, dehydration, and colic. If not treated promptly with the appropriate antibiotic and supportive care, complications of severe laminitis may develop or the horse may lapse into shock from dehydration, and die.

A vaccine has been available to protect horses against this disease but it is currently thought that the vaccine has limited efficacy. Two intramuscular injections are given, 3 to 4 weeks apart.

Choke

Horses can choke on their food, but rather than an obstruction blocking the airway as in people, food is lodged somewhere along the esophagus, making it impossible for any food to pass to the stomach. Upon first impression, a choked horse suddenly turns away from his food and stops eating, acting as if he is colicky.

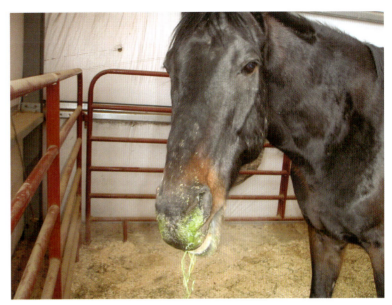

11.18 *A horse with choke often has green-tinged saliva mixed with feed streaming from one or both nostrils. A choked horse cannot swallow food due to an obstruction in the esophagus. This is a true emergency since there is a potential for him to inhale this material into the lungs, resulting in pneumonia.*

Initially, a choked horse appears distressed and agitated. He stretches his neck to relieve the pressure, or paws, sweats, or rolls on the ground, similar to what might be seen with colic. Saliva foams from the mouth, but with a choke there is a greenish froth coming from the nostrils, often accompanied by gagging and coughing (photo 11.18).

PROBLEMS ASSOCIATED WITH CHOKE

Aspiration Pneumonia

Choke is a true emergency, requiring immediate veterinary attention. Food, mucus, and saliva that are regurgitated from the mouth and nostrils may be inhaled into the lungs as a horse struggles to relieve the esophageal obstruction. Material inhaled into the lungs and airways leads to an *aspiration pneumonia*.

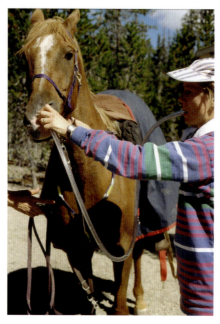

11.19 *One method a veterinarian uses to relieve choke is by passing a nasogastric tube to methodically remove the food impaction in the esophagus. Passage of a nasogastric tube is also used to medicate a horse with colic (see p. 302).*

Electrolyte and Fluid Loss

A choked horse suffers serious electrolyte imbalances, as well as dehydration. Not only does an esophageal obstruction prevent drinking, but also the horse loses saliva as he drools from the mouth. Saliva contains large quantities of sodium and chloride, and is essential for recycling these salts through the intestinal tract where they are reabsorbed by the body. A horse experiencing a prolonged episode of choke is unable to swallow the saliva, and needs intravenous fluids and electrolytes.

TREATING CHOKE

With immediate veterinary attention, the majority of chokes are easily resolved without complications. While awaiting a veterinarian, it is helpful to place the horse on an incline with the head facing downhill. Such a small change in position helps drain regurgitated material out of the mouth and nose and lessens the chances of it being inhaled into the airways. Remain calm and talk soothingly to help control the horse's anxiety. If the ball of lodged food is visible on the left side of the neck as a bulge, very gentle massage may help break it down.

Sedatives administered by a veterinarian position the head and neck downward, while sedatives and oxytocin relax muscles that spasm around the food mass. A stomach tube is passed into the esophagus to the level of the obstruction, and a gentle stream of water breaks it up (photo 11.19). Nonsteroidal anti-inflammatory (NSAIDs) drugs minimize scar tissue formation once the obstruction is dissolved. Broad-spectrum antibiotics prevent infection of the esophageal lining and protect against aspiration pneumonia.

FEEDING AFTER A CHOKE CRISIS

Following a choke crisis, management strategies are essential. Withhold food from a sedated horse until he is fully recovered, because both the cough reflex and swallowing apparatus are depressed under the influence of sedatives. In some cases, it is necessary to entirely withhold food for the first 24 to 48 hours. For a horse to safely swallow food, it must be adequately chewed and softened liberally with saliva. Presoaking pellets in ample water for 20 to 30 minutes breaks apart and softens them. A gruel slips easily down an irritated esophagus, allowing the esophagus to heal, and inflammation to subside. When it is safe for the horse to eat again, feed the gruel in small amounts, several times daily for up to two weeks after the episode. During this time, a horse is highly susceptible to a recurrent episode of choke, so care must be taken to remove all coarse or dry feed from the diet.

PREVENTING CHOKE

Implementing certain management procedures prevents choke, or prevents a reoccurrence in a previously choked horse. Most chokes are caused by large pelleted concentrate, or by coarse hay. These feeds are easily eliminated from the diet. If pellets are fed, they should be the small variety. Dental problems may cause a horse to swallow food before it is chewed properly. Teeth should be checked and floated regularly. Grass pasture and hay cubes rarely cause choke; however, competition with herd-mates may make a horse bolt his feed. Such a horse should be separated at feeding time to encourage him to eat slowly. If a greedy horse seems to "inhale" grain or pellets, place smooth rocks (2 inch minimum size) in the feed tub with the concentrate. The rocks slow intake because the horse must rummage around them.

Inadequate water intake can result in choke. Drinking plenty of fresh water ensures ample saliva, and adequate water for intestinal digestion. During transport, it is important for a horse to drink enough to limit dehydration. Some horses stressed by trailering may snatch and gobble hay or grain. It is best to withhold feed from anxious horses.

Introduction of new or palatable bedding materials, such as straw or wood shavings, should be monitored carefully to ensure a horse does not eat them.

Some instances of choke are unpreventable if caused by tumors, space-occupying abscesses, or scar tissue from an old injury. These problems decrease the functional diameter of the esophagus. A veterinarian can diagnose these problems with an endoscope, or by contrast radiography that injects radio-opaque dye into the esophagus, followed by X-ray films of the area.

Colic

Colic is not a disease in itself, but rather it is the word used to describe abdominal pain. It is a symptom indicating a digestive disorder. Colic must be differentiated from other problems not directly related to the gastrointestinal tract. Examples of pain related to non-intestinal causes include:

- Ovulation (see p. 538)
- Foaling (see p. 557)
- Tying-up syndrome (see p. 166)
- Bladder stones
- Laminitis (see p. 74)
- Fever (see p. 429)

The horse has a unique intestinal system. The distinctive anatomy of the intestines predisposes to a variety of syndromes that cause pain. Pain of colic is a result of excess tension or stretching of the bowel lining (*mesentery*) that serves as a supportive sling of the intestines within the abdomen. Spasms of the bowel lining, due to irritation or a decrease in blood supply, also result in pain.

The incidence of colic in the horse population of the United States is 4.2 colic events per 100 horses each year. Of these, 1.4 percent went to surgery, and 11 percent of all colic events ended with a fatal outcome. Colic has financial and emotional impacts on a horse owner so any strategies that minimize colic risk are of benefit to horse and owner.

SIGNS TO WATCH FOR

Sensitivity to a horse's changing mood can detect subtle and early stages of colic. Rather than waiting for a horse to exhibit marked signs of pain, a veterinarian should be summoned immediately upon finding a horse that is depressed (photo 11.20), off feed, or lying down at odd times, or in odd postures. Obvious or persistent expression of pain by a horse affirms a need for veterinary help.

A colicky horse may paw the ground, kick or bite at his belly, roll his upper lip (*flehmen*), yawn repeatedly, or grind his teeth (photos 11.21 and 11.22). He may stretch as if to urinate, yet discomfort in his abdomen prevents him from applying an abdominal press to empty his bladder. As pain progresses, a horse may lie down, get up, only to lie down again to

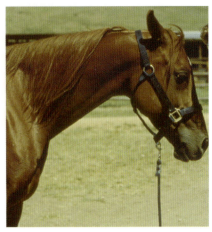

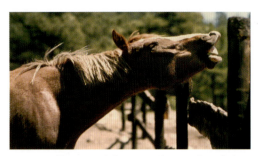

11.21 *Rolling up of the upper lip is referred to as flehmen, a behavior a horse exhibits when he smells an interesting odor; this is also a behavior displayed with abdominal discomfort and colic.*

11.20 *A horse that displays signs of depression and/or a lack of appetite may be showing early stages of colic.*

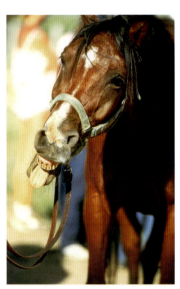

11.22 *Another typical colic sign is when a horse yawns repeatedly.*

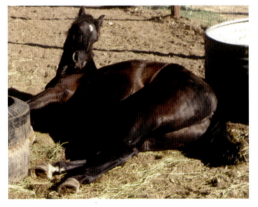

11.23 *A horse that persists in lying down may not be feeling well, or may be showing early signs of colic. Intermittent turning toward and looking at one or both sides of his abdomen is typical behavior of a horse with abdominal pain.*

relieve the agony in his belly (photo 11.23). Vigorous rolling on the ground, self-inflicted trauma, or a soaking sweat are signals of severe distress (photo 11.24). Prompt recognition of a problem, with immediate administration of medical therapy, can often correct a colic crisis before it turns into a surgical condition.

INTERPRETING A HORSE'S PAIN

While waiting for medical help to arrive, there are a few things that help a horse ignore his discomfort. In initial stages of colic, trotting a horse on a longe line for 10 or 15 minutes may relieve the crisis if it is a gaseous or spasmodic episode. The trotting horse may pass gas; following this brief exercise, the crisis may abate. If the horse is still painful after trying this strategy, a horse in mild pain should be allowed to rest quietly if he will do so, either standing or lying down. In the old days, horse owners thought there was value in walking a bellyaching horse for hours. In fact, prolonged forced movement can be counterproductive: walking or trotting a horse for lengthy periods saps valuable energy reserves needed to combat the crisis, for both horse and owner, except in the situation described on p. 299.

Although each horse has a different threshold in response to pain, intestinal pain is overbearing to any individual, making symptoms and mental attitude valuable diagnostic aids. If a mildly painful colic persists for more than 8 to 12 hours, or if it recurs intermittently during that time, or if intravenous fluids and pain-relieving medications are not correcting the problem, it is probably time for surgery. If a horse has experienced

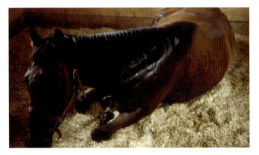

11.24 *Colic pain often causes a horse to sweat heavily, as seen here with this recumbent horse.*

repeated episodes of colic with no specific diagnosis attained, it may be time for exploratory surgery of the abdomen to identify the source of a recurrent problem. Severe or unrelenting pain despite the presence of pain-relieving medications makes a strong argument for the need for surgery.

A horse in colic distress is sometimes difficult to handle as he throws himself to the ground, rolling violently in an effort to relieve his plight. Such a horse may require forced walking to keep him distracted and somewhat controlled until help arrives. Due to the unpredictability and uncontrollable nature of an extremely violent colic, stay as clear of the horse as possible. Be attentive to the danger of being wedged in a stall corner with the horse. Get him on his feet if feasible, and move him to a large area or grassy spot where he is least likely to inflict injury to himself and people.

VITAL SIGNS

Some physical exam parameters can be monitored throughout a colic ordeal. The horse's degree of pain and mental attitude are noted. Rectal temperature, respiratory rate and character, heart rate, pulse rate and its strength are obtained. Color and capillary refill time of mucous membranes are carefully assessed (see below). Moistness of mucous membranes and skin elasticity provide a rough estimate of dehydration. Quality and frequency of intestinal sounds in all quadrants are evaluated by listening with a stethoscope.

Of these parameters, each is important to the overall clinical picture. With practice, you can learn to examine a horse and recognize when signs differ from those found when a horse is in a normal state. A study conducted by the Morris Animal Foundation concluded that color of the mucous membranes has a significant relationship to survival. Because mucous membrane color and capillary refill time reflect blood perfusion through the body, they correlate well to development and progression of shock. Shock is closely associated with surgical colic syndromes, such as strangulating obstructions of the bowel or very serious "simple" obstructions. (For a complete list of vital signs, see "Normal Physiological Parameters," *Appendix A*, p. 567).

Mucous Membranes

A pink color to the mucous membranes of the gums, sclera of the eye, or of the vulvar lips of a mare is an encouraging sign. As fingertip pressure on the membranes blanches away the color, capillary refill time should be less than or equal to 2 seconds (photos 11.25 A & B). Pale membranes with slow refill time indicate inadequate cardiovascular circulation that may precede development of *shock*. (Shock is a profound depression of the body's vital processes as a result of reduced blood

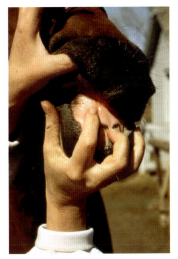

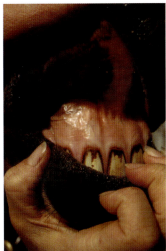

11.25 A & B One measure of the status of blood circulation is to evaluate mucous membrane color and the capillary refill time. This is done by blanching the gums with a fingertip and measuring how quickly the color returns. Mucous membranes should begin pink in color and color should return after blanching within 2 seconds.

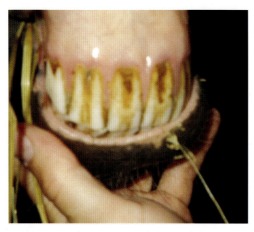

11.26 *A purple tinge around the tooth line, called* margination, *indicates endotoxic effects related to intestinal stasis and colic.*

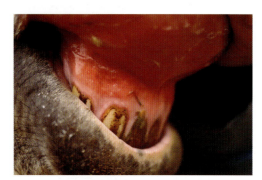

11.27 *Brick-red membranes with rapid refill time of less than 1 second reflect shock from dehydration, and bacterial or endotoxin circulation.*

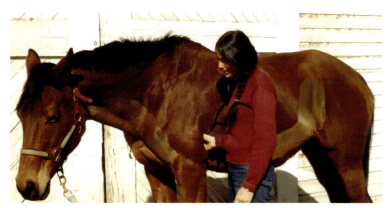

11.28 *The heart rate is most easily listened to with the bell of a stethoscope held on the body wall, just behind and at the level of the left elbow.*

volume and pressure.) A purple tinge around the tooth line, called *margination*, indicates endotoxic effects that may as yet be mild but in need of treatment (photo 11.26). Brick-red membranes with rapid refill time of less than one second reflect shock from dehydration, and bacterial or endotoxin circulation (photo 11.27). Horses in shock require rapid anti-shock therapy with drugs, intravenous fluids, and surgery. Blue or purple membranes foretell severe, irreversible shock with a grave prognosis. Horses in a state of advanced shock should be euthanized to ease them from their misery, as they will not likely survive anesthesia or surgery.

Heart Rate

The heart rate can be heard best through a stethoscope held on the body wall, just behind the elbow (photo 11.28). Elevated heart rates of less than 60 beats per minute (bpm) reflect pain. (Normal equine heart rate is 30 to 40 bpm.) If a heart rate persists between 60 to 80 bpm for more than 10 or 15 minutes, a horse may be severely dehydrated or in beginning stages of shock. A heart rate greater than 80 bpm implies a horse in shock and in immediate need of surgical intervention, if possible. Survival rates on these high heart-rate cases are about 25 percent. Heart rates over 100 bpm are associated with a grave prognosis and a very low survival rate of less than 10 percent. Peripheral pulse rate and character, taken under the jaw, should be the same as heart rate, and it should be bounding and strong.

Respiratory Rate

The respiratory rate in a normal horse ranges from 12 to 24 breaths per minute, depending on the ambient temperature. Rapid and shallow breathing may correspond to pain, fever, or severe alterations in metabolic status of the horse.

The Digestive System: The Oral Cavity, Dental Care, and the Intestinal Tract

Rectal Temperature

Normal rectal temperature of an adult horse ranges between 97 and 101° F (36 to 38° C). A fever may reflect endotoxemia, severe dehydration, or a septic condition within the abdomen or thorax. A low body temperature accompanied by cold and clammy limbs, and a cold muzzle signifies shock.

Intestinal Sounds

With a stethoscope, intestinal sounds are listened to on the upper and lower areas on both sides of the flank (photo 11.29 and fig. 11.30). Ideally, at least two *borborygmi* (waves of intestinal contractions) can be heard each minute over each quadrant. If no sounds are heard, corrective measures are needed to restore normal motility to the bowel. Gas in the bowel sounds similar to the tinkle of a pebble falling down a well. Squeaking noises indicate an attempt at peristaltic contractions with no progressive movement of material through the bowel. An excess amount of intestinal noise may indicate spasms or hyperactivity due to irritation in the bowel, or efforts to correct an obstruction. Sometimes it is possible to "hear" the movement of sand by placing a stethoscope on the abdominal midline at the level of the girth, near the sternum. Sounds heard are similar to the sound of roiling surf on a sandy beach, or sand moving in a paper bag.

OTHER VETERINARY DIAGNOSTIC TOOLS

Rectal Examination

A veterinarian will evaluate all these physical parameters upon arrival. To further assist in a diagnosis of what is causing the colic, a vet will perform a rectal examination. This procedure entails a careful, systematic palpation of segments of bowel for position, tone, and contents of each accessible loop of intestine. Gas-distended intestines may point to a surgical

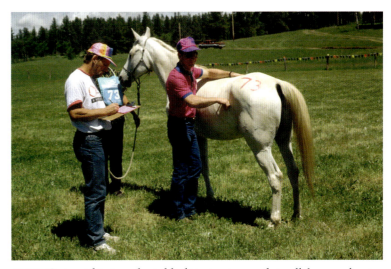

11.29 Gut motility is evaluated by listening to sounds in all four quadrants of both sides of the flanks. Here, the veterinarian is listening to the upper left quadrant in the area of the small intestines. Sounds in the lower left quadrant are heard from activity in the large colon.

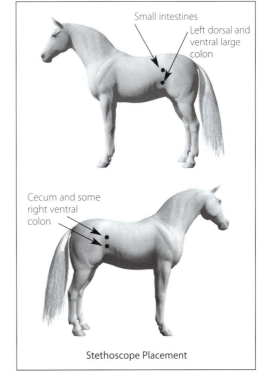

Stethoscope Placement

11.30 Placement of the stethoscope on each of these four quadrants in the flanks enables assessment of intestinal sounds representative of progressive motility. Both locations on the right side refer to the cecum, while on the left side, a stethoscope placed in the general location of the upper left dot will hear noises of the small intestine, and over the lower dot will hear noises of the large colon.

condition, particularly if loops of small intestine are abnormally distended. Displacement of portions of the large colon may be felt. Presence or absence of feces in the rectum is noted.

Manure, if present, is examined for information. Are the fecal balls of normal size and consistency, or are they firm or dry indicating dehydration? Are the feces coated with mucus, indicating gut stagnation (see photo 9.12, p. 237)? Is the manure soft or a diarrhea consistency? An easy check for sand in the manure can be done by placing 6 fecal balls in a plastic glove and adding water. If more than 1 teaspoon of sand settles out, that is significant. If no sand is found in that sample, that doesn't mean there isn't any. It is common to see sanded horses have intermittent diarrhea or soft stools (see "Sand Colic," p. 310).

If gas-distended loops of intestine are felt on rectal exam, if a displacement is obvious, or an impaction is found, a veterinarian can make a definitive diagnosis. The original cause may remain elusive, but the anatomical problem can be defined. Coupling the findings of a rectal exam with cardiovascular parameters and lack or presence of intestinal activity provides a vet with concrete information regarding the need for aggressive medical treatment or surgery.

Stomach Tube

With all data gathered thus far, the vet passes a nasogastric tube into the stomach (see photo 11.19, p. 296). Smooth muscle lining the bottom half of the esophagus does not allow a horse to burp or vomit, so large quantities of gas or fluid can accumulate within the stomach, contributing to pain and cardiovascular compromise. A stomach tube allows an avenue for escape of painful gas and fluid pressures in the stomach. This improves blood flow through distended bowel and to the heart.

Copious quantities of fluid (more than 2 to 4 liters) drained through a stomach tube indicate stagnation or obstruction of the small intestine, possibly (but not always) representative of a surgical condition. Not only does a stomach tube provide valuable diagnostic information, but it is also a means to administer intestinal protectants, laxatives, fluids, and electrolytes. Based on the presence of intestinal motility, the vet will decide if it is safe to administer something by stomach tube. What to give is determined from specific rectal exam findings and the thorough physical exam.

Belly Tap

If a horse poses a questionable surgical case, a vet may obtain a sample of *peritoneal fluid* by inserting a needle into the abdominal cavity. An *abdominocentesis* is a relatively painless procedure, a horse only responding to the needle prick as it passes through the skin. Examination of peritoneal fluid is not always a reliable test for a decision for surgery, but if the color is abnormal or the protein content of the peritoneal fluid is high, then surgery is indicated. Straw-colored peritoneal fluid is normal, whereas pink or orange peritoneal fluid signifies devitalization of an intestinal segment and the need for surgery or euthanasia (photo 11.31).

Abdominal Ultrasound

This is another diagnostic tool useful to determine position and content of intestinal parts, and to look for displacements of bowel that might necessitate surgery.

Undetermined Diagnosis

In three-quarters of all colic cases, a definite diagnosis is not achieved. Continual observation and monitoring of a horse with an unspecified source of colic by both owner and veterinarian is essential until the horse either responds to medical therapy, or a decision is made to go to surgery.

TYPES OF COLIC

Spasmodic Colic

Spasmodic colic is due to spasms of the smooth muscle of the intestines. Nervousness and excitability, sometimes induced by sudden weather or barometric pressure changes, may result in spasmodic colic. Stress from transport or athletic competition can upset normal nerve impulses to the intestine and alter intestinal movement. Toxic plants (see p. 320), or blister beetles in alfalfa hay (see p. 321), are exceedingly irritating to the intestines and can be fatal. Certain drugs such as *organophosphate dewormers* overstimulate intestinal motility with resulting spasmodic pain.

Severe changes in intestinal movement may cause a segment of bowel to telescope into an adjacent segment, called an *intussusception*. Without surgical intervention, an intussusception effectively acts as an obstruction, and the condition of the horse rapidly deteriorates with development of gangrene and bowel *necrosis* (tissue death).

Impaction Colic

On the flip side of too much fluid and water loss through the intestines with diarrhea, intestinal contents become overly dried out when intestinal motility is too sluggish or if there is insufficient intestinal water. This occurs with dehydration, from electrolyte imbalances that affect gut motility, or with an intestinal obstruction that prevents movement of ingesta through the bowel, leading to desiccation of the material.

Signs and Symptoms of Impaction Colic

Transit of feed through the large colon takes several days so what passes as manure today was ingested as hay or pasture at least three days ago. An impaction may take days to form and to reveal itself as a problem. It is not until a horse feels abdominal tension that he will feel discomfort and alert you to it.

When pain does develop, it usually starts out as mild and intermittent. An affected horse may at first appear depressed. He may look at his flank, may paw, stretch, kick at his belly, flehmen, or spend a bit of time lying down. He may still nibble at food, but tends to be more finicky about what he eats. One tip-off of brewing trouble is when manure production is scant or absent, although a horse with an impaction of the cecum may continue to pass manure. Any feces that pass are dry and diminishing in quantity. The feces of a stagnant bowel may be coated with mucus and fibrin strands in the body's attempt to lubricate dehydrated fecal material for passage. (A normal horse will pass at least 8 to 12 bowel movements in a 24-hour period.)

With an early-detected, simple obstruction, the horse's heart rate, temperature, and other vital signs are usually within normal limits, but the respiratory rate may accelerate related to the degree of pain (see *Appendix A*, p. 567, for normal vital signs). The body's attempt to correct the blockage may create a *hypermotile gut* with active and noisy intestinal sounds in an attempt to squeeze the impaction through the bowel. These gut sounds can be misleading since not all intestinal activity results in progressive movement of material down the tract.

As a horse's status deteriorates with an unrelieved impaction, there will be increasing distention and pressure on the bowel, lessened blood flow to the intestinal lining, and resulting degeneration of the lining. There may be a possible link of colon displacement to a preceding impaction.

How an Impaction Forms

Large colon impactions occur in 8 to 10 percent of all colic conditions. As food traverses the digestive tract, it enters several segments of

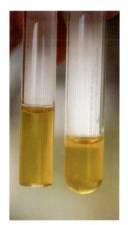

11.31 *Normal peritoneal fluid obtained from an abdominal belly tap is straw-colored and relatively clear with no sediment, as seen in the samples in these vials.*

large colon that narrow considerably before opening into a somewhat wider portion of intestine. Impaction may also develop in the cecum (less than 5 percent of all impactions) or in a portion of the small intestine leading into the cecum, called the *ileum* (see fig. 11.17, p. 291).

An important function of the large colon is to provide a reservoir from which fluids and electrolytes are absorbed. Normally each day, 30 to 40 gallons of fluid is secreted into the upper bowel, with about 90 percent of this efficiently reabsorbed in the cecum and large colon. High-fiber diets composed of strictly good quality hay have the advantage of increasing colonic water by at least 30 percent over diets that are comprised of grain products as well. Motility of the large colon is best stimulated by the volume of food and water introduced to the intestines. Delay or slowing of movement through the colon causes water to be absorbed out of the fecal contents.

There are many important mechanisms that contribute to intestinal transit, like viscosity of the food material, diameter of the "tube" through which ingesta flows, and pressures within the intestine that progressively propel materials toward the rectum while retaining them long enough to extract nutrients. In addition, offering a large meal only twice daily may interfere with activity of intestinal microbes that are responsible for efficient digestion of fiber.

Effects of Feeding Strategies on Intestinal Function

Twice-Daily Feeding

Feed intake is a major stimulus for gastrointestinal motility; fasting leads to GI hypomotility. There are times when fasting may be unavoidable or even desirable but management practices that mimic more natural conditions involve offering a horse the opportunity to have a continuous eating pattern. Horses evolved to graze small amounts of fiber-rich plants for 13 to 15 hours a day, and this style of eating avoids overfilling of the stomach. In today's fast-paced society, horse-keeping habits have altered to accommodate space and schedules. Not all horses have access to pasture, and not all horse owners can be present to feed small meals throughout the day.

Feeding large meals twice a day, particularly of grain, has profound effects on intestinal function. Horses that are fed a large grain meal twice a day experience a 15 percent reduction in plasma volume within 30 minutes of each meal. In contrast, there is no change in plasma volume in horses that are fed smaller amounts every few hours. Grain consumption reduces the amount of fiber in the diet, which decreases the water content of the colon and alters fermentation to produce more gas. Changes created by twice-daily feeding of grain set up conditions for extremes in fluid exchange in the colon, which can dehydrate ingested feed, potentially leading to impaction colic.

Water Needs for Digestion

For every pound of feed ingested, a horse needs 2 to 4 pints of water for digestion. Hence, a 1000-pound horse consuming 20 pounds of food each day needs a minimum of 7½ gallons (or 30 liters) of water to process feed material. This is the amount necessary solely for intestinal function; additional water is necessary for other bodily maintenance functions. Horses tend to drink when they eat; some even like to dunk their hay into water. A horse normally consumes 5 to 10 gallons of water each day in cool weather, and up to 20 gallons a day in hot weather.

Dehydration and electrolyte imbalances also contribute to GI hypomotility. Dehydration elicits drying of the colonic contents, and coupled with sluggish gut motility, there is a potential to develop an impaction. Inadequate intake of water for any reason causes dehydration and drying out of fecal contents. This may occur due to lack of water availability, or polluted or contaminated water. Frozen water or excessively cold water discourages drinking (see p. 345). In addition, dehydration occurs subsequent to protracted exercise, intense sweating, or hormonal changes that regulate body water balance.

Feed Type

Coarse feed materials or pelleted foods also require a lot of water for digestion, and have a potential to lead to impaction if water intake is restricted for any reason. Excessively dry or coarse feed can create an obstruction within the bowel, or it can irritate the bowel lining, causing diarrhea or constipation. Dental problems add further insult by interfering with adequate grinding of feed (see p. 284).

Feeding extra hay during cold weather generates internal heat as a by-product of fiber breakdown in the large colon (see p. 292). However, if a horse is not drinking enough, this practice compounds the problem by increasing intestinal bulk without adequate water to process it.

Consumption of Bedding

Shavings or straw bedding may seem palatable to a bored horse; these materials can form an impaction. A horse may consume bedding in excess to satisfy a fiber deficiency. Or, a horse may eat bedding when suddenly confined in a new environment for observation or rest from injury.

Life-Style Effects on Intestinal Function

Confinement or Limited Exercise

Events associated with the impaction can include recent management change within two weeks prior to signs, particularly when exercise is restricted due to a musculoskeletal injury. During cold or wet weather, horses used to being outdoors may be brought into a stall thereby restricting even low-level exercise.

One study reported that recent stall confinement was associated with 53.7 percent of impaction colic cases, while another study noted that 62.5 percent of colon impactions occurred within two weeks of significant management changes, such as stall confinement or transport. Confinement has multiple adverse effects on equine intestinal function. Stall-confined horses often experience inconsistencies in feeding intervals and amounts relative to their previous management habits. An owner may be unaware of the quality of hay that is fed in terms of its energy and protein content, yet there is a tendency to offer excess or high calorie feed to a bored, confined horse, a practice that is counterproductive to intestinal health. Any type of feed modification and diet change is incriminated in causing colic. During periods of confinement or transport, use of bran mashes or other diet alteration has not been proven to prevent impactions.

Exercise incurs multiple benefits by increasing metabolism and improving intestinal motility. Fiber digestibility increases by up to 20 percent in exercised horses, promoting greater retention of the fluid part of the diet and shortened retention of the more formed, particulate part of the feed. Progressive movement of particulate materials down the intestinal tract promotes efficient digestion while not allowing it to linger to form dehydrated intestinal contents.

Feeding During Rigorous Exercise

Yet, feeding in the period surrounding exercise is not without its own set of problems. Rigorous exercise just prior to feeding may decrease feed digestibility while blood remains shunted to working muscles, away from the intestinal tract. Strenuous exercise will shut down intestinal motility and feed should be restricted. However, during moderate or light aerobic exercise, forage can be fed safely if offered at intervals. Proper measures should be taken to adequately cool out a hot horse before feeding large meals, particularly grain.

Enteroliths

In certain geographic areas, most notably in California and the southwestern United States, horses that are fed high amounts of calcium and magnesium-rich and protein-rich hay such as alfalfa, may develop an intestinal "stone" known as an *enterolith* (photo 11.32). Such concretions of layers of salts develop around a small object like a speck of sand, a tiny pebble, or other ingested foreign material. High alkaline conditions in the intestines favor the formation of an enterolith, as does diminished motility in the large colon. Enteroliths can grow to obstructive sizes within the large colon, causing recurrent colic pain. In one-third of cases, intestinal rupture occurs as a result of pressure on the intestinal wall from the obstruction. Abdominal radiographs (X rays) of horses with chronic colic have identified 77 percent of enteroliths in the large colon and 42 percent in the small colon. Upon identification, these may be removed surgically before resulting in irresolvable consequences.

Although all breeds may develop enteroliths, for unknown reasons, Arabians, Morgans, American Saddlebreds, and American Miniature horses are reported with the highest incidence of enterolithiasis. Providing access to a high fiber diet and/or pasture, along with exercise are management strategies that reduce the risk of developing enteroliths. Elimination of alfalfa from the diet and monitoring of mineral content of the water are other means to reduce the risk. Some studies suggest that the feeding of apple cider vinegar may be helpful to achieve acidification of the bowel.

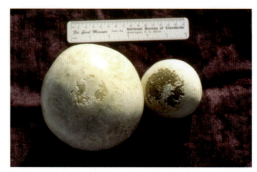

11.32 *An enterolith is an intestinal stone that forms from layers of mineralized salts that deposit around a small foreign body or grain of sand. These can grow to a large size, causing colic by putting pressure on the bowel and by acting as an obstruction to fecal flow. The larger enterolith seen here is about 4 inches by 5 inches, and the smaller one is half that size.*

Causes of Impaction Colic

Predominant Causes

Impaction colic can be caused by:

- Limited exercise
- Decreased water intake
- Coarse food
- Consumption of bedding or foreign materials
- Enteroliths
- Heavy parasite load (see p. 321)

Other Causes

A diet of coastal Bermuda grass (*Cynodon* spp.) common to the southeastern United States is known to elicit active intestinal contractions around a mass of feed, causing more water to be compressed out of the food material; this can lead to increased desiccation and firmness of the intestinal contents. Coastal Bermuda grass in its maturing state has a high, non-digestible, crude fiber content that increases its propensity to ileal impaction colic.

Overfeeding of indigestible material such as poor quality hay is thought to be a significant contributing factor to the development of an impaction. It is best to avoid mature grass or any feed composed of poorly digestible fiber.

Sand ingestion also has the potential to create an impaction, particularly in the right dorsal colon.

Tapeworm infestation has also been incriminated as a cause of ileal impaction.

Certain medications, such as phenylbutazone and flunixin meglumine, are often given to a horse for an injury or to reduce post-operative pain and swelling. Such nonsteroidal anti-inflammatory drugs (NSAIDs) may contribute to the risk of cecal impaction by diminishing smooth muscle contractility of the colon.

Significant orthopedic pain from hind limb injury or surgery is a risk factor in developing a cecal impaction. Activity of the sympathetic nervous system, such as results from pain, results in reduced GI motility; therefore pain should be controlled as best as possible.

Intestinal tumors or abscesses can mimic an impaction. The tumor or abscess pushes on the bowel lining, causing discomfort, or it reduces blood flow and alters normal intestinal motility, potentially leading to an impaction.

Effective Treatment of Impaction Colic

Prevention focuses on providing ample water, high quality feed, and exercise, and careful monitoring of character and quantity of bowel movements, water consumption, and a horse's general attitude. However, if an impaction forms, treatment objectives include pain relief, softening of the impacted feed material, and stimulation of intestinal motility to increase fecal transit. An effective strategy relies on overhydration of the horse with intravenous fluid therapy to add fluid to fecal contents. Overloading the blood vascular system with fluid increases secretion of intestinal water into the impaction to soften it, while also maintaining whole body hydration, and circulation to intestinal blood flow. IV fluid treatment may require 40 to 80 liters per day administered in an intravenous drip. Administration of laxatives or electrolyte-laced water by stomach tube is an additional useful strategy in many horses with impaction.

Pain-relieving medications, such as sedatives, elicit smooth muscle relaxation of the intestinal wall, thereby minimizing intestinal spasms around an impaction, and allowing gas and fluid to pass. The oscillations of a trailer ride also may be beneficial to evacuate gas and to stimulate intestinal motility.

It is important to stop a horse's food intake that might add to the size of an impaction. It may be necessary to apply a muzzle to prevent eating as he starts to feel better. Colon hydration is increased when fasted horses are fed hay. Although feeding may increase motility and oral water intake, a horse with an impaction should not be fed until there are obvious indications that the impaction is moving or is resolved. Only hay should be offered initially, without grain. Bran should also be avoided since it contains large amounts of carbohydrates, which reduces total fiber content with decrease of water content in the colon. The horse can be offered short periods grazing green grass, which is helpful by its laxative action and high water content. Care must be taken to avoid overconsumption of green grass as it is highly fermentable, and might contribute to gas distention of the bowel.

The majority of impaction colics respond to medical treatment. Although called a "simple" obstruction, some impactions may not be simply resolved with intense medical management or intravenous fluid therapy. Ongoing deterioration may necessitate surgical intervention due to a concurrent problem such as displacement of the intestinal loops or

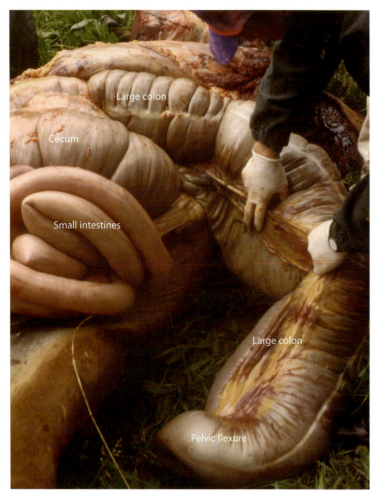

11.33 *A normal intestinal tract seen during a post-mortem exam on a horse that did not die due to colic. The entire bowel including the small intestines, cecum, and large colon is homogeneous in color and no twists or displacements are visible. The pelvic flexure has been removed from the abdomen and rests on the ground at the bottom of the picture. Photo: David Varra, DVM.*

bowel movements altogether is called an *ileus* (see p. 316). Fermentation continues, but gas does not move toward the rectum. As gas builds within the intestines, overdistention results in pain. Bacterial overgrowth occurs in the stagnant gut, and bacteria begin to die. The death of certain types of bacteria release endotoxins that can result in shock, laminitis, or death.

Building gas in a stagnant gut compromises the blood supply by exerting excess pressure and tension on the blood vessels. Portions of the bowel may be displaced as the segments balloon with gas and attempt to fully occupy the abdominal cavity. The left side of the large intestine normally floats freely in the abdomen with no supporting attachments to the body wall or other organs. The large intestine is therefore prone to great movement within the abdomen.

Intestinal Displacement or Torsion

A *displacement* refers to a colic that is associated with a loop or more of bowel that has moved into an inappropriate position. Many intestinal displacements will rectify themselves with medical treatment if bowel motility can be restored with intravenous fluids. In some instances, no matter how aggressive the therapy, the displaced bowel will go on to twist or become entrapped, necessitating surgical intervention.

Strangulation obstruction usually is accompanied by an acute and severe onset of pain. In these cases, *torsion* (large intestinal twist) or *volvulus* (small intestine rotates at least 360 degrees) involves twisting of a loop of bowel to completely block-off its blood supply (photos 11.33, 11.34, and 11.35). Another possible type of strangulation obstruction occurs if a piece of bowel is *incarcerated* (trapped) through an opening like a diaphragmatic hernia, an umbilical or scrotal hernia, or through a tear in the *mesentery* (a sheet of tissue that slings the intestines in the abdomen). An *intestinal lipoma* is a fatty tumor

compromise of bowel circulation. Obstruction of the large colon that persists for more than 24 hours may have an adverse effect on intestinal nerves, predisposing a horse to future impaction colic. Rapid identification and resolution of an impaction is key to a successful outcome.

Gaseous Colic

Any change in normal movement patterns in the intestines can cause problems. Cessation of

The Digestive System: The Oral Cavity, Dental Care, and the Intestinal Tract

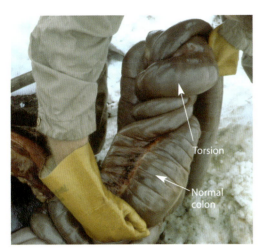

11.34 *One serious intestinal displacement involves a twisting of the large colon, referred to as torsion. Here the twisted portion is visible as a tightly coiled area at the top of the photo just below the person's left hand, while the normal large colon configuration rests beneath the person's right hand. This horse died due to impingement of blood supply and tissue death. Photo: David Varra, DVM.*

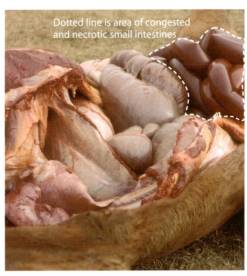

11.35 *A small intestinal twist that rotates at least 360 degrees is referred to as a volvulus, seen here as the dark congested portion of bowel in the far right-hand side of the photo. (The dead intestinal loops have a vague resemblance to sausage links.) A volvulus prevents blood flow to and from the small intestines, leading to swelling and blood congestion as seen here. The horse's head would be to the left and the tail to the right of this picture.*

on a stalk that may wrap around a portion of bowel, thereby strangulating it (see "Lipoma," below). The pelvic flexure (a portion of the large colon on the left side) can become entrapped behind the ligament of the splenic in a situation known as a *nephrosplenic entrapment*. A loop of bowel that telescopes inside itself is called an *intussusception*; blood supply is interrupted, and bowel begins to die.

Abnormal contractions, aided by gravity, may cause rotation of the intestine to result in an intestinal twist (intestinal torsion). Normally, the left side of the large colon is freely suspended in the abdomen. Gas distention coupled with abnormal peristaltic waves or an ileus can result in a displacement.

It is largely a myth that twisting of the intestines is a result of a horse rolling around in pain. Twisting can happen from rolling, but intestines can also twist in a standing horse with colic. Allow a colicky horse to lie quietly if he will, but prevent the horse from rolling so he does not hurt himself or the handlers (see p. 298 for more information).

Lipoma

An *intestinal lipoma*, as discussed previously, is a pedunculated, fatty tumor that develops in the mesenteric fat that cloaks the small intestines (photo 11.36). An overweight horse is predisposed to lipomas. As fat accumulates in the body, it builds into lumps within the

11.36 *An intestinal lipoma is a mass of fatty tissue that often hangs on a stalk, around which the small intestine may wrap to become strangulated by loss of its blood supply. Colic pain from this condition is violent and unrelenting, requiring immediate surgical intervention. Photo: David Varra, DVM.*

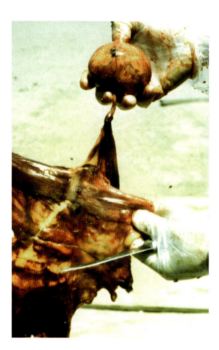

mesentery. Gravity may pull these lumps of fat into one large mass with a stalk attaching it to the mesentery. The stalk of such a tumor can wrap around the intestines resulting in strangulation of a loop of bowel. A horse with a strangulating lipoma presents with severe and unrelenting colic pain that requires surgery for its resolution. These occur most commonly in Arabian horses, geldings over 15 years of age, and in ponies, particularly those that are overweight from being fed too many groceries.

Sand Colic

Horses may eat as much as 2½ percent of their body weight in feed intake per day, equivalent to 20 to 25 pounds for a 1000-pound horse (see chapter 12, *The Digestive System: Nutritional Management*, p. 326). At least 50 percent of that feed should be in the form of roughage. This fiber component stimulates intestinal movement. A horse that is fed complete pelleted rations, condensed hay cubes, or a limited quantity of hay suffers from boredom.

His natural urge to chew finds him devouring fence boards, eating dirt and sand off the ground (photo 11.37), or consuming his manure. Over time, horses can consume a large amount of dirt or sand, which can weigh heavily in the gut and severely abrade the intestinal lining. Due to the insidious nature of this sanding syndrome, a long period may be required before it progresses to the point of overt abdominal pain.

Sand colic is not solely a problem in specific geographic areas, such as the West Coast, Eastern seaboard, Mississippi delta, or the sand hills of North Dakota. Anywhere there is sand, decomposed granite, or just plain dirt, sand colic can arise. Paddocks or arenas are often covered with sand or road base to improve footing, so although these soils may not be found naturally in the environment, they pose a threat.

Mechanics of Sand Colic

The design of the equine large colon, with its narrowing segments, encourages deposit and trapping of sand in constrictive areas. If excessive sand accumulates in the large colon, it obstructs passage of food materials (see photo 11.38). This immovable impaction causes gas to build behind it, with associated pain as segments of bowel distend and swell. Pain reflexes and spasms around an impaction may shut down movement. Abnormal peristaltic contractions in the gut can lead to a displaced or twisted intestine (see p. 308).

At the site of the impaction, the heavy and abrasive material can erode through the intestinal lining. Pressure necrosis on that portion of bowel causes the intestinal contents to leak into the abdominal cavity. Inflammation and infection of the abdomen (*peritonitis*), *endotoxic* and/or *septic* shock, and death can result. A similar situation occurs if a swollen or weakened bowel ruptures.

The Digestive System: The Oral Cavity, Dental Care, and the Intestinal Tract

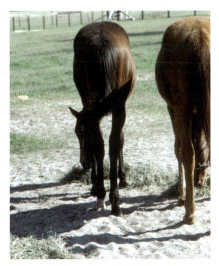

11.37 *A horse that is fed off sandy ground often accumulates quantities of sand and gravel in the bowel, leading to diarrhea, poor nutritional absorption, and/or colic.*

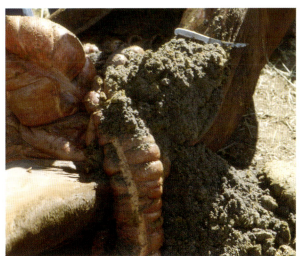

11.38 *This horse died due to severe sand colic. As seen here in this opened portion of bowel, the entire contents of the intestines were replaced with sand. This horse was fed a small ration of complete feed pellets each day with no other available roughage, and to satisfy the urge to chew, she ate the decomposed granite of the ground. Over time, the sand accumulated to this fatal state.*

Symptoms of Sand Colic

Several symptoms are tip-offs to a problem from excess sand ingestion. One indication is that 35 percent of afflicted horses will develop persistent diarrhea before the onset of painful symptoms. Sand abrasion of the lining of the intestinal tract impairs absorption of nutrients and fluids. As intestinal movement slows, diarrhea intensifies.

In some horses, the only signs may be depressed appetite and weight loss. Performance may suffer because of chronic discomfort or reduced nutrient efficiency. Other horses experience low-grade, mildly painful bouts of colic that appear as intermittent, but recurrent episodes. Sometimes a colic crisis starts during or after riding, possibly because the sandpaper-like abrasion stimulates painful spasms of the intestine. Imagine a sausage of concrete lining the gut, as the horse is subjected to extreme physical exertion. Necropsy results on horses that have died due to sand colic have revealed that up to two-thirds of the intestinal space was full of sand, wall to wall. In some places this material could be crumbled between fingers; in others it was so tightly packed that it could not be manually broken up.

Any horse that experiences chronic diarrhea or recurrent episodes of mild colic should be examined by a veterinarian. The key is to diagnose the problem early, before it becomes too advanced to rectify.

Diagnosing Sand Colic

Gut Sounds

Occasionally, a veterinarian can listen to the abdomen in front of the navel with a stethoscope and hear sounds similar to what one hears in a conch shell, that is, surf on sand.

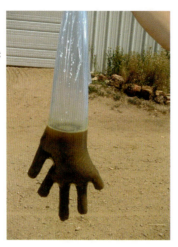

11.39 One means to identify if a horse is accumulating sand in his bowel is to place 6 fecal balls in a plastic bag, such as this plastic rectal sleeve, add water, and wait for the material to settle out over a few hours. Any sand in the bottom of the plastic bag indicates the presence of sand in the intestines; however, the absence of sand in the bag does not mean it is not present in the horse, just that it is not passing through at that time.

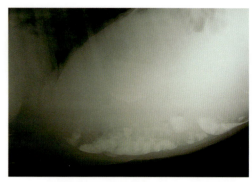

11.40 Abdominal radiographs taken of this horse with colic pain indicate a significant accumulation of sand in the bowel, leading to abdominal discomfort and distress. For orientation, the outlines of the ribs are visible as vertical white stripes on the left aspect of the X-ray film.

These sounds may also resemble the sound made by slowly rotating a paper bag partially filled with sand. Absence of these sounds does not mean absence of sand. For "sand sounds" to be heard, the bowel must be heavy enough to be lying next to the abdominal wall, and the bowel must be moving (see p. 301).

Sand in the Feces

Any sand or grit in the fecal material is significant. Lack of sand in the manure does not guarantee that it is not present in the gut. A simple test can be performed to monitors sand buildup. Take 6 fecal balls from the center of a fresh pile of manure where it has not contacted the ground. Mix the feces in a quart of water. Once the solid material separates out, measure the amount of sand in the bottom of the vessel: more than 1 teaspoon per 6 fecal balls is considered abnormal (photo 11.39).

Rectal Examination

Rectal examination of the intestinal tract does not always reveal definitive information. If a large amount of sand is present in the gut, it may collect in the intestines toward the bottom of the abdomen, and out of reach.

Belly Tap

A belly tap (abdominocentesis) involves inserting a needle into the abdomen to determine fluid character and volume (see p. 302). Sand may be obtained through such a tap because the weight of the sand pushes the intestines along the belly wall, and the needle may inadvertently penetrate the intestine. This technique is not generally used to diagnose sanding, but if such information is accidentally obtained this way, it clarifies a tentative colic diagnosis.

Radiography and Ultrasound

Radiographs (X-ray films) of the abdomen can positively diagnose sand in the intestines (photo 11.40). This procedure requires powerful X-ray equipment, often available only at a university veterinary teaching or private referral hospital. Diagnostic ultrasound is also useful for identification of sand in the bowel.

The Digestive System: The Oral Cavity, Dental Care, and the Intestinal Tract

Feeding Situations That Promote Sand Ingestion

- Feeding hay on sand or loose dirt
- Offering a pelleted feed as the full ration, with limited fiber availability
- Tasty, alfalfa leaves mixing in the dirt
- Boredom
- Overgrazed pastures

Preventing and Managing Sand Colic

Monitoring Feeding Habits

Monitor each horse for changes in eating habits, especially those that eat anything, or that search the ground all day. To prevent sand colic in these horses, feed more roughage, or feed more often, and provide more exercise to curtail boredom. An occasional individual may need a muzzle to prevent him from eating dirt. By not overstocking pastures, ample forage is available so horses do not consume dirt. A diet of free-choice grass hay, salt, and adequate water limits sand and dirt ingestion. A high fiber diet with high quality hay promotes movement of sand out of the intestinal tract.

Provide Clean Water

Check water tanks to see if sand collects in the bottom of the tank; this is a signal that a horse's mouth is full of sand that is rinsed into the tank with drinking. If the only available water source is a shallow, muddy, or sandy pool, dirt consumed in the water could precipitate within the bowel. Clean, fresh water encourages drinking, which promotes intestinal health and normal peristaltic movement.

Feeding Systems

Removal of hay from direct contact with the ground is essential for prevention. Feeding on rubber mats, concrete pads, or in the stall are strategic alternatives to remove hay from dirt contact. Overhead feeding arrangements, like hay racks or nets, present another problem, that of stimulating respiratory irritation. A horse fed from an overhead system that raises his head above his chest makes it difficult for him to clear debris and mold spores from the respiratory tract because his head is raised in an unnatural feeding position. Also, hay is pulled out of overhead feeders and scattered on the ground. Rubber tire feeders better ensure that feed material stays put while allowing safe, head-down feeding (photo 11.41). It is noteworthy that young foals can get trapped and injured inside tire feeders, and horses of all ages occasionally chew on the white walls and rubber of tire feeders with the potential to develop impaction colic.

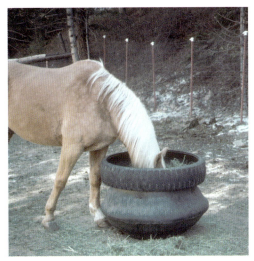

11.41 *Hay can be contained within large rubber tire feeders to minimize sand ingestion if a horse tends to consume every scrap when it is scattered across the ground.*

Preventive Medications

Psyllium is derived from the husk of the psyllium seed (*Plantago ovata*). Many commercial psyllium products (Equi-Aid®, Sand-Ex®, Sand-Lax®, as examples) are marketed as aids in eliminating sand from a horse. Some come as pellets, some as powders, some in both forms. The recommended treatment is to feed 1 scoop (supplied in the bucket) daily on consecutive days for a week per month. Psyllium was once considered to move sandy material out of the gut by lubricating it in a gelatinous material. Currently it is considered to stimulate motility of the bowel, and to pull "water" into the intestine to increase fecal water and bulk. Improved motility and mixing of ingesta may subsequently pull sand from the bowel.

An illuminating study (Colorado State University) used abdominal radiographs to illustrate that only two days of therapy with psyllium resolved chronic diarrheas attributable to sand. Because sand builds up over a long period of time, a lengthy time may be necessary for it to pass. Recommendations for treating seriously "sanded" horses include stomach tubing with psyllium for 2 to 5 days, followed by feeding ½ pound twice a day to adult horses, or ¼ pound twice a day to foals. This regimen should be carried out for 4 to 5 weeks. Sand is inconsistently found in the feces during psyllium therapy, so treatment should not be discontinued prematurely.

Feeding psyllium is not harmful in any way. A horse should not be offered an indefinite, continuous diet of psyllium as the microbes in the bowel will start to digest it as a fiber source and it will lose its effectiveness as a sand treatment.

There is some controversy surrounding the use of psyllium. A study (University of Illinois) examined elimination of sand from the large intestine by feeding psyllium. All 12 horses in the study had sand surgically placed in their cecum. Six horses were fed or stomach-tubed with psyllium while the other six control horses received none. The abdomen was radiographed on days 1, 5, and 11 to compare the control and treated horses for transit and evacuation of sand from the intestines. All were euthanized on day 11 and the amount of sand remaining in the intestine was weighed. The results of this study reported that there was no statistical difference between the treated and the non-treated horses with the conclusion that psyllium did *not* hasten the evacuation of sand from the bowel. However, a few points should be noted regarding this study: veterinarians in different parts of the United States have noted different degrees of success in treating sand with psyllium. It is possible that not all sand is created equal, and it is possible that not all sand/dirt throughout the United States is amenable to psyllium therapy. The variability in size of the grains that collect in the bowel may determine the effectiveness of psyllium as a treatment strategy. The other notable point is that it takes a while to clear sand from the bowel, and 11 days may not be an appropriate time frame upon which to base success or failure. A final conclusion is most telling: "When the intake of sand is prevented, the equine large intestine can reduce and possibly eliminate its sand burden."

A study (Finnish, 2001) concluded that laxatives using psyllium alone or with the addition of magnesium sulfate or mineral oil were ancillary in eliminating sand from the bowel in thirteen of fourteen horses in their study. The fourteenth horse managed to eliminate sand from his bowel when he was turned onto grass pasture rather than housed on a dry-lot with only hay being fed.

Another preventive "medication" is wheat bran, but contrary to popular myth, bran is neither therapeutic nor preventive for managing sand colic (see p. 329). Due to peculiar equine intestinal anatomy, by the time the relatively small amount of bran reaches the large intestine of the horse it can hardly exert any laxative effect. The equine gastrointestinal system is radically different from a human's. Bran encourages water consumption, which indirectly improves intestinal movement and passage of material through the bowel. If peristaltic contractions move feed along normally, then fecal contents will not stay in the bowel long enough for sandy material to separate out.

Surgery for Sand Colic

Surgery to correct sand colic may be the only alternative to physically remove the sand from the gut. A study (University of Minnesota) determined that horses undergoing surgery for sand colic experience a 50 percent survival rate. One study (University of Florida) revealed that those cases treated surgically had a survival rate of 92 percent, because of aggressive treatment before the bowel became gangrenous and necrotic.

Surgery for sand colic may be necessary if:

- There is a limited response to medical treatment within 48 to 72 hours.
- Vital parameters such as heart rate, capillary refill time, and mucous membrane color deteriorate.
- Pain persists and worsens.

Colic Caused by Diet or Management

Inappropriate dietary management often causes colic. An overabundance of excessively rich feed (grain, alfalfa hay, lush pasture) stimulates excess gas production within the stomach or large intestines. Sudden changes in feed are detrimental to the bacterial microflora in the gut and predispose to overproduction of gas or endotoxins. Moldy food, or rapid introduction of large amounts of grain or legume hay will upset the system. Cribbing behavior and stress from management issues can create colic (see p. 288).

Highest Risk Factors

One of the most prevalent findings in one study (Texas A&M) was that the risk of colic increased when anything changed within two weeks prior to a colic episode. If the horses changed their stabling, 18 percent colicked compared to 10 percent of those horses that stayed at home. If the activity level changed, 13 percent colicked compared to 10 percent of the controls.

But, most importantly, any change in diet resulted in a *quadrupled* increase in colic risk: 20 percent colicked as compared to 5 percent of horses kept on a steady feeding program. A study (Scott Equine Medical Center by Nat White, DVM) demonstrated that feeding grain increased the risk of colic as follows:

- If less than 5 pounds of grain is fed daily, there is no significant increased risk of colic.
- If 5 to 10 pounds of grain is fed daily, there is a 3.5 times greater risk of colic.
- If more than 10 pounds of grain is fed daily, the colic risk is increased 4.5 times.
- Any *changes* in grain feeding increase colic risk by 3.6 times.
- Changes in the type of hay fed double the risk of colic.

Other significant events were associated as colic risk factors as well. One such event included transport within the last 60 days. A nervous temperament or travel during hot weather most significantly affected the colic risk. Although a horse may be well adjusted to traveling, we have no control over the climate. Many horses arrive at a competition already somewhat dehydrated from hauling. Another colic risk factor included fever. An elevated body temperature may occur due to infectious disease or during protracted exercise.

Another interesting piece of information was discovered on the operating table. Many cases of intestinal torsion or displacement may be precipitated by an impaction in the right dorsal colon (a section of the large intestine—see fig. 11.17, p. 291). It is speculated that a large food mass may precipitate the descent of the colon in the abdomen, whereupon it can twist on its axis or tangle in a knot (see photos 11.33, 11.34, and 11.35, pp. 308–9). An impaction occurs for many different reasons, but one primary reason is attributable to anything that causes the intestines to slow activity for an extended period of time. Rigorous exercise coupled with dehydration that accompanies travel and competitive events can cause diminished gut motility.

Colic Related to Exercise

Feeding after Exercise

Feeding large amounts immediately after vigorous exercise can be risky (see p. 305). While blood is still circulating in the muscle tissue and shunted away from the stomach, emptying of food from the stomach is delayed, promoting excess fermentation. After the horse has cooled down, blood circulation is diverted back to the intestines, making it a safer time to feed. The time required for cooling a horse after exercise depends on his condition, environmental temperature and humidity, and the demands of the workout.

Cold Water after Exercise

Drinking excessively cold water after exercise may elicit spasms at the *pyloric sphincter* located between the stomach and the small intestine. Pyloric spasms delay movement of ingesta out of the stomach. Distention of the stomach with gas is quite painful, causing a sudden and violent colic.

Dehydration Effects with Exercise

During sustained exercise, as much as 80 percent of the blood flow is diverted to the muscle tissue for muscle contraction and to the skin for heat dissipation. This detracts from intestinal circulation, reducing it to minimum function. At the same time, a horse engaged in extended exercise needs to continue eating and drinking at every opportunity. This nutrient intake must be digested and absorbed to replenish losses of fluids, electrolytes, and energy used. Because of some detour of blood flow away from the gut, intestinal activity diminishes but should not cease altogether. We expect to hear less vibrant motility sounds when all quadrants of the flanks are listened to with a stethoscope. But, there should be consistent and plentiful activity.

As a horse becomes increasingly dehydrated with exercise, the remaining available circulating blood volume still must be shunted to the muscles to drive locomotion. Blood flow of some organ systems is reduced with continued fluid losses, and one of the first systems to feel this lack will be the intestinal tract. So in effect, quiet or quieter-than-expected gut sounds reflect a declining hydration status of a horse. Electrolyte imbalances, particularly of potassium, calcium, and magnesium, also contribute to shutdown of intestinal activity. As part of the "exhausted horse syndrome" complex, reduced gut sounds are a warning sign of dehydration and electrolyte imbalances that potentially could deteriorate to a point of crisis.

Besides the effects of fatigue on appetite suppression, hard-exercising horses may be experiencing serious electrolyte aberrations that further depress the normal thirst reflex. A horse may stop eating because of a feeling of intestinal "fullness" due to gas and fluid sequestration in a stagnant bowel. At times, the intestines become hypermotile in an attempt to "squeeze" out a forming impaction. Initially, it may seem that gut sounds are active. Yet with time and further dehydration and electrolyte depletion, intestinal sounds become absent altogether, a dangerous condition known as *ileus* (see p. 308). This adds to decreased absorption of intestinal water and electrolytes, worsened dehydration, devitalized bowel lining, increased fermentation of intestinal contents, more endotoxin and exotoxin uptake, a drying-out of intestinal contents, and a cycle of deterioration continues. Guts that cease motility set up conditions for intestinal displacement or twists to occur in addition to the metabolic complications encountered by endotoxin circulation and ongoing dehydration.

The Effects of Reduced Bowel Function

Gut sounds may only diminish in one portion of the abdomen rather than being absent altogether. Stagnant intestinal activity reduces the absorption of intestinal water and nutrients from the bowel. Then, vital fluids are sequestered in the gut and dehydration worsens. Feces may become sparse in frequency or amount. In occasional instances, the bowel may be irritated sufficiently to result in diarrhea. Or, mucoid strands may coat firm fecal balls, indicating stagnation of the large intestine, which could later lead to impaction colic (see photo 9.12, p. 237).

What Happens as Intestinal Sounds Diminish?

Besides being a measure of whole body hydration, intestinal sounds represent the mixing of intestinal contents and its progressive movement down the tract at a controlled rate. Depressed bowel activity is accompanied by diminished intestinal sounds. Then, instead of being digested, the feed sits and ferments, setting off a domino effect of problems. Although in most cases there may not necessarily be a physical blockage of intestinal contents, a quiet bowel experiences a functional obstruction created by lack of effective intestinal motility. In a stagnant bowel, fluid is leached from intestinal contents, potentially leading to an impaction. In addition, the pH change of the bowel caused by stagnant, fermenting feed kills off normal intestinal flora, allowing for overgrowth of intestinal bacteria. With overgrowth of some comes death of others, with release of *endotoxin*.

The outer membrane of the cell wall of Gram-negative bacteria is composed of endotoxin. Death of these organisms accompanies bacterial overgrowth, releasing large amounts of endotoxin. This particular toxin is absorbed easily from a devitalized intestinal lining that results from reduced circulation subsequent to disease or dehydration.

Endotoxin itself is not poisonous, but it elicits a chain reaction of activity of other inflammatory chemical mediators in the body that deteriorate the system. Some visible effects are appreciated as an elevated respiratory rate, accelerated heart beat, poor heart rate recoveries during exercise, and shut down of intestinal function. Body temperature may also elevate to further aggravate the heat-load a horse must lose while exercising, adding to increased fluid and electrolyte losses. Energy supplies are used up more rapidly. The effects of endotoxin elicit constriction of blood vessels throughout the body, including those of the intestinal tract, the kidneys, the heart, and potentially of blood flow to the feet. Alteration in blood flow exacerbates an already compromised circulatory system and furthers dehydration.

It is the effects of dehydration and endotoxin on blood flow to the distal (lower) limbs that are thought to contribute to laminitis. Research (Dr. Chris Pollitt) suggests that an overgrowth of *Streptococcus bovis* in the cecum creates a release of exotoxin and enzymes in the blood stream that upsets the attachment of the laminae within the hoof capsule to precipitate laminitis (see "Laminitis," chapter 3, *The Hoof,* p. 74). In an extreme case of a continual downward spiral, endotoxin can lead to cardiovascular shock and death. However, it is usually the effects of overall dehydration and electrolyte imbalances that create a life-threatening crisis in a sick horse rather than a direct effect by endotoxin.

Gastric Ulcer Syndrome

Gastric ulcer syndrome (GUS) is recognized in all types of sport horses despite the fact that most competitive athletes adjust and cope to their changing environment with minimal problems. Through endoscopic examination of the stomach, it has been found that 60 percent of performance horses experience GUS. A competitive horse is subjected to a variety of stressors: strange surroundings, long distance transport, changes in feed, the adrenalin induced by competition, and changing routines on a periodic basis.

As many as 85 percent of racehorses examined by endoscopy of the stomach have evidence of gastric lesions, with the ulcers worsening in the face of progressive training. Racehorses live a far different life than other types of competition horses and their diets vastly differ, as do management strategies, putting them more at risk.

Subtle Indications of Gastric Ulcer Syndrome

Many cases of gastric ulcers in the adult horse are seemingly asymptomatic, at least until one looks deeper. Often, the clinical signs associated with gastric ulcers relate to poor performance and/or declining physical condition. A horse's hair coat may appear dull, or he may appear lethargic and depressed at times. Some affected horses show behavioral changes and may become irritable and cranky. A horse with gastric ulcers may have trouble holding his weight despite ample food availability. His appetite may be less vigorous than normal, and he may even show signs of intermittent diarrhea or colic.

None of these symptoms points directly toward gastric ulcers, but this syndrome should be considered any time a horse seems not quite right. Ideally, it is best to catch a problem long before it develops into a more critical condition. Blood profiles of horses with chronic bleeding gastric ulcers may reveal anemia and low proteins, but performance and appetite issues would be noted long before you were stimulated to pursue laboratory work.

Areas of Concern within a Horse's Stomach

There are two different areas within a horse's stomach:

- The gastric *squamous mucosa* develops erosions due to an excessive amount of gastric acid production, with ulcers developing here in as quickly as 48 hours.
- The gastric *glandular mucosa* develops erosions due to a defect in the protective mechanisms of the stomach lining: any reduction in blood flow to the stomach or reduction in prostaglandins (specifically PG E2) will reduce the protective mucous barrier.

Any situation that causes a delay in the time it takes for the stomach to empty its contents or any event that prolongs stomach contractions will adversely affect the stomach environment with the likelihood that erosions may develop. With protracted exercise, blood that is diverted to the working muscles is diverted away from the gastrointestinal tract, leading to reduced blood flow and less active intestinal motility. This sets up conditions that contribute to gastric ulcers. In addition, horses that gallop at high speeds experience compression of the stomach between the intestines and the diaphragm, thus exposing the stomach lining to acid.

Currently there is limited evidence that the bacterial organism, *Helicobacter pylori*, which is associated with maintaining active human peptic ulcers, has any relationship to the development of equine gastric ulcers. So, there must be other reasons why these erosions exist. Intestinal parasites may play a role in eroding parts of the gastrointestinal tract: bot fly larvae invade the stomach epithelium, while tapeworms inhabit portions of the small intestine (see p. 461). Erosions can develop in any of these areas to create a poor-doing horse.

Dietary Considerations

In adult horses, most of the problems seen with gastric ulcers are related to the squamous mucosa as a result of excess acid secretion rather than problems that develop in the glandular portions of the stomach. Even when a horse is not eating, the stomach continues to secrete a lot of acid. It has been demonstrated unequivocally that horses on a diet of free-choice hay or pasture have less gastric acidity than horses fed at fixed intervals as occurs with two- or three-times-a-day restricted feedings. A hay diet (particularly legume) has a buffering effect on stomach acids, so horses on unrestricted access to fiber less commonly develop gastric ulcers. In addition, grain supplements elicit greater acid secretions within the stomach and thereby compound the problems related to a diet that limits roughage intake.

Misconceptions about Grain

As explained in detail in the next chapter, grain, although like candy to a horse, is *not* the most efficiently used food material, and it can create problems. Oats, corn, and barley are only some of the many types of grains available as horse feed. Grain contains abundant starch that needs to be digested in the small intestine to produce simple sugars. Oats may be 84 percent digestible, while corn may only be 29 percent digestible unless it is processed (ground, crimped, rolled) to improve its digestibility. Any grain that is not fully digested in the small intestine then passes on to the large intestine to be fermented there by bacteria. Too much starch fermentation results in production of lactic acid, which is irritating to the intestinal lining and also modifies the intestinal pH to a more acidic environment. When that happens many of the normally present gut bacteria die off, releasing endotoxins and exotoxins (poisonous substances produced and released by bacteria) into the bloodstream. Furthermore, within the four hours following a grain-fed diet, insulin surges to drive blood sugar into the cells, making less available for use by working muscles. The suggestion for athletic horses, particularly those facing protracted exercise, is to feed a large grain meal no less than four hours prior to work ("large" meaning more than 1 or 2 pounds of a grain product). At rest stops, offer plenty of hay plus a beet pulp mash that contains as minimal an amount of grain as necessary.

A wise general rule is to feed a horse as little grain as possible to maintain body condition, using fat supplements in substitution for grain to provide energy density to the ration. Fat is available in the form of vegetable oil, powdered animal fat, or rice bran products. Never feed more than 5 pounds of grain at a single meal. If it is necessary to feed grain, it is better to split the total daily amount into small and more frequent feedings. (For more detail, see chapter 12, *The Digestive System: Nutritional Management*, p. 329.)

Prevention of Gastric Ulcers

Dietary management is critical to maintaining gastrointestinal health of the horse. Treatment of gastric ulcers is best left to an individualized approach to each horse's needs based on conversations with a veterinarian. *Omeprazole* has been an invaluable medication for treating and managing gastric ulcers in horses. Some over-the-counter antacid products are also available and may be advantageous to use to buffer the acid secretions of a horse in high stress situations such as encountered during competition.

One antacid product is aluminum hydroxide buffer (Maalox TC®, Mylanta II®, or extra strength Maalox®) that can be added to electrolytes to ease the potential of GI and oral irritation associated with frequent oral salt supplementation. These antacids need to be given in large amounts (8 ounces) to accomplish a temporary decrease in stomach acidity lasting about two hours, but smaller amounts can be added to syringed electrolytes to provide a little relief.

Another buffer is a product called Neigh-Lox® (Kentucky Equine Research) that buffers stomach acid by coating the stomach lining. This product is not meant to replace treatment, but may be useful as an aid in prevention.

A product that may have value in managing *ulcerative colitis* (ulcers of the large colon) is *germinated barley foodstuff* (GBF). This is spent brewer's grain and can be obtained as a by-product from a local brewery. Storage relies on freezing since it has a limited shelf life. The insoluble nature of this fiber source is useful for increasing fecal bulk by pulling water into the intestinal contents, as does psyllium (see p. 313). GBF is also rich in *glutamine,* which is a non-essential amino acid that improves intestinal health and immune competence. GBF may be fed at a dose of ½ pound, 3 times a day.

Adverse Effects of Nonsteroidal Anti-Inflammatory Medications

An adult horse may have trouble with the glandular mucosa subsequent to chronic use of nonsteroidal anti-inflammatory drugs (NSAIDs) like phenylbutazone, flunixin meglumine, ketoprofen, or aspirin, which are prostaglandin inhibitors (see *Appendix B,* p. 568). Their role as anti-inflammatory drugs is to reduce the production of inflammatory mediators, specifically prostaglandins, but activity of favorable prostaglandins, like PG E2, are also inhibited by these drugs. A sport horse is often exposed to doses of these medications to ward off soreness created by hard work. Be judicious in the use of these medications, and only use them when warranted and under advisement of a veterinarian.

Plants That Affect the Digestive Tract

Some plants exert varying effects on the intestinal system leading to abdominal pain, colic, diarrhea, and/or impaction situations. Two members of the heath family, rhododendron and mountain laurel, possess a toxic compound (*andromedotoxin*) that affects muscle tissue, the heart, and the nervous system, while also stimulating abdominal pain, diarrhea, and excessive salivation. Leafy spurge (*Euphorbia esula*) is another instigator of gastrointestinal irritation.

The tannin found in oak trees and acorns can irritate a horse's abdominal tract causing abdominal pain, constipation or bloody diarrhea, and severe weakness. Persimmons (*Diospyros virginia*) contain tannins that bind with soluble proteins in the intestinal tract. Inhibition of activity of digestive enzymes and absorptive functions of the bowel can lead to impaction colic. Fresh leaves of the avocado tree (*Persea americana*) create swelling of the chewing muscles of the head, the tongue, and around the throatlatch. Occasionally a horse will colic from avocado poisoning, but most times an affected horse is not interested in eating or drinking because of related facial pain. This problem responds well to medical therapy and to removing the horse from access to the fresh avocado leaves (see "Avocado Toxicity," p. 283).

The Kentucky coffee tree irritates the gastrointestinal tract while simultaneously depressing the central nervous system. The seed of the mustard plant (*Brassica* spp.) is known to create colic. Similarly, bindweed (*Convolvulus arvensis*) seeds have been reported to cause colic.

Pound for pound, the black locust tree (*Robinia pseudoacacia*) and the castor bean (*Ricinus*) may rank at the top as being some of the most toxic of all plants. Symptoms caused by ingestion of the bark and sprouts of the black locust include diarrhea or constipation, depression or stupor, staggering, labored breathing, cardiovascular collapse, and laminitis. (For a comprehensive list of toxic plants, see *Appendix C, p. 571*).

GI Irritation by Common Household Plants

Some common household and garden-variety plants can also make a horse sick, even if eaten in small doses. An example includes members of the nightshade family: thorn apple (jimsonweed) and nightshade species, as well as tomatoes, potatoes, and eggplant. The fruits and vines of these plants can create gastrointestinal and nervous system effects. Generally, the bitter taste of these plants discourages a horse from eating them. Other garden plants and herbs can have lethal consequences: chives have been documented to cause fatal liver and kidney degeneration; horseradish inflames the stomach lining.

Prevention of Plant Toxicity

- Don't overstock pastures or allow pastures to become overgrazed.
- Supply hay when pasture forage is limited, especially in early spring and late summer and fall, which are the most favorable times for horses to seek out poisonous plants due to limited forage.
- Feed a good quality and balanced diet.
- Clean pastures and paddocks of dead fall from trees, particularly after storms and wind.
- Fence horses away from ornamental shrubs and plants.
- Discard all garden and plant cuttings or prunings out of reach of horses.
- Advise neighbors not to feed your horses anything without discussing it with you first.
- Buy hay and bedding from reputable sources, and carefully scrutinize the quality.
- Well-maintained pastures are generally weed-free, as are dry paddocks, whereas horses kept near stream banks, bogs, marshes, or in the vicinity of disturbed ground from building, logging, burning, or tilling are exposed to a greater likelihood that weeds or poisonous plants will flourish there.
- Identify the kinds of trees and shrubs cohabiting a pasture with your horses, and fence horses away from potential hazards like red maple, oak, black locust, buckeye, black walnut, plum, peach, apricot, oleander, yew, Kentucky coffee trees, black cherry, magnolia trees, and chokecherry bushes.
- Learn to recognize potential plant hazards in the pasture and around the house.
- Have a vet or a local county extension agent or plant specialist periodically investigate your property for potential plant toxins.

Blister Beetle Toxicity

Blister beetle poisoning creates a serious and often fatal colic crisis. Blister beetles particularly congregate in legume hay pastures wherever grasshoppers abound. The beetle produces a toxin called *cantharidin,* and horses that consume even as few as 5 to 6 beetles will get sick, and may die.

Clinical signs occur rapidly with depression, fever, excess salivation, elevated heart rate, and other signs of colic. Decreased circulating calcium concentration associated with cantharidin toxicosis accounts for some of the clinical symptoms. Because the toxin also creates blisters throughout a horse's intestinal tract, there are usually oral ulcerations in the mouth. An affected horse makes multiple attempts to urinate, and urine that is passed is often bloody. Death usually occurs within the first day of ingestion, but illness and mortality are dependent on the number of beetles consumed.

Colic from Parasites

In previous decades, postmortem exams of colic deaths revealed that 90 percent suffered from damage to intestinal blood vessels due to migration of larvae of *Strongylus vulgaris* worms. Occlusion of blood vessels by larvae and clots created by their presence resulted in a syndrome known as a *non-strangulation infarction*. In these cases, blood supply to the bowel was obstructed, although initially, the bowel itself was in normal health. As blood flow ceases, intestinal motility is disrupted to affected loops of bowel. The end result mimics a strangulation obstruction due to accumulation of gas, fluid, and toxins as bowel degenerates and shock develops. Due to a vast education program and implementation of effective deworming drugs at frequent intervals, parasites are a far less common cause of fatal colic in horses today. (See "Internal Parasites and Control," chapter 15, *Preventive and Mental Horse Health*, p. 459.)

Internal parasites such as *small strongyles* create areas of inflammation and irritation as they encyst in the intestinal lining. *Large strongyles* (bloodworms) migrate through the blood vessels supplying the intestines, interfering with circulation and intestinal movement. *Roundworms* form obstructions within the cavity (*lumen*) of the bowel. Blood flow interruption diminishes oxygen to bowel loops, and interferes with nerve input to the intestines. Waves of contractions then become disorganized, or may cease altogether. Other internal parasites damage and erode the bowel lining, causing leakage of fecal contents into the abdomen. Resulting infection and inflammation are called *peritonitis*. This condition is painful and potentially lethal.

The role of parasites in colic cannot be overstated. Adequate cleaning of corrals and stalls, along with an aggressive parasite control program at least every two months, markedly reduces this cause of serious colic.

THE BEST COLIC THERAPY IS PREVENTION

Despite all the advances in modern veterinary medicine, it seems that colic is still a number-one killer of horses. In an attempt to provide our horses with the best, we have inadvertently interfered with an efficient digestive adaptation that developed over millennia. Horses are at their digestive best when foraging on dried grasses scattered over arid ground, roaming in search of sustenance. The horse evolved to intermittently snack throughout the day, yet we place them in confined spaces and twice daily supply them with abundant food that is dried and in a relatively concentrated form.

It is agreed that the most effective way to prevent colic is to minimize changes in management practices. Horses are creatures of habit; both mentally and physically, they thrive on routine. Apply excellent preventive management strategies such as:

- Provide clean water *always*, and ensure that it remains unfrozen in winter.
- Keep a horse's diet consistent, and feed at least 60 percent of his diet (by weight) as roughage (hay or pasture), remembering that high grain diets increase colic risk by 3.5 to 4.5 times.
- Avoid changes in feed when possible since there is a quadruple increase in colic risk when diet is changed.
- Feed good quality hay, not too coarse and not too fine, and avoid dust and mold.
- Feed *grass* hay free-choice, supplementing with *legume* hay only as needed.
- Keep the source of hay constant throughout the year, and buy excellent quality.
- Minimize access to fermentable feeds like rich pasture, alfalfa, and grain.
- Use vegetable oil or rice bran as a caloric

The Digestive System: The Oral Cavity, Dental Care, and the Intestinal Tract

- alternative to excessive grain concentrates.
- Keep grain supplements to a minimum, and only as needed.
- Provide a salt block at all times.
- Supplement with electrolytes during intense exercise or in hot or humid conditions.
- Use feeding systems that minimize eating directly off the ground: one technique is use of a tire feeder that prevents a horse from spreading hay through the dirt.
- Feed psyllium products for 5 to 7 consecutive days each month to move dirt and sand through the bowel.
- Implement an aggressive deworming program every 6 to 8 weeks, dosing appropriately to a horse's body weight and ensuring that all the medication is ingested.
- Pick up manure in paddocks at least twice a week to minimize load of infective parasitic larvae.
- Have yearly dental exams and teeth filing performed by your vet to enable your horse to adequately grind the feed well.
- Allow the horse ample exercise, either in turnout or under saddle.
- Pasture turnout is ideal particularly if into a *non*-irrigated pasture.

The Digestive System: Nutritional Management

12

The equine intestinal tract is highly developed to extract nutrients from the digestion of plant matter. Horses need to consume energy, protein, vitamins, minerals and salts. Roughage comes in the form of hay or pasture, providing many of these necessary nutrients. The high fiber content of roughage is essential to normal intestinal function and health, and serves as the foundation upon which to build a feeding program. (For a detailed list of preventive management strategies for intestinal health, see p. 322.)

Basic Nutritional Requirements

Energy

Energy is a critical requirement for a performance horse's daily diet, yet misconceptions persist about how horses obtain energy. A primary source of energy is carbohydrates, which are found in the fiber components of hay and grass, and also in a concentrated form as grain. By weight, grains provide more energy than hay but are not necessarily the safest forms of energy to offer. Carbohydrates from concentrated feeds (see p. 329) are easily digested to glucose, which is readily absorbed in the bloodstream for availability to working muscles, or is stored as fat in *adipose* (connective) tissue or as glycogen in the skeletal muscles and liver. Metabolism of roughage in the large intestine, and fermentation and breakdown of fiber generate large amounts of *volatile fatty acids* (VFAs). These, along with glucose, can be used immediately, or are stored as fat or glycogen (see p. 139). Conditioning encourages the use of fatty acids as an energy source, saving glycogen for later. Performance fatigue is directly linked to depletion of energy stores.

When considering energy needs of a horse for exercise demands, the following recommendations by the National Research Council (NRC) may be used to tailor a diet. If a horse is exercised for 2 hours per day, different exercise demands increase energy needs as follows:

- A slow walk increases energy needs by 12 percent.
- A fast walk increases energy needs by 18 percent.
- A slow trot increases energy needs by 46 percent.
- A fast trot or slow canter increases energy needs by 97 percent.
- A medium canter increases energy needs by 138 percent.

Combining various proportions of high quality roughage as *fiber* (see below), high calorie *concentrates* (see p. 329), energy-dense fat (see p. 330), and protein (see p. 332) in a sensible manner allows control of a horse's energy intake and customizes a ration for each horse's special energy needs. Guidelines create a safe diet that best meets a horse's nutritional requirements:

- In general, a horse can only consume as much as 2½ percent of his body weight per day in feed. If a horse weighs 1000 pounds, his daily feed intake limit, grain and roughage combined, is a *maximum* of 25 pounds.
- At least half of the daily ration, by weight, should consist of roughage in the form of hay or grass, or a combination of the two: a 1000-pound horse with a maximum daily ration of 25 pounds should consume at least 12.5 pounds of that in roughage, and although this amount does not provide the entire daily supply of essential nutrients, it is a starting point at which to incorporate substitutions for hay as necessary.
- The higher the proportion of roughage, the safer the diet; the more concentrate fed, the greater the risk of metabolic disease, colic, laminitis and various orthopedic problems.
- Measure all feed by *weight* and not volume, as the weight of bales of hay or different grain products vary; weighing the food provides consistency at each feeding.

Roughage

The gastrointestinal tract of horses evolved to efficiently process dietary fiber in the form of roughage, which includes pasture or hay. As a general rule, a horse should be fed a minimum of 1 pound of roughage for every 100 pounds of body weight each day. As just mentioned, a horse may consume between 1½ to 2½ percent of his body weight each day. This means on a diet of exclusively hay, a 1000-pound horse should eat 15 to 25 pounds of hay in a day. Feeding adequate amounts of hay, or feeding at frequent intervals can decrease aberrant behavior such as licking the ground or dirt eating, called *pica*. If lacking in fiber, a horse will seek it in the form of board fences, weeds, or dirt. A fiber deficiency also limits normal stimulation of the large colon, resulting in more sluggish intestinal motility that might allow sand to precipitate out into the intestine (see p. 315). A fiber deficiency also makes a horse prone to developing gastric ulcers (see p. 318). The most effective means of limiting the development of colic is to feed plenty of good quality hay to promote efficient intestinal activity. Careful pasture management assures ample forage so horses are not forced to consume dirt.

Availability of clean and fresh water encourages drinking which is vital to gastrointestinal health and motility.

HAY

Because horses evolved to graze at frequent intervals throughout the day and night, they prefer to graze over a long period than to eat only a small portion of grain that disappears quickly. If a horse cleans up his feed and looks for more, offer grass hay while he stands idle in the stall or paddock, or turn him out to pasture.

There are two means to achieve abundant glycogen stores: conditioning muscles to use fat resources first, and by a high intake of fiber. High roughage diets supply the fiber necessary to support prolonged aerobic exercise; low fiber diets correlate with an increased risk of failure in performance. The type of hay consumed (alfalfa or grass), the amount, and the quality are important factors.

Nutritional Value of Hay

Nutritional value of hay depends on the stage of harvest and the state of preservation. Most of hay's nutrition (⅔ of the energy and ¾ of the protein value) is contained within the leaves. Good quality hay is leafy and soft, rather than stemmy and coarse. If hay is stemmy because it was harvested late in the maturation process, or if the leaves have turned to powder and fallen off because it was poorly cured, its nutritional value must be discounted proportionately.

Moisture content should be less than 20 percent to prevent mold and spoilage. However, leaves that are excessively dry will fall away with loss of nutrient value. Shake a flake of hay to see how many leaves fall out, or if they crumble to dust. Smell it for mold, and break it apart to look for discolored areas. If the hay is green, smells sweet, holds together well, and is not irritating to handle due to sticks, stems, or weeds, then it passes the test for freshness and palatability.

Protect the haystack and feed storage areas from excess moisture that would promote proliferation of mold. Routinely clean feeders to remove spoiled or old hay so a horse's appetite remains keen. Check that hay palatability is adequate, and that the hay smells fresh and sweet. To preserve vitamin A content of the hay, protect it from sun scorch.

Grass Hay

An exclusive diet of quality grass hay provides nearly adequate nutrition for a mature, idle horse, meeting his needs for protein, energy, and fiber, but may need to be supplemented with other energy sources for a horse in work. In addition, grass hay is relatively low in calcium, and high in phosphorus. Therefore, the diet may need calcium supplementation to satisfy an adult horse's mineral requirement for a calcium-to-phosphorus (Ca:P) ratio of no less than 1 part calcium to 1 part phosphorus, or 1:1 (see p. 337).

Grass hays vary depending on geographic locale and a nutritional analysis should be run to enable proper balancing of dietary components.

Cereal Grain Hay

Cereal grain hays, such as oat hay, are similar in nutritive value to grass hays in many respects. However, once the grain heads have fallen from this type of hay, most of what remains is straw, which is reduced in energy value.

Legume Hay

Legume hays, such as alfalfa or clover, are 20 percent higher in energy, twice as high in protein, three times as high in calcium, and five times higher in vitamin A than good quality grass hays. Legume hay, therefore, gives greater nutrient value than grass hay. Depending on the amount of legume hay fed, its high calcium content may need to be offset with a phosphorus supplement.

Preferably, legume hay should be used as a supplement to a diet of grass hay to improve condition. Feeding a diet of exclusively legume hay is fraught with problems. These include the development of gaseous colic (see chapter 11, *The Digestive System: The Oral Cavity, Dental Care, and the Intestinal Tract*, p. 308), laminitis (see, chapter 3, *The Hoof*, p. 74), and myositis (see chapter 6, *Muscle Endurance*, p. 166). Also associated with legume hay is the need for a horse to drink more water to excrete the high nitrogen load that comes from metabolism of the high protein content of the legume. This may lead to dehydration issues in a performance horse in summer. And, increased urination elicited by high protein adds to ammonia buildup in the stall, which potentially injures a horse's airways and creates respiratory problems.

Growing horses are very sensitive to calcium and phosphorus imbalances created by the exceptionally high calcium content of legume hay. Such mineral imbalances, along with the high protein and high energy content of legume hays potentially lead to developmental orthopedic diseases such as *osteochondrosis* (OCD), *epiphysitis*, *contracted tendons*, or *wobbler syndrome* often seen in potential young athletes fed a rich diet (see chapter 5, *Joints*, p. 133).

When feeding alfalfa hay, a safe general rule for any age horse is to feed no more than one-third of the hay ration as alfalfa. This provides calories, but does not overload the body with excess calcium, protein, or energy.

PASTURE

The nutritional content of pasture forage varies not only according to plant characteristics, but also by season. Energy and mineral content depend on soil type, but certain general rules help determine how to supplement pasture during different seasons. During rapid spring growth, grasses are high in protein, minerals, and vitamins, and sugars known as *fructans*. Sprouting plants are also high in water content. Pasture loses water content as it matures, and it also loses protein and mineral value as its fiber content increases.

OTHER ROUGHAGE ALTERNATIVES

Because hard-working equine athletes are often unable to consume as much feed as necessary to maintain a high level of exercise, concentrated feed is useful to provide nutrition and calories without the bulk or intestinal fill. Concentrates come in many forms: complete feed pellets, beet pulp, wheat bran, grain, and fat. Any of these components are considered *feed supplements* since they are intended to augment the larger portion of the diet that is offered as hay and/or pasture.

High Fiber Feed Supplements

Complete Feed Pellets

Concentrated supplements that are high in fiber yet provide more calories than hay include compressed alfalfa pellets or complete feed pellets, which are largely alfalfa based. Complete feed pellets also contain about 25 percent grain products along with added vitamins and minerals. When pellets are fed as the sole ration, horses finish them quickly, with boredom and a desire to chew causing them to turn to eating the barn, fences, or dirt (pica). Offering pelleted feed in combination with hay and/or pasture facilitates extra calorie intake while minimizing boredom. When feeding compressed alfalfa pellets, offer the small size pellet to avoid choke (see chapter 11, *The Digestive System: The Oral Cavity, Dental Care, and the Intestinal Tract*, p. 295). Pelleted feeds are useful to make soft gruels or mashes for horses with significant dental problems and to increase water intake when desired.

Beet Pulp

Another useful high fiber pellet that is highly digestible and has more energy than grass hay is *beet pulp*. As a substitute for some amount of hay, a horse's need for fiber can be satisfied by feeding up to 2 pounds of beet pulp per day. Beet pulp is a good roughage substitute because it is relatively high in fiber (18 percent), yet low in protein, thereby avoiding problems that occur with legume hay. Also, beet pulp is digested efficiently in the large intestine without the concerns related to carbohydrate overload that arise from grains.

Wet beet pulp swells to many times its original volume. To ensure that it won't swell inside a horse and cause colic, it should be soaked in ample water for many hours before feeding. A one-pound coffee can of dried beet-pulp pellets will absorb 5 gallons of water to form a mash. Warm or hot water hastens soaking of the pellets to 6 hours while cold water requires a soaking time of 8 to 12 hours. To introduce beet pulp to a horse's diet, start with a dry measure of ½ cup and then soak this in water until it swells to full volume. Slowly introduce increasing amounts, building up to 2 cups of dry beet-pulp pellets per feeding that is then soaked to volume.

Wheat Bran

Another low nutritive, but filling, grain product commonly fed is wheat bran. Bran is high in fiber, low in energy, and about 15 percent protein. By weight, wheat bran has 12 percent less energy than oats and 25 percent less energy than corn. By volume, corn has four times more energy than wheat bran, while oats have double the energy as wheat bran. So to use this product as an energy substitute would be false logic.

Not only is wheat bran extremely high in phosphorus, but it also binds calcium in a horse's body so caution should be used to avoid dietary imbalances of calcium relative to phosphorus. This characteristic makes bran useful to counterbalance high calcium diets of legume hays. Consumption of too much bran by any age horse without balancing the diet can lead to *nutritional secondary hyperparathyroidism* (see chapter 4, *Developing Strong Bones*, p. 107), or developmental orthopedic disease (DOD—see chapter 5, *Joints*, p. 131).

Although there is no direct laxative effect from wheat bran, it may improve a horse's water consumption, especially when fed as a wet mash. Too much bran may be constipating, so should be limited to a volume less than a one-pound coffee can each day.

CONCENTRATES

When a horse is burning more energy than he is able or willing to eat in forage, adding a concentrated feed supplement like grain is an efficient way to increase energy intake. Per pound, grain has 30 to 50 percent more digestible energy than hay. As mentioned, an important general rule when feeding concentrates is to feed *at least* 50 percent of the diet as roughage to maintain healthy gastrointestinal function. Grains offer a concentrated source of energy, but are relatively high in phosphorus and low in calcium, necessitating balancing of the ration. There is no evidence that processing grains improves digestibility more than 5 percent. The heating process involved in cracking, rolling, crimping, steam flaking, or micronizing grains may improve how well a horse chews the feed, making it easier for digestive processing.

When more than 5 pounds of grain is fed at one meal, the carbohydrate content may not be digested completely; then starch enters the large intestine. There, excess fermentation develops, leading to overgrowth of bacteria that might set up conditions for laminitis (see p. 74) or colic (see p. 297). A preferred general rule is to feed minimal grain only as necessary for additional calories. This strategy maintains normal function of the intestines, and keeps the intestines from developing too acid an environment that could lead to ulcers or colic. Less grain also keeps a horse from becoming "hyper," and reduces the risk of laminitis, or tying-up syndrome. Many horses do well on as little as 1 or 2 pounds a day, but if more is needed, do not exceed 6 pounds of grain in a day. Split grain feedings into smaller amounts fed more frequently, like 3 to 4 times per day, instead of offering a large amount twice daily.

If a horse is putting on too much weight from an enhanced diet, then more exercise is called for, and/or concentrate feeding should be reduced. Initially, adjustments in the diet are necessary to find the correct amounts of extra feed that will keep a horse comfortable and happy while muscle builds through exercise.

Oats and Corn

Oats and corn are two popular feed grains. Oats are higher in fiber content and lower in digestible energy than other grains due to a fibrous hull surrounding each oat kernel. Corn is twice as high in digestible energy as oats, thereby providing more calories for an equal volume. For example, ½ scoop of corn is equivalent in energy to 1 scoop of oats. It is safer to feed by *weight*, not volume. A one-pound coffee can holds 1 pound of oats, yet it holds 1½ pounds of corn; although both measures fill the same size scoop, corn has three times more energy than the same volume of oats. Another difference between oats and corn is the protein content with oats containing 12 percent protein, while corn has 9 percent. Both have acceptable values of protein for mature horses (see p. 332).

Rye and Barley

Rye and barley fall between oats and corn on the energy scale. Rye, when fed alone, is unpalatable. Barley must be processed to remove its indigestible outer hull. These grains are usually fed in combination with other foodstuffs, in the form of a mixed grain or pelleted feed.

Sweet Feed

Sweet feed is a grain product that is a highly palatable combination of corn, oats, and barley (COB) bound together with a light coating of molasses.

FAT FOR ENERGY

Feeding fat to a working horse has been proven as an excellent source of energy with minimal side effects. Fat is a great source of calories for improving body condition, and an additional benefit is enhanced luster of the haircoat. Many forms of fat are palatable and efficiently digested and metabolized to fuel aerobic activities. During aerobic exercise, horses preferentially burn fats and VFAs, thereby sparing glycogen reserves in the muscles and liver for use in anaerobic activities like sprinting or jumping (see p. 141). This delays the onset of fatigue that accompanies glycogen depletion to give a horse a competitive edge. Short-term adaptation to a fat-supplemented diet has little effect on gastric emptying thus enabling horses in protracted aerobic work, like endurance athletes, to absorb energy and nutrients when fed fat supplementation along with hay at rest stops.

Not only is fat more than 85 percent digestible, but also its absence of carbohydrate content minimizes the risk of colic or laminitis. A high fat diet improves a horse's tolerance to exercise in hot weather as metabolism of fatty acids generates 30 percent less heat than seen with high protein diets (see p. 343). And, a high-fat diet increases a horse's calorie intake without increasing the volume he must eat.

Vegetable Oil

As much as 8 to 12 percent of the concentrate diet can be fed in the form of fat. A horse can safely consume up to 1½ cups of oil twice a day, with excellent results. Vegetable oil is not as filling in the digestive tract as grain or hay, and less fat is required to supply a similar amount of calories and energy as found in grain. By feeding fat, less other concentrate needs to be offered; this enables a horse to eat more hay, making the ration safer for intestinal health. Vegetable oil can be substituted for some or most other concentrate supplements, like grain.

As a relative comparison of the energy content of fat, consider that a cup of vegetable oil (240 grams of fat) is equivalent to 1¼ pounds of corn or 1½ pounds of sweet feed. Any type of vegetable oil can be fed, and particularly any of the long-chain unsaturated fats such as corn, soybean, coconut, peanut, canola, or sunflower oil. Corn and soybean oils are the most palatable, although most horses accept any type when it is top-dressed on small amounts of grain or complete feed pellets. To ensure quality and palatability, vegetable oil should be stored properly in a cool, dark place so it won't spoil or become rancid. Oral vitamin E supplementation provides an antioxidant effect to protect against rancidity effects of fat when subjected to lengthy storage.

Oil should be introduced gradually into the feed so a horse becomes accustomed to the taste, and so diarrhea doesn't develop from a sudden feed change. Start with about ⅓ cup fed twice a day, building up to the desired amount over a 2-week period. Too much oil is unpalatable and may interfere with mineral absorption.

Fat is also available in powdered form. Pace® (Morgan Manufacturing Co., Inc.) is powdered animal fat and sugars, which is digested well by horses and does not freeze in winter. Another powdered fat product is Fat Pak 100® (Milk Specialty Products).

Rice Bran

Rice bran products are invaluable as an energy-dense feed and useful as a fat supplement. A horse can safely consume 1 cup (about 1 pound) of rice bran twice a day. Rice bran is 20 percent fat as compared to the 100 percent fat of oils so a horse won't derive as many calories as compared to vegetable oils. However, horses readily accept rice bran mixed in with grain, and it is less messy and less difficult to handle, particularly in cold climates. Rice bran is typically high in phosphorus so pay attention to balancing the calcium/phosphorus ratio for the total diet. Some commercial rice bran products (Equi-Jewel®) are prepared with calcium and phosphorus in balance, so check the labels.

The comparative caloric value of rice bran relative to other products is worthy of consideration: 1 pound of rice bran is comparable to 1⅓ pounds of oats or 8 fluid ounces of corn oil. The fat in rice bran products is at least 85 percent digestible, but the product purchased should be heat stabilized so it does not go rancid.

PROBIOTICS

A *probiotic* is a feed supplement containing live microbial organisms. It is thought that these products exert beneficial effects on a horse by inoculating the gastrointestinal tract with active microbes to aid digestion. Favored microorganisms used are lactic-acid bacteria, such as *Lactobacillus*, and some strains of yeasts. *Lactobacillus* strains commonly found in yoghurt do not necessarily possess probiotic properties, nor do they retain activity with extended shelf life. Commercial products do not always list the organisms in the preparation, so one has to guess if anything of value is being given.

There is general skepticism about the value of feeding such microbes to a horse: these organisms must be able to survive transit through the acidic environment of the equine stomach and then also be resistant to digestion by bile salts in the small intestine. Once having passed these obstacles, the microbes must be able to colonize the intestinal tract. There, they must exert favorable effects, such as inhibiting pathogens that flourish in the GI tract. It is a tall order to expect probiotic organisms to achieve all these ends at an appropriate dose of viable organisms. In addition, not all products contain the organisms listed on the label in sufficient quantities to have any effect. Thus far, objective research has not been available to ascertain scientific value; as yet, favorable testimonials remain only anecdotal.

Probiotic products most likely do little harm, and so have been tried in a multitude of conditions:

- Show horses stressed by competition and travel
- Hard-keepers that have difficulty holding weight
- Sick individuals
- Older horses

- Horses with poor appetites
- Chronic diarrhea cases
- Horses on long-term antibiotic therapy
- Neonatal foals

Of greatest benefit to the health of the equine colon is provision of sufficient dietary fiber and B vitamins. There is also a valid argument to be made that *psyllium*, as a dietary fiber, promotes microbial growth in the large intestine, and accomplishes some of what one sets out to do in feeding commercial probiotics. (For more on psyllium, see p. 313.)

Protein

Because humans have a high demand for dietary protein, people assume horses have a similar need. Therefore, protein is commonly overfed to horses. Horses use it as an energy source only if they lack carbohydrates in hay and grain, or fats. Protein is metabolically inefficient for a horse to process and excrete when fed in excess.

Every horse needs protein, but a mature horse, even one in regular work, requires only moderate amounts of 8 to 10 percent of his ration. Growing horses, pregnant and lactating mares, and aged horses need up to 16 percent. Supplemental protein can be provided with legume hays, or with concentrated grain mixes of higher protein levels. With regular exercise, a horse's appetite normally increases to ingest more energy. With greater feed consumption, additional protein needs are usually met.

Corn and oats provide 8 to 12 percent protein. Grass hay or pasture are variable in protein content, and for exact values should be analyzed at a laboratory. Generally, good quality grass hay contains at least 8 percent protein. Alfalfa products provide 15 to 28 percent protein. Protein is a metabolically expensive form of energy. Feeding high amounts of protein as an energy source is analogous to walking clear round to the back of the house and coming in the back door when you could come directly up the steps through the front door. Both routes get you in the house, but the direct approach through the front door requires fewer steps and has greater efficiency. The front door approach uses fat as an energy source, while the back door route feeds high protein, like legume (alfalfa or soy) products.

SOY PRODUCTS

Extruded soy or soybean meal has been used as a caloric supplement. As for caloric content, soy meal products (extruded or powdered or pelleted) are similar to rice bran. The usual amount fed is ½ to 1 cup of extruded soy per day. One advantage in using soy is that it is easier to handle than oils, especially in winter, but soybeans are only 18 percent fat (relative to 100 percent fat content of oils) thus making soy a less efficient fat supplement. In addition, soy products are 40 to 46 percent protein, which is not only far in excess of requirements for any age horse, but there are similar disadvantages to that explained in the section on feeding legume hay (see p. 327).

Water Requirements

Ample quantities of fresh water should always be available to a horse to ensure efficient digestion and to replenish losses from sweat. The more hay provided in the diet, the more water a horse needs for digestion, with horses on a hay diet needing to drink up to twice as much water as horses on a grain-supplemented diet.

PELLETS

Pelleted and extruded feeds contain small particles that pull body water into the large intestine during digestion. Feeding pellets results in softer manure, but pellets require more water for adequate digestion. Feeding a pelleted ration as a sole feed source may be unwise in a hot climate, because dehydration is a limiting factor of performance.

ROUGHAGE

Roughage (hay and pasture) is excellent for retaining water in the intestinal tract. Within reason, water lost in sweat is immediately replenished from a reservoir of water in the digestive tract. During prolonged competition, roughage also supplies energy (and fluids and electrolytes) to an exercising horse long after intake of a meal. The presence of fiber in the intestines also maintains circulation to the bowel, and efficient GI function.

Electrolyte Supplementation

Horse sweat contains a high concentration of body salts, making it uniquely different from human sweat. These chemical components of body salts are referred to as *electrolytes*, and individually include sodium, chloride, potassium, calcium, and magnesium. The first two components (sodium and chloride) are contained in the saltshaker that sits on the dinner table; a horse only obtains these in his diet as ingredients of salt blocks. A salt block should be available at all times to pastured horses. Most horses will lick about 1 to 2 ounces a day off a salt block. Hay and grass contain abundant quantities of potassium, and all hays contain calcium and magnesium, with alfalfa hay being particularly rich in these minerals.

WHAT ELECTROLYTES DO

Electrolytes serve essential functions that are key to a horse's peak performance:

- They mediate electrical impulses to stimulate muscle contraction and movement and efficient interaction of nerves and muscles.

- They regulate the balance of body water within the various tissue compartments.

All body functions depend on electrolytes, but in the working equine athlete, electrolytes are important for maintaining normal intestinal function, adequate blood circulation, normal heart rhythm, and muscular strength and coordination.

A horse may lose as much as 5 to 10 percent of his body weight in fluid loss, amounting to 25 to 50 liters, with long duration exercise even at low intensity. In general, a horse exercising at low intensity (5 to 8 mph) will lose 5 to 10 liters of sweat each hour of work. At high intensity exercise demands (13 to 16 mph), up to 15 liters of sweat may be lost per hour. Along with loss of body water is a loss of electrolytes. Because a horse's sweat is so concentrated in electrolytes, as much as a teaspoon of salt may be lost with each cup of sweat. A horse undergoing protracted, low-intensity exercise potentially may sweat away 5 ounces of electrolytes during each hour of work, particularly in hot and humid climates. (The need for electrolyte supplementation is discussed in chapter 6, *Muscle Endurance*, p. 162.)

ELECTROLYTE DEPLETION

A major effect of electrolyte imbalance or depletion is its influence on excitable, nerve-rich tissues, such as found in skeletal muscles, the cardiovascular tissues, and the nerves themselves. Muscle function is compromised and intestinal function diminishes in a horse with electrolyte depletion. In addition to losses of electrolytes in sweat, a horse is also losing valuable body water, leading to complications associated with dehydration. Myositis (tying-up syndrome), thumps (synchronous diaphragmatic flutter), colic, and diarrhea often stem from electrolyte imbalances and dehydration (fig. 12.1).

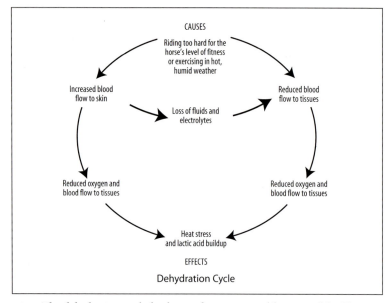

12.1 *The dehydration cycle leading to heat stress and lactic acid buildup.*

WHO NEEDS ELECTROLYTE SUPPLEMENTATION?

A horse that sweats during a mile-long track race loses lots of body water and some small degree of electrolytes, but then the exertion is quickly over; in a short time he easily replenishes what was lost. The same is true for a sprint horse like a roping, reining, barrel racing, or a cutting horse, or for other high-intensity sport horses like show jumpers. These horses have sufficient electrolyte reserves in the intestines to replenish such daily losses. But in sports that require a low-to-moderate intensity for long durations, such as endurance-related sports, a horse sweats throughout hours of effort and loses abundant, valuable water and electrolytes. Not only does a distance trail horse or an event horse exercise for many hours, but in some cases for 2 or 3 consecutive days. In considering the effects of fluid and salt depletion on these sport horses, consideration must be taken of the losses a horse experiences on the trailer ride to and from an event. Electrolyte deficits have a significant impact on a horse's performance even before a competition begins, and certainly affect how a horse feels while doing his work.

Most horses require electrolyte supplementation if used strenuously and especially for long periods, while others in light work may not need any supplementation. Some horses take care of themselves by eating and drinking well. These individuals may easily adjust to the stress of travel and performance and manage fine with access to loose or block salt, or free-choice electrolytes provided in a bucket. All horses are individuals in their metabolic response to exertion. Similarly, climatic conditions vary at each event and in different geographic parts of the country. Fitness of a horse for the intended sport is an important element in evaluating the amount and frequency of supplemental electrolytes. The more fit the horse, the less exertion needed to get the job done. The faster the speed and/or the longer the duration, the more intense is the effort. Horses exercising for protracted periods in high ambient temperatures, high humidity, difficult terrain, or high altitude are at risk of losing significant quantities of body fluids and electrolytes. These are situations where it is always prudent to supplement. It is noteworthy that in low humidity (arid) climates, horses still sweat, but the sweat evaporates so quickly from the skin that it is difficult to appreciate just how much sweat is lost. These horses also need salt supplementation in hot weather.

In any equine athletic discipline, electrolyte supplementation is an adjunct to proper conditioning and preparation, to an intelligent riding strategy, and to proper nutritional management. Electrolyte supplementation is not a substitute for fitness, but it is a useful strategy to derive maximum and safe performance from a well-prepared mount. This strategy does not enable a horse to be a more brilliant competitor or to surpass his inborn capacity, but it does allow a horse to perform with less risk of metabolic collapse or danger to his health.

HOW MUCH AND HOW OFTEN?

A horse's body will not store electrolytes given in excess. Usually the kidneys excrete any excess through the urine, provided that kidney function is not compromised by dehydration. A horse drinks better when supplemented with salt as this maintains a more normal sodium level in the bloodstream to trigger the thirst center in the brain. Electrolytes given orally don't immediately enter the bloodstream and find their way to the body tissues. There is a lag time of at least an hour or two after administration of the salts for them to do any good.

In sports where there is an anticipation of prolonged or intense sweat losses, it is preferable to give small amounts (an ounce or two) of electrolytes frequently throughout an event. In distance trail events, a safe general rule is to pre-load prior to competition (2 ounces the night before and 2 ounces the morning of) and then to administer 2 ounces of electrolytes for every 10 miles of competition or training, or every 2 to 4 hours, depending on speed and climatic conditions. To maximize the beneficial effects of salt supplementation it is best to give doses in smaller amounts at more frequent intervals, as for example each time a horse drinks (photo 12.2). An event horse would benefit from electrolyte supplementation the morning prior to and just following the cross-country phase of a horse trial. This strategy enables a horse to maintain a relative electrolyte balance, rather than having to play catch-up during rest periods.

Salt is mixed in a syringe with water and administered by mouth or added to a mash (photo 12.3). Minimize feeding copious amounts of molasses, sugar, grain, or fat supplements when providing electrolytes since high sugar or high fat has the potential to slow gastric emptying and delay absorption of electrolytes. Following a competition, provide a dose of electrolytes and then top-dress 2 ounces over each of the next several meals. For sports that are less rigorous in duration, it is not necessary to syringe electrolytes; instead, you can offer your horse a bucket of electrolyte-laced water in addition to plain water.

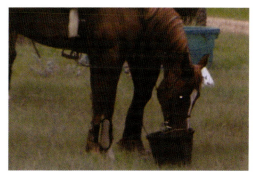

12.2 *The best time to administer electrolytes to an exercising horse is immediately after he has had a good drink.*

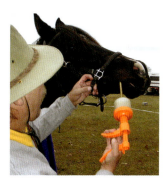

12.3 *Administration of electrolytes is facilitated by using a dose syringe to squirt a salt-water mixture into the horse's mouth.*

WHAT KIND OF ELECTROLYTES TO USE

A commercial electrolyte mix should be purchased that is specifically formulated with a balanced blend of salts. Not all electrolytes are comparable, with many commercial preparations consisting of nothing more than a lot of sugar with a little salt. Purchase commercial electrolyte supplements that are rich in salt ingredients rather than being bulked up with dextrose, sucrose, or other unimportant additives. No more than 10 percent sugar content is necessary to achieve electrolyte absorption. If a product tastes salty, it probably contains a reasonable amount of salt; if it tastes sweet, it is most likely more sugar than salt, so find a salty alternative. A useful commercial product is one that provides a readily utilizable source of calcium in an acetate form that is rapidly absorbed from the bowel.

Alternatively, an inexpensive mix is made by combining several ingredients: 3 parts Lite® salt (potassium chloride and sodium chloride) to 1 part calcium acetate, or 2 parts table salt to 1 part Lite® salt to 1 part calcium acetate. Table salt is a mixture of sodium and chloride, while Lite® salt is a mixture of potassium chloride and sodium chloride.

In addition to electrolyte supplementation, it is important to provide free-choice quality hay to horses prior to, during, and following participation in low-intensity exercise of prolonged duration. The high fiber content provided by hay within the intestines provides a reservoir of electrolytes, energy, and water from which to draw upon throughout an event.

Cautions and Precautions

Horses engaged in protracted exercise should not be supplemented with any electrolyte product that contains bicarbonate! This "basic" substance exacerbates problems related to an alkalotic (high pH) bloodstream that develops due to losses of potassium and chloride in the sweat. Prolonged aerobic exercise alters a horse's acid-base balance, leading to muscle cramping, thumps, colic, fatigue, and heat exhaustion. Administering bicarbonate further alkalinizes the bloodstream and worsens metabolic problems (see more discussion on p. 163).

Some horses back off food and drink when electrolytes are force-syringed into the mouth. Electrolytes may be irritating to the stomach or mouth so it is helpful to buffer the mixture with an antacid like Maalox® or Mylanta®. Maalox®, applesauce, or yoghurt mixed in the syringe make salt more palatable.

(Note: some buffering products contain calcium *bicarbonate* and should not be used.) One recipe suggests mixing 5 pounds of of an electrolyte product with 12 ounces of Maalox®. (You need not mix up this total quantity at one time; mix the appropriate proportion of each to make an amount that will be used during an event.) Also, offer a choice of a bucket of electrolyte-supplemented water along with plain water to give a horse the opportunity to selectively replenish his salt needs.

There is a potential, especially in arid climates, for excess electrolyte supplementation to cause diarrhea from bowel irritation. However, in hot and humid climates, a horse loses great quantities of salts in his sweat. With that in mind, it may be necessary to supplement with as much as 4 ounces (120 cc) of electrolytes every 10 to 15 miles of riding in hot and humid conditions. After an event, a salt block should be available to the horse or salt can be added to the feed for a few days. If losses are extreme during rigorous exertions, it may be necessary for a veterinarian to administer fluids and electrolytes by stomach tube or intravenously.

There are no hard and fast rules of how much electrolytes to administer, as each horse is an individual. Some horses need more; some need less. These suggestions are guidelines for an average situation and should be fine-tuned to each horse, the work effort, the terrain, the speed, and the climate.

Sodium Bicarbonate

In the racehorse industry, it is common to treat a horse with a sodium bicarbonate (baking soda) drench, called a "milkshake" in an attempt to counteract lactic acid accumulations, and to enhance race performance. The idea behind this practice is that a horse is "drenched" (at a dose of 0.4 grams of sodium bicarbonate per kilogram of body weight) to achieve neutralization of lactic acid 3 to 4 hours following bicarbonate administration. Studies report no statistical differences in racing times of horses receiving milkshakes before racing, particularly in studies with Quarter Horse or Thoroughbred racehorses. Sodium bicarbonate should never be administered to a distance horse, as losses of electrolytes in the sweat for several hours tend to excessively alkalinize the bloodstream.

Minerals and Trace Microminerals

CALCIUM/PHOSPHORUS

A quality, well-balanced diet probably provides a horse with necessary vitamins and trace minerals, including copper, zinc, molybdenum, sulfur, manganese, iron, and selenium. Calcium and phosphorus and other microminerals must be present in a horse's diet, not only in sufficient amounts, but also in the correct ratio, and this may require some adjustment. A veterinary consultation best manages mineral balances in a horse's diet.

Grains and grasses tend to be high in phosphorus; legume hays provide excess calcium. The ideal ratio of calcium to phosphorus (Ca:P) for a mature (working or idle) horse is between 1.2:1 and 2:1. (The maximum Ca:P ratio tolerated by a mature horse is 5:1, while a growing horse has a critical need for a ratio of about 1.5:1. A legume diet often provides a 5:1 ratio.) If calcium is in excess of phosphorus, musculoskeletal problems may develop, and a horse is prone to muscle cramps (tying-up syndrome) while exercising.

MICROMINERALS: COPPER, ZINC, IRON, IODINE, AND SELENIUM

There are many microminerals important to a horse's diet; however, some have more significance than others.

Copper is an important element for proper function of elastic connective tissue, to mobilize iron in the body, to maintain mitochondrial function, and for synthesis of melanin. Copper deficiency contributes to anemia and hair depigmentation. Studies have implicated copper deficiency with a higher risk of DOD, specifically osteochondrosis lesions in joint cartilage (see p. 133) or epiphysitis (see p. 132). Also, copper interacts with other microminerals, and excesses of these, such as zinc, sulfur, or molybdenum, may cause a functional deficiency of copper. Copper is present in adequate amounts in most equine feed.

Zinc has a role in activity of *metalloproteinase enzymes* (see p. 42). Zinc is also important for skin health and bone integrity. Excess zinc may interfere with the absorption of copper and calcium to create an absolute deficiency of either of these minerals, with resultant DOD problems.

Iron is commonly found in most forage products eaten by horses. Iron is important as a constituent of hemoglobin (oxygen-carrying substance in red blood cells) and myoglobin (protein of muscle tissue). It is rare to see iron deficiency in a horse that has not experienced acute blood loss. A deficiency would contribute to anemia, whereas excess iron affects zinc concentrations.

Iodine is important for thyroid hormone function. Iodine is found in salt, mineral supplements, or seaweed-containing products. Toxicity of iodine may lead to chronic respiratory disease, skin problems, and to *goiter* (enlargement of the thyroid gland).

Selenium is important to enzyme detoxification of components that are toxic to cell membranes. Its role is to stabilize cell membranes and counter the anti-oxidant effects of free radicals. Feed varies in content of selenium and some geographic areas may have too little in the roughage, whereas other geographical areas have excess. Toxicity creates problems in the hair, skin, and hooves (see p. 57), and as an acute form may cause blindness. Selenium deficiency causes muscle problems such as white muscle disease or tying-up syndrome (see p. 173).

Vitamins

VITAMIN A

Vitamin A is normally found in its precursor form, *beta-carotene*, in sufficient quantities in green hay, and particularly in legume hay. A deficiency is a problem only if the hay source being fed is of marginal quality, and is brown or sun-bleached. Excesses of vitamin A can lead to bone or tendon disease, while deficiencies lead to eye, skin, and reproductive problems, and infections. Vitamin A is stored in fat and the liver, so excess amounts fed can become toxic.

VITAMIN B

B vitamins play an important role in energy metabolism, and so contribute to performance. Not only does a horse obtain ample B vitamins in hay or pasture, but a horse with normal gastrointestinal function will produce ample quantities of vitamin B in his hindgut, particularly when fed an adequate supply of roughage (at least 50 percent of the diet). Intestinal disease, a lack of appetite, or a long-term course of antibiotic therapy may hinder production of B vitamins by the intestinal tract, and a horse with this issue may need supplementation. Anecdotal reports claim that B vitamins, particularly *thiamine*, help to calm anxious or nervous horses. Brewer's yeast (50 grams per day) can supply a portion of the B vitamin requirement. The kidneys excrete excess intake of B vitamins.

VITAMIN C

Vitamin C, also called ascorbic acid, is usually manufactured in plentiful supply in the liver by horses. Generally, it does not need to be supplemented except when a horse is stressed, as with training, competition, and transport, or is affected by respiratory problems. One supplement form, *ascorbyl palmitate*, is well absorbed at doses of 20 to 40 grams per day. If ascorbic acid is used, 10 to 20 grams should be fed per day. Vitamin C is water-soluble so the kidneys excrete excess amounts.

VITAMIN D

Vitamin D is important for calcium and phosphorus absorption and metabolism that is critical to bone, muscle, and tendon health. Horses ingest adequate amounts of vitamin D in quality hay, and they produce ample vitamin D if exposed to a few hours of daylight each day. Oral supplementation with excess vitamin D can lead to signs of toxicity: *dystrophic calcification* (deposition of bone in areas of soft tissue where there normally isn't bone) in the heart, blood vessels, and kidneys. Bones and joints may also develop calcium deposits, with resulting lameness and DOD.

VITAMIN E

Vitamin E is recognized as a useful antioxidant to stabilize cell membranes. Vitamin E is helpful to treat wounds (topical as well as ingested), to improve immune function, and for treatment of some neurologic conditions. Vitamin E is usually present in good quality, green roughage, especially in summer pastures. High doses (4000 to 6000 IU/day) of *alpha-tocopheryl* are generally supplemented for disease situations, whereas 500 IU/day is effective for managing selenium or fat supplementation. Vitamin E is fat-soluble and excess is not excreted but probably causes no harm.

Meeting Nutrient Requirements

By recognizing an evolutionary need for horses to frequently eat small amounts of good quality fiber, feeding practices can be modified to improve the health of the digestive system, and a horse's mental happiness. A horse performs best if his urge to nibble is satisfied with free-choice grass hay, and by supplementing only hard-working individuals or difficult keepers with extra calories.

The Idle and Lightly Worked Horse

An idle, mature horse that is not currently in training needs no special dietary considerations other than maintaining correct weight and body condition. Idle, mature horses fulfill their energy needs effectively with good quality roughage (hay or pasture), and need only be supplemented with free-choice salt and a balanced mineral mix.

When running a hand along a horse's ribs, only the last two should be felt. Usually, an idle horse thrives on a maintenance diet of 1¾ pounds quality grass hay per 100 pounds body weight. (In this example, a 1000-pound horse would receive about 18 pounds of hay per day.)

LIGHT TRAINING

When reintroducing a horse to a light training schedule of 3 to 4 days a week of trotting and cantering, feeding demands need only provide 15 percent more energy than maintenance. To provide a lightly exercised horse with the fuel he needs, feed up to 1½ pounds of grain for each hour of exercise, not to exceed 6 pounds a day, in addition to quality grass hay. Protein needs do not increase with light exercise, so a diet of 8 to 10 percent protein is sufficient for an adult horse.

The Hard-Working Athlete

The goal of a feeding and conditioning program is to improve muscular efficiency and provide fuel reserves for working muscles. The mental and physical stress of hard exercise on an athletic horse significantly increases energy and trace mineral demands. An equine athlete must be supplied with a quality ration that can be consumed within his intestinal limits (approximately 15 to 25 pounds of feed) while providing fuel for locomotion.

Horses in the endurance sports (endurance racing, long-distance competitive trail rides, and eventing) need large amounts of energy to sustain them through the rigors of prolonged athletic output, in both training and competition. At speeds less than 10 to 12 mph (a fast trot), horses work within aerobic limits, with ample oxygen supplied to working muscles.

Horses involved in sports requiring intense bursts of speed (racing, polo, hunting, gymkhana, roping, and cutting) will use aerobic metabolism, but they will also rely on fuel supplied under anaerobic conditions in the muscles (see chapter 6, *Muscle Endurance*, p. 141). Horses exercising at high speeds (more than 12 to 15 mph) rely primarily on anaerobic metabolism that does not burn fat efficiently. Without ample fuel supplies, a horse will lose his competitive edge as he tires.

REPLENISHING ENERGY

The diet of an equine athlete must not only fulfill normal metabolic function, but it must replenish energy supplies depleted in strenuous daily workouts. Hay does not offer enough energy to meet the fuel demands of an athletic horse, even if he eats his full intestinal limit (2½ percent of his body weight) every day. The sheer bulk of hay limits a horse's necessary intake.

Although it is difficult to maintain body fat on a hard-working horse, there are ways to maximize a horse's caloric and energy intake without jeopardizing his health or digestive function. To compensate for energy expenditures of rigorous athletics, it is helpful to supplement with beet pulp (see p. 328), concentrates (see p. 329), and fat (see p. 330). Up to half the daily intake (by weight) of feed can be supplied in a concentrated form.

FREE-CHOICE HAY

An active performance horse thrives best on free-choice hay so he can eat whenever the urge. A horse can consume more dry-matter nutrients from hay than he could from pasture, because more than 80 percent of hay's water content evaporates during the curing process. Good quality grass or oat hay is usually sufficient, but when necessary, about one-third of the roughage can be provided as a legume source (see p. 327). Pasture may be a sufficient roughage source provided a horse has ample time to graze and the pasture has adequate and balanced nutrients.

As mentioned earlier, roughage in the intestines provides a continuous energy source for an exercising horse, and serves as a reservoir to hold water in the intestines, restoring sweat losses and avoiding dehydration.

ELECTROLYTE SUPPLEMENTS

Although electrolytes are not technically considered "food," they are essential to a horse's well-being. During training and competition, an athlete may need electrolyte supplements besides a salt block (see p. 333).

Effects of Feeding on Gastrointestinal Function

Feeding encourages blood flow to be distributed to the digestive tract at the expense of other organ systems, like the muscles (see pp. 305 and 316). Cardiac output of fasted ponies at rest distributes 20 percent of blood flow to the intestines, while feeding increases this to 27 percent. Not only does the digestive tract become more active in the presence of feeding, but its bulk and weight increase as well. Saliva and intestinal juices necessary for digestive processes extract fluid from the plasma volume. This shift in hydration throughout the body drives the thirst reflex to make up for the demand.

The high-fiber diet of a horse is instrumental in holding water in the large intestine, conveniently making this a reservoir to draw upon during protracted exercise. However, there is a trade-off between added intestinal bulk and weight in an exercising horse as related to energy value of foodstuffs eaten. A study (Dr. Stephen Duran) summarized that the more fiber fed in the diet, the more fluid contained within the digestive tract, and hence the horse carries more internal weight. For endurance-type exercise, the weight and bulk of intestinal contents may not have as adverse an effect on performance when traded off with the ability of the guts to act as a reservoir to hold fluid. Yet, greater intestinal weight and bulk may have more of a negative impact on speed horses that exercise at high intensities for short periods of time, like racers, steeplechasers, or event horses. These horses may benefit by reducing the amount of fiber fed and supplementing with grain and oil prior to an exercise effort. A study (Dr. Kronfeld) determined that a mixed diet of forage plus grain and vegetable oil reduces feed intake by 22 percent, fecal output and gut fill by 31 percent, and the water requirement by 12 percent over horses fed a straight forage diet. Horses fed a strictly forage diet drank 33 percent more water than the horses fed a mixed diet thus adding to the weight and bulk of intestinal contents a horse must carry while exercising. If the objective is to maintain a horse in protracted work for hours at a time, then greater water intake is a good thing.

Moderate intensity exercise for medium duration describes a horse working at 50 to 75 percent of maximum capacity for hours where speed is not an important variable. This might be a show horse scheduled in numerous classes, or a recreational trail horse. The best strategy for this kind of horse would be to feed small but frequent meals of hay and high fiber feeds. Grain should be eliminated in the eight-hour period preceding exercise in order to minimize blood glucose fluctuations associated with the high carbohydrate content of grain.

Hot Climate Feeding

In the summer, horses are usually exercised more than during winter months. Although exercise burns calories and energy supplies, ironically, many horses reduce feed intake by 15 to 20 percent during heat spells. Water requirements vastly increase. Without ample water, a horse may stop eating when he actually needs to replenish his fuel resources.

A horse dissipates heat from actively working muscles through sweating, or evaporative cooling. As a horse sweats, loss of water and electrolytes leads to dehydration and diminished performance unless he can replenish those losses. To compensate for reduced feed intake and loss of electrolytes, it is important to increase digestibility of the diet, and to supply adequate nutrients to an exercising horse. A fit and properly nourished athlete with no excess body fat sweats efficiently. Conservation of body water and electrolytes delays the onset of fatigue or performance failure.

Heat Increment

Diet plays an important role in keeping a horse "cool" during exercise. Just as working muscle produces internal heat, so does digestion. The body metabolizes each foodstuff at a different level of efficiency. Digestion and metabolic processes, and muscular activity involved with eating and digestion produce a different kind of heat. This amount of heat is a food's *heat increment* (HI). Understanding which foods have low heat increments allows dietary manipulation to improve a horse's cooling ability during hot weather. The lower the heat increment, the less internal heat digestive processes generate, and the less heat a horse must dissipate in a warm climate.

GRAINS VERSUS ROUGHAGE

Grains are substantially lower in their heat increment than fibrous roughage feeds. Roughage, such as grass hay or pasture, has a heat increment value of 33 percent, while oats, barley, and alfalfa hay have HI values ranging from 15 to 18 percent. Corn has a HI of 10 to 12 percent. Compare these values to fat at a HI of 3 percent.

Because it is important to limit heat production in hot climates, and because high environmental temperatures reduce a horse's appetite, the grain portion of a ration may be increased to accommodate special needs. Grains are mostly digested and absorbed in the small intestine with little heat generated by metabolism, whereas bacterial fermentation of roughage in the cecum and large intestines generates heat. (This is one reason why extra hay should be fed to horses in wintertime, as large intestinal fermentation generates heat from within.)

Excess Grain

The proportion of grain fed should *never* exceed 50 percent of the ration. At least 1 percent of body weight must be consumed as roughage each day because fiber is essential to healthy equine digestive processes. Grain fed at more than half the ration may overwhelm the ability of the small intestine to digest the high starch content of grain. Excess fermentation of rich carbohydrates can lead to colic, gastrointestinal ulcers, laminitis, or tying-up syndrome. Grain concentrates provide calories to burn during exercise, but too much grain contributes to deposits of body fat. Insulating fat deposits slow heat dissipation to an extent greater than any value gained by overfeeding grains for their low heat increment.

Corn versus Oats

Contrary to popular myths, corn is not a "heating feed." This mistaken impression may be earned from the fact that corn is double the digestible energy as oats. If corn is substituted for oats at the same *volume* as oats, a horse will receive twice the energy. The result is a very "high" or "hot" horse that may become difficult to handle. An overly energized horse fusses and frets, and bad behavior patterns develop. References to such horses have dubbed corn with the misnomer of being a "hot" food. When substituting corn for oats, cut the volume in half. It is best to *weigh* the feed so there is no question as to how much energy a horse receives. (For more information, see p. 329.)

The HI of corn is one-third less than the HI of oats. This difference is due, in part, to the indigestible fibrous hull of oat kernels. As the large intestine breaks down this non-nutritive fiber, internal heat is generated from its metabolism.

Feeding corn instead of oats increases energy supplies. The amount of roughage a horse must eat can then be reduced as long as it still is offered as more than half of the ration, and only half the volume of corn needs to be fed as oats. A low HI and its high-energy content make corn a reasonable carbohydrate to feed in hot summer months when an individual requires additional calories.

FAT FOR ENERGY

Since the heat increment of fat is only 3 percent, it contrasts dramatically with other foodstuffs. Feeding 1 to 2 cups of vegetable oil each day provides a valuable source of digestible energy in the form of fat. Vegetable oil is efficiently digested and metabolized, while minimizing heat production in the body.

For horses that voluntarily limit feed intake during hot environmental temperatures, adding fat to the diet overcomes the difficulty of supplying ample energy. Fats are 2¼ times greater in energy density than an equal weight of grain. With fat supplementation, it is possible to reduce amounts of other foods and still meet daily energy needs. Feeding a cup of vegetable oil 2 times a day to a 1000-pound horse reduces the amount of grain required to maintain body weight by as much as 25 percent. There is also a decreased risk of laminitis or tying-up syndrome by feeding fat because less grain needs to be fed (see p. 330 for further explanation).

Protein Requirements in Hot Weather

Another mistaken belief of dietary folklore is that exercising horses need extra protein. Protein does not serve as a major fuel source during exercise efforts. Normally, an adult horse thrives on a diet of 8 to 10 percent protein. Supplementing protein greater than 15 percent may be detrimental to an exercising horse. Any slight increase in protein-need as a response to exercise is usually compensated for by an increase in both appetite and intake of food to fulfill energy demands. During high environmental temperatures, horses that voluntarily limit their food intake need only minimal protein supplementation by adding small amounts of alfalfa pellets or alfalfa hay to the ration. Legume hay has a relatively low HI value of 18 percent, whereas grass hay has an HI of 33 percent. Nonetheless, the high protein content (as much as 28 percent) of legume hay stimulates other adverse effects on an exercising horse.

PROTEIN'S ROLE IN SWEATING

An insignificant amount of protein is lost in sweat during exercise. Proteins act as "detergents" within sweat glands to disperse sweat "water" evenly along the hair shaft, resulting in more effective evaporative cooling. In early stages of training, proteins contribute to the "lather" of sweat (photo 12.4). As a horse is exercised daily in a conditioning program, proteins are not restored to the sweat glands between exercise periods. Therefore, as fitness improves, sweat thins, and less protein is lost during exercise.

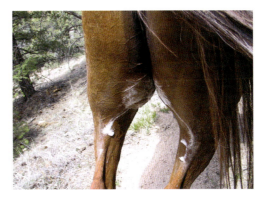

12.4 *The lather of sweat is created by proteins that act as "detergents" within sweat glands to disperse sweat "water" evenly along the hair shaft, resulting in effective evaporative cooling. As a horse becomes more fit, sweat becomes less lathered as the proteins are used up.*

EXCESS PROTEIN IN HOT CLIMATES

Protein-rich alfalfa hay tends to generate heat by metabolism, and indirectly affects a horse's performance by interfering with his cooling ability. Many horses easily tolerate this metabolic heat, while others do not. Too much protein fed to horses results in the need for more water, placing a performance horse at a disadvantage in hot climates. Similarly, feeding excess mineral supplements on a regular basis also promotes urination, resulting in the loss of more body fluids.

Muscle Fatigue

Muscle fatigue during performance is directly related to a buildup of excessive lactic acid, glycogen depletion, and heat in the muscles. In addition to greater metabolic heat production, high protein in a legume diet increases blood and muscle ammonia levels, resulting in an increased production of lactic acid in the muscle tissue. In turn, this may lead to fatigue and tying-up syndrome (see p. 166).

Increased Water Requirements

Nitrogen is a component of ammonia by-products from digestion of protein. Excess nitrogen in the body is toxic, and the body eliminates it through the urinary tract. A horse on a high-protein diet needs to drink more water to replace additional urinary excretion of nitrogen; increased body water loss compromises an exercising horse in a hot climate.

Respiratory Problems

Besides increased urine production, nitrogen in urine produces ammonia. Accumulation of ammonia fumes in stalls injures the respiratory tract, compromising how well the respiratory system can oxygenate the tissues, and potentially limiting performance (see p. 254). The respiratory tract also helps dissipate heat from the body. While evaporative cooling dissipates most of the heat, respiratory cooling contributes 20 percent to the cooling process. The healthier the respiratory system, the more an athletic horse benefits in all ways.

Electrolyte Supplements

Electrolyte losses through sweat are unavoidable. It is unnecessary to supplement light working or idle horses with electrolytes even in hot weather. Such individuals replenish their own needs from a free-choice salt block and good quality hay. However, horses in transit for hours in a hot trailer, or those performing short-duration speed events or lengthy periods of exercise in hot weather will sweat more than you may think. A distance athlete benefits from a dose of electrolytes the night before and the morning of the competition, in addition to continued replenishment throughout the event (see p. 333). These individuals may need 1 to 2 ounces of salt top-dressed on the feed at the end of the traveling or working day.

Improving Performance in Hot Weather

Manipulating meal times and quantities can increase the opportunity for internal heat (generated by digestion and metabolism) to be dissipated throughout the day. Small meals at frequent intervals optimize body-cooling mechanisms. During hot weather, feed the largest proportion of roughage at night. While a horse is resting during these cool hours, he metabolizes and ferments the fibrous portion of the diet. With less fiber in the intestines during exercise on hot days, heat produced from feed is not a limiting factor to performance.

In implementing a dietary program for a horse, there are no hard-and-fast rules. Each horse must be fed according to his individual needs. Not all horses need grain in their diet, while others require large amounts. Athletic pursuits and exercise regimens vary between horses, and from day to day for any individual. Genetics and age considerably influence the efficiency of nutrient use. By following some basic principles about which foods are "cooler" than others, and by discarding obsolete myths about feeding requirements, a horse's diet can be modified to improve mental and physical performance in all climates.

Cold Weather Feeding

A horse's nutritional needs increase about 5 to 10 percent for every degree below freezing. For every 10-degree-Fahrenheit drop below the *critical temperature* (the temperature below which a horse begins to burn calories to keep himself warm), a horse may require up to 20 percent more feed. The less flesh a horse has on his frame, the less insulation to fend off cold temperatures. Consider how it feels to go out in the cold weather wearing no more than a thin jacket: your body works harder to stay warm than it does when wearing an insulating down coat.

Roughage for Warmth

Offer good quality grass hay free-choice, which through fermentation by the microflora in the large intestine will generate heat from within, much like an internal combustion chamber. During cold, wet snaps, it is best to feed more hay to help a horse stay warm rather than to load him with extra grain. Over time, grain is helpful to put weight and fat on a horse's frame but does little for an immediate need for warmth. An exclusive diet of hay may not be enough to support additional climatic demands. Roughage is filling, so a horse may only consume a limited amount. Estimation of how much hay a horse consumes each day must also account for wind losses and any loss from trampling of hay into the ground or spreading it around so it's rendered unpalatable.

Provide Ice-Free Water

A major concern during wintertime is to ensure that a horse has plenty of fresh, clean, and ice-free water available at all times. A horse that stops drinking is more likely to suffer from impaction colic (see p. 303), or may decrease his feed consumption. If a dominant herd member won't allow others access to the trough for extended periods, then add another water tank to ensure equal opportunity.

A horse consumes 5 to 10 gallons of water per day in cold weather, and more when exercised. A warm bran mash may increase water consumption. If necessary, use stock-tank heaters to prevent ice formation, but beware of electrocution possibilities from floating heaters. Those heaters with heating elements that are totally immersed are safest. Check to make sure a heater is not shorting out in the water and thereby discouraging drinking. (If you see a horse standing near the tank, seemingly interested in drinking but not doing so, there may be an electrical short that is shocking him when he touches the water.) Protect electrical cords by running them through PVC pipe so a horse doesn't accidentally chew on the cord.

Assess Body Condition

A furry winter coat can mistakenly hide a gaunt frame. Run your fingers across a horse's thorax periodically to make sure he is holding flesh on his body. Ideally, the last two ribs should be barely felt when fingers are run lightly across the rib cage. If greater caloric intake is needed to maintain or increase body condition, supplement grass hay with alfalfa hay, beet pulp mash, and/or fat, and/or grain.

Body Condition Scoring System

One report concluded that racehorses have an optimal racing weight within a range of plus or minus 16 pounds. This range is a finely tuned balance, considering a horse can drink or urinate almost 16 pounds in a matter of moments. An average pleasure horse is considered overweight if he carries an excess of 100 to 300 pounds of body flesh. Body condition can be evaluated to determine the correct weight for an individual, regardless of breed or conformation. Use of a *condition scoring system* accurately estimates stored body fat more effectively than does measurements of weight, height, or heart girth.

Thickness of fat over the rump and back correlates well with total body fat. Also evaluate rib fat; although it is not as reliable an indicator, it should be considered as part of the whole picture. Feeling the fat cover and visually appraising areas over the back, croup and *tailhead* (top of the tail), ribs, behind the shoulder, and the neck and withers, enables assignment of a numerical condition value to each individual. This scale offers a *body condition score* (BCS) from 1 to 9, ranging from least body fat to most body fat (fig. 12.5).

Emaciated to Very Thin

An emaciated horse in poor condition has a BCS of 1 (photos 12.6 A & B). A very thin horse has a BCS of 2 (photo 12.7). The *spinous processes* (bony knobs on top of the vertebrae), ribs, tailhead, and hipbones project prominently. The bone structure of the neck, withers, and shoulders are pronounced, and no fatty tissue is felt.

Thin to Moderately Thin

A thin horse has a score of 3, and a moderately thin horse has a BCS of 4 (photos 12.8 and 12.9). There is some fat covering the spine about halfway up the spinous processes, but they are still easily seen. The ribs are visible but have a slight fat covering. The hipbones, tail-

BODY CONDITION SCORING SYSTEM

Score	Description	Back	Neck	Ribs	Shoulder	Withers	Tailhead
1	Emaciated	Vertebrae prominent	Extremely thin	All ribs show prominently	Little to no covering	Prominent	Projects prominently
2	Very thin	Vertebrae prominent	Very thin	Prominent	Very thin	Prominent	Very prominent
3	Thin	Vertebrae still visible although some fat half-way up	Thin	Ribs are visible but with thin layer of fat	Prominent	Prominent	Prominent
4	Moderately thin	Vertebrae slightly raised	Moderately thin	Slight outline still visible	Still lean appearance	Still lean appearance	Small layer of fat
5	Moderate or optimal condition	Back is level	Blends smoothly into the body	Ribs not visually distinguished but last two ribs can be felt	Rounded	Blends smoothly into the body	Feels spongy
6	Moderately fleshy	Back is level but full	Fat deposits	Fat covering is spongy	Some fat deposits	Some fat deposits	Fat is soft around tailhead
7	Fleshy	Crease down the back	Riddled with fat	Noticeable fat between ribs	Riddled with fat	Riddled with fat	Riddled with fat
8	Fat	Crease and ripple with fat	Thick and cresty	Cannot feel ribs at all	Ripple with fat	Ripple with fat	Ripple with fat
9	Obese	Rain-gutter-like crease down the back	Thick, cresty, and bulging with fat	Patchy fat over the ribs, and the flank lacks definition	Bulging fat	Bulging fat	Bulging fat

12.5

head, withers, shoulders, and neck are more full, but are discernible. Thin to moderatley thin horses do not have enough body reserves to support protracted or rigorous performance. They also chill easily in inclement weather.

Ideal Condition

A score of 5 corresponds to a "moderate" condition: the back is level, and the ribs are not visually distinguished but are easily felt when running a hand across them. Fat around the tailhead begins to feel spongy; the withers appear rounded over the spinous processes, with the neck and shoulders blending smoothly into the body. This condition is considered *ideal* (photos 12.10 A & B).

Moderately Fleshy

A horse with a body condition score of 6 is considered "moderately fleshy" and has certain features: fat around the tailhead is soft, fat over the ribs is spongy, and there is fat deposited along the withers, shoulders, and neck (photo 12.11).

Although this is not the best condition score for an athletic horse, such a plump condition is often seen in show horses. On occasion, it is appropriate for a horse to develop a moderately fleshy body condition. When a horse is continually exposed to inclement weather in harsh climates with no access to shelter, a thin layer of fat "traps" heat within the body. Also, a lactating mare needs plenty of body reserves to manufacture and provide enough milk for her foal, and she should not be maintained too lean.

Overweight

Many overweight horses tend to be fleshy, with a BCS of 7 (photo 12.12) or fat with a BCS of 8 (photo 12.13). Although individual ribs may be felt in a fleshy horse, there is noticeable fat between ribs, there is a crease down the back, and the withers, neck, and areas behind the shoulders are riddled with fat. It is difficult to feel the ribs at all in a fat horse, and the neck is noticeably thickened and "cresty." Shoulders, croup, and buttocks ripple with fat.

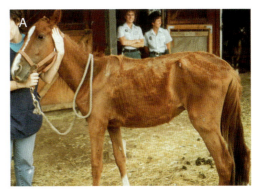
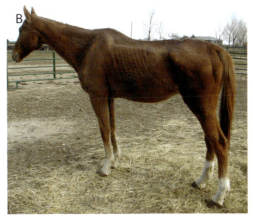

12.6 A & B *An emaciated horse with a body condition score of 1 has no flesh on his bones and is severely malnourished (A). Another BCS score of 1 is what should be a 1250-pound horse that weighs only 826 pounds (B).*

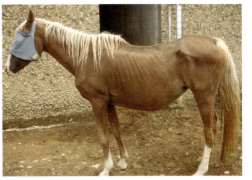

12.7 *This scrawny horse has a body condition score of 2.*

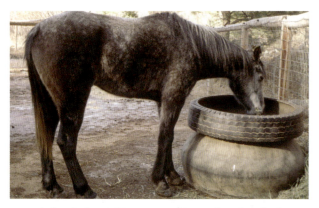

12.8 A thin body condition score of 3 or 4 describes this horse that has some flesh covering his frame, but the bones of the hips, ribs, tailhead, and withers are visible. A fuzzy fur coat sometimes makes it difficult to assess true body condition so it is important to use your hands to palpate what lies beneath.

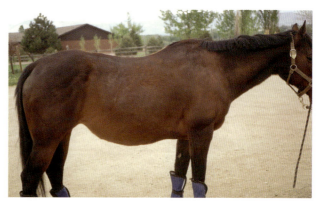

12.9 This horse is a lean body condition score of 4 with a thin layer of flesh over his ribs, but still not an optimum condition for athletic demands.

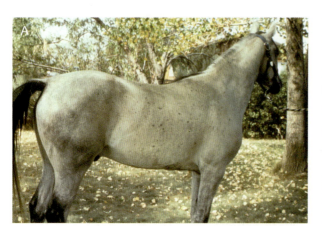

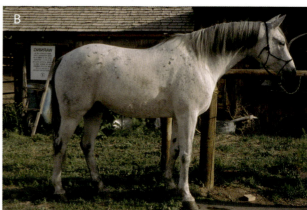

12.10 A & B Both these horses demonstrate variations on a desirable body condition score of 5. (A) is a relatively young horse, age 7, while (B) is an adult, teenage horse with bulkier muscling.

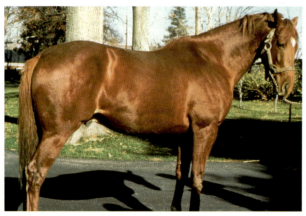

12.11 A body condition score of 6 describes a horse that is moderately fleshy, with ample fat over the ribs, tailhead, withers, shoulder, and neck.

The Digestive System: Nutritional Management 349

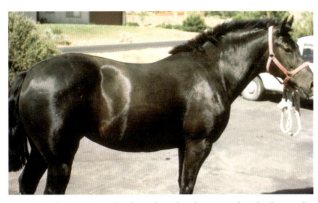

12.12 *A bit overweight describes this horse with a body condition score of 7. The ample fat coverage makes her appear soft and round, and slightly plump.*

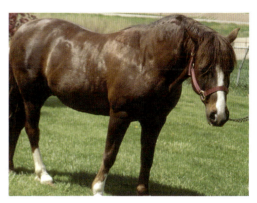

12.13 *A horse with body condition score of 8 is simply fat, with deposits of fat between the ribs, and along the withers, neck, and shoulders. This very fat horse developed laminitis as a result of overabundant caloric intake.*

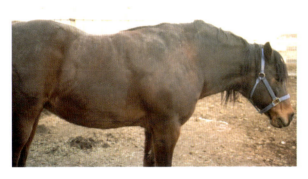

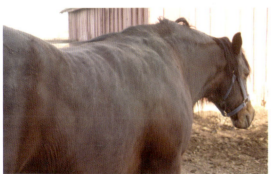

12.14 A & B *These images are of the same obese horse, which tops the scales with a body condition score of 9. Fat pads riddle her body in every location, the cresty neck, shoulder, and buttock fat pads representative of too much food and too little exercise.*

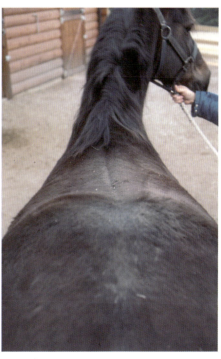

12.15 *This horse with a body condition score of 8 or 9 has a visible rain-gutter crease down his back due to fat deposits along the side of the back, buttocks, and shoulders.*

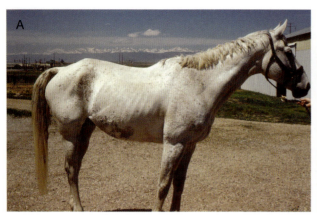
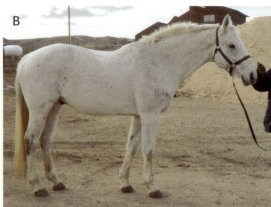

12.16. A & B *Photographs taken at intervals help to objectively assess a horse's body condition. This horse started with a body condition score of 3 (A), then after dietary modifications and 18 months, this same horse plumped into a condition score of 6 (B).*

Extremely Fat

An extremely fat horse tops the scale with a score of 9 (photos 12.14 A & B). Such a horse has a pronounced rain-gutter like crease along his back (which, in fact, will hold water), and patchy fat over the ribs (photo 12.15). Fat also bulges around the tailhead, along the withers, behind the shoulders, and along the neck. The flank lacks definition and is filled in with flesh. Ample fat along the inner buttocks causes them to rub together. Serious metabolic problems threaten such a horse if a weight-loss program is not begun immediately.

Monitoring Condition

Combining a scoring system with conventional methods, such as weighing a horse or measuring heart-girth, achieves fine-tuned control of body condition. Gradual weight gains are difficult to appreciate with daily observation. Weight tapes are not always accurate, but are useful to evaluate changes over time. Snapping a photograph of the horse at intervals permits an objective, visual comparison of body condition (photos 12.16 A & B).

Nutritional Diseases

Obesity

The subject of a malnourished horse conjures images of an emaciated rack of bones. However, malnourishment has another extreme: obesity. An overweight horse is a statement of dietary imbalance, one that is overabundantly supplied with energy.

EATING BEHAVIOR

A horse accumulates fat for the same reasons people do. Either too many calories for his level of exercise are provided, and/or a bored or greedy horse eats more than he needs. Eating behavior in horses evolved in an environment where survival of the "fittest" depended on a well-nourished and robust individual. A wild horse does not have the leisure or opportunity to become fat, whereas domesticated horses do.

Free-Choice Diet

Natural range forage is relatively low in energy, with variable nutritional content, depending on season and terrain. In the wild, horses consume moderate amounts of forage at frequent intervals, each meal being about 1 to 3 hours long. Unlike humans, the amount of food consumed is not governed by signals conveyed to the brain of stomach distention, or "feeling full," unless the distention approaches pain. A horse with free-choice food stops eating before the stomach is fully distended. Therefore, in the wild, stomach distention does not usually occur.

The amount of food a horse eats is governed by the rate of emptying food from the stomach, or the nutritive value of food in the stomach. Cues are sent to the brain from hormonal and nerve receptors that are integrated throughout the gastrointestinal tract and the body. These receptors recognize satisfaction of nutritive needs, and accordingly regulate hunger or fullness by an appetite-control center in the brain. In a natural state, these integrated signals do not influence the amount or length of a particular meal. Instead, these cues affect the time until, and the amount ingested at the next meal. A horse with normal control eats only enough to maintain good body health.

In an artificial environment where humans dictate when and how much a horse eats, this natural control of eating no longer plays as significant a role. Knowing this fact, feeding practices can be modified to advantage.

Meal Intervals

Horses with free-choice food do not voluntarily fast longer than 2 to 3 hours at a time. A horse receiving only two meals a day feels psychologically "starved" by the next meal because of imposed and lengthy fasting between meals. The horse then consumes large amounts rapidly at each feeding, rather than "grazing" throughout the day. If free-choice food cannot be arranged, it is best to feed a minimum of 3 times per day.

Palatable Foods

The actual presence of food induces a horse to eat, but how much he eats is determined by the food's palatability and how easy it is to obtain and eat. A horse's perception of smell, taste, and texture decides palatability of the food. With today's plethora of commercial feed choices, like grains and pellets, plentiful amounts of tasty and easily consumed feed are available without a horse having to seek it. Many horses eat until all the food is gone. Access to abundant or appealing foods may override normal "regulatory cues" from the gastrointestinal tract and metabolic pathways. A horse that continues to eat even though he is physiologically sated in energy and nutrients then stacks up the extra pounds.

Seasonal Effects

An extensive layer of fat beneath the skin protects horses from the elements. This insulation diminishes the penetrating effects of wet and cold. Insulating fat deposits maintain a precise body-temperature range, and they serve as a readily available source of energy when food is scarce.

Equine feeding behavior evolved in adaptation to an environment with ample nutrition in the summer, and sparse supplies in the winter. During mild months, horses store sufficient body fat and energy to last through a winter of limited forage. Horses have not yet adapted to the constancy of modern feeding practices that carry them through winter without need of surplus fat depots.

Competition

Competition within a herd stimulates dominant horses to run others away from the food. Assertive individuals may then have access to more food than they need. Coupling an evolutionary tendency to "plump" up, with easy accessibility to highly palatable and energy-

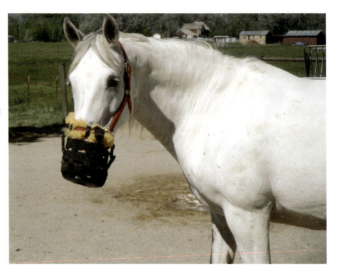

12.17 *A grazing muzzle is an excellent tool to limit nutritional intake when a horse is turned out to pasture. The muzzle should be attached to a halter that will break when the muzzle gets snagged on an object. Fleece over the noseband prevents facial abrasion. The horse is able to drink with ease, and a small hole in the bottom of the muzzle bucket allows him to work at cropping small amounts of grass so he "feels" as if he is actively grazing.*

dense food, results in an overweight horse. If exercise is restricted and a horse remains relatively idle, instead of building muscle, he continues to put on fat.

The Human Factor

It is much too simple to blame equine obesity on a tendency to overeat; the human factor is important. In some cases, the physiologically ideal body weight a horse carries may not correspond to ideal as viewed through an owner's eyes. Sometimes, human desire improperly plumps up a horse to "show" condition. It is our role to learn what constitutes healthy body condition so we do not overindulge a greedy individual. One of the greatest health hazards for horses is obesity.

A diet must be continually retailored to accommodate a horse's exercise demands and the weather. It is helpful to take photographs periodically to compare body condition from month to month. A horse owner sees a horse each day, so it is easy to lose perspective. A picture really is worth a thousand words. Although not exactly accurate, weight tapes also provide a useful comparative measure of how much a horse is gaining, or losing.

GRAZING MUZZLE TO CONTROL OBESITY

A grazing muzzle is helpful in controlling dietary intake of a horse, particularly when turned out to pasture (photo 12.17). A grazing muzzle allows a horse to drink, but restricts consumption of grass or hay. The horse can still self-exercise with pasture turnout, but he can only obtain a limited amount of roughage through the holes in the muzzle. Horses do extremely well wearing these for an entire spring and summer season. It is helpful to apply fleece over the noseband to prevent chafing of the face. Attach a muzzle only to a halter (leather or a BreakAway® halter) that will break if snagged.

Obesity-Related Diseases

Obesity is a systemic disease that can lead to serious consequences and metabolic problems in the horse. A list of these problems includes:

- Colic (see chapter 11, *The Digestive system: The Oral Cavity, Dental Health, and the Intestinal Tract*, p. 297)
- Exercise intolerance
- Myositis or tying-up syndrome (see chapter 6, *Muscle Endurance*, p. 166)

- Heat exhaustion (see chapter 13, *The Skin as an Organ*, p. 359)
- Musculoskeletal injuries
- Intestinal lipomas (see chapter 11, *The Digestive System: The Oral Cavity, Dental Health, and the Intestinal Tract*, p. 309)
- Insulin resistance (see chapter 3, *The Hoof*, p. 79)
- Equine metabolic syndrome (see chapter 3, *The Hoof*, p. 78)
- Laminitis (see chapter 3, *The Hoof*, p. 74)

Obesity also contributes to developmental orthopedic diseases such as malformation of joint cartilage (*osteochondrosis*) or inflammation of the growth plate (*epiphysitis* or *diaphyseal dysplasia*) in a growing horse (see chapter 5, *Joints*, p. 109). Pregnant mares may have difficulty foaling due to reduced muscle tone attributable to lack of exercise associated with obesity. Although they are listed here as a group, each individual syndrome is a separate debilitating condition, potentially resulting in permanent lameness or death. At the very least, an overweight horse cannot perform to potential.

The Skin as an Organ   13

Besides being an emblem of shining condition, a horse's skin is considered an important organ to maintain inner health (photo 13.1). Not only does the armor of the skin protect as a physical barrier against environmental irritants and trauma, but it also serves other important functions.

The Role of the Skin as an Organ

- Skin and the overlying hair coat provide a photo-protective barrier against ultraviolet rays from the sun.
- The hair coat and the layer of fat beneath the skin provide insulation against winter cold.
- Skin is important as an immune barrier by its ability to recognize foreign proteins (*antigens*) such as bacteria, fungi, and viruses; the skin responds to these potential invaders by secreting immunoglobulins to neutralize their dangers to a horse's health.
- Skin also serves as a metabolic barrier against topical exposure to toxic compounds encountered in the environment.
- A critical role of the skin is its ability to regulate internal temperature of the body: skin contains sweat glands that function to dissipate heat generated by working muscles.

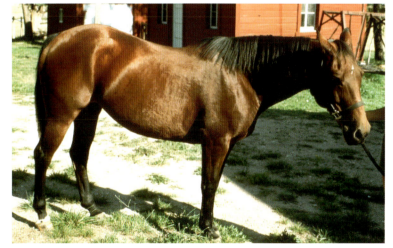

13.1 *A shiny hair coat reflects inner health.*

Skin's Role in Thermoregulation

As a mammal, an internal set point is regulated in a horse's midbrain to maintain body temperature within a very narrow range. Working skeletal muscles generate a lot of internal heat. Part of the body-temperature-control process relies on losing heat generated by working muscles and normal digestive metabolism. A racehorse running 1 mile in 2 minutes can lose as much as 2½ gallons of sweat as he "cools" his body. A well-conditioned horse loses as much as 2 to 3 gallons per hour in the face of protracted exertions under conditions of high heat and humidity.

One primary means a horse has to dissipate this heat is by evaporative heat loss through sweat. Blood flow is used as a conduit for heat transfer from working muscles to the skin. Some proportion of heat is lost from the inner body by rapid respiration and panting, but the bulk of heat dissipation depends on an efficiently functioning sweating mechanism. A horse's hair coat acts as an insulating layer that deters effective heat dissipation through the sweat. Fat also insulates against heat loss from the body core. In winter this is useful, but in the heat of summer, it can challenge an exercising horse. Too much fat or hair elicits a greater sweating effort with the attendant result of increased losses of fluid and electrolytes in the sweat.

Sweat glands have a nerve supply in close association with them. "Body water" lost in equine sweat is *hypertonic* (more salty) relative to equine plasma, and is in contrast to less salty human sweat. Equine sweat particularly loses sodium, chloride, and potassium salts. Low-intensity yet prolonged exercise, associated with some equine endurance-related sports, results in sustained losses of fluids and electrolytes leading to dehydration and to electrolyte imbalances (see p. 316). No amount of training or competition will alter the concentration of electrolytes lost in the sweat; however, training and fitness improve the efficiency and strength of working muscles, making each effort less difficult. A horse sweats slightly less when fit. Equine sweat also has a high concentration of proteins that are seen as a foamy lather on sweating skin (see photo 12.4, p. 343). These proteins help spread and evaporate the sweat over a larger surface area to further dissipate internal body heat.

DISSIPATING THE HEAT

With each stride, muscles of an exercising horse flex and strain from the effort. Vast amounts of heat accumulate from the metabolism of working muscles: over half of the energy used for muscular activity and locomotion in a horse is converted to heat. If no thermoregulatory mechanisms were active in an exercising horse, metabolic heat could increase by 1.8° F (1° C) for every 5 to 8 minutes of exercise. Fortunately, the equine system has developed useful mechanisms to rid the body of this metabolic heat load. As body temperature in the core elevates during exercise, heat dissipation mechanisms are triggered. The extent of this triggered response is relative to the degree of elevation of the core body temperature. A specific core temperature initiates sweating as a valuable reaction; this changes in response to the heat load accumulated within working skeletal muscles. Such a complex and interactive feedback system is important for maintaining stable body temperature innate to mammals.

In order for body temperature to remain within a constant range, the rate of heat production must equal that of heat loss. Any factors that limit the ability of the horse to dissipate heat will increase temperature within working muscles. Elevated muscle temperature is an irritant to muscular contractions and can precipitate spasms or tying-up syndrome (see p. 166).

As exercise proceeds, muscles continue to store heat, which is then transferred slowly to the core; there, thermoreceptors are activated to directly increase blood flow to the skin for sweating. Blood flow increases by as much as ten-fold to working muscles to improve oxygen supply in the muscles and to remove heat and metabolic waste products from the muscles.

Heat is transferred to the skin by circulating blood. Under normal circumstances, increased temperature in the skin drives evaporation of sweat, while increased blood flow supplies the fluid to create sweat. Blood vessels are well developed in a fit horse to facilitate heat dissipation (photo 13.2). With fitness and training, more capillary beds develop in the skin. These are visible on the skin surface, and particularly stand out when a horse is hot and the vessels are dilated. With heat as a driving force, arterioles and *arteriovenous anastomoses* (AVAs) dilate to increase blood flow through the skin. (AVAs connect arterioles and veins; opening of these vessels bypasses the capillary beds so more blood is flushed through larger areas of skin to release heat more quickly.)

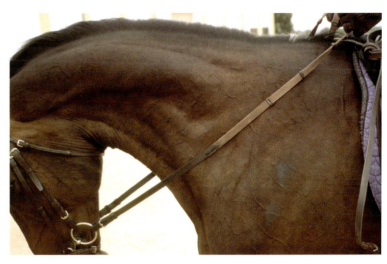

13.2 *Blood vessels are well developed in the skin of a fit horse to facilitate heat dissipation by bringing internal body heat to the surface for the evaporative cooling of sweat.*

Wherein Lie the Problems?
An efficient cooling process is dependent on sufficient blood circulation and so is dramatically and adversely affected by dehydration. A dehydrated horse selectively recruits blood flow at the expense of various organs, including the skin and the gastrointestinal system. Along with a highly developed vascular network within the skin, cardiac output increases to the muscles and skin of a working horse, with as much as 15 percent of the cardiac output being diverted to the skin. With preferential circulation to those organs actively involved in maintaining locomotion, blood flow is diverted away from other organ systems. In humans, blood flow to the kidneys and intestines decreases by 25 to 40 percent; it is possible that this is the case in horses as well. Decreased intestinal blood flow may be associated with impaction colic, intestinal displacements, and reduced uptake of nutrients, electrolytes, and fluids from the bowel.

NATURAL COOLING METHODS
The body dissipates a vast amount of heat produced by muscle metabolism through evaporation. A smaller amount of heat is lost through respiration.

Evaporative Cooling
Hours of protracted exercise or high intensity exercise for short periods are conditions that particularly tax the ability of a horse to move heat out of the body as quickly as possible. To remove muscular heat, a horse sweats, pulling heat from the interior of his body to the skin in a process known as *evaporative cooling*. Water vapor on the skin, produced from the sweat glands, pulls heat from the blood vessels and the outside air evaporates the warm skin water (photo 13.3). Around 70 percent of the heat of locomotion is normally dissipated from the body using this process of evaporative cooling. Along with heat loss, evaporative cooling also releases large quantities of fluid and electrolytes.

Respiratory Cooling
As internal body temperature rises, sweat is not the only means to dissipate heat. Another, but

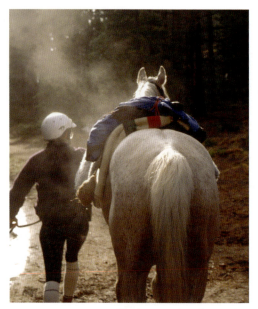

13.3 *Water vapor on the skin, produced from the sweat glands, pulls heat from the blood vessels, and the outside air evaporates the warm skin water. On a cool day, heat dissipated from body sweat is visible as steam.*

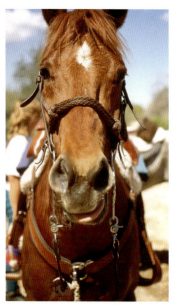

13.4 *Rapid breathing is a contributory mechanism to eliminating heat load in a hot horse. The flared nostrils of this horse are typical of one that is rapidly moving air because he is overheated.*

less-effective mechanism can eliminate up to 15 percent of the heat load: just as a panting dog moves air across his hanging tongue, a horse breathes rapidly to cool his body (photo 13.4). Warmed blood flowing from heated skeletal muscles circulates to the heart and through the lungs. With each incoming breath, cool air (and oxygen) is exchanged for warm, exhaled air.

EXTERNAL COOLING METHODS

Cool Water Application

Repeatedly drenching the neck, chest, and legs with water creates a similar evaporative effect as sweating. Copious bathing of a horse's head, neck, armpit, and legs with cool water assists cooling. Large blood vessels in these locations flush heat to the skin surface. Rapid evaporative cooling is achieved by continual sponging of these areas. Draping wet towels over the head and neck may be counter-productive to cooling as towels serve to insulate, particularly if the water on them remains warm. Continuously apply and scrape water away until the horse's skin feels cool to touch. The respiratory rate should settle down as internal body temperature is brought back within a normal range (see *Appendix A*, p. 567). All exercised horses need some assistance with cooling in the summer months even if the respiratory rate is not inverted or elevated.

Ideally, the body temperature of an overheated horse should only be decreased by 1° F (0.5° C) every 30 to 40 minutes by bathing head and neck areas with water. Cooling a horse down too rapidly leads to chilling. In hot and humid climates, cold or ice water may be applied to the entire body with less risk of muscle cramping.

The danger in cooling these large muscle groups too rapidly lies in the tendency of blood vessels to constrict away from the surface while retaining metabolic by-products (heat, lactic acid) that need to be carried out from deep muscle tissues. Diminished blood flow to the skin surface is an effect of too rapid cooling; this further allows heat to persist within deep muscles, causing heart and respiratory rates to remain elevated. Besides exhibiting poor metabolic recovery, the horse might develop tying-up syndrome, with sudden cramping and muscle spasms (see chapter 6, *Muscle Endurance*, p. 166). Such an affected horse refuses to move, and may exhibit signs of "colic" due to pain akin to a severe "charlie-horse." Heart and respiratory rates further climb in response to pain. As muscle fibers spasm and contract, more heat is generated in already overheated muscles.

Continue to monitor rectal temperature and muscle tone while cooling out a horse. Once the rectal temperature reaches 101° F (38° C), see if the horse stabilizes without further cooling assistance. Walking and natural cooling mechanisms further dissipate heat from muscles. Suppleness of the muscles can be assessed, as well as tenderness to hand pressure along the large muscle groups of the back or hindquarters (see p. 168). A normal horse has a fluid stride in contrast to one that is beginning to tie-up. Tight or excessively firm muscles, or obviously cramping muscles indicate fatigue and electrolyte abnormalities.

Cool Drinking Water

A bucket of water should be offered to a horse following exercise. If the horse has been galloping, only offer small, frequent drinks initially until he has cooled down a little bit. If the horse has been working aerobically for protracted periods, he should be encouraged to drink as much as he desires at every opportunity, during and after exercise.

Shade and Air Currents

Find an area of shade for the overheated horse, and one where there is decent air circulation, preferably with a light breeze. An enclosed space with stagnant air adds to heat retention. Fans are helpful to amplify *convective cooling*: as air flows across the horse's body, it pulls heat off the skin. Periodic, short walks help the muscles pump heat out of deeper tissues.

A dangerously overheated horse may need to be dunked into an available pond, or soaked entirely by hose or with buckets of water. Intravenous (IV) fluids are often necessary for treatment of a horse suffering from severe heat stress. IV fluids not only treat dehydration and shock to maintain circulatory health, but they also cool internal organs and muscles.

Heat Stress

Initially, as internal body temperature rises, the bulk of blood from cardiac output is diverted to the skin away from working muscles to facilitate heat dissipation. Internal heat continues to rise if surface evaporation (sweating) is no longer able to keep pace with the heat buildup. As muscle temperature elevates, contractile function of the muscle fibers is impaired, further contributing to fatigue and exhaustion (see p. 169). Loss of vital fluids through the skin causes a steady state of dehydration unless this "water" is replenished. Blood flow diminishes to the subcutaneous layers of the skin, further limiting sweating action in an effort to conserve body water. Heat continues to build within the horse with no outlet.

Heat stress occurs when body temperature climbs above 105° F (40.5° C) and the body cannot efficiently cool itself. Heat stress generally develops from overexertion leading to overheating rather than to external heating by the sun's rays. A bright, sunny day contributes to high ambient temperatures. Exhaustion or heat stress may develop if weather conditions have overtaxed a horse's ability to dissipate heat, or have interfered with proper fluid and electrolyte levels of the body.

HOT WEATHER

Hot weather limits a horse's ability to shed heat from the body. The horse sweats, but sweating is not always enough to stay ahead of the heat buildup. As either environmental temperature or humidity increase, evaporative cooling of sweating becomes less efficient. Training during hot and humid weather, especially interval training or prolonged workouts, can cause heat stress. The horse should be monitored closely for signs of heat stress on hot, humid days. Workouts should be less intense or shorter to prevent heat buildup in working muscles.

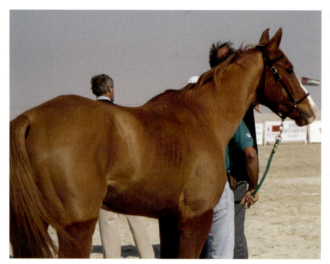

13.5 *A full body clip provides the greatest surface area for evaporative cooling and dissipation of heat generated by working muscles.*

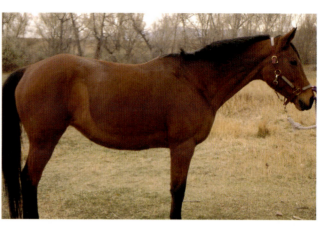

13.6 *A trace clip is useful when weather conditions vacillate between cool at night and hot during the day. The horse can relieve a good deal of heat in the areas of large blood vessels on the neck, chest, and abdomen, yet still retain enough of a fur coat to insulate against the cool of night.*

A horse sporting a full fur coat is at risk of overheating since the hair coat that keeps him warm in cold climates serves as an insulator to heat dissipation. Hairy horses should be clipped to accommodate taxing weather conditions (photos 13.5, 13.6, and 13.7 A & B). Heavily muscled horses, such as warmblood breeds and Quarter Horses, are at greater risk of retaining heat in the working muscles than leaner breed horses such as Arabians or Thoroughbreds. Wetting the neck, chest, and forelegs of the horse before and during exercise can delay heat buildup on a hot day.

LEVEL OF CONDITIONING

Hot weather is not the only factor contributing to development of inversions, dehydration, or signs of heat stress. A horse that is ridden too fast for his level of condition produces excess body heat. An overweight horse with abundant fat layers beneath his skin cannot dissipate heat effectively. A horse being asked to climb a particularly intense hill or mountain, or to put forth an extraordinary work effort in jumping or galloping will tend to overheat. A horse that is ridden for too long without a rest may also build up an excess heat load in the muscles.

Not only does excess body weight interfere with normal cooling processes, but it also reflects a lack of fitness. Adequate preparation and training develop a horse into a sleek physique, building muscle where once there was fat. Conditioning expands capillary beds and blood flow within skin and muscles to improve circulation of oxygen in the tissues and flushing of heat to the skin surface.

TRANSPORT ISSUES

Transport of a horse in an enclosed trailer in hot weather can also contribute to dehydration and heat stress. (For more discussion, refer to "Transport Stress," chapter 15, *Preventive and Mental Horse Health,* p. 478.) A horse that has shipped from a distance away and has not been acclimated specifically to exercise in hot and humid conditions is ill-prepared to deal with the added stress of the environment no matter how fit the athlete. Most horses need at least three

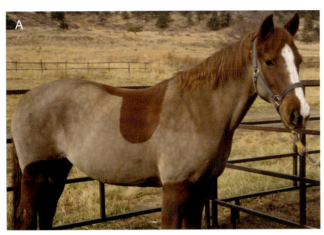 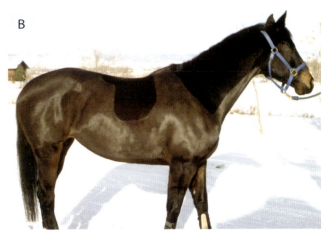

13.7 A & B *These horses each have a "shave job" that is more than a trace clip, yet not an entire body clip. In (A) hair is left in the area of the saddle to prevent chafing, and on the legs, while the horse in (B), with a blanket clip, has fur on her neck so she does not need a neck blanket for cool nights.*

weeks in a warmer climate to allow their bodies to learn to dissipate heat most efficiently.

EXCESS SWEATING

One of the more challenging environmental conditions to an exercising horse occurs in hot and humid climates. High heat and humidity limit the ability of heat loss through evaporative cooling of sweat because there is less temperature differential between the hot air and the hot skin to facilitate evaporation of sweat. This results in persistently higher temperatures in the working muscles. In addition, many overheated horses continue to pour off enormous amounts of sweat, and in so doing will continue to lose significant amounts of body fluids and electrolytes. The entire skin surface of such a horse remains soaked in his sweat; sweat drips into his eyes. Such sweat losses may not contribute sufficiently to cool the horse. Eventually, the horse may become so dehydrated that there is no longer a sufficient supply of body fluid to generate sweat.

ANHIDROSIS

In conditions of excess heat and humidity, a horse may cease sweating altogether due to a syndrome known as *anhidrosis*. In this case, the sweat glands cease to function and although the horse is hard at work, the skin remains dry and hot. A horse that does not sweat cannot cool himself. These horses tend to overheat rapidly. Performance suffers and dangerous heat exhaustion can occur if the horse's problem goes unrecognized.

Besides restricting all exercise, or helping such a horse to cool with soaks and fans, a suggested treatment for anhidrosis is the use of *clenbuterol* for its ability to stimulate sweat glands.

DETERMINING THE DANGER OF HEAT STRESS

A simple formula of *heat index* determines the danger of heat stress on any given day by adding the air temperature in degrees Fahrenheit to the percent humidity. If, for example, the temperature is 90° F (32.2° C) and the humidity is 80 percent, the sum is 170. At this level, evaporative cooling may not be enough to cool the horse. In order to know heat index, it is necessary to know temperature and percentage of moisture in the air. There are several tools for obtaining the moisture content of the air; among them is the *wetbulb thermometer*, which is also used to calculate dewpoint (interrelationship between temperature, moisture, and wind). Because these are difficult measurements to obtain without special equipment, a general rule for heat index can be applied as follows (fig. 13.8):

- If the sum of temperature and humidity is less than 120, normal cooling mechanisms are sufficient unless a horse is obese or has a long hair coat.
- If the sum of temperature and humidity is greater than 140, a horse relies mostly on sweating to dissipate body heat.
- If the sum of temperature and humidity is greater than 150, and especially if humidity contributes more than half of this amount, evaporative cooling is severely compromised.
- If the sum of temperature and humidity is greater than 180, there is no natural means for the body to cool itself; internal body temperature will continue to rise, resulting in heat stress.

PREVENTING HEAT STRESS

Whenever possible, employ effective cooling strategies so blood flow is also maintained in the muscles and intestines rather than being predominantly diverted to the skin. Sponge at every opportunity in hot weather, and soak a horse's body in humid conditions. Use a sweat scraper to remove residual water from the skin as the water that has just been applied quickly becomes warm and acts as an insulator on your horse's skin. Continually apply water until

Heat Index
Heat + Humidity General Rule

< 120	Horse can cool himself
130–150	Needs sponging or hosing
> 150	Difficulty cooling even with assistance
160–170	Must decrease speed and duration
> 180	Should not compete in these conditions

13.8

the skin feels cool to touch. Allowing a horse to drink at every opportunity is a helpful cooling strategy.

In addition to conditioning for the intended task, ride at a pace that is within a horse's ability to perform. Keep him steady and as calm as possible. When in a group, ride with horses that move at a similar speed and have a quiet disposition. Sweat losses can be minimized by routinely using cooling strategies and by maintaining a horse's most efficient gait.

Body water losses begin the minute a horse leaves home. Try to arrive several days before a competition that is a long distance from home. This gives a horse time to recuperate, relax, and rehydrate.

Use of a Thermistor

With increasing ambient temperatures, blood flow to the skin increases to conduct heat flow from the interior to the body surface. Skin temperature increases accordingly and this can be measured with the use of a *thermistor* sensor pad placed under the saddle blanket in front of the saddle pommel (photo 13.9). Surface skin temperature in a working horse should not exceed 101 to 102° F (38 to 39° C). In instances where blood flow is reduced to the skin due to dehydration or poor circulation, the thermistor may read surface skin temperatures

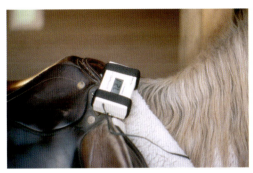

13.9 *A skin temperature gauge, called a thermistor, is useful to obtain a relative measure of internal body heat during locomotion. While a horse exercises, skin temperature exceeding 101° F (38° C) indicates overheating, yet a reading below 97° F (36° C) may indicate that the horse does not have sufficient circulation to the skin due to dehydration.*

below 97° F (36° C), which, for the skin of an exercising horse, is too low. Either too high or too low a reading can forecast problems for the horse. Both situations indicate that there is insufficient circulation to the skin to rid the body of its heat load, and this may be due to dehydration concerns. (For more discussion on dehydration and exercise intolerance, see chapter 9, *Cardiovascular Conditioning*, p. 235.)

Skin Diseases

Diagnosing Skin Diseases

AN ACCURATE DIAGNOSIS
The diversity of skin problems in horses is varied, and in many cases visual inspection of a lesion may not accurately diagnose the reason for the problem. The best means to identify what is wrong with a horse's skin is to have a veterinarian perform a skin biopsy. A biopsy takes a punch of tissue through all skin layers and gives a definitive diagnosis of the disease process, and often the source of the problem. In addition, a skin-scraping sample can be reviewed under a microscope to determine cell type or to identify parasitic organisms. A tissue sample can be submitted to a lab to culture for fungal or bacterial organisms when appropriate. These tests are simple to perform with minimal discomfort to a horse.

In the field of veterinary dermatology sometimes the disease cannot be positively identified, but rarely are skin diseases life threatening. Some questions to ask when investigating a skin lesion include:

- What is the horse's age and breed?
- In what season did the lesion appear?
- How long has the lesion been present?
- What is the location of the skin lesion(s) and where did the lesion first appear?
- Has the lesion spread?
- What does the lesion look like? Is there hair loss? Is it red? Is it scabby? Is it crusty or scaling? Is the affected area moist or dry? Any granular material?
- Are hairs broken, or do they pull out readily? Do hairs mat together?
- Is there a firm nodule, or a soft swelling?
- Is the skin of normal texture or thickness?
- Does the lesion bother the horse, i.e. does he scratch or bite at it?
- Is the area sensitive when touched or pressed?
- Are other horses on the premises similarly affected?
- Has the horse traveled to a different premise?
- Does the horse have other medical problems?
- Is the horse on any medication?
- Is the horse pastured and/or stalled?
- What is the horse's diet (including supplements or horse treats)?

By examining a horse carefully, and noting these particulars on the checklist, an owner can help portray a clinical picture to a veterinarian about the progression of a skin problem. A careful veterinary examination combined with further diagnostic aids facilitates rapid diagnosis. With an accurate diagnosis, therapy is best implemented.

Mechanical Skin Concerns

The inner and invisible workings of the skin are vital to a working horse, but horse skin as a protective barrier also plays an important role in successful performance. Even the slightest wound or trauma or photosensitivity reaction of the skin of the legs can elicit sufficient lameness to render a horse unfit for riding.

SADDLE SORES AND GIRTH GALLS

Causes of Saddle Sores

Poorly fitting girths and cinches can bunch up along the girth area and create a friction rub. Dirt or mats of hair wadded in the crevices of webbing or fabric of the girth or cinch similarly abrade tender skin. Poorly placed or inappropriate types of electrodes of heart rate monitors create stress points on the skin that are then subject to trauma (see p. 222).

There is no substitute for well-fitted equipment and diligent monitoring for problem spots. Even with a custom-fit saddle, problems can arise. Uphill climbs and downhill descents in steep terrain, or rapid movements created by jumping, reining, cutting, or roping sports may cause a saddle or girth to shift, creating friction points. Changes in body physique accompany changing seasons or varied levels of condition. A summer fat or winter lean frame changes saddle fit. A tired horse may subtly alter his gait, causing imperfectly fit tack to chafe in unlikely places.

Different breeds of horses are prone to saddle sores. Many accomplished athletic horses tend to have thin skin. Thin skin is an advantage for cooling the horse's core during exercise, but thin skin is also easily damaged. Thoroughbreds are known for their thin, tender skin, as are Arabians.

Sweat and caked-on mud that remain on a horse after a workout might irritate the skin, creating conditions that favor bacteria, such as *Staphylococcal* organisms that normally live on the skin. Bacterial infection is easily avoided by rinsing hair and skin after a workout to remove accumulated sweat and debris.

Signs of Saddle Sores

Sometimes it is hard to detect problems that occur with saddle fit until an obvious soreness or wound develops. Not all horses provide clues that tack is ill-fitting. If a horse shows progressively poor behavior such as wringing his tail, humping his back, or acting cranky or sluggish when asked to move forward, then look for saddle sores. A self-preserving individual may demonstrate less subtle behavior changes: he stops in his tracks, refusing to move until an offending article is removed.

Signs of impending saddle sores include subtle behavioral changes, or raised, swollen areas of the skin. Swelling is caused by serum leaking beneath the skin, along with edema due to poor circulation beneath a pressure or friction point. These spots often are tender to finger pressure, and are red, inflamed, or ulcerated (photos 13.10 and 13.11). Other warning signs are isolated spots of missing hair with a pinkish tinge to the skin, indicating mild abrasion at a friction point. Note isolated dry areas under the saddle after a workout. Dry heat builds under pressure points where the skin cannot sweat and breathe.

Hair follicles and pigment-producing cells (*melanocytes*) may succumb to localized heat

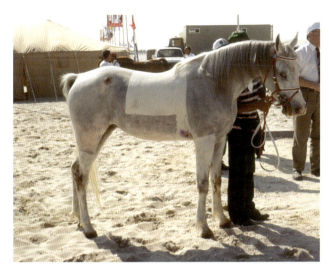

13.10 *This horse has been shaved to leave fur in the saddle and girth area, yet he has developed a significant sore on the right side of his girth.*

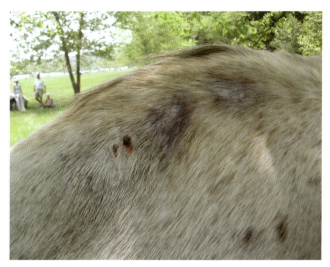

13.11 *Saddle movement or compression can create a serious withers' sore, as seen here, with the potential to deeper infection as fistulous withers (see p. 214). This horse, with high withers, needs to be rested from work to heal, and he should be fit with an appropriate saddle and light rider in future.*

production, resulting in growth of black hairs on a gray horse, or white hairs on any other colored horse (photo 13.12). This destruction of melanocytes results not only from heat injury to the skin, but from any form of physical trauma.

Prevention of Saddle Sores

Prevention of saddle sores is based on common sense and attention to detail.

Equitation

Rider expertise is important. When a horse must carry an unbalanced rider, tack should be checked frequently. A rider sitting off-center may grip more with one side of the body than another, or may dig in with calves or heels. Sores may be found under the leg skirts or stirrup leathers.

Selecting the Proper Saddle

The type of athletics pursued is critical when selecting a saddle. Using a dressage saddle on

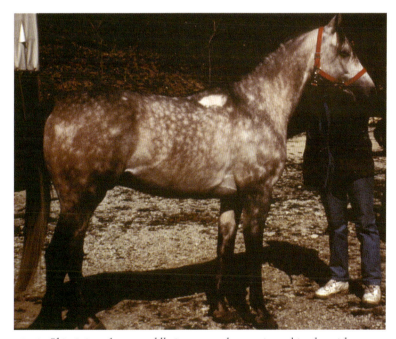

13.12 *Skin injury from a saddle is commonly experienced in the withers area with a loss of pigment, as seen by the white spot on this grey horse. As this horse turns whiter with maturity, subsequent injury to the hair follicles will likely leave dark discoloration to the coat.*

a trail horse invites problems with sore backs, for both horse and rider. Although a heavy-duty roping saddle may fit a horse's back well, its added weight can hasten fatigue. When a horse exerts an extended work effort, a heavy saddle contributes to heat buildup.

Grooming

Before saddling, carefully curry and brush the horse so grit does not embed in the skin. Dirt particles abrade protective hair from the skin, contributing to skin chafe. Saddle blankets should be cleaned of matted hair and sweat-caked dirt before each use so no friction points develop under the saddle.

Saddle Pads

Use saddle pads that wick away excess moisture from the skin and pads that won't trap heat beneath the saddle. The best way to avoid saddle sores is to make sure the saddle fits well (see p. 209). There should be no pressure points, and the saddle shouldn't shift fore and aft, or side to side. Saddle pads should be uniformly thick and smoothed out so there is no material bunching up. When saddling, put the saddle blanket on the horse's neck, and slide it backward into position in the same direction as the hairs lay to flatten the hairs beneath the pad.

New technology has provided materials for saddle pads that have not been previously available. One such product is the Supracor® pad, which is made of synthetic material favored in wheelchairs and hospital beds (photo 13.13). This pad has been successful in minimizing pressure points from saddles that do not fit perfectly. However, a pad will not make a poorly fitting saddle fit any better; all it can do is eliminate some small areas of pressure points.

Girths, Girth Sleeves, and Breast Collars

Girths and cinches come in smooth leather, in neoprene, or in cotton webbing or cords.

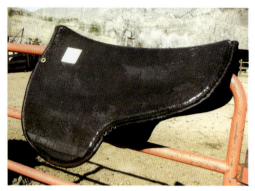

13.13 *The material in a Supracor® pad is used to cushion bedridden hospital patients or wheelchair-bound people, and it serves as an excellent padding to protect a horse's back from a saddle. Saddle pads should not be used as a substitute for good saddle fit, but a pad such as this can improve a horse's comfort.*

Fleece girth sleeves are useful to pad a cinch so it slides easily across the skin, particularly when lubricated with sweat. The fleece also absorbs moisture and prevents pinching of the skin between the elbows and the girth. Cord girths configure more exactly to skin contours as a horse moves, and an English figure-eight girth also conforms better than a straight piece of leather. The girth or cinch shouldn't be too loose or too snug. A loose girth allows a saddle to shift side to side with the girth rubbing similarly in that direction. Too tight and the girth pinches and compresses thin skin, creating bruises and chafed areas.

Some horses develop fat rolls or loose skin around the girth area. Once the saddle is on and the girth or cinch tightened, stretch each forelimb forward to relieve pinching of loose skin rolls that could become trapped.

Neoprene Equipment

Tack made of rubber neoprene prevents chafing in areas commonly rubbed by conventional equipment. Neoprene breastplates, girths, and girth covers are useful for horses worked under saddle for many hours. Skin beneath the neoprene does not overheat from contact with the equipment. Neoprene tack slides over sweaty skin and fur with ease. Cleaning neoprene tack is a horse owner's dream: it is hosed off after each use to remove sweat and mud, and then hung up to dry.

Electrode pads for heart rate monitors are available as relatively flat, neoprene rubber material to minimize pressure points.

Treatment of Saddle Sores

The key to treating girth or saddle sores is to give the tissue some rest. That means, remove the inciting cause, like the saddle and girth, and "park" tack in the tack room or trailer. Given time, the skin will heal. The primary objective is to relieve inflammation and discomfort from the chafed area. Most superficial skin abrasions heal rapidly within 10 to 21 days provided reinjury does not occur. If a girth or saddle sore is discovered and treated immediately, it remains in the most superficial tissue layers, capable of healing in 1 to 2 weeks. If deeper tissues are injured, the wound may not fully heal for up to 3 to 6 weeks.

Hygienic cleansing with antiseptic scrubs removes debris, grit, and serum that ooze from a girth gall. Applying cold packs or ice to a fresh wound reduces inflammation, but after a day or two, warm packs relieve residual swelling and make the horse feel better. Just as one would dry up diaper rash on a baby's bottom, a girth gall can be treated using Desitin®. Or, the skin can be kept soft and pliable by applying useful water-soluble ointments, like Horseman's Dream®, triple antibiotic salve, or Silvadene® cream. Some have had success using Vitamin A & D® ointment, aloe vera creams, vitamin E salves, or Thuja zinc® ointment. The type of wound ointment used is not as critical as keeping the skin supple and protected, and making sure that flies don't feed on the traumatized area.

Toughening the skin with caustic powders or drenches generally leads to thickened scar tissue in the area, setting up conditions for more girth galls to occur in the future. The goal is to have the skin heal up as good as new, just like the tissue that was there before it was injured. Patience is important so the tissue isn't prematurely stressed before it has had a chance to heal.

Scratches

White markings on a horse's legs add flash to his overall appearance. Beneath the white fur lies pink skin, which under most circumstances poses few problems as the hair coat protects pink skin from sunburn. Yet, legs marked with white socks or stockings are prone to irritation. Irritation creates *dermatitis* (skin inflammation) of vulnerable tissues at the back of the pastern. The syndrome has many names, each a description of either the cause or symptoms of the problem. Commonly called *scratches*, other descriptive terms include *grease heel, mud fever, cracked heels, white pastern disease,* and *dew poisoning.*

CAUSES OF SCRATCHES

Trauma and Poor Hygiene

Under the right conditions, any horse can develop scratches. Some cases result from persistent irritation to the skin that produces a situation similar to what we experience with chapped hands. Caked-on manure or mud, sandy or abrasive soil, grit of training surfaces, and rough stubble in a field are possible irritants to skin on the lower legs (photo 13.14). Unsanitary conditions of urine-soaked and dirty bedding cake on the feet and pasterns of stalled horses, creating chemical and bacterial

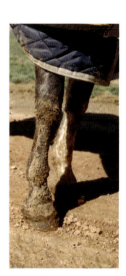

13.14 *Poor hygiene, especially mud-caked limbs, creates conditions for development of dermatitis such as scratches.*

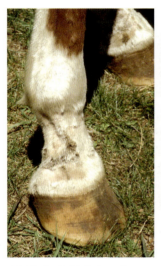

13.15 *An initial sign of scratches is the presence of scabs in the pastern and/or cannon region with underlying skin that is painful and sensitive to touch.*

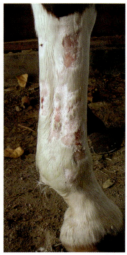

13.16 *Any area of a white limb can be affected by scratches due to lack of skin pigmentation and limited protection from ultraviolet light. This horse has weeping, raw sores beneath the fur, clearly visible once the overlying scabs and fur are removed.*

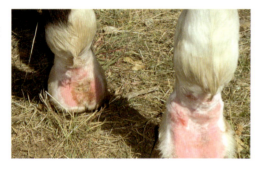

13.17 *Removal of hair and scabs related to scratches reveals raw, irritated skin beneath. This is painful and often causes lameness.*

scratches occur even under the best conditions. Long hair traps moisture and debris, which are prime conditions for dermatitis. In some portions of the western United States, alkaline soil "burns" the skin on the lower legs and poses a peculiar problem to horses ridden in these types of soils.

Like chapped hands, the skin is painful and is often accompanied by localized swelling and lameness. Initially, there is no visible evidence of an inflammatory crisis, but in a short time scabs develop and hair loss occurs, along with weeping, red skin at the back of the pasterns (photos 13.15, 13.16, and 13.17). Constant motion of the pastern causes the skin to crack and form fissures. Ulcerated and raw sores persist beneath the scabs. A cracked skin surface that is caked with dried and moist serum appears greasy, hence the name "grease heel."

Photosensitization

In many cases, scratches is often more accurately described as a condition called *photoactivated vasculitis*, a tongue-twisting term that describes what happens to the skin when it is exposed to the ultraviolet of sunrays. This syndrome may be caused by ingestion of certain plants (like clovers, legumes, and other photodynamic plants such as ragwort, buckwheat, vetch, St. Johnswort, or horsebrush) that cause mild liver damage (see *Appendix C*, p. 571). Usually only white-marked limbs are affected, and swelling and lameness are out of proportion to the mildness of the skin lesions. As a case of scratches progresses, swelling may encompass the entire lower limb. Lesions weep and ooze serum. Sores develop not just on the back of pasterns, but also on the sides and fronts of pasterns and fetlocks. If pink skin ascends the leg, the dermatitis may spread to the cannon area. Photosensitization ("sunburn") reactions often include other white areas of the body, such as the face and muzzle.

irritation to skin. Sand and abrasive dirt trapped beneath leg boots can abrade and irritate the skin, creating conditions for scratches to develop. In horses with particularly long hairs down the back of the legs, such as the feathering common to certain draft breeds,

Plants That Cause Photosensitivity of the Skin

Certain plants contain photoreactive pigments that are absorbed into the blood and these then react in areas of non-pigmented skin in the presence of ultraviolet light from the sun. The horse's skin then sunburns. Two main plants are culprits in this situation: St. John's wort (*Hypericum perforatum*) and buckwheat (*Fagopyrum esculentum*). Other plants create a photosensitivity response secondary to damage in the liver caused by alkaloids in the plants. Examples of these include: *Senecio* spp. (tansy ragwort, groundsels), hound's tongue (*Cynoglossum* spp.), horsebrush (*Tetradymia* spp.), and alsike clover (*Trifolium hybridum*). Generally, the horse has to consume these plants over a period of a couple of months before the liver effects are severe enough to allow accumulation of a by-product of the breakdown of plant chlorophyll in the blood. This compound is called *phylloerythrin* and its accumulation in areas of non-pigmented skin intensifies the effects of ultraviolet sunrays (photos 13.18 and 13.19).

SYNDROMES CONFUSED WITH SCRATCHES

Fungal Infection

Fungus proliferates in dense hairs or in an unsanitary skin environment common to the lower limbs; this may be mistaken for scratches. However, a fungal infection may also occur on a darkly marked limb or on other parts of the body. Skin scrapings grown on a special nutrient medium can identify a fungus (see p. 372).

Chorioptic Mange Mite

In breeds with fetlock feathering, it is possible to find an infestation of *chorioptic mange mites* that causes severe irritation, crusts, and scabs on the pasterns and lower legs. Draft horse breeds are particularly susceptible. This mite causes intense itching in the invaded area, and horses will stomp or bite at their legs in agitation. The mite is diagnosed by analyzing a skin scraping under a microscope.

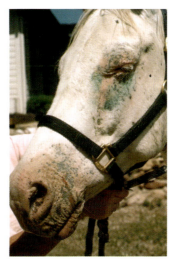 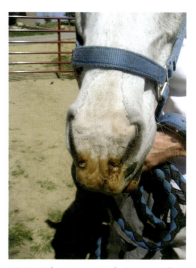

13.18 *Photosensitivity or sunburn can occur in any area of non-pigmented skin, such as on the face and muzzle.*

13.19 *Photosensitive lesions on the face may begin as symmetrically located raw spots near the nostrils. This horse, recently moved to a new pasture, may be ingesting a plant that causes skin photosensitivity.*

Rain Scald

In moist areas of the United States like the southeast, or during warm and rainy spring months in any region, a common problem is infection with the *Dermatophilus congolensis* bacteria (for more details, see p. 375). Lower limbs are affected in areas of moist terrain, earning it the name *dew poisoning*. Dermatophilus dermatitis that is limited to pastern areas is often mistaken for scratches.

White Pastern Disease

Bacterial organisms, such as S*taphylococcal* bacteria, can cause or complicate a case of white pastern disease. Unlike scratches, only one limb may be affected.

RECOGNITION OF SCRATCHES

Various remedies exist, each providing varying degrees of success. Perhaps the most critical remedy involves early recognition of a problem so immediate steps can be taken to stop the painful skin inflammation. Some initial signs to watch for include:

- Red or tender areas on the back or front of the pasterns or heel bulbs
- Amber beads of moist or dried serum resulting from seepage from inflamed skin
- Cracked skin with or without raw ulcerated spots
- Dried crusts or scabs that tightly adhere to the skin
- Swelling in the lower portion of affected legs

Also, look for any sign of skin irritation around white areas of the face or muzzle. This gives a visual clue that the problem may stem from localized skin irritation due to contact with a particular substance or plant, or there may be an underlying systemic response.

One means of early recognition depends on understanding the type of situations that generate a case of scratches. If a horse is exposed to any of the following, then monitor for signs of irritation, or change the management to eliminate these sources:

- Alfalfa or legume hay
- Clover or legume pasture
- Pasture with the presence of photosensitizing plants, such as ragwort (groundsel), horsebrush, St. John's wort, or buckwheat
- Wet, marshy ground or irrigated pastures
- Alkaline soils
- Poor hygiene, including urine-soaked bedding or mud

TREATMENT OF SCRATCHES

Remove the Inciting Cause

The first line of treatment or prevention involves removing the inciting cause:

- Remove the horse from the offending pasture, and/or remove legume hay from the diet.
- At first notice of a problem with scratches, bring the horse inside during the daylight hours, and turn out at dusk.

The horse can remain outside during the day if the lower legs are covered with bandages, tube socks, or other material to block sun exposure of the skin

Anti-Inflammatory Treatment

The above suggestions not only prevent a case of scratches, but they also are methods used to treat an active case. In addition, appropriate treatment should include the following:

- Shave or clip away fur overlying the inflamed area of skin to remove residual particulates, crusts, and contaminants along with clinging hair.
- Gently scrub with antiseptic soaps (Betadine® or Nolvasan®) to cleanse the skin and remove as much scab and crust as possible.
- Towel-dry the skin before bandaging.
- If crusting tissue adheres tightly to underlying, ulcerated skin, forceful removal of the scabs worsens the skin injury so it is better to apply salve to matted areas beneath a bandage for a day or two to soften crusts, mats, and scabs; then they'll peel away easily from the skin without further trauma.
- Apply skin salve medication to all lesions, for example, corticosteroid ointment, Silvadene® cream, triple antibiotic ointment,

aloe vera gel, Desitin®, or Vitamin A & D® ointment.
- Apply a light support bandage to reduce inflammation and swelling, to protect the leg from ultraviolet radiation, to reduce tissue edema, and to maintain healing warmth under the bandage.
- Change the bandage every 5 to 7 days until all reddened areas return to normal skin color and weeping tissue is dry and non-painful to touch; tube socks can be used at the final stages of healing to protect the limbs from the sun (photo 13.20).

People struggle for months using ineffective home remedies, such as sauerkraut poultices, trying to rid a horse of scratches, to no avail. There is no substitute for cleaning affected legs and shaving away the hair so appropriate topical salves and bandages can be applied in contact with irritated skin.

If a case of scratches has developed beyond a local irritation to a larger extent, apply zinc sulfate (contained in white lotion) or calamine lotion to suppress serum production and weeping. After a day or two, apply an antibiotic/corticosteroid cream and bandage as above. The tissues should never be dried out with astringent products, such as copper sulfate or lime, because that worsens the dermatitis and substantially slows healing.

Inflammation and tissue swelling impair circulation to the area, and must be controlled for healing to advance. This goal is accomplished with nonsteroidal anti-inflammatory drugs (NSAIDs), like flunixin meglumine or phenylbutazone ("bute"). In severe photoaggravated vasculitis cases, systemic corticosteroid medications may be necessary.

Sensible Hygiene

Frequent attention to cleanliness and hygiene prevents environmental situations from adversely affecting a horse's skin. During periods of heavy rain or pasture irrigation, move a horse to dry ground as poor hygiene sets up conditions for bacterial infection with *Staphylococcal* sp., *Streptococcal* sp., or infection with *Dermatophilus congolensis* (rain scald). If a horse has particularly thick feathering on the lower legs and has a propensity to develop scratches, clip away excess hair on the back of the fetlocks. Fungal infections can invade any area of a horse's skin, including the lower legs. Clean leg boots well and often and make sure the legs are clean before reapplying.

Managing Sunburn

Just as one would throw on a long-sleeved shirt and slacks over sunburned body parts to protect from further damage, the same can be done for a horse. The torso can be covered with a flysheet and the lower legs with bandages or tube socks. More difficult is a means to cover the face, and especially the muzzle, which usually suffers the worst effects of sunburn.

Some salves help to a degree. The most common example of a sunblock product is zinc oxide ointment. Another product (although rose in color) is called Thuja zinc®, which contains a mixture of zinc oxide, scarlet oil, and other soothing ingredients. This product works as a sun block and an antiseptic and seems to repel flies as well. Desitin® ointment also provides a protective barrier to the sun. One shortcoming of gooey ointments is that they collect dirt. Nonetheless, a horse's skin will remain protected from the sun until the salve rubs off. Other human sunblock creams can be used with good success but some horses are

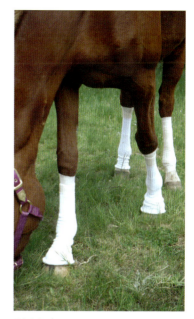

13.20 *An inexpensive way to protect non-pigmented skin on the lower legs from the photosensitizing effects of ultraviolet sunlight is with the use of tube socks.*

sensitive to PABA-containing products. A face dunk in the water trough also removes a lot of the sun block protection. Aloe-containing products or steroid creams are soothing to alleviate the inflammation of sunburnt skin, but neither will protect it from further burning. Few salves or medications are appropriate for use around the eyes as their chemicals could cause eye irritation.

Commercial fly masks are available with a mesh extension that covers a large part of the lower face and muzzle while still allowing a horse to breathe, eat, and drink. Another sun-protection strategy relies on a piece of dangling terry cloth secured to the noseband of a Breakaway® or thin leather halter that will break if snagged; the fabric remains over the muzzle whether a horse is standing with his head up or has his head down grazing.

Tattooing of areas of pink skin on the face can provide a slightly longer-lasting solution to the problem. This is not a permanent solution and will need to be repeated frequently. Another possibility is to use dyes on a weekly basis that are formulated to treat pink eye in cattle. Others have tried the use of mascara or eye makeup around the horse's eyes with limited success.

Certain breeds, like Paint horses and Appaloosas, are at risk of sunburn of non-pigmented areas around the eyes, vulva, and sheath. Some Arabian horses have an inherited syndrome known as *vitiligo* (Arabian fading syndrome) in which they lose pigment around areas of the face, inguinal area, and perineum (around the anus and vulva). The big danger for these horses is that *mucocutaneous* junctions (where the skin meets the mucous membranes) in these non-pigmented areas are prime for developing skin cancer known as *squamous cell carcinoma*. The problem may begin in the early years of a horse's life although the cancer may not visibly develop until many years later.

Meshed fly facemasks reduce ultraviolet radiation by up to 70 percent around the eyes and a large portion of the face, so these provide an effective means of prevention of cancer and sunburn. Snow glare is just as likely to irritate mucocutaneous tissue as is intense summer sun, so horses at risk of eye cancer should wear a mask year round. Most horses negotiate well in the dark with the mask in place so it is possible to leave it on day and night. A horse can be ridden in the mask if necessary. Do a daily check to make sure no debris has collected beneath the facemask, and to check that all is well with a horse's eyes.

In serious cases, the most obvious solution is to house a horse inside out of the direct sun during the day, and turn him out at night. Schedule training rides before the sun hits its daily peak, or more toward the hours of dusk.

Fungal Infection

Small, firm, pea-sized bumps in the skin, flaking skin, or loss of hair are suspect signs for fungal infection. A fungus cannot grow in living tissue, but produces toxins to create an environment in which it can thrive. These toxins cause an inflammatory reaction in the skin, with resultant edema, necrosis, or an allergic hypersensitivity reaction. Because fungus weakens the hair shaft, the hair easily breaks off.

RINGWORM

A fungal infection of the skin is referred to as *dermatophytosis*. A skin fungal infection is also called "ringworm" since the lesions are often oval or round in appearance (photos 13.21 A & B). Fungi thrive in dark, damp barns, particularly in autumn and winter months. Once the fungus gets established on a horse's skin, a long winter hair coat helps maintain an infection. The time of year should not rule out the presence or absence of this as a skin disease. Fungal infec-

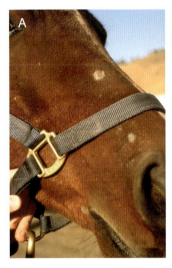
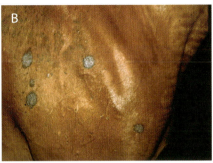
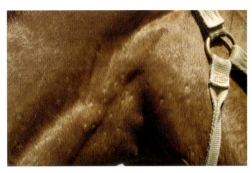

13.21 A & B *Circular skin lesions devoid of hair are typical of a ringworm infection as seen here on a horse's face (A) and a horse's shoulder (B).*

13.22 *In early stages of ringworm infection, all you may see are small oval or round spots of missing hair, such as seen on this horse's neck.*

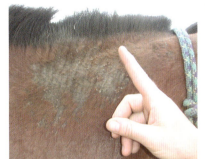

13.23 *Some strains of ringworm cause intense itching. The circular lesions coalesce into large areas of alopecia (missing hair). In this picture, you can see broken hairs caused by the horse scratching against firm objects.*

tions also become established in warm, humid climates, particularly during fly season.

Lesions are commonly seen around the area of the girth and saddle, the hindquarters, or along the chest, neck, and face. Fungi are highly contagious and are transmitted between horses by shared tack and equipment. The incubation period for fungal infections takes from 1 to 6 weeks. An infection may start with a hive-like lesion that then becomes circumscribed in an oval shape (photo 13.22). The skin lesions look scaly and crusty, and are accompanied by hair loss (photo 13.23). Sometimes the edges of the lesions have frayed, broken, or distorted hairs just prior to the hair falling out. Usually a ringworm infection is not itchy or painful to the horse, but it can be. Young horses, or those with a compromised immune system may develop a generalized form of ringworm (photos 13.24 A & B). Children are susceptible to catching the disease from petting an infected horse.

Diagnosis is best made by fungal culture, however it can take as long as six weeks for growth of a positive culture. In the meantime, it is best to treat the horse as if he has ringworm. Treatment requires diligent attention to

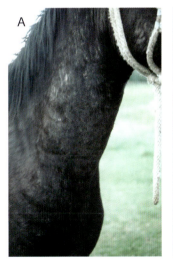
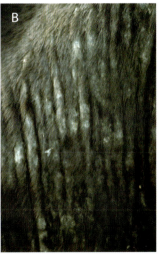

13.24 A & B *A young or immunocompromised horse may suffer a generalized fungal infection that requires full body shampoos as well as systemic anti-fungal medications (A). This is a closeup of the corrugated and thickened skin seen on the same horse (B).*

hygiene. All saddle pads, brushes, girths, and cinches must be washed and disinfected, and each horse should have his own designated equipment to reduce chances of transfer from horse to horse. Remove contaminated bedding from stalls. Disinfect stalls and equipment with bleach, chlorhexidine, or benzalconium chloride. Isolate infected horses from others.

Daily bathing for the first week and then once or twice a week is helpful to control the infection. Weekly baths should be administered until at least two weeks following resolution of all of the lesions. The best disinfectants include povidone iodine (Betadine®) shampoos, chlorhexidine shampoos, dilute-bleach (0.5 percent solution) rinses, 5 percent lime-sulfur solutions, and a fungal orchard spray (Captan®) as an effective rinse. During bathing, work the medicated shampoos well into the skin, and allow them to remain for at least 15 minutes before rinsing.

Topical salves and ointments can be applied to small lesions. Useful products include miconazole (Conofite®), clotrimazole (Lotrimin®), and thiabendazole (Tresaderm®). In extreme cases that occur in immunosuppressed or very young horses, systemic antifungal medication may be warranted to help the horse's immune system eliminate the disease. In most cases, ringworm is self-limiting once a horse's immune system has had a chance to recognize and process the infection. With the help of good hygiene, exposure to sunlight, and frequent antiseptic baths, most horses clear the infection within about six weeks.

Skin Problems Associated with Hair Loss

SKIN SCALD

A common cause of hair loss on the lower legs is a result of poor hygiene in the stabling or pasture area. Urine or manure scald on the legs will cause hair to fall out from chronic inflammation within the skin. Usually this is accompanied by crusting and scabs in the areas of patchy hair loss. The environment should be cleansed of caustic irritants like urine, manure, soaked straw or shavings. Daily cleansing of the lower legs will clear up most of these without too much trouble. In some cases, systemic antibiotics may be necessary. If you cannot point to damp or dirty environmental conditions, have a veterinarian check the horse for the presence of a bladder or urinary stone. Partial blockage of the urinary tract may cause an abnormal urine stream that scalds the skin where urine contacts it.

PATCHY SHEDDING

In the spring, horses may experience seasonal *alopecia* (hair loss) in which large patches of hair shed out before entry of the new hair growth, leaving a bald patch of skin. The area of naked skin appears normal. Given patience, hair will reappear within the month.

SELENIUM TOXICITY

Horses grazing on plants that accumulate selenium or horses fed hay that has been grown in selenium-rich soils may suffer from toxicity. Selenium poisoning, referred to as *alkali disease,* often takes a chronic form with the hair coat, mane, and tail obviously thinning. Horizontal hoof-wall cracks resulting from selenium toxicity are a serious concern as an advanced form of this leads to laminitis and sloughing of the hoof capsule (see chapter 3, *The Hoof,* p. 57).

Hair, serum, or feed can be analyzed for selenium content. If selenium toxicity is a suspected problem, an affected horse should be removed immediately from the offending pasture, or the hay should be substituted with that from a reliable source.

Plants That Are Selenium Accumulators or Indicators

Plants store all kinds of nutrients, but in certain soils and geographical locations of the country, certain plants store too much selenium. Some plants can only grow if high levels of selenium are present in the soil. Known selenium-rich areas include the central United States and semi-arid states, around the Rocky Mountains, for example. (On the flip side, both coasts of the United States usually have selenium-deficient soils.) Finding specific selenium-indicating plants is a tipoff that excess selenium is concentrated in the soil, and subsequently in the plants. Species that require selenium to grow include: milk vetch (*Astragalus* spp.), prince's plume (*Stanley pinnata*), and the woody aster (*Xylorrhiza* spp.). Others that indicate the presence of selenium but do not require it to flourish include: gum weed (*Grindelia* spp.), snakeweed (*Gutierrezia* spp.), and paintbrush (*Castileja* spp.), as a few commonly recognized examples. Selenium especially accumulates in these plants during periods of drought when the plants set their roots deeper to find water and then contact pockets of selenium.

RAIN SCALD OR DERMATOPHILUS INFECTION

Another cause of hair loss can be attributed to an organism known as *Dermatophilus congolensis,* which elicits a condition referred to as *rain rot, rain scald*, or *dew poisoning* (see p. 369). Spores are continually present in the environment and are activated by moisture. Activated spores infiltrate skin traumatized by insect bites, abrasions, or constant inrritation by frequent rain exposure that softens the skin, particularly along the topline. When seen along the back, loins, and croup, dermatophilus is called rain scald. When the lower limbs are affected, dermatophilus is referred to as dew poisoning. Initial lesions are seen along the rump, lower limbs, face, muzzle, withers, and in the saddle region. This organism lives in the soil as well as in the scabs of infected horses. Horses may also be "infected" with dermatophilus without showing outward signs of disease, yet they still remain as carriers to susceptible individuals. Young or older horses with poorly developed immune systems are at higher risk.

Rain-scald lesions are crusty and scaling and the hair often pulls away with crusts still attached, revealing ulceration beneath. Initially these may start as raised tufts of fur with crusts. These lesions are usually painful. Unfortunately, crusting and scaling abnormalities in the skin accompany many types of skin problems, so the best way to diagnose dermatophilus is to review cells obtained by a scraping under a microscope, and to culture the organism from a scraping. A biopsy of the tissue also reveals a diagnosis.

Control and prevention are important to limit the severity of the disease. Horses should be provided with a run-in shed or a stall to shelter them in rainy climates. Adequate insect control minimizes trauma to the skin from bites. Once a horse's skin has been infected with dermatophilus, a course of antibiotics such as trimethoprim-sulfamethoxazole or procaine penicillin may be necessary to eradicate the infection. Systemic antibiotics are essential if the weather prevents daily bathing. In warm climates, the hair should be clipped away from the lesions, scabs removed, and then the horse should be bathed with povidine iodine shampoos which are lathered into the fur for at least 10 minutes, then rinsed thoroughly.

External Parasites

FLIES AND GNATS

Psychological Attack

Horses that live with others have a great advantage in their numbers. They can sidle up to each other to form body blocks on one side and fly-swatting protection from front and rear with active tails. They can groom each other and scratch the itchy spots. If turned out to large acreage, horses will seek a comfort zone where fewer flies prevail, moving to accommodate the time of day and insect preferences.

A horse housed alone or in a small confinement bears the brunt of fly attacks. Some of the most easygoing horses, particularly thin-skinned individuals, turn into demons when repeatedly bitten and pestered by flies. Nerves strung tight, muscles exhausted from continual foot stamping and flickering of skin, these horses can't seem to concentrate on their work. A horse with a normally placid demeanor may suddenly behave poorly under saddle, refusing to accept the slightest command or reprimand. You may look for esoteric reasons behind the sudden behavioral change when in fact, a horse feels like you do, irritated by the flies. It is not always easy to appreciate the degree of a horse's discomfort since not all flies are as attracted to human skin as they are to horse fur and flesh. Horses may invite injury when kicking at flies, particularly if they kick out when next to a fence. In odd instances, biting flies may become so annoying that horses may be inspired to flee, potentially injuring themselves while running in the pasture.

On a less obvious level, flies actually create sufficient stress and anxiety to disrupt normal feeding patterns. You may see a horse drop weight not only because of lessened feed intake but also due to the physical effort expended by stamping and stomping at the annoying creatures. There is a possibility of flies creating considerable blood loss over a period of time to cause anemia, leaving a horse feeling tired and looking unthrifty.

Horseflies and Deerflies

One fly that causes troublesome skin irritations is the *horsefly*, *Tabanus*; another is the *deerfly*, *Chrysops*. These bites are painful, creating nodules on the skin. The most commonly affected areas are along the neck, withers, back, and legs. These large flies can transmit disease due to transfer of relatively large amounts of blood from horse to horse. One such transmissible disease is called *equine infectious anemia* (EIA), a viral infection related to the human HIV virus; in this case EIA infects horses with a chronic, wasting disease (see p. 241).

Face Flies and Houseflies

Face flies (*Musca autumnalis*) and *houseflies* (*Musca domestica*) prosper in the corners of the eye where they feed on eye secretions stimulated by their presence. A horse's eye weeps persistently in response to the inflammation. Intense itching created by eye discharge stimulates a horse to rub his face on various surfaces, potentially scratching the cornea to form a corneal ulcer (see p. 494). Chronic eye discharge due to fly irritation often causes the skin around the eye to loose its pigmentation, creating a cosmetic blemish. Face flies also can transmit eye worms (*Thelazia*), but these are responsive to oral treatment with *ivermectin*, a deworming product.

Stable Flies

The *stable fly* (*Stomoxys calcitrans*), similar to the common housefly, pierces the skin with its mouthparts. The stable fly bites a horse just about anywhere on the body, but mostly on the legs, belly, chest, and back. Often, this results in a nodular swelling at the bite site that may be uncomfortable but normally resolves quickly. When the bite occurs where the tack or girth sit, it becomes more of a functional problem as tack persistently irritates the lesion. Stable flies have also been found to transmit *Corynebacterium pseudotuberculosis* bacteria that cause dryland distemper infection (p. 174).

Stable flies are poorly named because they really prefer light and sunny areas, only going inside during rainy weather. They lay eggs in decaying urine-soaked straw and manure.

Black Flies

Black flies (*Simulium*), commonly known as ear gnats, feed on blood drawn from the flat surface (*pinnae*) inside the ear (photo 13.25). Black flies are also called *buffalo gnats* due to their humpbacked appearance. These tiny insects reach a maximum length of 5 millimeters, about the size of an apple seed. Black flies are found throughout the United States, particularly near running water, which is a breeding ground for the pest. Because adults travel great distances, up to 100 miles, control is nearly impossible.

As black flies feed on the delicate lining of the ears, toxins secreted in their saliva increase permeability of capillary beds, improving access to blood meals. Oozing and blood-encrusted scabs form where black flies have fed. The discomfort from an intense inflammatory response may cause a horse to become headshy. What begins as an instinctive response to avoid pain and discomfort may develop into an aversive habit even after the ears are healed.

Allergic Reaction

Some horses respond to black fly bites with a severe allergic reaction. Horny growths, or *plaques,* develop inside the ear (photo 13.26). These cauliflower-like plaques can be peeled

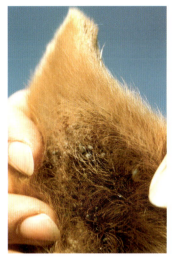

13.25 *Black flies, or ear gnats, feed on the inner surface (pinna) of the ear, creating irritation and pain. These gnats prefer to nest in thick hair so one method of control and treatment is to shave the inner surface of each ear.*

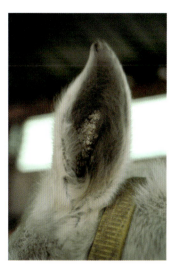

13.26 *The saliva of the black fly creates an allergic response in some horses, leading to growth of cauliflower-like lesions inside the ear pinnae.*

away by rubbing with a thumbnail or a piece of gauze, providing the horse allows them to be touched. (Such relatively easy removal distinguishes them from more tenacious sarcoid tumors also often found in the ears.) Once black fly plaques are removed, application of a topical corticosteroid ointment reduces the severity of the allergic response. A horse can be encouraged to accept daily topical medication inside the ears by quickly applying ointment while he is distracted by a bucket of grain.

Pigmentation Loss

A persistent inflammatory response to black flies causes a horse to permanently lose skin color inside the ears (photo 13.27). This white patch is only of cosmetic significance, and does not interfere with the skin's return to function or health.

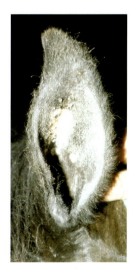

13.27 *Some horses react to black flies with a loss of pigmentation to the skin of the inner ear.*

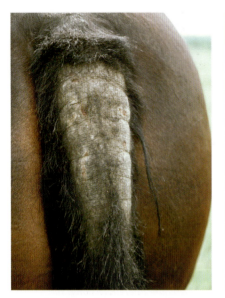

13.28 *The rat tail appearance is due to an allergic response to the Culicoides gnat that creates an intense pruritus (itching) along the horse's topline and abdomen. The malady is called sweet itch, and an affected horse will traumatize his own skin by rubbing vigorously on any solid object he can reach.*

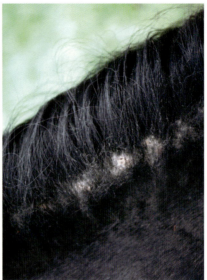

13.29 *Culicoides hypersensitivity causes the mane to be rubbed out and the skin to be rubbed raw.*

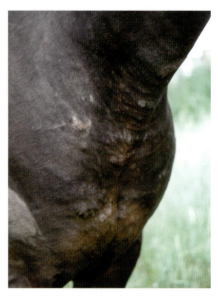

13.30 *A horse with sweet itch will also rub his chest, another characteristic sign of Culicoides hypersensitivity.*

Culicoides Gnats

One of the most common causes of *pruritus* (itching) is an allergic dermatitis caused by hypersensitivity to biting gnats (*Culicoides*), popularly known as biting midges or "no-see-ums." The gnats create a skin problem in the horse known as *Queensland's itch* or *summer itch*, seasonally associated with periods of high insect activity. The surrounding environment has a large part to do with presence of these gnats. Culicoides gnats prefer breeding in slow or still water such as found in ponds, small creeks, or springs.

These pests tend to feed on the sensitive skin of the belly, inner thighs, poll, mane, withers, and tailhead. Intense irritation created by these insects stimulates a horse to frantically scratch on anything in sight: a post, the side of the barn, the feeders, trees and bushes, or the ground. An initial hint that something is amiss will be the glaring sight of a worsening "rat tail" appearance of a horse's tail (photo 13.28). Often, the mane is also mutilated and bald (photo 13.29). Usually the rubbing starts out lightly, and then progresses as the allergic response progresses (photo 13.30). There is a hereditary predisposition to Culicoides hypersensitivity. Usually it surfaces in horses over 2 to 3 years old, and the allergic response worsens with age. Not only does a horse destroy his hair coat and skin with this behavior, producing a scruffy appearance, but he also becomes depressed and irritable, and may become belligerent with handlers. If the horse can be ridden, his performance likely suffers.

Management of this condition is possible. This ailment is seasonal, showing up from late spring through late fall as it coincides with warmth and the fly season. Affected horses should be stalled during dawn and dusk when the gnats are most active in feeding. Screens on the stalls are helpful, but the mesh should be small enough to prevent passage of the gnats. Insecticide spray-misters also help in reducing the numbers of gnats. Fly/mosquito sheets help to some degree, but these bugs prefer the abdomen and thigh areas, which are not covered well by a flysheet. Insect sprays containing *permethrin* should be applied regularly to susceptible areas of the horse. In many cases the gnats may feed on the belly, but the systemic allergic response creates itching all over, specifically over the topline of the horse.

Treatment for the condition relies on excellent management and insect-control strategies, but some horses may require systemic administration of corticosteroids and/or antihistamine (*hydroxyzine*) medication to control the allergic response. Supplemental feeding of flaxseed may reduce the hypersensitivity response. In extreme cases, a severely affected horse may need to be relocated to a different property away from standing water and gnat breeding grounds.

Confused with Pinworms

Initially, Culicoides hypersensitivity is confused with pinworms (see p. 463) due to a horse's tendency to rub away hair on the tailhead (photo 13.31 and see photo 15.6, p. 464). However, Culicoides hypersensitivity progresses along the topline of the horse, whereas pinworms or a normal estrus cycle causes a horse to concentrate on rubbing the rear end only. Scotch tape applied to the skin around the anus can be analyzed under a microscope for pinworm eggs.

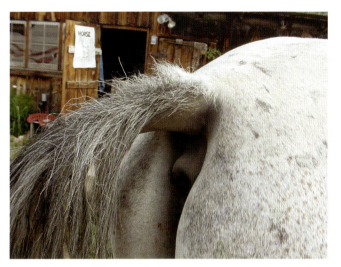

13.31 *A horse with pinworms typically lifts his tail and rubs his buttocks, or he may back up to a fence and rub out the hairs on the tailhead. This kind of itching is often confused with sweet itch; however, with pinworms, the horse does not traumatize himself to raw skin, but merely scratches away a light layer of fur or tail hair.*

Bot Flies

As bot fly (*Gasterophilus intestinalis*) larvae mature and travel from the stomach of the horse to the rectum and anus, they spend a short time attached to the lining of the rectum. These parasites also can cause itching of the tailhead. If there is any doubt about the possibility of infection with either bots or pinworms, administer an appropriate deworming paste to see if the itching disappears in about a week.

Horn Flies

To make matters even more confusing, another fly-bite-hypersensitivity reaction is easily confused with Culicoides hypersensitivity: *focal ventral midline dermatitis*. As the name suggests, skin irritation is found only on the undersides of the horse, particularly the belly. The skin around the navel or on the underside

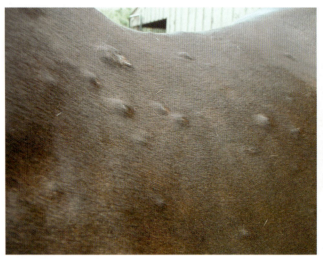

13.32 *Firm nodules such as seen here are referred to as nodular necrobiosis, a condition created by an allergic response to fly bites, or to fibers in some saddle pads.*

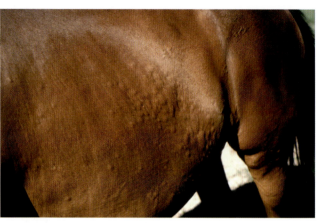

13.33 *Mosquito bites can cause great irritation to a horse, and if plentiful enough may coalesce into a swollen mass on a horse's sides, neck, and belly. Mosquitoes carry neurologic viruses, so efforts should be made to cover the horse with a flysheet and to apply insect repellents to exposed skin.*

of the neck is scaly, crusty, ulcerated, and lacks hair *(alopecia)* and color. This reaction is due to the horn fly, *Haematobia,* which prefers to obtain a blood meal along a narrow strip on the abdominal midline. The horn fly can be recognized by its peculiar feeding position with the head pointing toward the ground. Horn flies require cattle manure to propagate so only horses housed with or near cows will be affected. Horn flies may be one vector for pigeon fever infection with *Corynebacterium pseudotuberculosis* (see p. 174). Strategic fly-control measures are important, while anti-inflammatory corticosteroid ointments control localized irritation and hair loss.

Warbles

Fly bites from *Hypoderma* spp. may create a large single nodule with an opening, located on a horse's back. The opening in the nodule is most likely the breathing pore of a *warble* or grub laid by the *Hypoderma* fly. The warble, also called a *heel fly,* lays eggs on a horse's hairs. Once these eggs hatch, *Hypoderma* larvae migrate through the skin, arriving at the back about 4 to 5 months later during the fall and winter months. On rare occasions, the warble could migrate to the brain instead of the back, resulting in severe neurological problems. Fly warbles tend to infect horses only when they are kept in proximity to cattle, which are the preferred host.

Other Causes of Nodules

If no breathing pore is present, the nodule may instead be a *nodular necrobiosis,* which is the result of cell death and scar tissue buildup. Such a nodule is caused by reaction around a particle of synthetic material from a saddle pad, or from a fly bite. These firm lumps are easily seen and felt in areas along the withers, back, thorax, or belly (photo 13.32). They are not usually painful and there is no skin ulceration or reddening over the lumps.

Application of a topical corticosteroid cream may cause the knot to disappear. If not, it can be treated by a corticosteroid injection into and under the lump. The nodule then regresses in about 3 weeks. During the healing period, it is important that no tack pressure is placed over the lesion. If the nodule persists, or if it is constantly aggravated by tack, it may be necessary to surgically remove it. The nodule does not grow back, but healing takes longer than treatment with corticosteroids.

Mosquitoes

Not only are mosquitoes annoying to horses and people, creating small, itchy welts (photo 13.33), but they also transmit neurological diseases such as *equine encephalitis* (Eastern, Western, and Venezuelan forms) and *West Nile Virus*. (See chapter 17, *The Neurologic System in Health and Disease*, pp. 504 and 508.)

Bee Stings

Bees will attack a horse that ventures into their area, leaving painful welts. Horses are susceptible to an allergic reaction from too many bee stings (photo 13.34).

FLY AND INSECT CONTROL STRATEGIES

Environmental Management

The most effective management kills the infestation at its source. Poor hygienic conditions such as manure, urine-soaked bedding, or dirt create breeding grounds for flies. The environment can be rid of favored larval habitats by cleaning paddocks and stalls daily, and removing decomposing material away from a horse's living quarters. Compost this debris to kill insect eggs, parasite eggs, and weed seeds.

Knowledge of preferred habitats helps wage war on flies. If a horse is housed near boggy, wet areas or a pond where insects proliferate, consider moving the horse to a more distant location. Black flies prefer areas with standing water, and gnats (no-see-ums) prosper in areas of stagnant water, while horse and deerflies abound in wooded areas. Drain standing water where possible, clean water

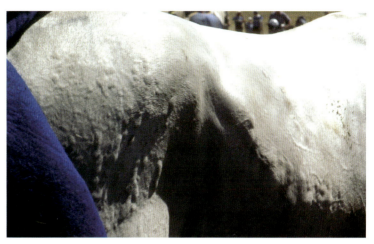

13.34 *If a horse encounters a bee or wasp nest, he may be stung repeatedly. Such a number of stings can create an adverse systemic reaction requiring treatment with antihistamine and anti-inflammatory medications.*

tanks to remove decaying matter, and clean raingutters of rotting vegetation, as well. Some species like horn flies and face flies require cattle manure to propagate so isolate horses from the vicinity of cows.

Physical Protection

Fly Sheets

Use a fine-mesh fly sheet to cover the body and torso to minimize irritation caused by flies settling on the back, chest, and thorax. In extreme situations, a fly "hood" can be built to additionally cover a horse's head, neck, and upper chest (photo 13.35).

Fly Masks and Ear Nets

A fly facemask keeps face and house flies away from sensitive eye structures and improves a horse's comfort during turnout. To minimize ear damage from black flies, coat the ears with a petroleum-based gel, or use roll-on insecticides. The thick coating of gel on the inside of the ears creates a mechanical barrier to fly bites.

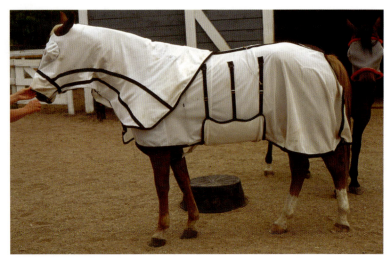

13.35 A fly sheet is made of fine mesh material that allows air to circulate, but protects against noxious biting insects and some percentage of ultraviolet light. This horse suffered from a severe hypersensitivity to biting insects so his owner had a full body suit built to cover him from head to tail. Leg wraps of mesh material are also available to protect the lower limbs.

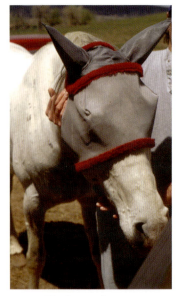

13.36 Fly facemasks protect a horse's eyes from fly attack and block about 70 percent of ultraviolet rays. These masks come with optional ear mesh, which is particularly useful for horses with ear-gnat hypersensitivity.

Some facemasks also have built-in meshed earpieces to protect the ears from fly attack (photo 13.36). Mosquito net material forming the mask covers the face, eyes, and extends over the poll and ears to keep insects off all structures of the head.

Hair Removal in the Ears

Normally, hair in the ear protects the deeper ear canal from collecting dirt or debris, and keeps insects or ticks from crawling into the ear canal. Trimming or shaving away fine hairs lining the ear pinnae obliterates hair that invites black flies to nest in the ears. Wads of cotton should be inserted into each ear before clipping to prevent particles of hair or debris from falling into the deep ear canal where they can stimulate an infection. It may be necessary to sedate a horse for this procedure. Removal of hair inside the ears allows thorough inspection of scabs or sores. Without hair for scabs and oozing serum to cling to, tender skin inside the ears heals quickly. Without the presence of blood to attract black flies to a "banquet," it is easier to provide relief for the horse. Anti-inflammatory corticosteroid creams or topical roll-on insect repellents are easily applied to hairless skin. Spray insecticides into the ears with caution, taking care not to accidentally spray an irritating substance into an eye.

Once ear hair is removed, a light layer of petroleum-based salve smeared inside the ears further deters flies from accessing the skin for feeding. Only products intended for use in the ear should be used, or a veterinarian should be consulted.

Stall Confinement

Determine the worst time of day for emergence of flies on a property. House horses inside during that time period, aiming fans at the stall to create sufficient air movement to turn back the flies. No-see-ums cannot fly in the face of a breeze. Stable flies, horseflies, deerflies, face flies, houseflies, and horn flies, favor daytime hours for flying and feeding, so for relief from these pests, turn horses out at night and stall them inside during the day. Black flies are most active in the mornings and evenings, while no-see-ums generally emerge at dusk to feed at night. No-see-ums are so tiny they can pass through mosquito netting. To prevent their entry into the stall, use fine-mesh screens (32 by 32 mils) on the stalls and additionally spray the screens periodically with pesticides.

The Chemical Arsenal

Unfortunately, flies have been exposed for years to insecticide poisons and have developed a resistance for many of the common products, rendering them ineffective. Some insect repellents work for a short time (hours) to keep flies off the lower legs. To have any effect at all, insecticides must be applied at least daily, if not more frequently. Skin-So-Soft® (Avon) is fairly effective against no-see-ums and mosquitoes when mixed half-and-half with water, or when mixed in equal proportions with vinegar and water. Adding a little citronella oil also is effective in repelling insects.

More toxic compounds that are somewhat effective against flies include the *pyrethrins* and *pyrethroids*. Not only do these products act to repel insects, but also contact with the chemical often kills insects. These chemicals are available in spray or gel form, as well as wipe-on and pour-on formulations. Sprays and wipe-on products seem to work for insect control, with best results when applied to favored feeding areas of most flies, like the belly, back, tail and mane. Pour-on products work by dribbling a little along the horse's neck or spine from where it will eventually migrate to other areas of the body. Pour-on products don't work effectively on horses that are exercised to a sweat. Oil-based formulations have a more prolonged residual effect than water-based compounds simply by continued presence on the hair and skin. Water-based or alcohol-based repellents are more quickly removed when a horse walks through water, rolls in the mud, sweats, or stands in a rain.

No matter what is used, don't spray insecticides around the eyes; use roll-on products and keep a wide berth away from the eye. Wash your hands after applying any chemical to your horse.

Automatic spray misters in the barn can be timed to periodically deliver a fine misting fog of an insecticide chemical like a pyrethrin or pyrethroid compound. While these chemical fogs keep adult insects to a minimum within a barn, they'll exert no harmful effects on a horse's lungs or intestinal tract. However, an occasional individual may develop a mild allergic skin response from carrier chemicals that are mixed with the insecticide chemicals to deliver the spray. Keep in mind that pyrethrin/pyrethroid compounds are extremely toxic to fish, acting to paralyze them. It is important to be environmentally responsible and keep these chemicals away from sources of water that serve as habitat to living creatures other than just pesky flies.

Many diseases caused by flies respond to the deworming product, *ivermectin* (see p. 466). *Habronemiasis* is no longer a common problem because of ivermectin, which kills the larvae embedded in the skin. Likewise, skin infestation with the *Onchocerca* parasite that is transmitted by flies is also diminished by ivermectin, as are skin warbles. Ivermectin is effective in killing stomach larvae of the bot fly and in obliterating eye worms (*Thelazia*) transmitted by face flies.

Feed-Through Fly Control

A fly-killing chemical (*tetrachlorvinphos*) is available as a feed-through fly-control product. It is supposed to pass in an inert form through the gastrointestinal tract to the feces where the chemical kills flies as they emerge from the manure. Previously, it was believed that the active ingredient in this product was not absorbed so did not affect a horse, but there are cases where toxicity has occurred. Consult your veterinarian before using this product.

Biological Control

Commercial sources sell packages of non-stinging wasps called *parasitoids* that feed on insect larvae. This significantly reduces the number of flies hatching to adult form. These wasps need to be released on a monthly basis throughout the fly season from spring until the first killing frost to effectively control the fly population. Fewer flies hatched means fewer flies mature enough to lay eggs, which means fewer flies around the property the next season. The best place to sprinkle the wasps is near manure. Keep in mind that insecticides used to kill flies also kill these "friendly" wasps.

Chemical and biological control strategies work best when all horses in a general locale are similarly treated. Otherwise, flies continue to proliferate across the neighbor's fence, flying to adjacent premises.

Fly Traps

Another useful insect control strategy relies on the use of traps or insect lures, using pheromones (scent hormones) or stinky baits to lure them in. Sticky traps use color to lure and trap flies.

MANGE MITES

Mange is not a very common condition in horses in the United States, but should always be considered in a horse that is very itchy and losing hair. *Psoroptic* mange mites like to inhabit the mane, forelock, base of the tail, or long feathers on the legs of draft-type breeds. *Chorioptic* mange also has a predilection for those long, feathered leg hairs. *Demodectic* mange is unusual in horses and is seen mainly in immune-compromised individuals. *Sarcoptic* mange has been altogether eradicated in horses in the United States.

Mites are usually transferred by direct contact of horse to horse, or by contaminated grooming tools, blankets, and tack. Identification of mange in horses requires examination of skin scrapings under a microscope. The use of ivermectin is recommended in treating mange mites, along with topical application of potent chemicals, which should be obtained through your veterinarian.

Scabies

Scabies or *Psoroptic* mites prefer areas of skin folds, the throat, and even the ears. Intense itching may cause the skin to thicken and the horse to self-mutilate affected areas. In the United States, it has been more than 40 years since equine scabies has presented a major problem.

Sarcoptic Mites

Sarcoptic mites can be a moderately serious skin ailment in the horse, beginning around the head, neck, and shoulders, accompanied by intense itching. This type of mange mite is contagious to humans but fortunately this disease has been eradicated in North America.

Demodectic Mites

Demodectic mites produce nodular lesions of the head, neck, withers, and hinquarters. They burrow deeply into the skin to the base of the hair follicles causing patchy hair loss. Consequently, a very deep skin scraping is necessary for microscopic identification. There is no itching associated with this infestation. Demodectic mites may inhabit the skin of up to 50 percent of normal horses, but usually elicit no disease symptoms unless a horse suffers from immune suppression or deficiency.

Chorioptic Mites

Chorioptic mites are a problem in winter, involving the abdomen or the lower limbs, especially the hind legs. Due to the cracked, greasy appearance of the skin of the lower leg, a case of chorioptic mites may be confused with a dermatitis called "scratches" or "grease heel" (see p. 367). Normally, scratches is caused by a skin irritant, or a bacterial and/or fungal infection around the back of the pastern. Its symptoms include painful, itchy, weeping, red, and inflamed skin. Some or all of these symptoms may be present, depending on the cause. If a case of dermatitis does not respond to conventional treatment with antifungals, antibiotics, and anti-inflammatory topical ointments, chorioptic mites may be the cause.

Straw-Itch Mites

The *straw-itch* mite causes small raised areas of edema on a horse's skin. They are non-itchy, crusty eruptions. The straw-itch mite normally parasitizes grain-insect larvae and is commonly found in alfalfa hay or straw. Humans are also affected with intense itching by this mite.

Chiggers

Infestation with *chiggers,* or *harvest* mites, is called *trombiculiasis*. It is the larvae that invade horse skin, rather than the nymphs or adults. In the southern Midwest and eastern states, chiggers can be a problem in late summer and fall. Horses pastured in fields and woods may develop crusty *papules* (elevated areas with a defined border) on the face, neck, thorax, and legs. Commonly, the lips and face are involved, with scaly, scabby areas lacking color. It is easy to mistake affected lesions around the muzzle as areas of *photosensitization* (see p. 368). Chigger sites may or may not itch. On the face, these mites may cause headshaking (see p. 515).

OTHER EXTERNAL PARASITES

Onchocerca Worm

An itchy condition that causes *alopecia* used to be quite prevalent before the advent of ivermectin: *Onchocerca cervicalis*. This parasite enters the horse from a bite by an infected gnat. Infective *Onchocerca* larvae migrate to the nuchal ligament along the top of the neck where they develop into adults. Then they release *microfilaria,* which infiltrate the skin of the horse. Dead and dying microfilaria cause a mild pruritus and associated hair loss, usually seen along the belly, withers, neck, chest, and on the face (photo 13.37). Dying microfilaria may also cause depigmentation, seen around the muzzle or along the belly. This skin problem is common during warm weather due to transmission by Culicoides gnats and more active

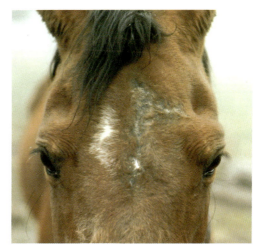

13.37 *One area that loses hair related to migration of microfilaria larvae of the Onchocerca worm is the face. The belly, neck, withers, and chest may also be affected. Photo: David Varra, DVM.*

microfilaria production by the Onchocerca adults, as they are stimulated by longer daylight hours. Diagnosis of *Onchocerciasis* is made by microscopic examination of affected tissue obtained by surgical biopsy, or skin scraping. Seeing microfilaria through the microscope positively identifies the skin ailment.

Moon Blindness

If microfilaria migrate through the eye, *periodic ophthalmia,* or "moon blindness," can result. Moon blindness is accompanied by chronic attacks of *anterior uveitis,* which is an inflammation of structures surrounding the pupil (see chapter 16, *The Eyes,* p. 497). Uveitis is painful, and symptoms include tearing, squinting, and sensitivity to bright light *(photophobia)*. Corneal ulcers develop subsequent to swelling of the eye's internal structures.

Fortunately, ivermectin has all but eliminated this skin syndrome in horses. This oft-used deworming medication kills the microfilaria and larvae, but not necessarily adults in the skin.

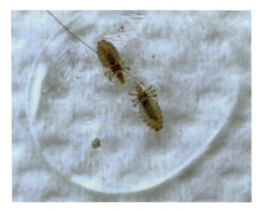

13.38 *Lice are visible to the naked eye as "walking dandruff," and when viewed with a magnifying glass will appear as in this photo. Photo: David Varra, DVM.*

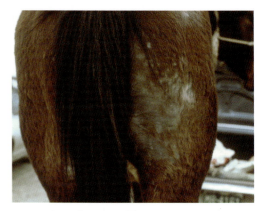

13.39 *An infestation of lice creates intense pruritus, and the horse will rub out hair anywhere lice may be. Commonly, lice inhabit the thick hairs on the mane, neck, shoulders, back, and buttocks. Photo: David Varra, DVM.*

Use of ivermectin 2 or 3 times a year provides an effective control, and is available over-the-counter where deworming products are sold.

Pelodera Strongyloides

Pelodera strongyloides is a microscopic parasite that affects the skin of the thighs and belly. The symptoms may be mistaken for urine or manure scald. This parasite causes *rhabditic dermatitis*, which is itchy and painful. Usually, sanitation of the environment controls this problem. Diagnosis often is only accomplished by a skin biopsy.

Lice

Onchocerca and *Pelodera strongyloides* are invisible to the naked eye. But carefully brushing the hairs the wrong way may lead to the discovery of more obvious skin predators, such as *lice*. Infestation with lice is called *pediculosis*. Typically, this parasite is a problem in winter, because the eggs (*nits*) thrive in the deep layers of a fuzzy winter hair coat. Lice are host specific, meaning that a horse louse will not infest a person, dog, or cat. Lice cannot survive more than 1 to 3 weeks off their preferred host.

The louse spends its entire life cycle on the host. It can be seen along the topline as a "walking dandruff." Pay particular attention to areas beneath the mane, the shoulders, the back, and the base of the tail. Part the fur and look for dandruff-like particles that move. These would be biting lice, moving rapidly away from the light. Sucking lice move more slowly, and a more critical look may find their heads embedded in the skin. The nits are cemented to the hairs, and should not be mistaken for bot fly eggs. Nits are white and more oval than the yellow bot fly eggs normally found on the legs. Using a magnifying glass aids identification (photo 13.38). Lice cause intense itching, and a horse self-mutilates to satisfy the itching. The hair coat may appear moth-eaten in places, and large areas of hair will be rubbed out, especially over the buttocks, thighs, neck, and head (photo 13.39).

Treatment involves bathing with appropriate medicated shampoo products specifically targeted for louse therapy. The biggest problem with this strategy is that louse infestation most commonly occurs in winter or early spring when the horse sports a thick coat; this is a difficult time of year to bathe a horse. Lice cannot reproduce or survive high body surface temperatures that are prevalent in warmer times of the year. Topical pyrethrin or permethrin products applied 2 weeks apart are effective against lice, as is ivermectin given as 2 doses, 2 weeks apart. Also, clean tack and grooming equipment with insecticides so the horse is not reinfected after treatment. Tack and equipment should be soaked in a bleach solution of at least 4:1 dilution (4 parts water to 1 part bleach).

Healthy horses with adequately functioning immune systems seem to be less affected by infestation with lice. Situations of over-crowding, poor nutrition, or poor environmental hygiene are stressors that set up conditions for lice to flourish. They are transmitted directly from horse to horse, or by brushes, blankets, and tack. Ample sunlight and regular grooming are effective tools in minimizing the risk of louse infection.

Ticks

Spinous Ear Ticks

The *spinous ear tick*, *Otobius*, is a soft tick that inhabits the ear canal (photo 13.40). These ticks remain attached for up to seven months, feeding off lymph secretions, causing irritation and headshaking. Sometimes a horse may droop a particularly affected ear, or rub his head incessantly on a post. Intense inflammation caused by these ticks makes their attachment sites susceptible to bacterial infection. This tick may elaborate a toxin that elicits severe muscle spasms. (See chapter 6, *Muscle Endurance*, p. 171 and chapter 17, *The Neurologic System in Health and Disease*, p. 515.) It

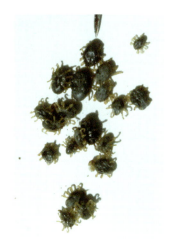

13.40 *The spinous ear tick prefers to inhabit the ear canals. This can contribute to headshaking, and at times these ticks may secrete a toxin that elicits muscle spasms. Photo: David Varra, DVM.*

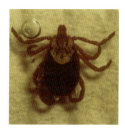

13.41 *This is a typical example of a hard tick, Dermocenter, common throughout the United States. Such ticks can cause tick paralysis.*

is often necessary to sedate the horse to properly examine the ear canals and apply topical treatment to remove the ticks.

Hard Ticks

Another type of tick, *Amblyomma*, is a hard tick common to the southeastern United States. It prefers to feed on blood deep within the ears. The bite is quite painful. These ticks are also found along the mane and tail, withers, and flanks. Another hard tick, *Dermocenter*, can be found throughout the United States (photo 13.41). Ticks irritate soft-skinned areas around the groin, under the tail, around the anus and vulva, and under the throat and belly. Ticks burrow their heads into superficial skin layers (photo 13.42). Secondary bacterial infections around these bites can occur, and occasionally edema and soft tissue swelling result even after the tick has dropped off. A neurotoxin in the saliva of Dermocenter ticks also can cause an ascending paralysis, particularly in a very young or small horse. The paralysis rapidly resolves once the tick is removed. (For further discussion, see "Tick Paralysis," p. 515.)

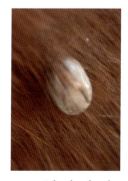

13.42 *This hard tick has imbedded itself into the neck skin and is engorged with the horse's blood. Care must be taken when removing these ticks to also remove the head and mouthparts.*

Disease Transmission by Ticks

Providing they do not carry disease or create paralysis, ticks generally cause little harm to the horse, although a heavy infestation indicates a suppressed immune system. With a heavy tick load, a horse could develop anemia from blood loss. Ticks, such as the *deer tick* (*Ixodes*) can transmit serious diseases such as *Lyme disease* (see chapter 5, *Joints*, p. 136), or *equine granulocytic ehrlichiosis*.

Ehrlichia Equi

A tick-borne disease that affects horses is called equine granulocytic ehrlichiosis, attributable to *Ehrlichia equi*, renamed *Anaplasma phagocytophila*. (This organism is *not* the same one that is responsible for Potomac Horse Fever: *Ehrlichia risticii*.) Ticks transmit *Ehrlichia equi*, with an incubation time of 10 to 20 days. Infection causes fever, depression, weakness, poor motor coordination, and limb edema, rather than the life-threatening intestinal diarrhea experienced with Potomac Horse Fever (see p. 294). Also seen with this infection is a loss of platelets and subsequent *petechiations* (small blood spots), which are visible as tiny red spots on mucous membranes. On rare occasions, a transient heart arrhythmia may develop. Treatment is not always necessary as the disease is usually self-limiting, but it is responsive to oxytetracycline. Humans also contract this disease from ticks, but it is not transferred from horses to people, or vice versa.

Tick Removal

Once a tick is identified on a horse, it should be removed immediately:

- Grasp the tick with fingers or tweezers, as close as possible to its point of attachment, the mouthparts.
- Exert gentle, steady pressure to remove the tick, and do not use heat, alcohol, or chemicals to stimulate removal.
- Avoid squeezing or crushing the tick with bare fingers as disease may be transmitted to humans through abraded skin or mucous membranes.
- Destroy the tick by flushing, freezing, or burning.
- Wash hands and tick bite thoroughly following tick removal.

Summer Sores

A syndrome caused by abnormal larval migration of the stomach worm, *Habronema* (see p. 463) or *Draschia*, is called *summer sores* or *cutaneous habronemiasis*. During warm months when house or stable flies are active, larvae from the stomach worm are passed in the feces and ingested by larvae of these host flies. Once fly larvae hatch and begin feeding on the horse, they are deposited at feeding sites. If worm larvae are deposited in areas of moist skin, such as the mucous membranes of the lips, eyes, vulva, or prepuce (sheath), or on wounds or traumatized skin, they migrate beneath the skin, causing a severe allergic hypersensitivity reaction.

The lesions that develop appear ulcerated, raw, and bleeding, and are very painful and itchy. A horse may bite at and traumatize the lesions. Although they may regress during winter, the lesions reoccur the next year at the same time and in the same place.

Summer sores resemble proud flesh, *fibroblastic sarcoids* (see p. 394), or a *squamous cell carcinoma* tumor (see p. 399). A biopsy differentiates a summer sore from these other problems. Surgically cutting away dead and dying tissue, along with nonsteroidal anti-inflammatory drugs (NSAIDs) and antibiotics, helps control tissue proliferation. Ivermectin is 100 percent effective in killing the worm larvae but may need to be administered every 2 to 4 weeks to maintain an effective blood level of the drug during warm seasons. Fly sprays should be used to prevent reinfection.

Black Widow Spider

An unusual creature that can bite the horse is the *black widow spider*. The horse responds quickly to the spider's poison, developing a severe and enormous swelling, along with considerable pain, illness, fever, depression, lack of appetite, or hives.

Normal wound management such as cold or hot soaking and administration of antibiotics and anti-inflammatory drugs are the treatments for this noxious bite.

Allergic Skin Reactions

THE ROLE OF THE IMMUNE SYSTEM

The world teems with invisible organisms. Under the right conditions, these microbes colonize the body, afflicting an animal with disease symptoms. Normally, the immune system keeps the organisms at bay. Disease-producing organisms are comprised of proteins. Inflammatory cells recognize these proteins, called *antigens,* as foreign, and wage invisible battles when they attempt to invade the body. Antigens then stimulate the body to launch an immune response. The immune system responds by manufacturing other proteins, called *antibodies,* which are weapons against a specific antigenic target. Preprogrammed antibodies set off a cascade of biochemical events. Localized inflammation starts within minutes.

Normally the immune system works in harmony with other biochemical responses to keep a horse disease-free, healthy, and vital. Occasionally, the body rebels and an immune response is blown out of proportion. Such a hypersensitive response is called an *allergy.* It can range from a serious, life-threatening reaction within the respiratory tract to mild, but

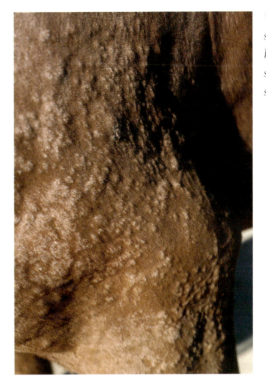

13.43 *A severe hypersensitivity response with hives may appear as a skin rash. Hives may sometimes itch.*

disagreeable skin reactions, called *hives* or *urticaria* (photo 13.43).

HIVES

Hives, or *urticaria*, are areas of edema (swelling of cells with fluid) that begin as small bumps. Then, they grow together into large, elevated, round, flat-topped bumps with steep sides, about the size of a fingernail. Pressing one leaves an indented impression of a fingertip, and is called *pitting edema*.

Hives can develop anywhere on the body, but most often start on the neck and shoulders and along the thorax (photo 13.44). As an allergic response progresses, the entire body may become involved, especially the upper hind limbs (13.45). An affected horse appears depressed as the immune system wages a silent war.

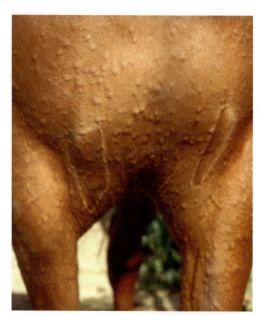

13.44 *Hives develop due to an allergic response. Hives are areas of edema (swelling of cells with fluid) that begin as small bumps that coalesce into large, elevated, round, flat-topped bumps with steep sides.*

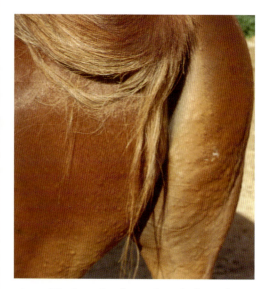

13.45 *This horse has hives along the buttocks and thigh from an intense allergic reaction. Pressing a finger into these coalesced areas of hives leaves an indented finger impression, called "pitting edema."*

Hives usually appear 12 to 24 hours after exposure to foreign protein, and resolve as quickly. Because hypersensitivity reactions take months or years to develop, a sudden onset of hives is not always a result of a very recent change, making it difficult to locate the source of the problem.

Causes of Hives

Most hives are caused by an allergic response to a plant, food, or drug, although the specific cause is isolated less than half the time. Blood transfusions, ingestion of certain plants or feed additives, or vaccines or other medications can be responsible for hives. Liver disease is sometimes associated with recurrent hives; in those cases once the liver heals, hive episodes abate. Autoimmune diseases can also cause hives.

Drug Allergies

Medications such as nonsteroidal anti-inflammatory drugs (NSAIDs) like flunixin meglumine or phenylbutazone, and *procaine penicillin* may cause allergic reactions. Hives can also occur after administration of equine influenza vaccine or tetanus antitoxin.

Food Allergies

Certain food substances, particularly those high in protein, cause hives in some horses. Small, raised areas, or *wheals*, that itch intensely and cause the horse to rub his tail, accompany an allergic response.

Pollen and Mold

Inhaled allergens, such as pollen or molds, are common sources for hives. Antigens inhaled into the lungs stimulate swelling in the respiratory tract, similar to asthma in people.

Topical Applications

Not all incidents of hives are caused by intake of a foreign substance. Topical application of povidone iodine scrub, which contains soap, or liniments, insecticides, or contact with certain bedding, may also spark an allergic reaction.

Insect Bites

Insect bites often stimulate an outbreak of hives. Isolated groups of bumps that appear rapidly, especially in thin-skinned areas, may be allergic reactions to mosquito bites, Culicoides gnat bites, or *Onchocerca* parasites. Most insect-bite reactions resolve without treatment within 12 to 72 hours. The wheals are mildly tender and flat. Insect bites rarely cause hives on the entire body unless the bite toxin is overwhelming. Usually the wheals are confined to one area.

Other Causes of Hives

Purpura Hemorrhagica

An allergic response to the bacteria responsible for strangles (*Streptococcus equi*) can cause *purpura hemorrhagica* (see p. 277). A month or two following a bout of *Streptococcal* respiratory infection, like strangles (see p. 273), or influenza (see p. 267), a horse may appear stiff from muscle soreness. The limbs are stocked up, edema extends into the belly and prepuce, and the horse is reluctant to move.

Hives often appear on the entire body in a case of purpura, due to a breakdown in blood vessel walls as a consequence of an immune response to the *Streptolysin O* toxin that remains from a strangles (*Streptococcus equi*) infection. Small blood spots (petechiations) are visible on the mucous membranes of the gums, eyes, and inside the vulva. As the syndrome progresses, swelling increases in the legs, and the skin begins to ooze serum.

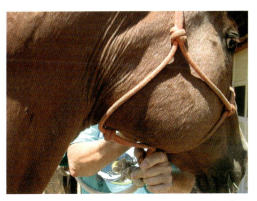

13.46 *One form of an allergic response is for the throatlatch area and face to swell, as seen in this horse. If the swelling is allowed to continue unchecked, the horse's airway could also swell, turning this into a life-threatening situation.*

To combat an allergic response to the *Strep* toxin, high doses of penicillin and anti-inflammatory agents are administered for weeks until the symptoms abate.

Angioedema

Profound hypersensitivity allergies, as seen with accidental administration of some drugs, may result in a syndrome called *angioedema*. This reaction is more severe than simple hives. The head and respiratory tract swell, and respiratory tract swelling migrates downward (photo 13.46). Hives is often a precursor to angioedema. Angioedema is a life-threatening condition; it can rapidly progress to *anaphylaxis* and death.

Anaphylaxis

Anaphylaxis can occur rapidly and progress to an irreversible condition within a few minutes. There is not always the opportunity to see an allergic response before it becomes a death warrant to a horse. The horse initially may appear anxious or colicky, or may experience muscle tremors and patchy sweating. Respiratory distress quickly follows, due to pooling of blood and fluid in the lungs. The horse collapses and may convulse before death.

Preventing Hives

When purchasing a horse, question the seller about previous allergic responses the horse may have experienced. Inform the veterinarian, trainer, and barn manager about these allergies. A big sign in red writing should be placed outside the horse's stall describing known allergies.

Determining the Cause of Hives

If a horse erupts in hives, discontinue new medications or food supplements immediately. To determine if hives is a result of a food allergy, change the grain and hay ration for at least two weeks. Slow reintroduction of a feed product may stimulate reappearance of the hives, which will determine that a particular food sparks an allergic response.

If hives occur as an isolated incident, the cause may never be discovered. However, if hives is a recurrent problem, tracking down the source includes intradermal skin testing for allergens like pollen (plants, bushes, and trees), molds, grasses, weeds, dust, and farm plants such as corn, oats, wheat, and mustard. After identifying the source, hyposensitization injections (injection of miniscule amounts of the allergen into the skin to desensitize the horse) may prove successful over the long-term. Treatment must be continued for life. Most horses affected with a case of hives recover uneventfully with little cause for concern. Pay attention to recent changes in diet, environment, medications, vaccinations, or stress factors that may cause the immune system to overreact.

Hyperelastosis Cutis

Hyperelastosis cutis, or more correctly called *Hereditary Equine Regional Dermal Asthenia* (HERDA), is a heritable disorder of skin connective tissue mostly seen in Quarter Horses, Paints, and Appaloosas descended from Poco Bueno/King bloodlines. This form of collagen defect is characterized by wrinkled and overly extensible skin, similar to Ehlers-Danlos syndrome seen in humans. When tented, the skin does not return to its original position (see photo 9.10, p. 235). Skin is easily traumatized whether bumped or beneath a saddle, with wounds occurring far more often than would be expected. Not only is the skin fragile and prone to tearing, but wounds are also difficult to heal. Pain is often pronounced around the wound margins. There is no treatment for this condition. Horses should be confined in areas where they are not at risk of wounding or likely to have physical interaction with other horses. DNA testing is not currently available to identify affected carriers of this genetic disease.

Skin Growths

Horses do develop skin growths, sometimes in the form of a *benign* process, and occasionally as a *malignant* cancer. A benign growth is only of cosmetic significance, and does not spread to other organs. If malignant, cancer spreads to internal organs. Cancers of the skin are rarely life threatening in horses as they are in dogs or people, but skin growths do detract from a horse's appearance. A veterinarian should examine any skin growth that appears suddenly or enlarges rapidly.

WARTS

Warts, or *papillomas,* generally occur on young horses, less than 3 years of age, or on a horse with a compromised immune system. The common places to find warts are on the muzzle, lips, prepuce, vulva, eyelids, and in the ears (photos 13.47, 13.48, and 13.49). Warts are usually self-limiting, meaning they will resolve on their own, but may take as long as a year to do so. Because they may be transmitted from a virus, warts are considered communicable. Care should be taken to avoid sharing of tack, or direct contact of a wart-affected horse with others. Flies feeding within the ear can aggravate ear warts.

EQUINE SARCOID

A common skin growth found on horses is the *sarcoid*. It is a benign tumor unique to equine skin. The term "tumor" is misleading since a sarcoid growth is usually localized to a small

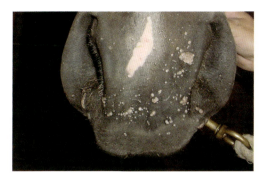

13.47 *A young horse with a naïve immune system may develop warts, most commonly seen on the muzzle. These usually resolve spontaneously when the horse's immune system eliminates the inciting virus.*

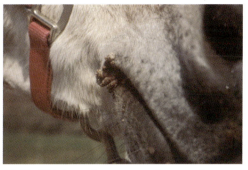

13.48 *This horse has warts at the commissures of the lips, another common location. Warts are potentially contagious to other horses with young or poorly functioning immune systems.*

area and does not invade underlying tissues or lymphatic vessels. Unlike malignant and life-threatening growths, sarcoids do not spread to internal organs. They remain an external, cosmetic blemish, but may occasionally interfere with tack or skin mobility and if traumatized, a sarcoid can become ulcerated or infected. Over 50 percent of horses with a single sarcoid ultimately develop multiple sarcoids.

Sarcoids are thought to develop from an infective virus that enters a break in the skin, or as a transformation of cell components as an abnormal response to trauma. Areas of skin subjected to trauma are predisposed to sarcoids. These tumors can be transmitted from one part of a horse to another by biting, rubbing, or contaminated tack.

Almost half of all sarcoids are found on a horse's limbs (photo 13.50), while 32 percent are located on the head and neck, especially the ears, eyelids, and mouth. Other locations for sarcoids include the chest and trunk, the abdomen and flanks, and the prepuce. In general, sarcoids do not pose a major health hazard to a horse. Because it is a common ailment of the equine skin, monitor any skin growths so benign tumors can be differentiated from dangerous ones.

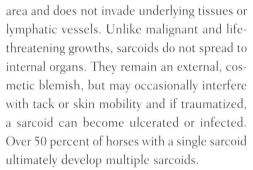

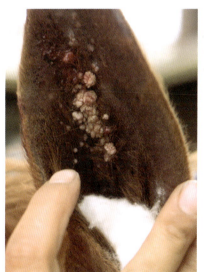

13.49 *Another common place to find a wart invasion is along the inner surface of the ear. It is important to differentiate warts from sarcoid tumors or gnat hypersensitivity, as treatment will be different for each condition.*

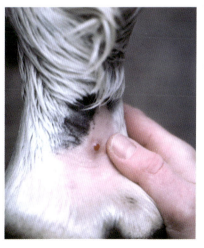

13.50 *Over half the sarcoids found are on a horse's limbs, such as seen here as a small lesion on the back of the pastern.*

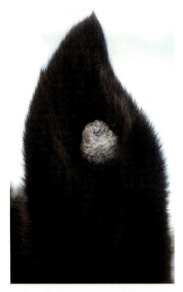

13.51 A verrucous sarcoid is a dry, horny mass, resembling a cauliflower, not too dissimilar in appearance to that seen in the ear with black fly hypersensitivity or warts.

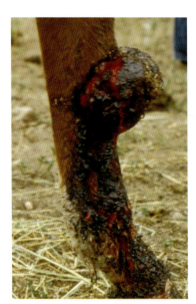

13.52 A fibroblastic sarcoid typically develops over a wound, giving the appearance of proud flesh that will not respond to treatment.

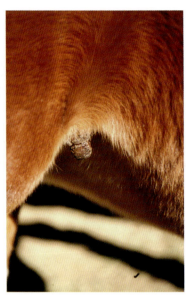

13.53 This pedunculated sarcoid is a mixture of verrucous and fibroblastic sarcoid forms.

Types of Sarcoids

Verrucous Sarcoids

Verrucous sarcoids are wart-like, dry, horny masses, resembling a cauliflower (photo 13.51). They are usually less than 2½ inches in diameter. Verrucous sarcoids can appear spontaneously without any prior trauma or wounding of the skin. They are difficult to distinguish from warts except that verrucous sarcoids tend to lack hair, partially or totally, while warts have hair growing up to the edges, and often regress spontaneously. Verrucous sarcoids do not regress.

Fibroblastic Sarcoids

If a verrucous sarcoid is traumatized, it can develop into *a fibroblastic sarcoid* (photo 13.52). Fibroblastic sarcoids often develop subsequent to a wound, and are difficult to distinguish from normal granulation tissue. These masses are like *proud flesh* (see p. 416), and may enlarge and expand to sizes greater than 10 inches in diameter. A fibroblastic sarcoid may remain as a small lesion for years, and then suddenly erupt into a nasty-looking sore. Or, it can start as a rapidly and aggressively growing tumor. A wound that refuses to heal and is repeatedly ulcerated and infected may be a fibroblastic tumor.

Mixed Sarcoid

Both the verrucous or fibroblastic types are further classified as broad-based (*sessile*), or with a stalk (*pedunculated*). A mixture of verrucous and fibroblastic forms represents, the third type, a *mixed sarcoid* (photo 13.53).

Occult Sarcoid

A flat tumor represents the fourth type, the *occult sarcoid* (photo 13.54). It is usually flat or

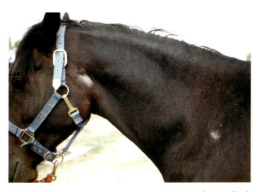

13.54 *The most common type of sarcoid is called an occult sarcoid, characterized by its flat, scaly, and hairless appearance. This is sometimes confused with a bite wound or ringworm but does not resolve with time or anti-fungal treatment.*

very slightly raised, the skin is thickened, and the surface roughened. It may resemble ringworm (see p. 372), or skin crusting from a bacterial infection or poor skin health. Occult sarcoids typically appear around the head, especially the ears and eyelids. If aggravated by rubbing, trauma, or by a surgical biopsy, it may convert to the fibroblastic form.

Recognizing Sarcoids

It is virtually impossible to determine the exact nature of many growths based solely on appearance. Complete or partial biopsy of an enlargement will reveal if abnormal cells are present. *Fibrosarcomas, neurofibromas, neurofibrosarcomas,* and *squamous cell carcinomas* are all different malignant tumor types easily confused with a sarcoid; these different cell forms are fairly invasive into the tissues. *Fibromas* are non-malignant growths, and although mistaken for sarcoids, they easily shell-out and are well-defined, while a sarcoid infiltrates around its margins, without a neat border. Summer sores caused by *Habronema fly* larvae also develop ulcerated masses not readily distinguishable from sarcoids (see p. 388). *Keloids* (see p. 420) are comprised of collagenous, connective tissue that may resemble a sarcoid. Warts in the ears also appear like sarcoids (see photo 13.49, p. 393).

Treating Sarcoids

Unless a sarcoid obstructs performance or tack, is an ulcerated mass, or its location causes a horse to become headshy, it is best to leave it alone. Carefully monitor the sarcoid for any growth or change.

If treatment is necessary, various techniques are available for different types and locations of a sarcoid tumor. The most difficult sarcoids to remove are those on the limbs. If multiple sarcoids are present, a complete cure is less likely. In conjunction with treatment, the bulk of a growth should be surgically removed. With surgery alone, 50 percent recur within three years, often within six months. By combining surgery with another treatment, such as cryosurgery, immunotherapy, or hyperthermia, greater success may be achieved.

Cryosurgery

A successful therapy to use along with surgical removal is *cryosurgery*. It is up to 80 percent effective if performed correctly. The lesion is frozen rapidly to -4° F (-20° C), and then allowed to thaw slowly to room temperature, whereupon it is refrozen, followed by a slow thaw. It may be frozen a third time.

Before a cryosurgical site has healed, it normally develops a noticeable inflammatory reaction with swelling, edema, and discharge. This reaction may last for a week. Complete healing may take up to two months for the body to reject dead tumor tissue.

Drawbacks

Although cryosurgery is a preferred treatment, it does have some drawbacks. It is not useful

13.55 A & B *This occult sarcoid on the chin was treated with repeated Bacillus Calmette-Guerin (BCG) injections (A). The same horse six months after the last BCG treatment (B).*

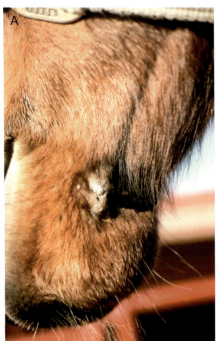
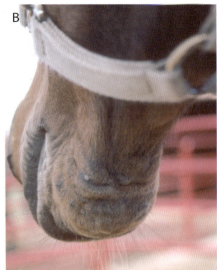

in locations around the head and ears, the eyelids, thin-skinned areas directly over a protuberant bone such as the hip, or points on the lower limbs over joints. In these locations, there is risk of injuring tissue beneath the sarcoid with freezing. Usually, scarring is minimal. The area loses hair color due to hair follicle and pigment-producing cell *(melanocytes)* destruction by freezing.

Immunotherapy

An alternative treatment is *immunotherapy*, which stimulates a horse's body to "reject" a sarcoid through normal immune mechanisms. Success of immunotherapy demonstrates that the health of the immune system plays a large role in the development and regression of the sarcoid tumor.

BCG Injections

The most successful treatment involves infiltrating the sarcoid with an immune-stimulating product called *Bacillus Calmette-Guerin,* or BCG. BCG is made from the cell wall of the organism, *Mycobacterium*, which causes tuberculosis. Success depends on a horse's ability to develop a delayed hypersensitivity response to activate the cellular immune system to destroy tumor cells. Success rates of 50 to 80 percent are achieved with BCG application combined with surgical removal. Over 90 percent of flat sarcoids on the head or neck regress with BCG therapy (photos 13.55 A & B).

Following injection of BCG, a local inflammatory reaction and swelling occur within the first 24 to 48 hours. Sites of BCG injection usually worsen before they improve. To achieve adequate regression of a tumor, 3 to 6 injections of BCG are required at two-to-three-week intervals. BCG injection of a sarcoid in one place may stimulate regression of sarcoids elsewhere on the body.

BCG is best applied to tumors less than 2½ inches in diameter. With multiple or excessively large lesions, injecting excessive amounts of BCG vaccine may be necessary to achieve the desired results. These excessive amounts can cause adverse systemic reactions, such as hives or anaphylaxis although purification of the BCG product decreases the risk of adverse systemic reactions.

Bloodroot Extract

A topical compound (Xterra®, Compound X, or Indian Mud) made with the extract of *bloodroot* (*Sanguinaria canadensis*) as its active ingredient has had favorable effects on triggering a horse's immune system to eliminate sarcoid tumor cells. This compound works best on the flat, occult form of sarcoid.

Other Chemotherapeutic Agents

Although non-malignant, equine sarcoids often respond well to two other chemotherapeutic agents, cisplatinin or 5-fluorouracil (5-FU).

Hyperthermia

A less common therapy for sarcoids is *hyperthermia*, which uses a radio-frequency current to heat the tissue to 122° F (50° C) for about 30 seconds. This technique may be repeated up to 4 times at one-to-two week intervals, depending on the size of the tumor. A cosmetic advantage of hyperthermia is that the hair follicles remain functional after treatment, and a natural hair color grows back.

MELANOMA

As horses tend to live outside under all sorts of conditions, skin pigmentation is advantageous to their survival. Melanin is a substance produced by pigment-secreting skin glands; it protects against "sunburn" of the skin from ultraviolet radiation. Horses with black hides are rarely bothered by sunlight. However, black skin can harbor a tumor of abnormal pigment-producing cells *(melanoblasts)*. The tumor, called a *melanoma*, forms when melanoblasts increase their metabolism and reproduce in localized areas of the skin. The black skin of a gray horse with excessive skin pigment can develop melanomas.

Of gray horses over 15 years old, it is said that 80 percent ultimately develop some form of melanoma. Most melanomas begin as slow-growing, encapsulated, and relatively benign growths. The tumors develop just under or above the skin with hair at first obscuring them until they become large enough to be visible. It can take years (as long as 10 to 20) for a melanoma to become hyperactive to the point of concern. Once a melanoma displays an accelerated growth rate, the malignant cells rapidly invade surrounding tissue.

Tissue around the tumor cannot keep pace with the consumptive tumor cells so it dies and ulcerates. Then the horse has bleeding or infected skin sores that fail to heal. Surrounding normal tissue may be displaced or replaced with the invasive melanoma.

Location of Growth

Melanomas develop around the anus, tailhead, vulva, or prepuce, and occasionally are found around the parotid salivary gland, head, and neck (photos 13.56 and 13.57). However, they can be found anywhere on the body, with a rare report of location within a hoof or spinal cord. Normally, melanomas take a long time to spread to internal body organs, such as the spleen and lungs. It usually takes years to wreak detrimental changes on the body and metabolism. It is not usually life-threatening, but when a tumor aggressively invades tissue around the anus or urinary tract, it may interfere with a horse's quality of life. In these cases, the humane option is to euthanize the horse to end pain and discomfort caused by ulcerated skin masses or obstructed bowels.

Treating Melanoma

If the tumors are isolated and single, it is advis-

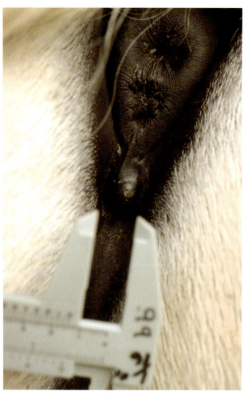

13.56 *A common site to find melanomas is in the perineal area around the anus and/or vulva. Usually they are not as severe as seen here, but some lines of certain breeds develop this aggressively invasive form. Sufficient tissue invasion can obstruct defecation or make it difficult for a mare to breed or foal. This is a typical presentation of size of a melanoma in the perineal region, or in the sheath or on the penis.*

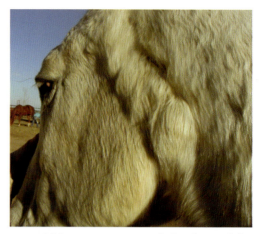

13.57 *Melanomas are commonly found around the parotid salivary gland in the throatlatch area, as well as on the inner surfaces of the lips and mouth (not shown here).*

Cimetidine

A form of chemotherapy for treatment of melanomas relies on the oral drug *cimetidine* (Tagamet®), commonly used for treating human stomach ulcers. The medication can be used by itself or along with surgical removal to halt progression or recurrence of melanomas.

Method of Action

It is thought that cimetidine modifies the immune system to control the cancer. Under normal circumstances, white blood cells called *suppressor T-cells* stop the attack of other white blood cells once an infection or "foreign" protein is defeated. This cellular check-and-balance system prevents an immune response from raging out of control. Cancer patients have an excessive number of suppressor T-cells that suppress the anti-tumor defense mechanism.

Histamine is a chemical that activates the suppressor T-cells. Therefore, histamine reduces the host's defenses against cancer. As an anti-ulcer medication, cimetidine blocks histamine pathways responsible for excessive secretion of gastric acid. By blocking histamine pathways,

able to leave them alone. Treatment by surgical removal tends to "anger" the skin. Not only do many of the tumors grow back, but they also become more aggressive than before. Multiple melanomas spread over much of the body are not solely a cosmetic problem. These melanomas are difficult to manage if they interfere with saddling, or the ability of a mare to breed or foal without discomfort.

occasionally spread to other organs, like the lymph nodes. Pink-skinned horses, like Appaloosas and Paints, are predisposed to squamous cell carcinoma around mucous membranes where there is no hair, and no melanocytes to protect the skin from ultraviolet rays. "Squames" mostly occur around the anus, vulva, prepuce, or eyes of pink-skinned horses. Ultraviolet radiation may cause normal cells to change into tumorous cells, but squamous cell carcinoma also develops in areas never exposed to the sun.

The only cure is surgical removal, or cryotherapy (freezing the tissue with liquid nitrogen). Horses with pink skin around the eyes benefit from fly facemasks to reduce the penetration of ultraviolet radiation. These mosquito-netted masks reduce ultraviolet rays by 70 percent. Zinc oxide or sunblocking agents can be applied to the face, reducing sunburn that may ultimately create tumors on the lips or muzzle (see p. 371).

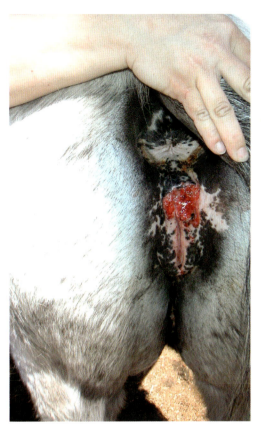

13.58 *Squamous cell carcinoma occurs in areas of non-pigmented skin near mucocutaneous junctions such as the eye, penis, prepuce, and vulva. This mare suffers from an erosive squamous cell carcinoma along the lips of her vulva.*

Sheath Cleaning

Cleaning the penis and prepuce within the sheath of a male horse is usually an annual process. It is not uncommon for a male horse with a dirty sheath to incessantly rub the tailhead. Routine hygiene maintains skin health of the penis and prepuce, and eliminates itching behavior. This procedure usually requires sedation to achieve relaxation of the penis. This allows an opportunity to inspect the prepuce and penis for development of small skin tumors that if left unattended could grow into life-threatening proportions (photos 13.59 and 13.60). Gray horses are at higher risk to developing melanomas in this region, while Appaloosas, Paint horses, or horses with pink skin on the penis or prepuce are at risk of developing squamous cell carcinomas.

During urination, many geldings and some stallions do not fully extend their penis, so not

cimetidine may also indirectly block activation of the suppressor T-cells. Then, normal antitumor defense mechanisms can function. *Macrophages* (specific white blood cells) battle against "foreign" cancer cells to eradicate them from the body without being suppressed by the suppressor T-cells.

SQUAMOUS CELL CARCINOMA

Horses with too little pigment in their skin can also develop skin cancer. *Squamous cell carcinoma* is a cauliflower-like growth that tends to ulcerate and bleed easily (photo 13.58). They

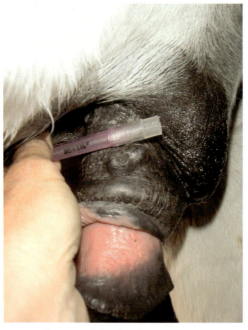

13.59 *Cleaning of the sheath is an opportune time to investigate for the presence of tumors like this penile melanoma.*

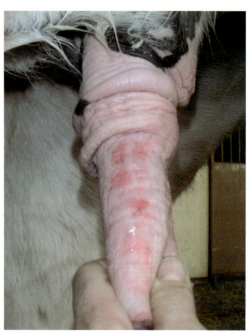

13.60 *This horse shows beginning stages of squamous cell carcinoma on the non-pigmented portion of his penis.*

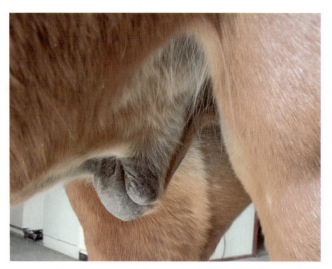

13.61 *A dirty prepuce is a favorite feeding area for flies, and irritation or bacterial infection can cause swelling.*

all the urine is voided from the urethra. Accumulations of *smegma*, dirt, and urine collect within the sheath over time. Smegma is an accumulation of natural oil secretions from skin glands, and is of a waxy texture. If allowed to accumulate, this material coats the inside of a horse's prepuce, and forms a scale along his penis. A particularly dirty prepuce may develop swelling (photo 13.61). Of significance is the balling-up of debris within a cul-de-sac (*urethral process*) at the end of the penis around the opening of the urethra. If the material that gathers is left to amass, it forms "beans" that can place pressure at the urethral process, potentially obstructing the opening through which urine is voided (photos 13.62 A & B).

If a horse allows handling without sedation, it is possible for a horse owner to accomplish this task. When cleaning a sheath, it is customary practice to stand at a horse's

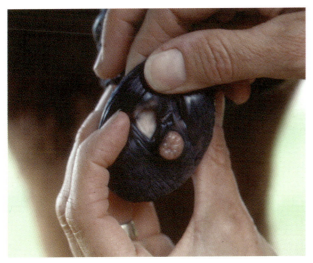
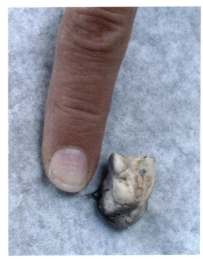

13.62 A & B *At the tip of the penis is a small cul-de-sac surrounding the opening of the urethra (A). This is called the urethral process, and it is here that "beans" of smegma and debris accumulate. The bean in (B) is typical of what is found in the urethral process. Often there are several of these, or one or two large ones that have formed from coalescence of dirt, sweat, and smegma (tissue secretions).*

shoulder, and to hook a leg around the front of the horse's forelimb. This prevents one from creeping back toward the haunches where a horse could make contact with a swift kick. Wear latex or rubber gloves to prevent chafing of the delicate mucous membranes of the penis. Wet gloves slide more easily within the sheath, eliminating irritating chafe. To loosen caked debris within the sheath, Ivory® soap is the lubricant of choice, or Excalibur®, a product intended for sheath cleaning. Other antiseptic soaps such as povidone iodine preparations are not recommended as they kill beneficial bacteria that reside within the sheath and on the penis. Such bacteria live in harmony on skin surfaces and have a direct role in preventing overgrowth of harmful (*pathogenic*) bacterial forms that cause infection. Ivory® soap is so mild that it does not interfere with normal bacterial residents. Remove all soap from within the sheath and penis when the washing is done, so that soapy residue does not cause a low-grade dermatitis.

Equine First Aid, Medication, and Restraint

14

Of the many medical incidents confronted by a horse owner or trainer, the most common are skin wounds. In most instances, a veterinarian is not present at the time of injury, and sometimes hours may pass before a veterinarian arrives to treat the horse.

Wound Management

Initial Treatment

Initial wound management greatly influences the outcome and duration of healing. It is often assumed that application of a topical salve is sufficient while waiting for the veterinarian, but this erroneous notion may do little to help. When the protective skin layer is broken open, environmental and skin contaminants are introduced into the wound along with dirt, gravel, and foreign materials like wood, paint, or hay. Certain soils, clay, and organic matter inhibit the immune action of white blood cells, antibodies, and antibiotics, and also interfere with normal antibacterial activity of serum. A wound should be cleansed of all foreign material as rapidly as possible to prevent bacteria from invading deep tissues. On a local scale, normal immune mechanisms effectively deal with up to one-million bacteria per gram of tissue. More than that will overwhelm the immune system, creating infection. Antiseptic ointments, creams, or sprays cannot reach into a wound obscured by devitalized tissue and foreign debris.

Assessing the Damage

Sensible hygienic techniques allow a horse's natural healing mechanisms to proceed undeterred, leading to rapid healing with minimal scarring. The first order of business when faced with any trauma is to gently hose away the bulk of dirt and contaminants before handling the wound. This not only cleanses the area, but also allows close inspection to determine the depth and extent of an injury. Some wounds appear superficial, only to reveal separation of underlying tissues that forms a tract leading into deeper layers (photo 14.1). A deep puncture can be serious if it enters critical structures or if an infection is allowed to simmer unchecked. It is not always possible to detect a puncture or deeper tissue involvement on cursory inspection, but a cooperative horse may allow handling of a wound to peer beneath a skin flap to see how deep it goes, and which structures may be affected (photos 14.2 A & B). Examination of a

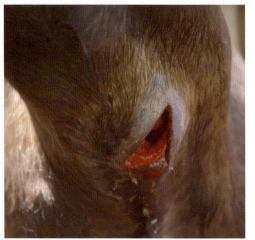

14.1 *A wound like this on the horse's neck may appear to have only impaled the skin and underlying muscle, but proximity to this horse's trachea, esophagus, and jugular and carotid vessels make it imperative to enlist professional veterinary evaluation.*

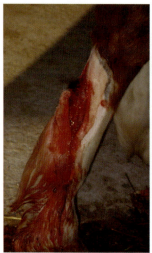 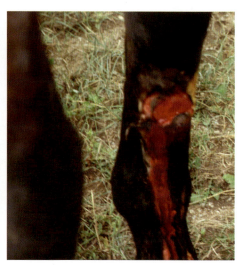

14.2 A & B *A laceration along the backside of the lower limb is considered an emergency due to proximity of flexor tendons, suspensory ligaments, and large blood vessels and nerves that could be injured (A). A laceration along the front surface of the lower limb is not as dire a situation unless the wound is over a joint. An injury to the front of a long bone typically runs into extensor tendon and/or bone and is easily managed with less threat of loss of use or loss of life (B).*

wound identifies its smell, if any, and the amount and character of the discharge *(exudate)*. Exudate may be nothing more than shedding dead and dying tissue, and white blood cells; it does not necessarily include bacteria. A bad odor, or a large amount of exudate is suspicious for infection, requiring immediate veterinary care. The best approach is to assume the worst and be moderately aggressive in treatment. With any wound, make sure the horse is up to date on tetanus prophylaxis (see p. 422).

A foreign body lodged in a wound needs to be extracted, and a skin flap should be removed or sutured to maintain adequate blood supply.

Debridement
Once the protective barrier of the skin's surface is broken, airborne, environmental, and skin bacteria contaminate the wound to colonize the wound margins with bacteria within 2 to 4 hours after injury (photo 14.3). If high bacterial numbers overwhelm the local immune system, bacteria proliferate and flourish, resulting in tissue invasion and infection. A wound that has been present for more than a few hours is likely so contaminated that a topical antibiotic does little to fend off infection. Extensive cleansing and *debridement* (cutting away of devitalized tissue) of the wound is necessary for successful treatment.

Shaving
When possible, surrounding hair should be trimmed and shaved away from a wound. Hair not only prevents proper evaluation of the damage, but it also interferes with thorough cleansing and hinders drainage from the

Equine First Aid, Medication, and Restraint

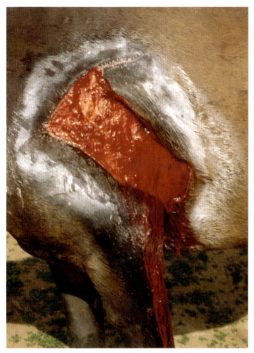

14.3 *Skin is a barrier to bacterial invasion, and within just a few hours after this barrier is breached, bacteria can colonize the wound, multiply in the tissues, and create infection, even in a relatively superficial wound.*

- The mechanical action loosens and removes dirt, debris, large particles, and dead tissue.
- Use of appropriate scrub solutions delivers an antiseptic layer to live tissue.

To kill bacteria, a wound should be vigorously scrubbed for a minimum of 10 minutes, alternately scrubbing and rinsing until it glistens and bleeds with healthy pink and bleeding tissue. If a horse does not permit scrubbing, hose the wound for 5 to 10 minutes while waiting for professional veterinary help. Gentle water pressure loosens adhered debris and grit to reduce numbers of contaminating bacteria at the wound site.

Lavage

To irrigate deeper regions of a wound, use a 35 cc (cubic centimeter) or 60 cc syringe filled with saline/antiseptic solution, or use a bulb pump on a bottle of salt solution (photo 14.4). Lavage a wound multiple times until the tissue appears clean and is lightly bleeding. The force of the fluid squirted from the syringe debrides away bacterial contaminants and pieces of tissue debris, and irrigates deeper tissues, leaving a wound in as clean a state as possible.

Antiseptic Cleaning Solutions

For cleaning a wound, prepare a homemade salt solution (saline) by mixing ½ tablespoon of table salt in a quart of water. This salt mixture approximates the salt content of body tissues, and is similar to commercial saline. Salt water is preferable to plain tap water for cleansing a wound. The higher salt content of the tissue tends to pull tap water into the cells, causing them to swell with edema, which interferes with blood circulation to an area and slows healing. On the other hand, a saltwater solution

wound. Hair itself acts as a foreign body to aggravate wound healing, and hair holds bacterial and particulate contaminants in the region of the wound. Before shaving, cover open tissue with moist gauze sponges to prevent shaved hairs from falling into the wound.

Scrubbing

One of the most effective techniques for minimizing the chance of infection is to rid the wound of dirt and contaminants as quickly as possible. Use gauze sponges and antiseptic soap, discarding debris along with the used supplies. Scrubbing the wound with an antiseptic cleanser accomplishes several things:

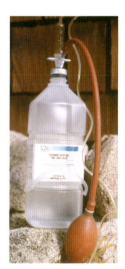

14.4 *A saline solution is optimal for wound cleansing. Irrigating the wound with a large syringe or pressurized bottle increases the pounds per square inch to loosen contaminants from the tissues.*

does not swell the cells with water since it approximates the same salt content of tissue. An antiseptic, such as povidone iodine or chlorhexidine, can be added to a saltwater solution to improve its antibacterial qualities for scrubbing and rinsing.

POVIDONE IODINE

Povidone iodine (Betadine®) has excellent antimicrobial properties. A commercial preparation of povidone iodine (0.5 percent) is made by combining iodine with a polyvinyl substance to decrease staining, stabilize iodine, and reduce its irritability to tissue. *Tincture of iodine* is an excellent antibacterial agent, but it is too strong for wound cleansing (see below).

To prepare a solution for wound cleansing, povidone-iodine (PI) solution is added to salt water to a concentration that visually approximates weak tea. To achieve this concentration, add 5 to 10 milliliters (ml) of the PI solution to 1 liter of salt solution. The best antibacterial and least tissue-toxic effect of PI occurs at concentrations of less than 0.1 percent. Too strong a solution (greater than 2 percent) is detrimental to wound healing. At a low concentration (less than 0.03 percent), white blood cells of the immune response are stimulated to migrate to the wound to perform their cleanup function. Conversely, at concentrations of 5 to 10 percent, iodine (tincture) dramatically hinders the immune function of white blood cells, increasing a wound's susceptibility to infection. Antibacterial activity of PI in a wound lasts for only 4 to 6 hours without any residual effect. Because a horse is so large, absorption of iodine into the body is insignificant. Humans, however, who must frequently apply this solution, should wear rubber gloves to avoid absorbing iodine in toxic amounts.

CHLORHEXIDINE

Chlorhexidine (Nolvasan®) is an excellent cleaning solution, effective against bacteria, viruses, and fungus. An ideal concentration of 0.05 percent for wound cleansing is prepared by mixing 20 to 25 ml with 1 liter of salt water, or 1:40 dilution. Not only does chlorhexidine work against a broad spectrum (many kinds) of bacteria, but its effects also persist in the tissues because it binds to skin proteins. Therefore, its antibacterial effects outlast those of PI.

Both PI and chlorhexidine are available as commercial antiseptic scrubs that contain soap, and should be diluted with a saltwater mixture when scrubbing a wound. Adequate rinsing is necessary to remove the sudsy soap from a wound once it has been thoroughly cleaned and investigated. Ideally, anything that is put into a wound should be so mild that if it were instilled into the eye it would not irritate mucous membranes or the eye itself. Following this principle avoids trouble.

Compounds That Slow Healing

Use of other types of soaps in a wound slows healing, and increases the susceptibility to infection. Most detergents and soaps are toxic to cells, causing them to swell and rupture; this adds to devitalized tissue. Only wound-specific, soapy antiseptics should be applied to equine tissue, such as chlorhexidine scrub, or PI scrub. If these are unavailable, Phisohex® soap (containing chlorhexidine) can be used with ample rinsing.

TINCTURE OF IODINE

Tincture of iodine (7 percent) is a strong antibacterial agent, however, it is so destructive to tissue that its only safe application is to the soles and frogs, to control thrush or toughen the feet. It is irritating when applied to intact skin, causing a rash or skin inflammation. Healing tissues are also negatively affected by tincture of iodine.

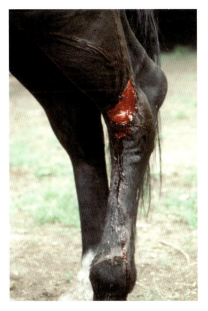 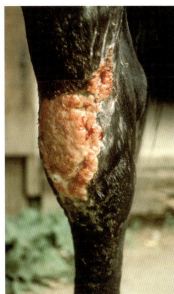

14.5 A & B *The initial injury to this horse's hock doesn't seem too deep (A); however, the lower legs tend to fill in with exuberant granulation tissue as seen in (B). Areas of movement, as over joints, are difficult to heal quickly because the bending motion of the joint continually disrupts migrating cells. The body continues to repair the area, laying down excessive granulation tissue, referred to as "proud flesh."*

HYDROGEN PEROXIDE

Hydrogen peroxide (3 percent) is useful on human skin for wounds with *anaerobic* (oxygen-free) bacterial growth because the foaming action increases the oxygen tension in a wound, which destroys anaerobic bacteria. Yet, hydrogen peroxide is toxic to equine cells, especially to migrating *fibroblasts*, the cells that produce *collagen* (connective tissue) to repair a wound (see p. 419). Peroxide also causes blood clots to form in microvessels, interfering with oxygen supply to the tissues. Reduced oxygen results in additional devitalized tissue, and delays healing. Hydrogen peroxide should be reserved only for cleaning off blood that has splattered the hair below a wound.

ALCOHOL

Alcohol (isopropyl or rubbing) should not be applied to open wounds because it destroys exposed tissue protein. It can be used to wipe around a wound perimeter to loosen debris, but should not contact open skin.

Promoting Wound Healing

Healing begins with fibrous connective tissue collagen, or fibrin strands, which are made of proteins (see p. 419). Fibroblasts, which manufacture fibrin, migrate into a wound by the third day. Budding blood vessels appear following migration of fibroblasts.

As *granulation tissue* (made of capillaries and fibroblasts) fills in a wound, it provides a surface along which *epithelial cells* (new skin cells) will migrate (photos 14.5 A & B). Regrowth of skin between wound margins is called *epithelialization* (photo 14.6). Not only do bacteria slow healing, but they also produce potent enzymes that destroy fragile and newly formed skin cells.

CONTRACTION

Wound size reduces through a process known as *contraction*. Adjacent, full-thickness skin at the wound margins is pulled toward the center of a wound by action of *myofibroblast cells* (specialized cells that convert from fibroblasts to act like muscle cells).

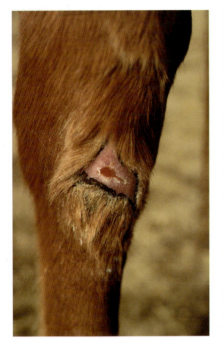 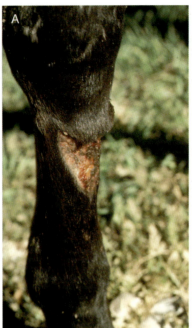 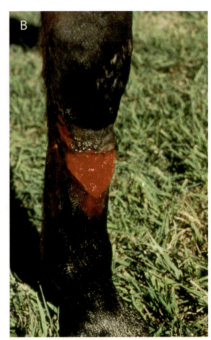

14.6 *This wound is healing nicely, with a pink border of newly forming epithelial cells, which will mature into skin. Only a small area of redder granulation tissue remains in the center of the contracting wound. Hair should regrow to occlude visibility of any remaining scar.*

14.7 A & B *A V-flap on even a superficial wound that is allowed to heal without first-aid intervention will often lead to a poor cosmetic result, as seen in (A) with a thickened wad of tissue and retraction of the flap. Infiltration of the wound with local anesthetic allowed surgical debridement of the scar tissue and flap with a scalpel. This turns a chronic wound into an active wound with a good blood supply, which can now repair with a more cosmetic and smooth scar (B).*

In a chronic wound, granulation tissue consists more of fibrous connective tissue, and is relatively sparse in myofibroblasts. Trimming this excess tissue away (*debulking*) with a scalpel removes a stagnant granulation bed, known as *proud flesh* (see p. 416) or *exuberant granulation tissue*. Fresh tissue replaces it, including myofibroblasts capable of reducing the size of the wound size by contraction (photos 14.7 A & B).

Factors Affecting Contraction Rate

Contraction rates of 0.2 millimeters per day during the first few months reduce a scar to half the original size (photos 14.8 A & B). Continued remodeling of a scar over the next 6 to 12 months further reduces its size (photos 14.9 A & B).

Skin Tension

The size of a wound does not affect contraction rate, but skin tension does. Lower-leg wounds tend to have taut skin edges so contract slowly (photos 14.10 A–C). Also, dry wounds are tighter and therefore contract more slowly than moist wounds. Excess tension, edema, or movement of a wound interferes with myofibroblast function. Then, contraction is limited, and may cease prematurely before wound edges meet.

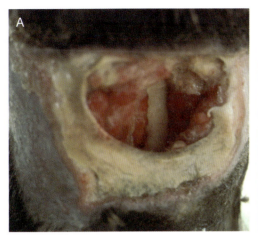 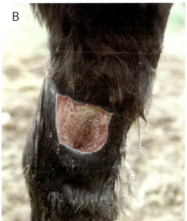

14.8 A & B At the time of initial injury, this deep thigh gash exposes muscle and bone (A). Within weeks, granulation tissue has filled in the gash, forming a smooth surface over which epithelial cells will form skin and hair (B). Injuries above the hock or carpus (knee) have a self-control mechanism to stop granulation formation and quickly heal the skin.

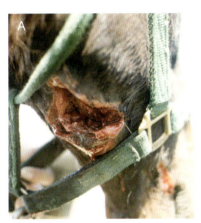 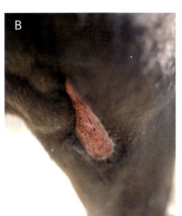

14.9 A & B The initial appearance of a gaping wound on the underside of the jaw (A). The same wound seven weeks later has filled in, contracted in size, and is epithelializing nicely on its way to full recovery with minimal scarring (B).

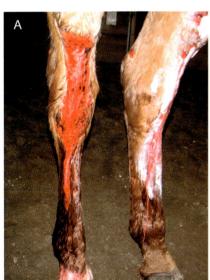 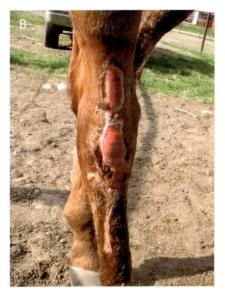 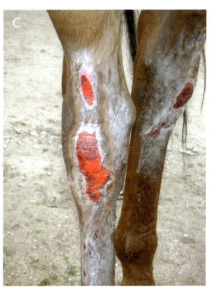

14.10 A–C This horse abraded away all the skin of the front surface of his rear limbs when he got his limbs tangled in a cable fence (A). At two months of healing, the wounds continue to contract in size and dimension. Bandages and topical medications throughout the treatment have controlled the development of proud flesh (B). The wounds at almost three months of healing (C).

14.11 A & B *Upon presentation, this forearm wound was dry, crusty, and contaminated, making it difficult to pull together with stitches due to excess skin tension (A). The appearance of the scar of this same wound years later (B). Had this wound been addressed with medical care at the immediate time of injury, it would have resolved with a more cosmetically pleasing scar, but it did heal well nonetheless.*

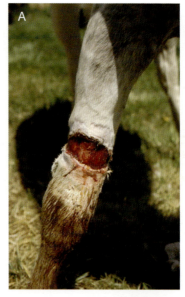
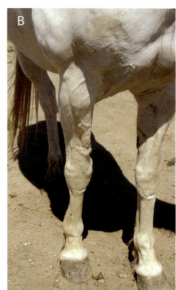

Hydration and Warmth

For the processes of skin repair and wound closure to advance, a wound needs to be maintained in a warm, moist environment, especially during the early stages of tissue repair. Because the mammalian body is made of almost 70 percent water, skin dehydrates if a wound is left open to air (photos 14.11 A & B). Dehydrated tissue eventually becomes devitalized tissue to compromise healing. Horse skin on the lower limbs lacks blood supply and warmth as compared to skin on the upper limbs or torso that overlies muscle, rather than mostly bone and sinew.

The length of time from when an injury occurs to when it receives medical attention affects the extent of tissue dehydration and onset of infection (photo 14.12). While awaiting professional care, apply a water-soluble dressing (triple antibiotic ointment or silver sulfadiazine cream—see p. 414) and a light bandage to a cleaned wound to limit tissue dehydration. A bandage maintains a moist environment, and retains a moderate amount of body heat at the wound site; both features enhance the early stages of healing.

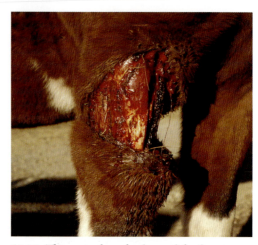

14.12 *This wound on the front of the forearm has been left unattended for several days, leading to drying of the tissue, skin contraction, and swelling with potential for infection.*

SYSTEMIC ANTIBIOTICS

Wounds that have penetrated into deeper tissues, or those that have suffered blunt trauma or shredding of tissue are best treated with systemic antibiotics. Blunt trauma, such as a blow from a kick, fall, or collision with a solid object damages surrounding tissues; in many

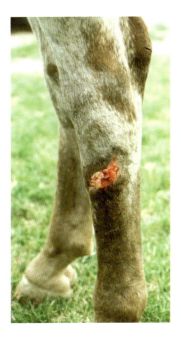 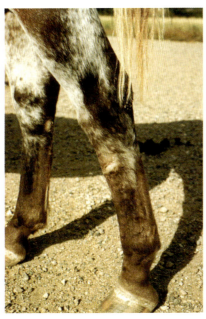

14.13 A & B *The cannon bone puncture on this horse was not addressed with veterinary intervention and was unable to heal for weeks due to infection trapped as deep as the bone (A). With proper wound irrigation, systemic antibiotics, and bandaging, the wound that had simmered along without showing any signs of healing resolved rapidly with only a small, remaining scar (B).*

cases tissue tears, resulting in jagged wound edges. Such wounds are at significantly greater risk of infection due to compression of blood vessels, an increased amount of devitalized tissue, swelling, and edema.

Taken orally or injectably, systemic antibiotics reach high concentrations throughout affected tissues, and so best ward off infection, especially following thorough wound cleansing and debridement. If a wound is deep or has been present for more than 1 to 3 hours, topical antiseptic ointments are unlikely to prevent infection.

Identification of Bacteria

Most wounds heal uneventfully within a couple of weeks following treatment. It is valuable to obtain a bacterial culture and antibiotic sensitivity on a wound that is heavily contaminated, or is accompanied by excess swelling and/or pain, or is not responding to treatment. A culture is taken by inserting a sterile swab into the wound depths before cleaning. The swab with the secretions is sent to the lab for cellular examination and bacterial growth.

Accurate identification of bacteria defines appropriate antibiotic treatment. While the lab grows the culture for a couple of days, the horse receives broad-spectrum antibiotics, which are selected by a veterinarian according to the greatest likelihood of success.

Drainage

Often, a "pocket" forms below a wound, necessitating a drainage hole at the low point of a wound so serum does not accumulate. A serum pocket slows healing because it prevents tissue connection, while also harboring bacteria. The size of the original wound, particularly a puncture, may need to be enlarged to allow healing from the inside out, without obstruction to drainage. Similarly, any scab that forms over the top of a wound should be removed; if a wound seals too quickly, trapped bacteria rapidly infect it (photos 14.13 A & B).

SUTURES

Since initial evaluation of a wound does not always determine if a wound can be surgically repaired and *sutured* (stitched), assume that a

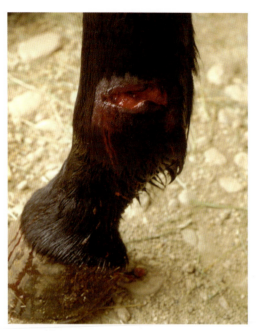

14.14 *This wound is well cleaned, and the skin margins are trimmed back to expose healthy, bleeding tissue; now the wound is ready for stitches. The location of such a wound over a joint necessitates careful exploration by your veterinarian to ensure the joint was not penetrated at the time of injury.*

wound will be sutured, and proceed accordingly (photo 14.14). Only water-soluble ointments or creams should be applied to a wound that will be sutured; sprays should not be used. Non-water-soluble medications stick to tissue, preventing the edges from touching when they are stitched together. Insoluble substances are also difficult to remove from deeper tissues of a wound; this interferes with how well sutures will hold. The decision to stitch a wound depends on:

- Location of the wound
- Skin tension at that site
- Configuration of the wound
- Degree of tissue damage
- Tissue contamination

Discolored tissue should be cut away since devitalized tissue contributes to an inflammatory response and provides nutrients for bacteria. A dark red or purple tissue color represents congestion and stagnant blood caused by bruising and crushing.

Facial wounds or wounds on the torso respond well to suturing efforts, even if discovered days after an injury (photos 14.15 A & B, 14.16 A & B, and 14.17 A & B). Depending on skin tension or degree of contamination, a limb wound may not be amenable to sutures even if evaluated within a few hours of injury.

SPRAY-ON PROTECTANTS

Antiseptic powders or sprays tend to obstruct drainage, leading to accumulation of exudate. Spray medications dry out the margins of a wound, leaving less tissue available to pull together with stitches. Dry tissue loses its blood supply, and needs to be trimmed back to fresh, bleeding tissue before healing can proceed.

One form of spray, Aluspray®, is useful over superficial wounds, or those that are in the final stages of healing and epithelialization. It is an aluminum-based spray that serves as a mechanical barrier to dirt and flies (photo 14.18).

TOPICAL OINTMENTS AND GELS

No matter what is applied to an equine skin wound, little can be done to *accelerate* healing. However, the natural healing process may be *delayed* by infection or tissue dehydration, or by inappropriate topical therapy.

Water-Soluble Ointments

Only *water-soluble* ointments should be applied to a wound that is to be sutured, or on open, contaminated wounds until the wound has filled completely in with granulation tissue. A list of commercially available wound preparations is exhaustive, many of which have beneficial effects, but it is best to consult a

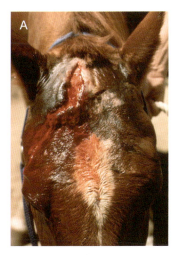 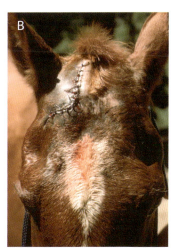

14.15 A & B This trauma, incurred in a horse trailer, is typical of a head wound (A). After cleansing, debridement, and stitching, this wound will heal with hardly a scar, and be invisible once the hair grows back (B).

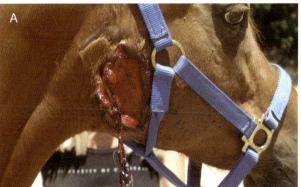 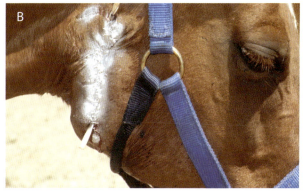

14.16 A & B Face wounds have an excellent blood supply and are readily amenable to suturing. The margins of this mare's wound are shredded and the injury deep enough so that a drain was inserted to facilitate drainage for a few days (A). The wound as it looked following surgical repair, with aluminum spray (see photo 14.18) to seal the stitches, and a drain in place (B). After two or three days, the drain will be removed, and by two weeks, the sutured wound will be healed, the stitches removed, and the mare's beauty restored.

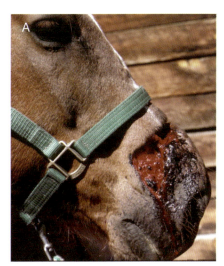 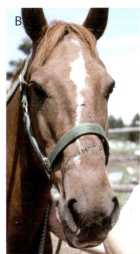

14.17 A & B As seen in the previous photos, the face lends itself well to full repair even with extensive injury. This horse was hit by a car and presented with a massive head injury (A). The stitches are ready to be removed three weeks later, and the wound is all but healed. Only a small scar will remain (B).

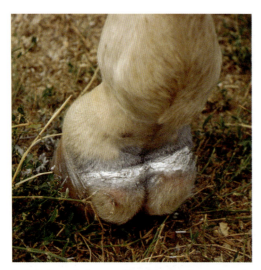

14.18 *A topical spray, like this aluminum-based product, is useful on superficial wounds to form a thin protective layer that creates a barrier against flies and dirt contamination.*

veterinarian before applying them to a wound. A short list of some examples of antiseptic products proven to be safe and effective on horseflesh includes:

- Silver sulfadiazine (Silvadene®) cream is a broad-spectrum, topical antibiotic that is water and tissue-soluble, proven to increase the rate of new skin growth (scientifically tested on pigs) by 28 percent, and has proven to be reliable on horses; it is particularly useful on rope burns, and silver ions in this preparation prevent the antibiotic from being inactivated by debris and discharge from a wound.
- Nolvasan® ointment is a water-soluble, broad-spectrum, topical cream that thwarts infection in deep wounds.
- Triple antibiotic ointment (containing polymixcin-B sulfate, neomycin sulfate, and bacitracin) provides broad-spectrum antibacterial activity, is nontoxic to fibroblasts, and increases new skin growth (in pigs) by 25 percent.
- Povidone-iodine (PI) ointment is broad-spectrum and tissue-soluble, and enhances rapid formation of granulation tissue.
- Vitamin A & D® ointment: vitamin A supports skin-cell health and counteracts the delaying effects of steroids on wound healing.
- Aloe vera has an antibacterial effect and stabilizes blood vessels in damaged tissue, reducing leakage.

USP-Petrolatum-Based Ointments

Petrolatum-based ointments are best used on normal skin that surrounds a weeping wound. They protect the skin from skin scald caused by protein-rich serum that drains from a productive injury. When applied directly to a wound, ointments with inappropriate pH ingredients interfere with healing. Petrolatum-based ointments may obstruct drainage while also attracting dirt and manure. Any product that contains USP-petrolatum as an ingredient slows skin growth, and delays wound healing. It is best to use tissue-soluble compounds that are not lethal to the cells.

Amount of Ointment

Only a very thin layer of antiseptic ointment is necessary to achieve a desired effect. Too much ointment has adverse effects, including:

- Impaired drainage to create excessive exudate and wound debris
- Reduced air circulation to the tissues
- Attraction of dirt and soil to a wound, which negates all positive effects achieved by scrubbing

Antibiotic Absorption of Ointments

Penetration of antibiotics in a wound is influenced by various factors. Inflammation increases blood circulation, which enhances antibiotic (both systemic and topical) penetration to a wound site. Dead and dying tissue and white blood cells elicit an acidic pH in the tissue. The presence of pus and serum, along with an acidic pH inhibits antimicrobial action of many topical antibiotics, such as sulfa-containing medications. After healing begins, fibrin or blood clots in a wound further block topical antibiotic penetration.

Ointment Contamination

Care must be taken not to contaminate large jars of ointments with dirt, hair, and debris, or these and associated bacteria will be deposited into a wound when applied. Tongue depressors, clean rubber gloves, or gauze are useful to remove medication from a jar without contamination. Note expiration dates on products containing antibiotics; discard outdated ointments that may be ineffective.

DMSO Gel

DMSO (dimethyl sulfoxide) is a powerful anti-inflammatory medication that is applied topically to resolve tissue swelling and edema around an injury (see p. 127). Care should be taken to wear gloves when applying gel and to not apply gel into an open wound.

OTHER TOPICAL WOUND DRESSINGS

Honey or Sugar

Granulated sugar and *unprocessed honey,* with high glucose concentrations, have antibacterial properties through osmotic action: water content is decreased in a wound, thereby inhibiting bacterial growth. White blood cells, most notably macrophages, are drawn to a wound for clean-up of bacteria. Devitalized tissue sloughs away in a natural process of debridement. *Lymph*, with its nutritive components, is pulled into a wound to advance tissue healing and regeneration. Topical application of these sugars deodorizes a wound by providing glucose as a substrate to infective bacteria rather than their reliance on protein metabolism that generates by-products with bad odors.

The antibacterial component in honey is called *inhibin*, which generates hydrogen peroxide at levels that are not harmful to tissue. Each hour, honey elicits hydrogen peroxide production at 1000 times less concentration than is found in commercial hydrogen peroxide solutions. Persistent presence of low levels of hydrogen peroxide in a wound is toxic to bacteria, while at the same time stimulating growth of fibroblasts and budding blood vessels. Honey also imposes antioxidant effects, and its acidic pH promotes wound healing and inhibition of bacterial growth. The honey must be unpasteurized and not heated past 98.6° F (37° C). [Some processes used to extract honey from the comb rely on temperatures of 102° F (39° C) or more.] Different types of honey possess varied antibacterial activity. About 30 ml (1 ounce) of honey is applied to a 10 x 10 centimeter (cm) wound dressing.

Granulated sugar should be applied to a wound at a thickness of 1 cm. Or, a mixture of povidone iodine with sugar at a ratio of 50:50 or 70:30 provides an antiseptic that resists bacterial growth. This solution is known as *sugardine*. Because wound secretions dilute the osmotic properties of sugar or honey, bandages should be changed once or twice a day, initially. If granulated sugar remains present on a wound at the time of a bandage change, then the frequency of bandage changes may be lessened. Sugar or honey can be applied to a wound until a healthy granulation bed forms. With the presence of granulation tissue, a wound is as resistant to infection as is intact skin.

Amnion Wound Dressing

An *amnionic sac* taken within six hours following birth of a newborn foal should be prepared immediately as a wound dressing. It is best if the amnion has not been contaminated with straw or debris, as it is difficult to clean. The amnion should be cleaned thoroughly by repeatedly rinsing it in a water solution of povidone iodine or chlorhexidine solution. Then, the amnion is cut into pieces and wrapped in plastic or wax paper along with a soaking layer of povidone-iodine water, or a 1:40 solution of chlorhexidine in water. Once frozen, it can be stored for up to a year for future use. Amnion is applied under a bandage, or superglued to the skin edges surrounding a wound. Application of amnion to a wound may improve rate of healing by 30 to 50 percent over the use of non-adherent wound dressings. It should be used only after a mature granulation bed has formed, to speed epithelialization.

MANAGING PROUD FLESH

When wound healing proceeds out of control, exuberant granulation tissue, also called *proud flesh*, forms an ever-growing mound of angry-looking tissue that bleeds easily with the slightest touch.

Corticosteroids

Corticosteroid medication acts as an anti-inflammatory drug to aid healing by controlling proud flesh. Corticosteroids stabilize the release of enzymes from white blood cells that initiate an inflammatory response, and they inhibit new capillary growth. By minimizing inflammation and overgrowth of surface blood vessels, granulation-tissue production is reduced. However, if applied for too long, corticosteroids eventually inhibit skin-cell growth and stop healing. Steroids should not be used in a deep wound before a granulation bed has formed because they depress normal function of the immune system and promote bacterial colonization.

Nitrofurazone

Certain compounds contribute to the formation of granulation tissue. *Nitrofurazone*, an antibacterial, petrolatum-based product, delays new skin growth by 30 percent when used on deep wounds. A thick scab forms over the wound surface, preventing healing from the "inside out." However, when used on a superficial skin abrasion, nitrofurazone keeps the skin moist and supple, so hair quickly grows back.

Caustic Chemicals

Other substances have been used to stop development of proud flesh, such as copper sulfate, bleach, lye, and similar caustic chemicals. By chemically cauterizing proud flesh, they also damage migrating skin cells, and ultimately slow healing.

Surgical Removal

It is better to surgically remove proud flesh than to resort to chemical irritants. Caustic substances cause tissue death, with redevelopment of proud flesh that persists as a non-healing, grotesque wound.

BANDAGING RECOMMENDATIONS

In most instances, limb wounds that have been bandaged will heal more quickly than those left exposed to the air (photos 14.19, 14.20, and see photo 7.22, p. 194). A wound that is not protected by a bandage forms hard, thick scabs that are persistently contaminated with dirt and bedding, resulting in increased local inflammation. In contrast, bandaged wounds are less inflamed, less dehydrated, and less contaminated than unbandaged wounds. Healthy granulation tissue forms more quickly under a bandage, with those wounds healing faster (63 days) than the wounds left open to the air (96 days). Faster healing is also dependent on reduced contamination or inflammation in early healing phases.

Wounds that are left unbandaged organize collagen more quickly, probably due to tension forces in surrounding skin that resulted from mild dehydration by air exposure. However, once a bandage is removed, wounds are prone to trauma and loosening of fragile, new skin.

In general, a wound should remain bandaged until an intact, healthy granulation bed is present. Once a layer of granulation tissue has filled in a wound, a bandage may do more harm than good by reducing oxygen to the wound, and by trapping an accumulation of inflammatory cells. Devitalized tissue and accumulated tissue debris lead to an acidic pH. To counteract these conditions, a wound produces more capillary buds to compensate for an oxygen deficit, while an acid environment stimulates fibroblasts to produce more collagen. The result is production of proud flesh. Although more granulation tissue may form beneath bandages than forms on unbandaged legs, bandaged wounds develop less scar tissue, with improved scar contraction.

Benefits of Bandaging

Bandaging a wound accomplishes several things at once:

- A protective bandage keeps the wound clean of environmental contamination, such as manure, soil, and particularly clay, that irritate the tissues and are counterproductive for wound healing.
- A bandage keeps tissues moist and warm, and serves like a layer of skin.
- Slight pressure from a properly applied bandage maintains contact of a loose skin flap with underlying tissue to restore blood supply.
- A light pressure bandage relieves local or gravitational swelling that may develop that would otherwise restrict circulation and oxygen supply to the tissues.

Moisture Retention

Covering a wound with a bandage reduces evaporative fluid loss from the tissues. If a wound surface on the lower limbs remains moist and oxygen-rich, new skin growth proceeds at a rate of up to 0.2 mm per day. On the torso, progress may be as rapid as 2 mm per day. If a wound dehydrates, decreased circulation deprives the wound of an internal oxygen source. Then, cellular migration proceeds at less than 0.1 mm per day in any area.

Although bandaging reduces a wound's uptake of atmospheric oxygen, by keeping a wound moist and by promoting unfettered circulation, a bandage compensates for this relatively minor deprivation of atmospheric oxygen. Bandages using cotton pads and breathable elastic tape (Elastikon®) improve accessibility of oxygen to a wound.

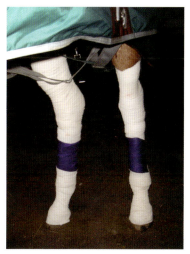

14.19 Full rear limb bandages provide tissue support and protection for a wound and/or swelling. Care must be taken to adequately pad over the Achilles tendon on the back of the hock when applying a bandage over the hock. Elastic stretch tape works best, as it is less likely to bind tendons than the vet-wrap-type tapes. The purple Vetrap® seen here is applied over a layer of cotton to minimize constriction of the circulation or tissues.

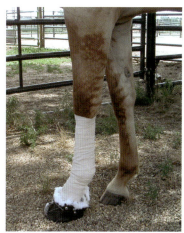

14.20 An injury to the lower limb may necessitate bandaging all the way beneath the heel bulbs. One means of keeping the bandage from rolling up is to apply an Easy Boot®, over the hoof and bandage (see p. 59). Here, elastic adhesive stretch tape (Elastikon®) is used over a layer of cotton padding.

Protection from Distortion

A bandage provides a stable support for migration of new skin cells across a wound. Distortion of a wound surface due to excessive movement, edema, or trauma disrupts myofibroblasts and epithelial cells that need to migrate across to bridge the gap. Collagen fibers and capillary buds are also disrupted by such distortions. A bandage protects a wound from further trauma and excessive movement, while also reducing edema swelling. Slight pressure exerted by a bandage reduces the development of proud flesh. Care must be taken to not wrap a bandage so tightly as to interfere with limb circulation.

Retaining Body Temperature

Application of an insulating bandage over a wound retains body temperature to provide the healing benefits of warmth. Temperatures around 86° F (30° C) promote wound healing, while temperatures less than 68° F (20° C) result in a 20 percent reduction in tensile strength. Cooler temperature at a wound site constricts superficial vessels to the skin, reducing blood and oxygen supply to a wound and its healing connective-tissue components.

Poultice

Local swelling may be reduced through application of a poultice or "sweat," using commercial products. If there is not an open wound, a sweat can be made using nitrofurazone and DMSO gel beneath a bandage (see p. 415). Warm water Epsom salt soaks, 2 to 3 times daily, serve a similar purpose (see p. 195).

Applying a Bandage

Lower leg wounds lend themselves well to bandaging. Apply a non-adhesive sterile dressing (Telfa pad®, Surgipad®, or Combine pad) to a wound. Use conforming roll gauze (Kling®) to hold it in place. Apply a layer of cotton or quilting around the limb before wrapping with Elastikon® or Vetrap®. Ample padding prevents accidental bandage constriction of the tendons and blood supply.

A bandage should not be applied too tightly or it could impair drainage. Wound dressings should be absorbent to clear exudates from the opening so drainage is not hindered. Bandage changes should be frequent enough to assess healing and to remove encrusted material. Initially, bandages are changed at least every 2 to 3 days. Once healing is under way, it is possible to leave bandages in place for 1 to 2 weeks.

Removing a Bandage

The appropriate time to leave a wound unbandaged is determined by examining the color of the skin cells. While newly formed skin is yet a thin layer, there is an apparent color difference between the thicker, outer margin and the thin, skin layer covering the granulation bed (photos 14.21 A & B). Once skin has thickened uniformly, it is the same color, indicating that it may be time to remove a bandage. As a general rule, when a wound has contracted down to the size of a nickel, it is appropriate to leave it open to the air unless flies will bother it (photo 14.22).

Slow Healing

If a horse persists in traumatizing a wound, or a wound is persistently irritated by manure, mud, or flies, a protective wrap allows healing to continue to completion. Wounds located over moveable surfaces, such as joints, heal slowly and have the potential to produce proud flesh, which retards healing (see p. 416). Skin cells that should migrate across a wound will layer themselves at the base of a mound of exuberant granulation tissue, which then grows without restraint rather than covering over with epithelial cells. A light pressure bandage often deters formation of proud flesh.

Equine First Aid, Medication, and Restraint

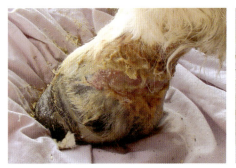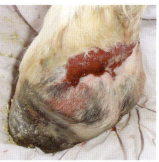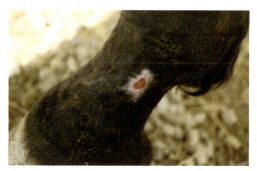

14.21 A & B When a bandage is removed, there is usually a layer of sloughed tissue debris overlying the wound that may smell vaguely odd. Any odd or significant odor may be cause for concern of infection (A). After wiping the debris away with clean gauze sponges, this pastern wound looks clean and healthy and is ready to be bandaged again (B).

14.22 The process of epithelialization is apparent in here by the pink-skin-appearing tissue on the margins of a small area of remaining granulation bed. If there is a possibility for contamination from dirt, feces, or flies, it is best to leave a wound wrapped; otherwise, it can be left unbandaged when the granulation bed is smaller than the size of a nickel, as seen here.

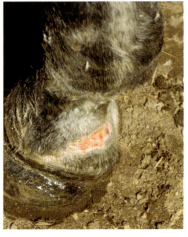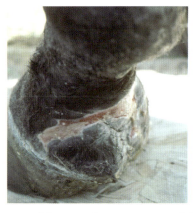

14.23 This pastern wound is healing rapidly, as visualized by the healthy pink epithelial tissue that has migrated over the granulation bed.

14.24 This wound was extensive and deep on its initial presentation. After radical tissue debridement, cleansing, bandaging, and systemic antibiotics, the pastern and hoof were placed in a lower limb cast to accelerate healing. A healthy epithelial layer covered the granulation bed, as seen here; the wound quickly contracted and resolved, leaving a minimal scar, and a pleasing cosmetic result.

REMODELING OF A WOUND

Tensile Strength

The ultimate tensile strength of a wound allows tissue to sustain normal mechanical stress so it does not tear or break open. Complete remodeling and contraction of a scar proceed rapidly for 3 to 6 months, reaching maximum tensile strength up to 1 year after injury (photos 14.23 and 14.24). Collagen, rapidly manufactured by fibroblasts during the first 2 to 4 weeks, is responsible for tensile strength of a wound as it organizes. By 40 to 120 days, skin regains 50 to 70 percent of its original strength. Epithelial cells and fibroblasts produce enzymes to break down existing collagen. Newly deposited collagen fibrils tightly interweave, with a corresponding increase in tensile strength and flattening of a scar. Collagen continues to remodel for 1 to 2 years.

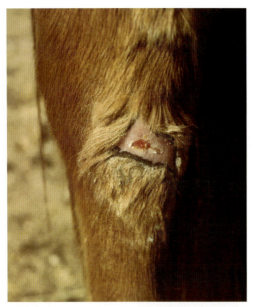

14.25 *This wound has all the appearances of a practically healed injury, with only a tiny spot of granulation tissue remaining in the center of margins of pink, healthy epithelial tissue that is forming new skin. For a while, the new skin will be fragile and subject to bleeding so care should be taken to minimize trauma to the wound. Hair should grow back over this wound with no problem.*

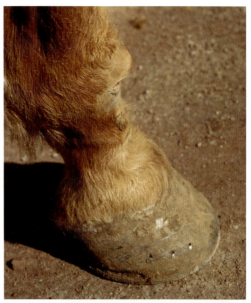

14.26 *A keloid is an exaggerated scar that protrudes above skin level, and may present as a skin-like covering over proud flesh. This type of scar requires surgical debridement with a scalpel, and appropriate bandaging and topical treatment.*

Scar Tissue Characteristics

Despite a horse's apparent tendency to self-destruct, regeneration and repair of skin wounds usually return an injury to almost as good as new. Usually, wounds that do not penetrate all the way through the skin form tissue identical to the original skin, without scar formation. However, large connective tissue and collagen components may not regenerate to their original pattern. Although "healed" epithelial tissue appears identical to original skin, new connective tissue is functionally less efficient (photo 14.25). Even under ideal conditions, scar tissue remains 20 percent weaker than the original tissue.

Keloid Formation

A *keloid* may develop as a skin-like covering over proud flesh (photo 14.26). This exaggerated scar protrudes above skin level. The wound surface resembles skin, but it remains fragile, dry, and crusty, and lacks elasticity and strength derived from an underlying skin layer. Such wounds may require skin grafts to replenish a skin layer, or they are subject to chronic cracking and bleeding.

HYPERBARIC OXYGEN THERAPY

A noninvasive treatment of a non-healing injury relies on exposure of a horse to high pressure and an oxygen-rich atmosphere as found in a hyperbaric oxygen tank. The objective is to saturate the tissues and body fluids with oxygen so that an injured area need not rely solely on delivery of oxygen through blood vessels, which may be damaged or located at too great a distance due to swelling. Treatment with *hyperbaric oxygen therapy* (HBOT) increases the amount of dissolved oxygen in the plasma that reaches all tissues. Application of this procedure has been helpful in healing of long-standing infections, internal abscesses, tenacious wounds, crush trauma, circulatory problems, osteomyelitis, and fractures, to name a few. HBOT is used in conjunction with traditional surgical, medical, and antibiotic therapies, and is meant as an adjunctive therapy, not a replacement.

Puncture Wounds

A superficial-appearing abrasion may disguise a deeper, penetrating hole through the skin (photo 14.27). Long hairs, mud, and dirt mask the extent of an injury, while bacteria introduced into a wound may quickly overwhelm the local immune response to create infection. If it is difficult to see if there is a puncture tract beneath the skin, prepare the wound for further evaluation with thorough scrubbing to remove all surrounding contaminants so they won't be carried into the wound. Gently insert an antiseptic-soaked cotton swab into the wound to see if a hole or pocket is present. Do not attempt to completely probe the hole with the cotton swab; cotton fibers or broken swabs discourage healing. This procedure is meant to evaluate if a wound is more than a superficial abrasion. A veterinarian should be summoned if the wound has any depth or if any swelling, pain, or heat accompanies it.

TENDON OR JOINT PUNCTURES

A puncture into a joint, tendon sheath, or bone

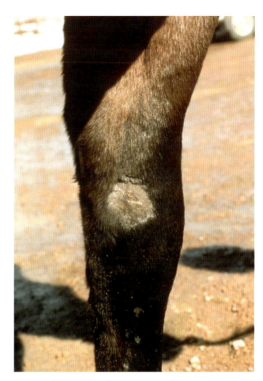

14.27 *A superficial-appearing abrasion may disguise a deeper, penetrating puncture through the skin. Sometimes these occur due to blunt trauma (like a kick injury), which causes a separation of the tissues with a break in the skin and an underlying tunnel tract. Puncture-type wounds seal over quickly, trapping bacteria and infection, and resulting in swelling, pain, and lameness. Proliferation of anaerobic bacteria can lead to life-threatening consequences.*

is considered a true emergency situation, requiring immediate veterinary expertise to prevent crippling consequences. Any wound or puncture that is suspected as having entered a tendon sheath or joint space should be evaluated by a veterinarian, and probed for foreign bodies such as wood, plastic, glass, or metal fragments. Special X-ray films, called *fistulograms*, can be taken to show the extent of injury: injection of a sterile, radio-opaque dye into a wound is immediately followed with

14.28 *Tissue infection with anaerobic bacteria, as in this case from Clostridial organisms that cause malignant edema, leads to extensive tissue sloughing, and a pronounced scar. This infection occurred following an intramuscular injection.*

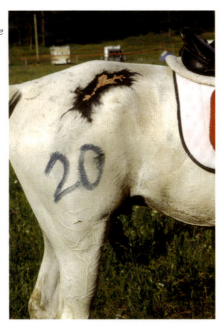

radiographic exam to outline the depth of the puncture tract with the dye. Dye surrounds and outlines foreign bodies such as wood, plastic, or glass that don't show on regular survey films because of their similar density to soft tissue.

ANAEROBIC BACTERIA

If left unattended, puncture wounds have serious consequences, despite a mild appearance. Of the many kinds of bacteria introduced into a wound, potentially life-threatening organisms include those that live in an anaerobic environment. When skin is punctured, a small portal of entry through the skin often seals over, providing an oxygen-depleted environment ideal for growth of anaerobic spores. As a wound festers, devitalized and dead tissue in the wound encourages anaerobic bacteria to prosper. *Clostridium* spp. is one such family of anaerobic bacteria, commonly found as inhabitants of the intestinal tract. They are passed as spores into manure, soil, and decomposing organic matter. The spores can survive in the soil for years, so any wound is at risk of contamination. These bacteria are inactivated with only 20 minutes exposure to oxygen.

Tetanus

One of the most common anaerobic bacteria associated with equine wounds is *Clostridium tetani*, the organism responsible for *tetanus* (see chapter 17, *The Neurologic System in Health and Disease*, p. 513). In the decades before vaccines were available, tetanus infected an alarming number of horses, causing a prolonged and painful death. Today, such an unfortunate demise from a wound is rare. A wounded horse that has not received a tetanus toxoid booster in the past 8 to 12 months should be boosted with tetanus toxoid to stimulate sufficient immunity in the face of increased risk. If a horse is injured, but has not been on a yearly tetanus toxoid immunization program, prophylactic tetanus therapy might be considered, using tetanus antitoxin, which neutralizes exotoxin circulating outside the nervous system. However, there is risk of a fatal liver reaction (*Theiler's disease* or *serum hepatitis*) from administration of tetanus antitoxin, so it should be used only after taking all factors into consideration. On the other hand, tetanus toxoid is a different formulation that is a safe form of tetanus protection, particularly if an injured horse receives concurrent systemic antibiotics.

Malignant Edema

Another life-threatening anaerobic bacteria is *Clostridium septicum*, which is responsible for a syndrome known as *malignant edema* (photo 14.28). This organism produces a large amount of gas in muscles, creating a "crackling" feel (*crepitation*) beneath the skin over a wounded area. The wound site is hot and painful, and swollen with edema and gas. An accompanying fever may spike to 106° F (41° C). Toxins

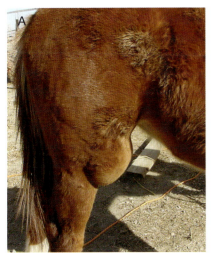 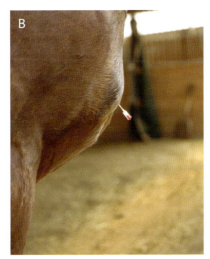 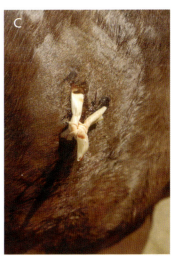

14.29 A–C *Blunt trauma, as from a kick, may create a seroma pocket (filled with serum) or hematoma (filled with blood) within a muscle or beneath the skin (A). These are best left alone initially, treated only with cold application, until any bleeding or oozing stops. After a couple of days, the swelling can be lanced and opened for drainage, and irrigated with antiseptic solutions (B). Otherwise, if the fluid is left in the swelling, the fluid may take a long time to reabsorb, all the while providing a site for bacterial proliferation and infection. Blunt trauma may necessitate insertion of a drain to promote continued drainage to prevent serum accumulation in the pocket space (C).*

released from the bacteria spread rapidly through the body, capable of killing a horse in less than two days.

Although infection with tetanus or malignant edema is uncommon, such possibilities cannot be ignored. A course of systemic penicillin injections kills anaerobic bacteria, and anti-tetanus prophylaxis protects the horse.

Blunt Trauma

KICK WOUNDS

Kick wounds are similar to puncture wounds because blunt impact from a hoof often causes a small break in the skin. Deeper connective tissue separates from the blow, leaving a tunnel along which bacteria can travel. If the blow is over a muscle, a wound heals with few complications when appropriately treated. If trauma is incurred over ill-protected bone, the bone may be cracked, or a piece of bone can be chipped off, or inflammation of the bone may interfere with blood circulation.

SEROMA OR HEMATOMA

Blunt trauma may separate tissue planes or tear muscle fibers, allowing accumulation of serum (*seroma*) or blood (*hematoma*) beneath the skin (photos 14.29 A–C and 14.30 A & B). A seroma or a hematoma feels like a water balloon, and when the swollen area is tapped with a finger, the inner fluid moves similarly. The best way to manage these is to use ice and time for serum and blood to stop oozing beneath the skin. After a few days, the swelling should be opened with a scalpel to permit drainage. The pocket should be irrigated, and any fibrin or blood clots should be removed.

14.30 A & B *This horse was kicked on the side of his haunch, and the resulting fluid-filled swelling moved like water in a water balloon when balloted with a finger (A). Placement of a needle allows drainage, which is seen here as a serosanguinous (blood-tinged) color. Then, a large incision was made through the skin to encourage continued drainage and to prevent the wound from premature closure that could trap more fluid inside. The wound was encouraged to heal from inside out by daily irrigation of the seroma pocket and cleansing of the incision site (B).*

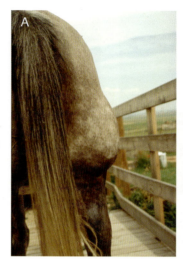
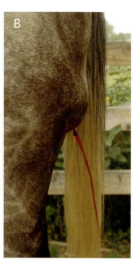

SEQUESTRUM

A wound that is deep or traumatic enough to affect underlying bone may create a *sequestrum* (photo 14.31). A sequestrum is a fragment of bone that has broken off with the initial impact of trauma, or has become devitalized due to reduced blood supply from infection. Such a dead bone fragment acts like a foreign body. A wound may heal initially, only to break open again. A chronic, draining tract persists until a sequestrum is surgically removed.

Rope Burns

A horse's hide is a tough but resilient structure, providing a thin, protective armor against perils in the environment, but it does not fare well when encircled by an abrasive rope. A horse caught in a rope usually panics, kicking and struggling to free his leg, without regard to himself. Living hide disappears, revealing muscle and sinew beneath.

CLASSES OF BURNS

Rather than classifying rope burns as first, second, or third degree, it is more informative to assess thermal injury in terms of depth of skin and tissue damage. Rope burns are classified as:

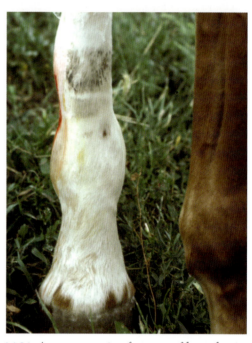

14.31 *A sequestrum is a fragment of bone that has broken off with the initial impact of trauma, or has become devitalized due to reduced blood supply from infection. Such a dead bone fragment acts like a foreign body and requires surgical intervention. The swelling seen here is typical of a splint bone sequestrum.*

- Superficial
- Partial thickness
- Full thickness

Superficial and Partial Thickness Burns

A *superficial* (minor) burn reveals only reddened, thickened skin. A *partial thickness* burn is accompanied by edema beneath the skin, intense inflammation, and pain. Damage to lymphatic vessels, along with increased leaking of capillaries, causes seepage of protein-rich fluids into subcutaneous tissues. This material provides the structural basis for fibrin clots that stop bleeding, repair a wound, and provide a scaffold for healing (see p. 407). However, a high protein concentration in damaged tissue also serves as a nutrient medium for bacteria, with the potential for infection.

Full-Thickness Burn

A *full-thickness* (major) burn results in extensive limb swelling, and tissue appears "tanned" and leathery (photo 14.32). Because pain fibers may be disrupted in a deep wound, the area may be numb. Although many rope burns are relatively minor and do not often progress beyond a partial thickness depth, any minor rope burn may become a full thickness wound if inappropriate topical medications are applied, or if a bacterial infection overwhelms the healing process.

CHARACTERISTICS OF ROPE BURNS

Rope burns exhibit unique characteristics. Initially, they are difficult wounds to manage, and require prolonged healing time. Although rope burns are similar to lacerations, they are considered burns due to the heat created by the friction of rope sliding across skin. If tissue is heated to more than 140° F (60° C), thermal injury results. A large amount of heat is necessary to raise tissue temperature high enough to damage tissue proteins. However, consider-

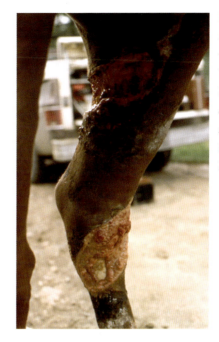

14.32 *A horse that entangles his leg in a rope, cable, or abrasive material suffers a "rope burn." These wounds become "worse before they become better" because of the thermal injury to deeper tissues. Extensive limb swelling and lameness usually accompany rope burns. Photo: David Varra, DVM.*

able time is required for heat to dissipate from the burned tissue and to restore the area to normal temperature. Because of this time lag, injury continues despite removal of a rope from the leg.

Inflammation

An intense inflammatory response to thermal injury changes the way cells flow into a wound. White blood cells stick to vessel walls, and red blood cells mass together (*agglutinate*). Toxins are released from dying cells, resulting in progressive tissue death. As blood vessels constrict in response to injury, oxygen supply is reduced to the damaged area, leading to more cell injury and death, resulting in a vicious cycle.

Eschar Formation

A coagulated crust of skin debris forms over the top of a rope burn. This crust is called an *eschar*. Not only does an eschar encourage harmful bacteria by providing nutrients, but it also delays penetration of antibiotics to deeper tissues. An eschar that appears brown-black in color is likely infected with bacteria.

Oxygen is important to cellular metabolism, particularly the processes involving wound healing. Oxygen enhances the activity of white blood cells responsible for cleaning up dead tissue and bacteria. An eschar prevents atmospheric oxygen from reaching the underlying wound. As a wound heals, fragile, newly formed skin cells compete with collagen-producing fibroblasts for oxygen. An eschar should be removed from a wound as often as possible, to allow healing from the inside out. Its removal maintains a moist environment, which aids the process of skin repair. Any remaining eschar usually separates from a wound as a granulation bed forms over a two- to four-week period.

TREATING ROPE BURNS
Wounds that appear minor may disguise extensive tissue damage caused by crushing and thermal injury when the horse struggled against a rope. The deeper the "burn," the longer will be the healing time, and the greater the possibility of tendon or ligament involvement. From the onset, rope burns should receive aggressive medical treatment to aid healing and limit scarring. Immediate application of ice (wrapped in a towel) to the injury for 20 to 30 minutes arrests persistent heat damage. Even a seemingly mild rope burn should be treated in this manner. What appears at first as a relatively superficial friction burn usually has a more serious appearance days later, accompanied by swelling and lameness.

Because most rope burns tend to worsen dramatically before they improve, it is impractical to suture them. Instead, they are allowed to heal by *second intention healing,* that is, as an open wound that will fill in with granulation tissue. The same principles applied to any open wound also apply to healing of rope burns.

Hemorrhage Control
Blood vessels in a horse's lower legs lie just beneath a thin, fragile layer of skin and connective tissue. Even a small, inconsequential limb laceration can sever an artery and result in profuse hemorrhage. Most hemorrhaging wounds occur on the lower legs, but occasionally other lacerations, like beneath the jaw, may sever a large artery. A cup of blood looks like a lot, especially when spread all over you, your horse, and the ground. At these moments, a cool level head can save a horse's life. As a measure of reassurance, consider that a 900 pound (400 kg) horse contains approximately 40 liters, or 10 gallons, of blood. Up to two gallons of blood can be lost with little problem.

CALM AND QUIET
One of the first things to do after summoning veterinary help is to confine an injured horse in a small area. This limits movement that elevates heart rate and pulse pressure. Find a safe space to minister to the horse. Speak in a soothing voice to calm him. No doubt he is frightened by whatever event caused him to injure himself in the first place.

PRESSURE TO STOP BLEEDING
Firmly press a clean compress directly over bleeding vessels. Pressing a finger on a pulsing artery is acceptable if nothing else is immediately available, but it is best to use bandaging materials for longer duration of compression. The first issue is to stop the bleeding, and later worry about bacterial contamination. Ignore the temptation to continually remove the pressure to see if bleeding has stopped. Normal clotting time in a horse is about 12 minutes for small-size vessels, but arteries and larger vessels take longer, an hour or more. If ice is available, apply it just above the wound to constrict blood vessels leading to the wound. These strategies thwart the development of shock

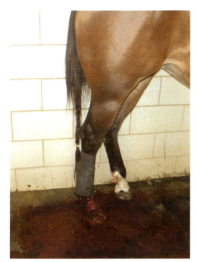

14.33 *This mare was kicked over the outside of her rear cannon bone, with a resultant laceration to a large digital artery that courses down the limb. The wound opening was about the size of an eraser; its small size, coupled with a large volume of hemorrhage, did not allow visualization of the spurting blood vessel to grab onto it to stem the flow. The next logical course of action was to apply a compression wrap, and then wrap ice packs around the compression bandage. The bandage was left in place for at least 15 to 30 minutes to allow clotting to begin.*

that results from loss of more than 3 gallons of blood. Once the bleeding is slowed somewhat, apply a clean, pressure bandage using an ace bandage or Vetrap® (photo 14.33). First, cover the gash with a nonstick dressing, like a Telfa® pad, or gauze, then firmly wrap with bandaging material (see "First Aid Kit," p. 428). A layer of roll cotton beneath a bandage diffuses the pressure. It is best not to apply cotton directly to an open wound as cotton fibers stick to the tissues and are difficult to remove. Don't excessively tighten the bandage over the tendons and ligaments.

TOURNIQUET

A controversial aspect of hemorrhage control is whether or not a *tourniquet* should be used. The concern is that soft tissue structures and tendons may be irreparably damaged with inappropriate application of a tourniquet. A tourniquet restricts blood flow and oxygen to tissues below it. This is good for controlling hemorrhage, but lack of oxygen may cause more damage than what occurred with the original wound. Unless an extremely large artery has been severed, try placing a pressure bandage over a wound for 20 to 30 minutes before resorting to a tourniquet. If the alternative is for a horse to lose large volumes of blood before professional help arrives, a tourniquet may be the only sensible option.

An ideal tourniquet is made of a soft, flexible, flat piece of rubber, surgical tubing and is applied smoothly around the limb just above the wound, without bunching or knots. But, the only thing available may be a saddle latigo, leather throatlatch, or a shoelace. After 20 to 30 minutes, slowly loosen the tourniquet to allow blood and oxygen flow back to the tissues.

An alternative to leaving a tourniquet in place is to quickly secure it above the injured area. Then apply a pressure bandage over the wound, slowly release the tourniquet over a period of a few minutes, and finally remove it. Continued digital pressure over a bandage further stems pulsing blood loss.

MONITOR VITAL SIGNS

Once an immediate crisis is past, monitor the horse's vital signs, like heart rate, mucous-membrane color and capillary refill (see "Vital Signs," p. 299). At first opportunity, offer a bucket of fresh water. He may instinctively drink in an attempt to replenish fluid losses.

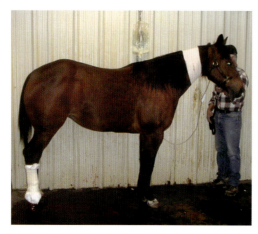

14.34 *Extensive blood loss from a hemorrhaging artery may necessitate replacement of intravenous fluids and hypertonic saline to prevent hypovolemic shock.*

Leave the pressure bandage in place even though it may be soaked with blood. Spurting vessels will clot beneath the bandage; disturbing fresh clots could start the bleeding again so resist the urge to peek. It is best to leave the wound covered until a veterinarian has a chance to examine it and properly clamp off bleeding blood vessels. Replacement of lost body fluids may be necessary through the intravenous route while hemorrhage is being controlled (photo 14.34).

First Aid Kit

It helps to be prepared for wound trauma, both at home and on the road. An emergency first aid kit is easily constructed. Start with a plastic container that will conveniently store the supplies. When emptied, this container makes a handy receptacle in which to mix a saltwater solution. Mark a line in indelible ink on the outside of the plastic container to denote a quart of water when filled to that line. Premeasured ziplock bags of table salt are stored in the kit and added to water at the time of need. The plastic container should hold the following first aid supplies:

- Disposable razor or scissors for shaving away hair from a wound
- Povodine-iodine (Betadine®) antiseptic wound scrub or chlorhexidine (Nolvasan®) scrub
- Povidone iodine or chlorhexidine solution to add to saline for rinsing and irrigating wounds
- Gauze sponges to scrub a wound
- Topical water-soluble antibiotic ointment: Silvadene®, Neosporin®, or Nolvasan®
- Desitin® ointment for saddle sores or rope burns
- Sterile, nonstick wound dressings: Telfa®, Combine pad, Surgipad®, or ABD dressing®
- Conforming roll gauze (Kling®)
- Self-adhesive stretch tape (3 or 4 inch roll of Elastikon® tape)
- Vetrap®, Equisport®, Flexus®, Medi-Rip® or an ace bandage for pressure bandaging
- Bandage scissors
- Oral broad-spectrum antibiotic tablets (Trimethoprim-Sulfa or doxycycline tablets)
- Oral syringe (60 cc catheter tip) to administer antibiotics
- Nonsteroidal antibiotic eye ointment for corneal abrasions or eye scratches
- Large (35 cc or 60 cc) syringe to irrigate wound or eye with saline/antiseptic solution
- Superglue®
- Flexible rubber tubing for an emergency tourniquet
- Rectal thermometer

In addition, other supplies are useful to include in a first aid kit:

- Extra towels or T-shirts to use as emergency dressings
- Stethoscope to obtain heart rate and to listen to intestinal sounds (see p. 301)
- Hemostat
- Nonsteroidal anti-inflammatory medication (NSAIDs) such as phenylbutazone, flunixin

meglumine, or ketoprofen to control pain and swelling
- Easy-Boot® or Old Mac® boot in case of a lost horseshoe
- Leatherman® tool
- Duct tape (to fix anything!)

These materials are the minimum supplies to have on hand until a horse can receive professional veterinary attention.

Fever

Sometimes a horse will act listless or go off his feed, but there is nothing in particular that seems to be wrong. When a horse seems "off" in any way, it is a good idea to check rectal temperature. A rectal temperature in an adult horse that reads higher than 101° F (38° C) is considered elevated and a *fever*. Foals may have a normal temperature as high as 102° F (39° C); anything higher is significant and bears further investigation. An overheated horse often has an accompanying elevated respiratory rate; heart rate may be elevated as well (see "Normal Physiological Parameters," *Appendix A*, p. 567).

Reasons for Fever

A horse develops a fever because of an alteration to the set point in the internal thermostat, the *hypothalamus* residing in the brain. A veterinary exam of a *febrile* (with a fever) horse may point to what is wrong. Situations that elicit a fever include the following:

- Viral respiratory disease
- Bacterial infection anywhere in the body
- Infection within the chest (*pleuritis*) or abdomen (*peritonitis*)
- A wound that has developed a *cellulitis* causing systemic illness
- Heat stress or heat exhaustion (see p. 359)
- Adverse reaction to medications or drugs
- An allergic reaction of any kind

Dangers of Fever

If a fever rises above 103.5° F (39.7° C), a horse needs active help in cooling down. In most cases, a fever is not in itself harmful unless it is prolonged or excessive. A horse with a fever often stops taking care of himself, going off feed and water, potentially developing dehydration or impaction colic. A fever over 106° F (41° C) may be life-threatening. Although uncommon, a very high fever has the potential to elicit convulsions or seizures. For every degree elevation in temperature, a horse's caloric requirements increase by 13 percent.

Cooling Techniques

Some simple techniques assist in controlling a horse's fever to make him more comfortable. Move the febrile horse out of direct sun into the shade or a barn. Ensure adequate ventilation. Remove any blankets or sheets he may be wearing unless there is a brisk wind or he has been body clipped. In inclement weather conditions or in winter, he might chill too quickly without the windbreaker effect of a sheet or blanket.

For immediate dissipation of abnormally high body temperature, cool the horse by taking advantage of evaporative cooling. Using a bucket of tepid water and a sponge or washcloth, soak the horse's neck and chest areas repeatedly until the skin feels cool to the touch (photo 14.35). Only soak areas in front of the shoulders as he may chill too easily if water is applied over his entire body. Monitor rectal temperature every 10 to 15 minutes to check progress. Fever reduction of a couple of degrees improves a horse's well-being. A febrile horse can be treated appropriately

14.35 *A horse with a fever over 103.5° F (39.7° C) should receive cooling assistance by soaking the neck and chest with tepid water. Soak areas in front of the shoulders repeatedly until the skin feels cool to the touch.*

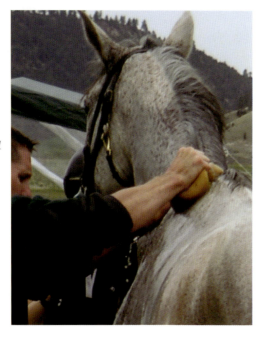

using nonsteroidal anti-inflammatory medications (NSAIDs) to bring down body temperature, and may possibly receive antibiotics if an infectious cause is the source.

Snakebite

Venomous Creatures

Within the continental United States, *pit vipers* and *coral snakes* make up the population of venomous snakes. Coral snakes are generally found in the southeastern United States, but due to their shy and reclusive nature, they are not commonly a problem to local horse populations. Pit vipers, on the other hand, live in areas more accessible to grazing horses, and are not as retiring as the coral snake. Snakes within the pit viper family include copperheads, cottonmouth moccasins, and rattlesnakes. Rattlesnakes represent the type of snake horses most commonly encounter.

A pit viper earns its name from the deep pit located between the eye and the nostril, which serves as a heat-receptor organ. Retractable fangs located within the triangular-shaped head of pit vipers bite a victim, but do not always inject venom into the wound. Human experiences with venomous snakes have indicated that about 20 percent of bites do not result in envenomation.

The Body's Response to Snakebite

When a snake does inject its venom, a rapid and profound inflammatory reaction occurs within half an hour, accompanied by pain. Severity of the tissue reaction is dependent upon how large a snake, how much venom is injected into a bite, the age and size of the horse, and where the horse is bitten. Bites on the head or nose or in the region of the neck are most common as a horse grazes near a snake. If bitten on the face, the entire head may swell, including nasal passages, eyes, eyelids, and the throatlatch region (photos 14.36 A & B). Dried blood is often present at the entrance to the nostrils as toxin damage to blood vessels precipitates abnormal bleeding from the nasal passages.

Snake venom elicits severe tissue destruction by its effect on the blood vessels, resulting in leakage of blood from capillaries and interference with normal clotting mechanisms; affected tissue "bleeds" into itself and swells with edema. Venom from pit vipers contains a mixture of proteins with enzymatic activities that contribute to local tissue destruction and impairment of circulation. Unlike the response seen in small animals and humans, horses rarely suffer from systemic effects of the pit viper toxin. Most of the damage occurs on a local level, with intense swelling and infection around a bite wound. A horse may be depressed and have a low-grade fever in response to the inflammatory reaction.

Equine First Aid, Medication, and Restraint

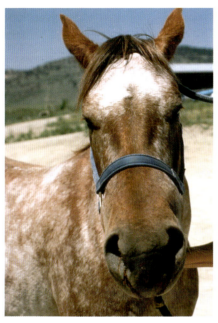
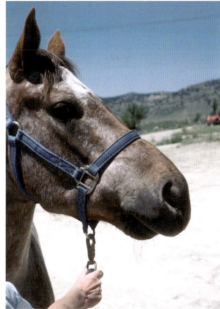

14.36 A & B *This horse demonstrates the typical appearance of one bitten by a rattlesnake on the muzzle. There is immediate swelling, and veterinary measures must be taken to limit swelling, limit infection, and enable the horse to continue to eat and drink.*

One of the biggest concerns about snakebite wounds in horses is the injection of *Clostridial* bacteria (see p. 422) into the tissue. Such bacteria thrive in an anaerobic environment such as is found in the presence of tissue destruction and injury to blood circulation. Venom also suppresses a normal immune response so broad-spectrum antibiotic therapy is indicated to prevent bacterial infection. Tetanus prophylaxis is essential just as with any puncture wound.

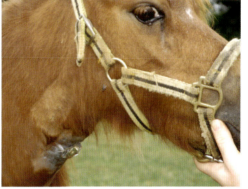

14.37 *In severe cases of swelling from a snakebite, a tracheotomy may be necessary to allow breathing. A surgical incision is made through the windpipe in the top third of the neck and a special stainless steel device is inserted to maintain this opening.*

Treatment

ANTI-INFLAMMATORY MEDICATIONS

Efforts are focused on controlling swelling and infection, using anti-inflammatory drugs such as corticosteroids or NSAIDs. Incisions made directly over the fang marks relieve tension on skin that has swollen with edema and also allow oozing of serum and toxin from the bites.

Maintain Airway

Being a creature the size that he is, a horse is not usually in mortal danger from venom unless swelling amplifies, unchecked. A bite on the face could elicit sufficient swelling and edema to impair breathing; a horse could die from suffocation as nasal passages swell closed. Emergency measures such as a *tracheotomy* (surgical opening directly into the trachea) may be necessary to ensure open airways (photo 14.37). A horse discovered in respiratory anxiety should be stressed as little as possible. In a dire emergency, a piece of garden hose or a large plastic syringe case can be inserted into the nostril as far as possible to provide the horse a breathing hole.

Ice Packs Contraindicated

Traumatic injuries accompanied by swelling are usually addressed with immediate application of ice packs to the area. However, such therapy worsens the damage incurred by snakebite; cold constricts blood vessels further adding to compromise of an already reduced blood supply to the area. Ice therapy, in this case, does more harm than good.

PROTECT FROM ULTRAVIOLET

Sometimes venom affects liver tissue in such a way that a horse becomes photosensitive and more prone to sunburn. It is a good idea to keep a snake-bitten horse confined to a stall during the daytime for a few days so that ultraviolet radiation from the sun does not further irritate swollen tissues.

ANTIVENOM

Commercial antivenoms are available and do have positive effects if administered within the first 4 to 6 hours. Yet, antivenoms are expensive and the amount necessary to give to a horse is fairly cost-prohibitive, especially when weighed against a relatively minor therapeutic advantage. In addition, antivenom is manufactured using horse serum as a component, which increases the risk of anaphylactic allergic reactions and death (see p. 391 and p. 439).

MONITOR FOOD AND WATER INTAKE

Swelling and sickness may render a horse incapable of drinking or eating. Take note of his water intake and appetite, since if he is not taking care of himself, it may be necessary to stomach tube with electrolytes and water, or to administer intravenous fluids to prevent dehydration.

ADDRESSING BITES ON LOWER LIMBS

Bites on the limbs do not swell as much as on the face because a minimum of soft tissue on the legs limits the extent of swelling. Snakebite on the legs is difficult to discern early on until lameness or swelling intensify. Such wounds should be treated aggressively as for any puncture wound, with particular care paid to combatting infection and improving compromised circulation and blood flow.

Once medical-emergency therapy has been instituted with anti-inflammatory medication and antibiotics, most horses respond quickly with resolution of the immediate crisis within a week. Swelling and mental depression improve within 24 to 48 hours of therapy with the horse back to eating and drinking. Tissue necrosis requires normal wound-care management over the course of a few weeks to minimize secondary infection and scarring.

Injectable Medication

Many pharmacological and biological products available for the horse come only in injectable form. As the number of available equine medicines increases with improved vaccines, antibiotics, and anti-inflammatory medications, more people are giving their horses injections. When a veterinarian prescribes a course of therapy, the following factors are considered before any medication is given:

- What is the therapeutic goal? Which disease process should be altered, and what medication will do that?
- Is there an oral alternative that effectively sidesteps the need for injections, or that is more cost effective?
- What dosage is appropriate for the individual, and how often must the drug be given to maintain effective blood levels?
- How long must therapy continue for therapeutic success?
- How does one evaluate response to treatment?

- Will one drug interact adversely with another that is given at the same time?
- Does the horse suffer from a liver or kidney problem that might prevent normal excretion of a drug from the body?
- Is the horse pregnant or lactating, thereby precluding use of certain drugs?
- What adverse or allergic reactions might be anticipated from the medication?
- Will a horse be monitored for adverse reactions, and can rapid control of an allergic response be initiated?

Consideration of these factors may best be left to a veterinarian's expertise. Safe principles should be followed whenever using injectable products. Any time a substance is injected into a horse, be well-advised and educated about what the product is, what it will do, and why it is necessary. Common sense should be applied regarding purchase and storage of drugs.

Equine insurance policies do not cover fatal accidents that occur from medication or drugs given without veterinary supervision.

The Label

GENERIC VERSUS NAME BRAND

Many products are available as both generic and a proprietary name brand. In many instances, a generic product is pharmacologically identical to the more expensive name brand. However, in other instances, the preservatives in a generic formulation, or the materials that suspend the active ingredients and carry them into the bloodstream may delay or reduce absorption of a generic drug as compared to the name brand. Unless cost is prohibitive, it is better to purchase the proprietary name-brand drug to ensure appropriate absorption and distribution of the active ingredient in the product.

ACTIVE INGREDIENT

It is important to carefully note the active ingredient of the drug or drugs to be sure the horse is receiving the intended product at the intended strength.

REFRIGERATED MEDICATION

Shipped products needing refrigeration should arrive in an insulated container with cold packs that remain frozen, or at least chilled. Many products, especially vitamins and vaccines, become unstable when exposed to heat, and are rendered inactive if they become warm for even a short period. It is best to deal with reputable sources like a local veterinary clinic. When dealing with mail order or over-the-counter medication, one cannot always know whether drugs have been handled properly during transport.

EXPIRATION DATE

Check the expiration date when purchasing an injectable product. Make sure there is enough time for the medication to be used before that date. When buying through mail-order supply centers for veterinary products, the expiration date cannot be evaluated until a product has been received. The date indicates that if a drug is stored in the recommended manner, and if given at the recommended dose, the product will be effective until that date. It is best to throw away a drug that is past its expiration date, especially antibiotics.

Outdated drugs do not often cause harmful reactions, but their effectiveness may be lessened. This is particularly important when using antibiotics against bacterial infection. Reduced effectiveness of antibiotics leads to antibiotic-resistant strains of bacteria and to severe infections. Outdated products do little to improve success of therapy.

TYPE OF DRUG

Intravenous drugs, like phenylbutazone, should not be injected into muscle because they may cause irritating muscle reactions, like skin sloughing and pain. Myoglobin released from muscle breakdown travels to the kidneys and may obstruct its filtering system, resulting in renal failure. Injection of *intramuscular* medications, such as vaccines or penicillin, into a vein can cause an *anaphylactic* (severe allergic) reaction and death (see p. 391 and p. 439). Read all labels, and consult a veterinarian if there is any question about drug type or usage.

Safe Storage

Injectable drugs come in many forms:

- Single-dose vials
- Multiple-dose vials or bottles
- Glass ampules
- Prepackaged, single-dose, plastic syringes

Most drugs come in liquid form, already mixed with a saline solution. However, some drugs and vaccines are unstable in solution and are prepared in a freeze-dried (*lyophilized*) form. These are mixed with a saline solution or sterile water immediately before injection so the active ingredient is not degraded by storage.

SEDIMENTATION

If bottles of vaccine or other drugs sit for long periods, sediments may form in the bottom. Sediment particles may be important molecules of active ingredient that are no longer equally mixed in the solution. These substances should not be injected into muscle as sediments may create a noxious reaction at the injection site. Sediment may return to solution with shaking; if it returns to solution, and is not past its expiration date, it is still acceptable to use. If it does not mix with shaking, or is past the expiration date, throw it away.

STORAGE

Any medication, whether in a bottle, vial, or syringe, should be stored carefully out of reach of children or pets, preferably in a locked cabinet or box. Medications discovered by children or pets are a hazard to safety, whether accidentally injected or ingested.

CONTAMINATED MEDICATION

Most injectable products have been heat-sterilized, or filtered through Millipore® filter systems to reduce the risk of contaminating bacteria or foreign proteins (*pyrogens*) that could cause fever or adverse reactions.

Vial tops often get dusty with lengthy storage. Clean the top of a bottle by swabbing it with alcohol before inserting a needle or withdrawing any medication. A dust-free cabinet or storage box reduces settling of grime and dust on the rubber stopper. If multiple-dose vials are used, as with flunixin meglumine, corticosteroids, hormones, tranquilizers, sedatives, or vaccines, beware of contamination of these bottles with dirt or used needles that can transfer blood or particles into the bottle. Any bottle suspected of such contamination should be discarded.

ENVIRONMENTAL STRESS ON MEDICATION

Chemical incompatibilities within some drug preparations may result in premature precipitation of sediment, color changes, gas formation, or *gelatinization* (residue clinging to the sides of the bottle). Changes occur due to interaction with preservatives or solvents in the drug, particularly if caused by pH changes, heat, or cold. A drug may be inactivated without any visible change. Storage of an injectable drug in a syringe for a lengthy time can result in injection of an inadequate dose as some compounds are absorbed into the plastic walls of a syringe.

Vitamin Storage

Injectable vitamin preparations are especially sensitive to environmental stress. Most vitamin preparations are stable at acidic pH, from pH 2.0 to 6.5. The higher the pH, the less stable the preparation. Many vitamin preparations are inactivated in the presence of ultraviolet rays of sunlight. Heat greater than 75° F (24° C), or aeration by shaking, destabilizes vitamins. Contact with certain metals, especially in the presence of light, heat, or aeration, promotes rapid oxidation of vitamins. Trace elements of iron, copper, or cobalt destroy B-complex vitamins in a vitamin-mineral mix, rendering it useless past its expiration date. Storage of a powdered mix in a metal container also inactivates vitamins.

To effectively maintain the recommended shelf-life of vitamins, store them in a dark, cool place, free from vibration. Throw away any outdated preparation, as it is probably ineffective.

Vaccine Storage

Heat stress is dangerous to vaccines. Only a small temperature rise is necessary to inactivate vaccines. They should be kept under refrigeration, and not stored on the dashboard or seat of a truck for even a short time. When transporting vaccines, it is best to pack them in a small ice chest to keep them cool. It is best to throw away a questionable product, and purchase a fresh batch.

Pre-Injection Procedure

READ THE LABEL

Before giving an injection, be sure the solution is well-mixed. Read the label several times to be certain it is the correct item. A wise practice is to read the label while picking up the bottle, read it again while withdrawing the medication, and once again while putting the bottle down prior to injection.

USE CLEAN NEEDLES AND SYRINGES

Use a brand-new, sterile syringe and needle when giving any injection to a horse. Needles should *never* be transferred from horse to horse because serious infections, such as equine infectious anemia or protozoan blood parasites like *piroplasmosis* may be transferred. Needles are inexpensive; there is no reason to save or salvage them.

Vials, syringes, and needles should be disposed of promptly and appropriately so children or pets have no access to them. Burning these items after use is the preferred method of disposal, especially for biological products like vaccines.

CLEAN THE INJECTION SITE

Alcohol

Proper technique is essential to ensure a safe and clean injection, and alcohol is not the best antiseptic to use on horses. Studies have shown that shaved or hairless skin must remain moistened in alcohol (70 percent ethanol or isopropyl) for at least 2 minutes before antiseptic action is achieved. Moreover, not all microorganisms are susceptible to alcohol. A quick squirt of alcohol on top of fur and skin may remove some debris and dirt, but it accomplishes little more.

Effective Antiseptic Solutions

Combining povidone iodine (Betadine®) or chlorhexidine (Nolvasan®) with 70 percent alcohol greatly enhances its antiseptic action, although the solution still must contact every microscopic particle of hair and skin for 2 minutes. Surgical scrubbing with povidone-iodine solutions before injection is impractical due to the length of time it would take, but certainly provides a less contaminated injection site. Horses are quick to learn about painful procedures, identifying the smell of surgical soap or

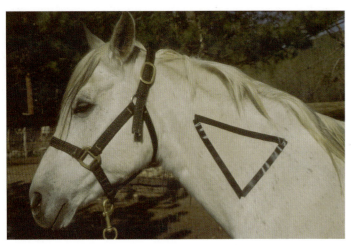

14.38 *The target for intramuscular injection of the neck is defined by a triangle formed by the front of the shoulder blade, the lower line of the nuchal ligament, and above the cervical spine and jugular furrow.*

Intramuscular Injection

Most of the time, a horse suffers no ill consequences from an *intramuscular* (IM) injection given by a knowledgeable person; however, there are risks and adverse side effects that should be considered. Some general rules should be followed. The objective is to perform the procedure as quickly and painlessly as possible.

INJECTION TARGET

Define the target for the injection in advance, to avoid blind stabbing. The anatomy of the horse provides many major muscle groups that are safe for IM injection. Intramuscular injections may be administered in the neck, rump, thigh, or pectoral muscles of the chest. Certain landmarks guide injection in each location.

Neck Injection

To avoid being kicked and hurt by a resentful horse, the neck and rump are the safest targets. If the neck is used, note the triangular-shaped area of muscle bordered above by the *nuchal ligament*, below by the cervical spine, and behind by the shoulder blade (photo 14.38). If an injection is deposited within the ligament, it is not absorbed appropriately. Avoid injecting near the spine or the bony shoulder blade. The jugular furrow (groove) sits in close proximity to the spine. Major blood vessels, such as the carotid artery and the jugular vein, lie within the jugular furrow. Vaccine or medication not intended for intravenous (IV) use should not be deposited in these vessels, or serious and potentially fatal reactions will occur. Drugs injected around major nerve branches running along the jugular furrow may also be harmful.

An IM injection in the neck that causes soreness may hinder performance. In addition, a horse with a sore neck is often reluctant to move his head up or down to eat or drink.

Rump Injection

The rump muscle is a large muscle mass located far from any vital structures. The target site for injection of the large rump muscles (*gluteals*) is defined by drawing a line from the top of the croup to the point of the buttocks, and another line from the point of the hip to the dock (photo 14.39). The intersection of these two lines is a safe spot for deposit of intramuscular medication. A disadvantage in using the gluteal muscles is the possibility of an abscess developing at the injection site. These muscle bundles are encased in a large, continuous sheet of connective tissue (*fascia*) so an abscess forming beneath the fascia may spread up the loin and back. This potentially leads to massive skin destruction and sloughing. Because the hip is located in an uppermost position, it is difficult to drain an infected injection site.

Thigh Injection

To avoid complications related to an abscess, a preferred injection site is one of two large strap muscles of the thigh, along the back of the leg (photo 14.40). These muscles are active in locomotion so exercise reduces soreness that may develop at the injection site. In the event of an abscess, infection in the thigh is constrained to a local area where it is easily lanced and drained.

Injections into the rump or thigh muscle may stimulate a horse to kick, so careful restraint procedures should be followed for safety (see p. 446).

Pectoral Injection

Another intramuscular location that is useful as an injection site is the pectoral muscles of the breast. It is easy to reach, has good circulation, and drains readily if infected. Any muscle soreness that develops there is usually short-lived but does not tend to interfere with eating or drinking.

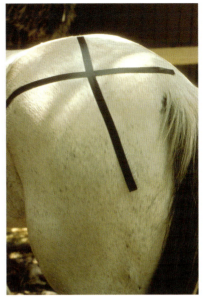

14.39 *The target site for injection in the large rump muscles is defined by drawing a line from the top of the croup to the point of the buttocks, and another line from the point of the hip to the dock, and inserting the needle at the point of intersection.*

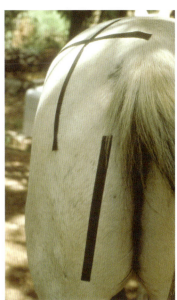

14.40 *Another area that is favorable for intramuscular injection is along the thigh muscles. Caution is key to prevent getting kicked when inserting the needle.*

CHOICE OF NEEDLE

Needle Size

Equine muscle is thick and profusely laced with minute blood vessels. A needle should be long enough to penetrate deep into a muscle-injection site to deposit the drug so the circulatory system can retrieve it from the muscle bed. A proper length of needle for most injections in the adult horse is 1½ inches long, and 18 or 20 gauge in diameter. Foals require no more than a 20-gauge, 1-inch needle.

Inserting the Needle

The needle should be inserted decisively, with a quick thrust, perpendicular to the skin. Punching the horse several times on the muscle before poking in a needle only alerts him to an oncoming prick. A quick thrust of the needle, with no warning to the horse other than a soothing voice and steadying hand, is all that is required. Pinching a fold of neck skin could distract a horse that is wary of needles. Then, thrust in the needle to its full length—up to the hub (the top part where the syringe attaches), just to the side of the pinched skin.

Regardless of where an injection is given, the needle should be inserted without the syringe attached. If a horse moves while a syringe is attached to the needle, its flopping scares and irritates the horse. A moving needle lacerates surrounding blood vessels and muscle tissue, increasing discomfort. Once a needle is in place and the horse is standing quietly, attach the syringe.

Always pull back on the plunger before injecting medication to confirm that there is no blood in the hub of the needle. Accidental administration of vaccines or penicillin, as examples, into a blood vessel can result in an anaphylactic reaction (severe allergic reaction) and death. If a needle has penetrated a vessel or capillary and blood returns with aspiration on the plunger, remove the needle, reinsert it, and start again. A needle that is bent in a struggle should be thrown away; start over with a fresh one. A bent needle could break and become embedded in deep muscle during a subsequent insertion.

ADVERSE REACTIONS

With careful selection of the compounds a horse receives, and with clean injection technique, over 80 percent of adverse drug reactions may be avoided. A new era finds more horse owners assuming the responsibility of their horse's care by administering vaccines and medicines. This do-it-yourself approach to health management is commendable, but it must be backed-up with comprehensive self-education. Knowledge of the risks and implementation of precautionary measures will ensure a horse's safety.

Abscess

Despite all precautions, some horses still experience adverse reactions to IM injections. A localized, firm, and tender swelling at the injection site may be a mild side effect, accompanied by muscle stiffness and soreness. However, if a swelling enlarges and softens, it may be developing into an abscess needing veterinary attention to lance, drain, and flush it. A fluid-filled abscess feels like a small water balloon, undulating when touched; it is usually warm and sensitive to finger pressure.

Cellulitis

Needle penetration invariably delivers a microscopic amount of bacteria to an injection site. Normally, the local immune system surrounding this needle prick cleans up introduced microorganisms. Only a tiny, localized swelling results, if anything at all. However, if an infection develops and is left to simmer within the muscle, *cellulitis* may result. An affected muscle becomes painful, swollen, and warm to the touch. The horse usually has a fever because of the systemic nature of such an infection. Cellulitis promotes growth of *Clostridial* spp. bacteria that prefer an anaerobic environment (see p. 422). These bacteria are rapidly lethal to a horse due to overwhelming toxin production. *Clostridial* spp. spores abound in manure, soil, and exist normally on a horse's skin. They enter the system as a horse eats, circulating harmlessly through the bloodstream. However, if *Clostridial* spp. bacteria seed themselves in muscle tissue that is inflamed or dying, within 2 to 5 days, the site is overwhelmingly painful, far out of proportion to the actual amount of swelling (see photo 14.28, p. 422). The area may feel crackly like tissue paper (crepitation) due to gas bubbles trapped beneath the skin.

Careful monitoring of an injection site for several days reveals a problem before it becomes serious. Watch for swelling, tenderness to finger pressure, lameness, or stiffness. Usually, a mild reaction at the site of an injection self-resolves after several days. Exercise, application of hot packs, massage, and topical DMSO hasten recovery. If swelling worsens, or seems abnormally enlarged or painful, contact a veterinarian immediately.

Fibrotic Myopathy

Subsequent to a muscle infection, previously inflamed tissue is replaced with scar tissue, to varying degrees. Scarring of the thigh muscle can result in a lameness syndrome called *fibrotic myopathy* (see chapter 6, *Muscle Endurance*, p. 173). On occasion, this syndrome can develop from an infection following an IM injection abscess.

Muscle Soreness

If multiple injections are necessary, use as many different muscle groups as possible on both sides of the body to limit soreness. Remembering "right at night" avoids confusion: a left-sided muscle group is used in the morning, and the right side at night.

Because many sport horses, like dressage, reining, and cutting horses, depend on engagement of the hindquarters to collect and perform symmetrical and rhythmic movements, some horse owners prefer to give IM injections in the neck, away from the hind end. This method prevents loss of several days' training if a horse becomes stiff or sore from an injection, although an adverse injection reaction in the neck will have similar performance consequences.

Sore Neck

An injection into the neck can cause a horse to become so sore that he refuses to eat or drink since these efforts require stretching of a painful neck muscle (photo 14.41). As mentioned, if a horse stops drinking, an impaction colic can develop, which is potentially life threatening. A sore neck might discourage a foal from nursing, resulting in weakness and stress.

Flu-Like Symptoms and Fever

Sometimes a horse reacts adversely to an intramuscular vaccine by exhibiting flu-like symptoms, such as aching muscles, fever, depression, or lack of appetite. For horses known to be sensitive to vaccines, light exercise improves muscle circulation, reducing swelling and inflammation, and hastening resolution of an adverse reaction. Nonsteroidal anti-inflamma-

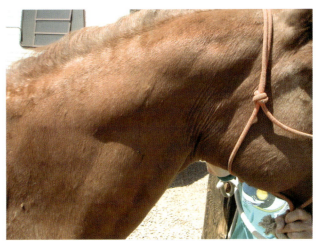

14.41 *An injection reaction may occur in the neck muscles, particularly if administered a little too high up in the neck, as was done here. This horse developed swelling and muscle soreness, making it difficult for him to lower his head to eat or drink. Ice packs, DMSO, and oral anti-inflammatory medications help to resolve this. Meanwhile food and water should be hung in a comfort zone so the horse can take care of these needs.*

tory medications (NSAIDs) may be administered concurrent with the vaccine. (Horses less than a year old should never receive an NSAID without first consulting a veterinarian.)

Anaphylactic Shock

A serious complication arising from an injection is an allergic reaction (*anaphylactic shock*) that can abruptly kill a horse (see p. 391). Penicillin, some vitamin injections, and many nonsteroidal anti-inflammatory drugs (NSAIDs) are implicated in these reactions, although any drug has the potential to cause anaphylaxis. The immune system of an individual that has previously been sensitized to a particular drug may react within seconds or minutes after the drug is administered. Airway spasm and throat swelling related to the allergic response may rapidly lead to asphyxiation and shock. Without an immediate injection of *epinephrine* (adrenaline), a horse may lapse into cardiac arrest, and die. Epinephrine opens the airways, allowing the horse to breathe. A horse experiencing an extreme anaphylactic allergic reaction may roll or convulse violently, making it difficult to inject counteractive medication. Epinephrine may be injected anywhere by any injection method to achieve an instant result (see p. 432).

Warning Signs

Often a horse shows mild allergic symptoms before developing a full-blown anaphylactic reaction. Watch carefully for hives *(urticaria)* that may or may not itch, located anywhere on the body (see photos 13.43, 13.44, and 13.45, pp. 389–90). Diffuse swelling of the limbs, head, or abdomen, an elevated respiratory rate, or behavioral changes, such as agitation or depression may signal an allergic response. Any combination of these problems may be warning signals that medication should be discontinued at once, and a veterinarian contacted. Profound hypersensitivity reactions may occur without warning; abrupt and fatal anaphylactic shock may be unavoidable.

Precautionary Measures

After administering a drug or medication to a horse, do not walk away immediately. Instead, monitor for an adverse reaction, which often peaks within 10 to 30 minutes. To prevent adverse reactions from intramuscular injections:

- Obtain a thorough drug history on each horse to identify previous allergic responses to certain medications.
- Affix a warning card on a horse's stall door to alert others of an allergy to specific drugs.
- Avoid mixing medications without first consulting a veterinarian.
- Properly dose a horse according to body weight and age to avoid excesses, and dose at appropriate time intervals.
- Read all labels to ensure that a drug is approved for IM administration.
- Dispose of outdated or improperly stored medicines.

Above all, avoid indiscriminate use of medication! If a drug is not really necessary or is not recommended by a veterinarian, do not give it. Oral preparations should be substituted for injectable medications whenever possible. Useful oral options exist for vitamins or nonsteroidal anti-inflammatory drugs (NSAIDs). It takes longer for a drug to be absorbed from the intestines than it would through a muscle, yet it may ultimately be safer.

Intravenous Injection

Intravenous (IV) administration of medication is a common means of injection in the horse. A horse's jugular vein is large and well-defined in the jugular furrow (groove), that runs parallel to the underside of the neck (photo 14.42). Brief obstruction with finger pressure toward the bottom of the jugular furrow causes the jugular vein to fill and swell (photo 14.43). Not only is the jugular vein used for administering IV drugs, but it is also the site for blood collection to run equine infectious anemia tests, complete blood counts, chemistry panels, blood typing, and drug testing (see p. 457).

Many medications are formulated for exclusive use as intravenous injections, such as phenylbutazone and *potassium penicillin*, but many substances may be given either intramuscularly or intravenously depending on how rapidly an effect is desired. Most sedatives and tranquilizers may be administered either way, but a relatively immediate therapeutic result is seen with IV injection. Any injectable medication should be a sterile preparation.

ADMINISTERING IV INJECTIONS

An IV injection can be accomplished with the needle inserted facing either toward the head or toward the heart. Blood flows through the jugular vein from the head to the heart. Once a needle is inserted into the vein, blood should flow through the needle hub as the vein is compressed with finger pressure. If blood spurts vigorously from the needle without compressing the vein, it is possible the needle entered the carotid artery. No medication should be administered in the carotid artery because it would go directly to the brain and central nervous system, and could result in convulsions or instant death.

Intravenous medication that leaks into surrounding tissue may create irritation that leads to loss of local skin or inflammation of the vein (*thrombophlebitis*). Phenylbutazone, sodium iodide, tetracycline, and guafenisin (a general anesthetic agent) are examples of irritating substances when given outside the vein.

Danger of Intra-Arterial Injection
Medication that is injected inadvertently into the carotid artery flows directly to the brain rather than to the heart via the jugular vein. In the vein, medication passes through the general circulation at a steady and consistent rate of tissue uptake. A dose of medication that travels through the artery directly to the brain elicits a seizure that generally only lasts a few minutes, but can be lethal. If the horse survives the intra-arterial injection and does not injure himself during a seizure, there should be no long-term effects since the medication is quickly eliminated from the bloodstream.

IV CATHETER
A need for frequent IV medication or large volumes of intravenous electrolyte solutions necessitates placement of an indwelling intravenous catheter. The insertion site over the jugular vein is clipped and scrubbed, and sterile technique is applied for catheter placement. An intravenous catheter is made of flexible, plastic material that may safely remain in the jugular vein for up to 72 hours.

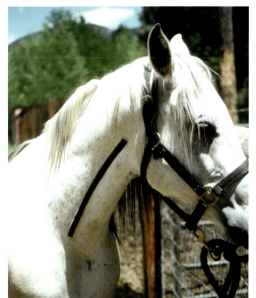

14.42 *The black tape on this horse's neck defines the jugular furrow. This is the site for intravenous injections, but it is important to note that the carotid artery runs alongside the jugular vein and is easily penetrated by a needle. No drug should be given in this artery.*

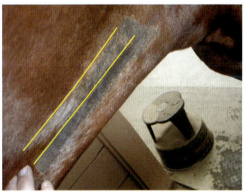

14.43 *When the jugular vein is occluded low down on the neck, it is well visualized as it fills with blood.*

Subcutaneous Injection
Most medications are intended for deep injection into a horse's muscle tissue, or directly into a vein. However, sometimes a therapeutic medication is given just beneath the skin into the subcutis. This is referred to as a *subcutaneous*, or *subQ*, injection. Loose skin behind the horse's elbow is useful for a subQ injection. The needle is placed just under the skin, but not into muscle, and the material is injected slowly.

The needle may be fanned in a semicircle to spread medication over a larger area. Medication or fluids given under a horse's skin are absorbed slowly, so a lump may be present at the injection site for several hours.

A common application for subcutaneous injection is infusion of local anesthetic to numb an area for suturing or for a scalpel incision. Fanning of anesthetic into the subcutaneous tissues increases the area of effect.

Intradermal Injection

An *intradermal* (ID) injection involves placing a needle inside the uppermost layer of the skin. It is not a common injection technique, but local anesthetic may be injected in this manner or injection of a corticosteroid into skin lesions, such as *nodular necrobiosis* (see p. 380), involves an ID infusion. Use of BCG to treat sarcoid tumors requires intradermal injection for best results (see chapter 13, *The Skin as an Organ*, p. 396).

Nonsteroidal Anti-Inflammatory Drugs

Equine athletic pursuits often result in sore muscles, swollen limbs, or mild lameness. It is not unusual for a horse owner or trainer to open the medical kit, and reach inside for a short-term anti-inflammatory solution to an ache or pain. In theory, this practice seems sensible, yet efforts to help a horse by numbing a problem with an anti-inflammatory drug may do more harm than good.

One highly overused and abused drug is that belonging to the class of nonsteroidal anti-inflammatory drugs, particularly phenylbutazone ("bute") and flunixin meglumine. Other, less commonly used NSAIDs include *dipyrone*, ketoprofen, and *naproxen*. (See also Appendix B, p. 568.)

Method of Action

An injury, a wound, a pulled muscle, colic, or arthritic problem stimulates the body to respond by producing substances called *prostaglandins*. Prostaglandins elicit a cascade of events involved in the inflammatory process. Prostaglandins are short-lived molecules, only produced at or close to their site of action. They are produced upon demand and are not stored by the body.

At the site of action, prostaglandins stimulate contraction and permeability of the cells lining the blood vessels, causing leakage of fluids into surrounding soft tissue. This results in tissue edema, and is seen as swelling. Prostaglandins also relax the smooth muscle of blood-vessel walls, causing blood to pool in localized areas, resulting in redness (*erythema*). Prostaglandins enhance the effects of other chemicals of the inflammatory cycle, such as *histamines* and *bradykinin*. These chemicals attract white blood cells, and increase blood circulation to the inflammation site. Warmth is noticeable due to increased blood flow and local blood pooling. In addition to eliciting swelling, redness, and heat at an injury site, prostaglandins super-sensitize pain receptors, contributing to an exaggerated pain response.

NSAIDs act as anti-inflammatory agents by inhibiting normal production of prostaglandins. As anti-prostaglandin medication, NSAIDs reduce the spiraling events that result in inflammation and swelling, and pain subsides. NSAIDs have no effect on prostaglandins produced prior to administration.

BENEFITS OF NSAIDS

NSAIDs are powerful drugs, capable of improving a horse's working capabilities by managing lameness and pain. NSAIDs help control leg swelling, or reduce fever caused by infection. They relieve spasms from muscle strain or a mild colic. They are helpful to an arthritic horse to enhance his quality of life and the longevity of his performance career. Yet, use of NSAIDs should be considered carefully.

INAPPROPRIATE USE OF NSAIDS

Colic

It is often a temptation to give a horse with colic an oral or injectable dose of flunixin meglumine or phenylbutazone paste. This is not necessarily a good idea for several reasons:

- These medications may mask symptoms of a surgical problem thereby delaying appropriate treatment.
- These medications can create kidney function problems in a dehydrated horse.
- Oral medication is poorly absorbed from the intestines of a horse with poor gut motility, as is often the case with colic.
- Oral medication requires several hours to be absorbed to full effect under normal circumstances so it is unlikely to help with the immediate pain.
- Injectable flunixin meglumine given intramuscularly is known for its ability to create *Clostridial* spp. infection, with life-threatening consequences.

Lameness

A lame horse that is asked for continued performance under the influence of pain-masking NSAIDs might aggravate a tendon or muscle injury (see p. 127 and p. 446).

Double-Dosing

A NSAID should not be repeated at less than 12-hour intervals unless specified by a veterinarian. Recommended dosing instructions per pound of body weight should not be increased. A common mistake is to give an appropriate dose of one NSAID, followed immediately by an appropriate dose of another NSAID. Toxic effects are additive, and this practice simulates a double-dose of any single NSAID. If relief is not achieved from an initial drug treatment, there is no reason to believe relief will come from an additional product with a similar mechanism of action. There is a time lag of several hours until clinical relief is seen. The prostaglandin cycle is blocked immediately, but existing prostaglandins need to be metabolized and removed from the system. Adding more NSAIDs will not alter or speed up this process.

NSAIDs and Foals

Foals less than 6 to 8 months old are extremely susceptible to gastric ulcer effects of NSAIDs. These are only given to a young horse, less than a year of age, if anti-ulcer medications are administered at the same time.

Cautionary Situations

PREPURCHASE EXAM

An unethical seller who wishes to mask a mild lameness problem may "improve" results of a prepurchase examination by using NSAIDs or other drugs. A drug-testing screen identifies these substances.

PROFESSIONAL ADVICE

Obtain professional veterinary advice before using NSAIDs. A treatment scheme that "worked" for one horse may have no application to another. What seems to be a mild problem may be serious, requiring medical attention and veterinary expertise.

WITHDRAWAL BEFORE COMPETITION

There are legal responsibilities involved with the use of anti-inflammatory agents. Drug levels are detectable in urine or blood up to 96 hours after administration. Rulings by the United States Equestrian Federation (USEF) state that a defined and limited amount of phenylbutazone or flunixin meglumine may be given in a daily dose to competition horses. To comply with these regulations, the maximum daily dose of phenylbutazone should not exceed 2 grams per 1000 pounds of body weight. The upper limit dose for flunixin is 500 mg per 1000 pounds body weight. Both drugs must be withdrawn 12 hours before competition, and should not be administered for more than 5 consecutive days. One drug or the other at the prescribed dosage is acceptable, but not both.

For track racing, each state has its own rules and restrictions. Check with the State Racing Commission (of the state where the race will be held) to ensure that a horse meets drug-withdrawal requirements.

There are a few sports and associations that strictly enforce "no drug" rules, forbidding use of any drug for competition: the Federation Equestrian International (FEI), the American Quarter Horse Association (AQHA), and endurance and competitive trail organizations. All NSAIDs must be withdrawn 4 days before a competition to avoid a positive drug test.

Types of NSAIDs

Understanding different pharmacological aspects of a drug is essential for its safe use. Manufacturer's labels and package inserts contain information about proper dosages and adverse side effects. Different products within the NSAID drug class act better on some ailments than others. For example, phenylbutazone is effective for musculoskeletal problems such as arthritis, a pulled muscle, or tendinitis. Flunixin meglumine is potent against gastrointestinal pain and endotoxemia (see p. 317).

COX-1 AND COX-2 ACTIONS

Cyclooxygenase (COX-1 and COX-2) enzymes are responsible for converting *arachidonic acid* to *prostaglandins*, one of the main mediators of the inflammatory cycle. Historically, NSAIDs have been used to interrupt the production of prostaglandins, and this in turn limits the inflammatory response by the body that elicits heat, pain, and swelling. The problem with blocking all prostaglandin formation is that some prostaglandins (COX-1) are beneficial to normal body functions, such as maintaining a mucous coating in the stomach to protect the stomach from the erosive effects of gastric acids, or maintaining blood flow through the kidneys. If this form of protective prostaglandin is reduced by administration of COX-1 inhibitors, then gastric ulcers or kidney damage are likely to develop. On the other hand, COX-2 enzymes selectively stimulate production of prostaglandins in inflamed tissue, but have only a small action in normal tissue. NSAIDs that contain only COX-2 inhibitors effectively block inflammation while not interfering with normal "house-keeping" body functions that are important to general health. Most currently available NSAIDs inhibit production of both COX-1 and COX-2 forms of prostaglandins, thereby affecting both good and bad processes in the body.

PHENYLBUTAZONE

One of the least expensive and more potent examples of the NSAIDs is phenylbutazone, or "bute." Following administration of an intravenous dosage of *phenylbutazone*, it takes about an hour to begin blocking prostaglandin production. Given in oral form as a paste, powder, or tablet requires 2 to 3 hours for absorption from the gastrointestinal tract. Peak effect occurs in 3 to 5 hours. This time lag is required for the body to break down previously produced prostaglandins. Total breakdown requires up to 12 hours, but phenylbutazone in the circulation prevents additional prostaglandins from being produced. If the blood level of phenylbutazone is not maintained at a therapeutic level, prostaglandins begin to accumulate again, and the inflammatory cycle repeats itself. Depending on the ailment, phenylbutazone protects against inflammation for 12 to 24 hours.

FLUNIXIN MEGLUMINE

Flunixin meglumine is useful for managing colic pain. It is also helpful against the effects of endotoxemia caused by an intestinal ailment, retained placenta, grain overload, or a pituitary disorder. Flunixin meglumine is more potent than phenylbutazone, and maintains its therapeutic effect for up to 30 hours.

ASPIRIN

Aspirin, which is excreted rapidly from the body, is only active for 6 to 8 hours. Because of its short duration, aspirin is a poor anti-inflammatory drug for musculoskeletal injury, or for anti-pyretic effects to reduce fever. Aspirin is a useful treatment for laminitis, navicular disease, colic due to obstruction of an intestinal blood vessel (*thromboembolic colic*), or anterior uveitis (see p. 497).

The primary value of aspirin in horses relies on its ability to alter the function of platelets. *Platelets* are a type of blood cell important to the blood-clotting mechanism. Aspirin alters platelet function for the lifespan of that platelet. The effect on platelets by a single dose of aspirin persists even after the bloodstream is cleared of the drug, lasting as long as 3 days.

COX-2 INHIBITOR NSAIDS

Currently a number of selective COX-2 inhibitors are being investigated for marketing to the equine industry. These could potentially minimize concerning secondary side effects like stomach ulcers, large colon ulcers, or kidney damage when using currently available forms of NSAIDs, like phenylbutazone or flunixin meglumine. Horses needing long-term (more than 10 days) anti-inflammatory medications to control pain and inflammation would benefit from such selective COX-2 inhibitors.

NSAID Toxicity

Toxic effects may occur with administration of excessive amounts of an NSAID over a short time (3 to 5 days), or by chronic dosing over months or years. Previously assumed safe doses in the horse can exert toxic effects if maintained at these levels too long. A lower-than-recommended dose of an NSAID may be toxic if given to a horse that is dehydrated, in pain, or stressed. Those horses respond to stress by internal production of corticosteroids, which in combination with NSAIDs amplifies toxic effects of both substances.

GASTROINTESTINAL SYMPTOMS

Excessive amounts of NSAIDs damage the gastrointestinal lining with subsequent leakage and loss of proteins. Symptoms of NSAID-induced toxicosis and protein loss include diarrhea, edema of limbs and abdomen, blood loss in the feces, and weight loss. Some horses exhibit depression, loss of appetite, or abdominal pain due to gastric ulcers or edema of the intestinal lining.

As mentioned, prostaglandin E2 (PG E2) protects the stomach lining by stimulating mucus production, and secretion of sodium bicarbonate by gastric cells to buffer stomach acid. Optimal blood flow to the stomach and intestinal tract is normally controlled by PG E2 activity. Without this protection, the stomach and intestines are prone to gastric ulcers (see chapter 11, *The Digestive System: The Oral Cavity, Dental Care, and the Intestinal Tract*, p. 318). Oral ulcers along the gums, palate, and tongue may accompany gastric ulcers. Mouth pain depresses appetite, and performance suffers.

KIDNEYS

Prostaglandins are responsible for maintaining normal blood flow, function, and water resorption abilities of the kidneys. Prostaglandins act as a protective device to dilate and enhance blood supply to the kidney. Irreversible, toxic effects may occur within 48 hours in dehydrated or blood-volume-depleted horses that are given a single dose of an NSAID. The syndrome is known as *renal papillary necrosis*, and is fatal. Even when administered at the recommended dose, NSAIDs may be toxic to a dehydrated horse.

JOINT EFFECTS

Another current area of investigation is looking at the effects of prostaglandins on joint metabolism. NSAIDs reduce concentrations of PG E2, which is known to sensitize nerve endings to mechanical stimuli and to chemical activation of pain receptors. By reducing pain "sensation" in an injured area, a horse is likely to do himself harm by not protecting the damaged part. It is also thought that PG E2 exacerbates lesions of osteoarthritis by encouraging cartilage and bone erosion and by stimulating release of inflammatory enzymes leading to cartilage degeneration. Some NSAIDs inhibit synthesis of cartilage components (proteoglycans) and may accelerate cartilage destruction. It is possible that some prostaglandins that are normally metabolized in the joints have protective effects much like those related to stomach protection.

ALLERGIC REACTIONS

Long-term use of NSAIDs (sporadic or consistent) may hypersensitize a horse to any drug in its class, resulting in allergic reactions. Reactions range from a mild case of hives or facial or limb edema, to a severe anaphylactic allergic reaction and death (see p. 391 and p. 439).

Alternatives to NSAIDs

Before indiscriminately using NSAID medication, explore other therapeutic alternatives such as rest, or hot or cold soakings (see p. 192). Apply DMSO to localized swelling, or massage sore muscles. Examine shoeing practices that might have changed limb biomechanics enough to bring on lameness. Re-evaluate training methods with a critical eye to the rate of increase in exercise difficulty. Look to management, parasite control, and feeding changes to decrease the incidence of colic.

Horses evolved to live on grasses, water, and salt. Anything else we put into their bodies must be evaluated for suitability and safety. Drugs are approved for animal use at specified dosages and frequencies to comply with research studies in safety and efficacy. NSAIDs have a role in the horse world, provided they are used intelligently and in moderation.

Safe and Effective Restraint

Building a partnership with a horse that is based on trust is a goal that takes time, but is full of reward. Unfortunately, not all events in a horse's life are free from unpleasantness or pain. Some examples are doctoring wounds, routine vaccinations, and administration of medications. For some horses, administration of deworming pastes, use of electric clippers, or horseshoeing are traumatic experiences. Other horses object to benign grooming procedures like bathing, or pulling and braiding the mane. The objectives of restraint are:

- To avoid getting hurt
- To prevent injury to the horse
- To get the job done effectively

Restraint of a half-ton animal obviously requires more than sheer human strength. A rearing horse can suspend a 200-pound man from the end of a twitch, and a horse recovering from general anesthetic can quickly flip two grown men off his neck. The brute strength of a horse should be addressed in a psychological arena, not in a physical showdown.

Understanding Horse Behavior

NATURAL INSTINCTS

By using our human mind we can outwit a horse at his own game of resistance. To do so, we must understand the motivating influences behind a horse's contrary behavior. Horses evolved survival mechanisms to protect themselves from predators, such as the big cats. Their immediate response when threatened is to flee from the area. A flighty horse is only responding to natural instincts to run from a fearful situation. A response to a painful or scary event is to move away from the stimulus by backing up, lunging sideways, or rearing. If backed into a corner, or prevented from fleeing, a horse then reverts to using his built-in defense weapons: his teeth and hooves. This fear translates to biting, kicking, or striking, all of which are unacceptable behavior from a human point of view.

By understanding normal equine behavioral instincts, we can capitalize on them, and modify their behavior to the task at hand. Horses evolved in a herd hierarchy, and they accept a single dominant herd member as the leader. Because a horse is able to distinguish between dominant and submissive individuals, and respond accordingly, it is logical for humans to achieve dominance to successfully fulfill the objectives of restraint.

Learn to read a horse's behavioral cues, such as flattened ears, or bared teeth that indicate aggression, or a tightly clasped tail and hollow, tense back reflective of pain or fear.

Other signals are subtle, but perked ears, a relaxed posture, or droopy lip and eyes should be positively rewarded, because they are signs of cooperation.

Creating Calmness

The temperament of an individual horse and his breed type are factors that may dictate a specific approach. However, certain fundamentals should be applied to restraint of any horse.

ENVIRONMENT

Make the situation appealing to a horse by working in a familiar environment that feels secure, and by using familiar equipment. Approach a horse quietly, and spend several minutes getting acquainted with his body language, while allowing the horse to become accustomed to the situation. Working off the near (left) side is comforting as most horses are accustomed to that. Talk in a quiet, calming tone of voice; a monotonous monologue exerts hypnotic effects upon a horse's psyche.

REASSURANCE

Spend a few extra minutes to reassure a horse rather than jumping right in and "mugging" him. The horse then begins to build confidence. Trust is gained by resisting the temptation to overpressure a horse. Proceed when he is ready to accept the situation with some degree of reassurance. Agreeable behavior should be rewarded with verbal praise while stroking the neck and face. Many horses like to be rubbed around the eyes or over the withers.

CONFIDENCE AND PATIENCE

Looking a horse in the eye commands his attention. Act decisively, because hesitation promotes the horse's suspicion and enhances his anxiety and distrust. Humans easily transmit fear and nervousness to a horse. Slow and deliberate movements build confidence. Be firm with commands, and discipline appropriately.

Many horses are not necessarily fearful of a procedure, but may only be displaying spoiled behavior. These horses often respect a firm reprimand. Human efforts at psychological domination are a positive learning experience for a spoiled horse. Sensitivity and patience teaches a horse about the necessity and benefits of submission to human will. Not only does this method make groundwork more enjoyable for a horse and his handlers, but a horse's response to riding or driving training also improves. With respect comes obedience and cooperation.

An essential ingredient in any restraint conflict is to restrain our personal fits of temper. Above all, stay cool and calm, and use a rational mind to command the situation. This advice sounds simple, but many know that self-restraint is not always easy during a battle of wills. It is better to back off, count to 10 (or 50 if necessary), and start over rather than embark upon a counterproductive physical match with the horse.

HORSE PSYCHOLOGY

A horse should always be reacting to people, rather than people reacting to the horse. This goal is not accomplished by threatening the horse verbally or physically, instead, be mentally one jump ahead of the horse. Anticipate what he will do. Before he has even started to make that move, take steps to counter him, converting the move to something else. Unwanted behavior is diverted, and this strategy also perplexes the horse, focusing his attention on the person. The horse looks to that person for a lead, accepting him or her as the dominant leader in the "herd."

This method of training requires empathy to individual equine personalities, and often is a gift with which one is born. Reading or attending seminars and clinics can teach about certain techniques, but it is best to trust in common sense and sensitivity. Recipes for psychological modification should only be used as guidelines. Each person should find what works with an individual horse and stick to it.

Restraint of a fractious horse is not about physical force. Instead it depends on a mental approach and understanding of each horse's unique response to any given situation. Figure out what makes a horse tick, and take strides to mold this knowledge into a plan of human design, without reacting to the horse.

Handling Procedures

SAFE WORK AREA

When approaching a situation that will be disagreeable to a horse, work in an area free of entrapments such as machinery, vehicles, rakes, wheelbarrows, low overhangs, nails and latches, and electrical cords. Find level ground with sufficient space for safe movement. Children, bystanders, and pets (dogs and cats) should be asked to leave or be removed from the working area. This practice ensures their safety, and prevents people from tripping over them while they work.

SAFE EQUIPMENT

Check the safety of all equipment, using intact, well-fitting halters and stout lead ropes. Be sure all buckles and snaps are functional, and are likely to remain so if stressed. Keep hands and fingers out of the halter, and never wrap a lead line around limbs or body. This prevents sprains, strains, or lost fingers if a hand entangles in a rope as a horse reacts suddenly.

Methods of Restraint

Because a horse's instinct to flee is so intense, removing the ability to flee often induces submissive behavior. Restraint of a horse's flight instinct is accomplished by either physical or chemical methods. Application of any form of physical restraint depends on psychological wit to ensure success. Learn which physical restraint method works best for each horse and recognize when a desired effect has been achieved. Some horses may object so violently to certain restraining measures, such as stocks or a twitch, that more cooperation may be achieved by quietly asking the horse to submit to a procedure without any physical restraint. Experience teaches which horses respond best to a "least restraint" technique.

Physical restraint begins simply when we place a halter and lead rope on a horse. Assuming a horse knows how to lead, he will go where we go. Once a horse is "in hand," more physical restraint can be applied as necessary. Placing a horse in a safe stall limits his ability to plunge and flee across a paddock or pasture. A horse can be backed into a corner where he has an impression of being controlled by a handler.

OPERATOR HANDLING

There should be at least two people involved in a procedure: the restrainer and the operator. The restrainer holds the horse while the operator performs the procedure. The restrainer should be a person who understands horses, and with whom it is easy to communicate.

Always untie a horse before giving medication or attempting any procedure. If a horse is tied and reacts violently to the insertion of a needle or handling of head or legs, he may lunge and throw himself against the rope. A horse's fright increases when he is unable to get free, potentially injuring himself or a person in the struggle.

Standing Positions

The best place for the restrainer to stand during any procedure is close to the horse, just behind the shoulder, out of the way of a striking leg. Far less impact is felt if the restrainer is knocked hard by a close horse as compared to the impact incurred if the operator is standing a few feet away. Never stand directly in front of any horse while performing a procedure. This position is hazardous as there are many ways for the horse to cause a problem, such as lunging, pawing, or rearing.

The restrainer should stand facing the same direction as the horse, with a good grip on the lead line; this position allows best control of a horse's head. If an injection is to be given in the rear end, the restrainer should stand on the same side as the person with the needle. Then, if the horse decides to kick, the handler pulls his head toward both people, automatically spinning the horse's kicking hind end away, in the opposite direction from the people.

Dedicated Restraint

The restrainer must be confident and stay with the horse, not letting go at a jumpy reaction by a fractious horse. Letting go increases the risk that the loose horse could hurt a restrainer or operator. A horse that runs past a handler can kick out and strike a person. Furthermore, letting go reinforces an adverse behavior and the horse now knows how to extract himself from the situation. Rather than submitting to the procedure, the horse intensifies his efforts to get away.

Cross-Ties

Cross-ties are a poor means of restraining a horse. Not only can a person be entangled in the cross-tie ropes, but a violently thrashing horse can also rear up and flip himself over in the cross-ties, fatally injuring his head or neck (see p. 522). If cross-ties are the only available

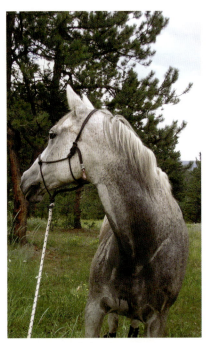

14.44 *A rope halter provides a measure of control, and applies more convincing pressure to a fractious horse than a leather or nylon web halter.*

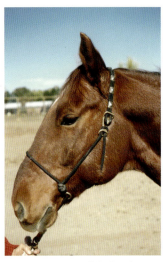

14.45 *A Be-Nice® halter has protruding knobs on the poll-piece that can apply pressure and discomfort to get a horse's attention.*

holding device, connect them with a quick-release buckle or with a piece of breakable baling twine. Never leave a horse unattended in cross-ties.

PHYSICAL RESTRAINT

There are a variety of techniques that produce submission in a horse. The best approach is to use the least restraint necessary. Overpowering a horse mentally and physically elicits more of a fight. The objective is to convince a reluctant horse to cooperate. Cooperation does not mean that he willingly complies. Sometimes, just standing still is a sign of submission. Accept small winning steps, and reward cooperation. If a tactic is not working sufficiently, then stop and regroup. Think the situation over. Try to figure out what exactly is troubling the horse. If necessary, seek professional help from a veterinarian.

Some restraint methods are more aggressive than others, and every horse responds differently to each strategy. They are discussed below from least physical or psychological intensity to most. Some restraints may be used in combination for the most desirable effect, with the least fright to the horse.

Rope Halter

An assertive type of halter is a *rope halter* (photo 14.44). When a sharp tug is made with the lead line, a horse is more likely to notice a thin rope braid of halter material than flat nylon webbing or leather straps.

Be-Nice® Halter

A *Be-Nice® halter* is a little harsher than a rope halter, and may be quite effective on horses that react negatively by throwing their heads or rearing (photo 14.45). The weight of the halter tightens the nosepiece and pulls down on the poll section. If the metal "prongs" are placed downward to contact the poll, negative reinforcement is asserted when the horse raises his head. Dropping his head (and body) causes pain to cease. A Be-Nice® halter can be an effective self-training device by punishing and rewarding a horse instantly at the time of the behavior.

Backing a Horse

Some horses prefer to go backward to flee an unpleasant situation. Unless there is a safe obstacle for a horse to back into, this flight behavior is incredibly frustrating. Forcing such a horse to rapidly back around and around a paddock may sufficiently fatigue his muscles so he willingly stops backing, and allows the procedure. At the same time, the restrainer has achieved psychological domination over the horse.

Equine First Aid, Medication, and Restraint

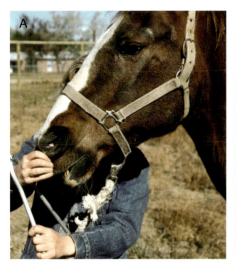
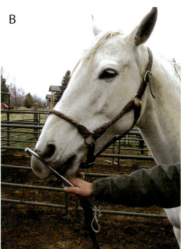

14.46 A & B *To place a twitch it is necessary to put it over your wrist, grab the horse's nose with a hand, and then gently squeeze the twitch on the nose while removing your hand (A). An easy twitch in place (B).*

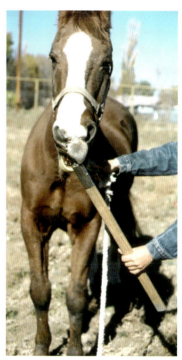

14.47 *A chain twitch applies more discomfort when the chain is wound around the nose. The long arm of the wooden handle provides added leverage.*

Distracting Noises

Sometimes jiggling a halter distracts a horse's attention as he listens to the jingling buckles. Knocking on his forehead in a non-rhythmical pattern also diverts his attention to the feel and sound. Knock in a random pattern so the horse does not know when the next tap sequence is coming. The horse may temporarily tune in to this distraction, long enough to give an injection or to apply a bandage.

"Earring Down" or Skin Pinch

Gently grabbing an ear and firmly pulling downward is another method of distraction. An ear should not be twisted or jerked. Downward traction is all that is required to achieve the necessary response. When performed properly, "earring" a horse rarely makes him headshy afterward; however, it is often difficult to grab hold of an ear on an already headshy horse. A similar distracting method is to grab a generous fold of skin on a horse's neck and pinch it tightly.

Twitch

An *easy twitch* is a piece of steel or aluminum clamped like a pair of pliers over a horse's nose (photos 14.46 A & B). A *chain twitch* is a device that winds a chain over the lip, with a long handle attachment to the chain for increased leverage (photo 14.47). It is uncomfortable enough to distract a horse's attention from other areas of the body. Caution should be taken to prevent the twitch from getting away from the restrainer because if a horse throws his head, a twitch can become a flying "billy club," capable of injuring nearby people. A twitch applied to a horse's nose should be held vertical to the ground, as twisting it sideways or upsidedown is painful enough to elicit violent reactions. It should not be used to lead or pull on a horse. Occasionally, a twitch is a fearsome device, causing a normally tractable horse to strike.

But, more typically, a twitch placed on the upper lip applies pressure to sensory nerves of the lip while also applying acupressure over calming points. In this manner, a nose twitch "sedates" and relaxes a horse while a mildly painful procedure is performed. A twitch stimulates release of chemicals, called *endorphins* and *enkephalins*, from the central nervous system; these chemicals are similar to mor-

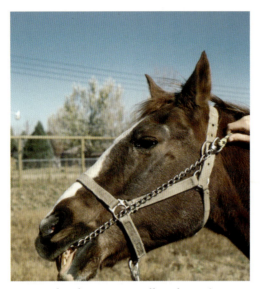

14.48 *A lip chain is an excellent device for control as dropping his head instantly rewards the horse, whereas pressure on the upper gum is amplified when he raises his head or pulls on the chain. The proper direction of gentle pull is upward toward the ear.*

phine in suppression of perception of pain, causing a horse to relax. Blood analysis (University of Utrecht, Netherlands) finds that endorphin levels increase by 81 percent during twitching, returning to normal within 30 minutes after removal of a twitch. Heart rates decrease by 8 percent while using a twitch, indicating lack of anxiety.

Lip Chain

A horse that fears and abhors a twitch may respond positively to the use of a *lip chain*. A lip chain is placed over the upper gum just under the lip (photo 14.48). Before applying the chain, run fingers under the upper lip and along the gums to provide a horse with a familiar taste of salt from the fingers and to encourage confidence. Then the chain is quietly and smoothly slipped into place. Not only is a lip chain less intimidating than a twitch, but it also serves as a self-punishing device capable of training a horse. When a horse exhibits undesirable behavior, the chain tightens over the gum and is painful, but as soon as he responds appropriately, he is instantly rewarded by release of pressure and pain. Rapid jerks on the chain by the restrainer are counterproductive and may elicit rearing. Light, steady pressure is all that is necessary to keep the chain in place; the horse's response automatically tightens or loosens it. In my hands, I find a lip chain to be the most acceptable and effective restraint method with least stress to the horse.

Stud Chain

Instead of placing a chain under the lip, it can be applied over the nose as a *stud chain*. A firm jerk on a chain in this position causes pain to the nose, enforcing a verbal reprimand.

War Bridle

Use of a "war bridle" is overly threatening and painful to a horse if it is applied incorrectly or with anger. The rope is passed over the poll and through the mouth as would a bit. This war bridle places painful pressure on the poll and at the commissures of the mouth and the gums.

Blindfold

Blindfolding a horse prevents him from fleeing. He is now completely subservient to the restrainer because he has no idea where to move. Occasionally, it is necessary to blindfold a horse to apply another physical restraint method such as a twitch or lip chain.

Hobble

Another means of removing a horse's ability to escape is to tie one leg in a hobble. The leg is flexed at the carpus (knee), and a leather strap or soft cotton rope is placed around the forearm and pastern. As one leg is held off the ground, the horse feels "crippled." His other limbs fatigue. Many horses hop around in confusion as they try to free their leg. Occasionally, a horse overreacts by throwing himself to the ground, yet other horses become subdued quickly.

The goal is achieved when the horse recognizes the human as his "savior" who removes the hobble from the leg. Now, the human is "The Good Guy" who presents the horse with the lesser of two evils: he can submit quietly with all four legs on the ground, or lose the use of one of his legs with a hobble.

Stocks

Use of *stocks* confines a horse and severely limits his movements (photo 14.49). Never be complacent about a horse in stocks because a determined horse is still able to kick or bite, or may attempt to jump out. A seat belt, snugly fit over the horse's withers, deters a tendency to leap upward.

Foal Restraint

Restraint of a foal requires a different technique than those used on grown horses. Foals often quiet down if the restrainer encircles the foal's chest with an arm, and runs the other arm around behind the buttocks. The tail can be pulled up gently, with no adverse effects, to stabilize the foal. Be sure the forward arm is not too high up on the neck so air intake is not impeded through the trachea. Pushing a foal against a safe wall, and placing a knee firmly into his flank while encircling him with the arms, usually holds him steady so the operator can perform a task. Do not be fooled by a foal's size; the littlest newborn can crack ribs or dent a head or shin.

CHEMICAL RESTRAINT

Fractious horses may respond best for procedures under the influence of chemical restraint. Chemical tranquilizers and sedatives diminish

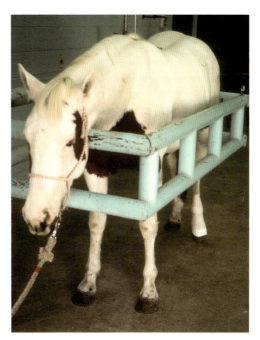

14.49 *Stocks create a restraining box around a horse to limit danger to the operator from kicks or unpredictable movements. A seat belt (not seen here) attached to the stocks and placed over the withers prevents a horse from rearing while in the stocks.*

stress to both the horse and operator and prevent a horse from injuring himself or others.

A *sedative*, like xylazine or detomidine, acts as a central nervous system, musculoskeletal, and cardiopulmonary depressant, rendering a horse fairly nonresponsive to noxious stimuli. He may lose his coordination and stability related to muscle relaxation from the drug. A *tranquilizer*, like acepromazine, is a generalized CNS depressant, with its predominant effect acting on a horse's mental state to modify his behavior. Acepromazine relieves anxiety and has a calming influence, with little effect on his motor coordination.

A horse that is excited and adrenalized prior to use of chemical restraint will probably not respond well to administration of a tranquilizer, and may require more sedative than usual to achieve tractability. Adrenaline speeds the heart rate and blood flow through the body, and results in flushing of drugs through the system too rapidly to affect the central nervous system. Anticipate whether it would be advantageous to start with chemical restraint rather than getting a horse excited first by unsuccessful attempts at physical restraint. Once a horse is excited and a decision is made to try a chemical approach, it is best to wait 20 to 30 minutes for all to calm down before administering the drug.

Adverse Reactions

Tranquilizers and sedatives should be used only under veterinary supervision, for although adverse reactions to these drugs are uncommon, they can occur. Prior to drug administration, the horse's heart should be monitored with a stethoscope to check for any murmurs or arrhythmias. These drugs exert cardiovascular effects that can adversely affect a poor heart condition.

Sedatives diminish the normal cough reflex, and so a sedated horse is prone to choke. Following sedation, a horse should not be fed until he is awake enough to eat safely.

Methods of Administration

Sedatives or tranquilizers can be administered either intravenously (IV) or intramuscularly (IM). Given IV into the vein, the effects are fairly immediate (within several minutes), but not as long-lasting as when given IM. An IM injection requires at least 10 minutes before the head drops and the horse's body relaxes. Different dose levels are calculated depending on whether the IV or IM route is used. The degree and duration of sedation is also dose-dependent.

ACHIEVING THE OBJECTIVE

Ideally, the goal is to train a horse to accept and tolerate a disagreeable event. In most cases, a horse will not simply submit to a painful or frightening procedure. Be satisfied with incremental successes, and build on these. Maintain a bright, optimistic outlook, and this attitude will be transmitted to the horse. Above all, stay rational and do not prematurely admit defeat. By drawing on all strategies of psychological, physical, and chemical restraint, there is always a way to get the job done, both effectively and safely.

Preventive and Mental Horse Health 15

The day-to-day details of managing a horse in his home environment create a template for physical and mental health. A group of horses is only as healthy as the individuals within the herd. Not only is daily management of each resident horse on a farm important, but so also are the details of introducing a new horse to the herd. It is exciting to bring home a new horse to the farm, his future bright and unknown. Although a new riding prospect may appear the picture of health, precautions should be taken before turning him into the pasture with the rest of the herd.

Herd Health

Health Inspection

Before any new arrival enters new premises, it is prudent to have a current health certificate and a recent (within the last 6 to 12 months) negative *Coggins* test accompany each horse (see "The Value of Blood Tests," p. 457). Every state requires a health certificate for interstate transport. Many states accept a veterinary exam for a health certificate that has been done within 30 days of entry into the state, although some require a health inspection to be done within 10 days. With a thorough physical exam, a veterinarian may detect a simmering infectious disease. Health certificates screen for horses that are carrying a transmissible disease, such as lice, fungal dermatitis, viral vesicular stomatitis, or viral respiratory illness, to name a few. A health certificate is also a safety precaution to identify a marginally or overtly sick horse that is about to be transported.

Some horse owners try to skirt the issue of health certificates and Coggins tests in order to save a few dollars. The objective of these regulatory procedures is to prevent an undetected sick or inapparent carrier of disease from slipping across state lines or to a horse event. The necessary health exam, lab tests, and paperwork improve health safety for all. Many horse show events and stables require negative Coggins tests and health certificates not to harass owners, but rather to help prevent outbreaks of an insidious disease.

A health inspection does not always uncover disease problems that are incubating within a horse that is not yet showing clinical signs. The biggest concern in introducing a new horse to a premise or to a horse event is that a horse may be incubating an infectious disease, like a virus, without exhibiting symptoms of sickness, and may never actually become sick. As "carriers," these individuals may initiate a viral infection of epidemic proportions by exposing other horses to a disease. Young and very old horses are particularly at risk as their immune systems are not as efficient as that of a horse in his prime.

Vaccination Status

The vaccination status of a horse should be current and appropriate not only for the environment from which the horse originates, but also for where he is going.

Horses in the herd at home should be vaccinated against respiratory viruses before bringing a new or traveling horse home. This ensures the strongest protective immunity possible. Ideally, vaccines should be boosted at least 10 to 14 days prior to exposure and maintained on a regular frequency throughout the year.

PRINCIPLES OF VACCINATION PROTECTION

Athletic horses depend on a huge lung capacity to fuel the muscles with oxygen to maintain performance. One of the biggest challenges to managing an equine athlete is maintaining respiratory health (see p. 254). Just as with humans, respiratory viruses readily circulate throughout a horse population. This becomes a greater risk the more a horse travels, the more stress he encounters, and the more horses to which he is exposed. To protect against respiratory viruses, a *minimum* program of twice-annual boosters of *equine influenza* and *equine rhinopneumonitis* ensures good antibody protection (see p. 265). Vaccines don't guarantee that a horse won't get sick from these viruses, but a high antibody titer in the bloodstream minimizes the degree of illness a horse experiences if disease is contracted. In highly trafficked barns and for horses that experience a lot of travel and stress associated with training and competition, vaccinate at least 3 or 4 times a year against influenza and rhinopneumonitis (see p. 270 and p. 272). These vaccines impart relatively cheap protection against the sniffles and coughs that pull a horse out of work for weeks at a time. Any viral infection of the respiratory tract also makes a horse susceptible to bronchopneumonia or to developing the allergic syndrome of *chronic obstructive pulmonary disease*, commonly referred to as COPD or *heaves* (see p. 259). Such secondary problems may have repercussions affecting performance far into a horse's athletic future.

Respiratory vaccinations are available in an intranasal form that has less risk of inducing adverse muscle reactions. The intranasal format may afford a high degree of protective immunity by blocking virus or bacteria at its site of entry, the lining of the respiratory tract.

MINIMIZING THE IMPACT OF VACCINATION

General rules apply to derive the most from vaccines for disease protection and the least inconvenience to training or competition schedules. Ideally, vaccine boosters given to a competition horse should be administered 2 to 4 weeks prior to travel or competition. This gives an opportunity to develop good antibody protection against worrisome diseases, while also giving a horse the chance to recover from transient muscle soreness or fever induced by an intramuscular vaccine.

Following vaccine administration, it is a good idea to turn the horse into pasture to continue to move his muscles, or exercise him lightly. There is no reason for a horse to stop all work for days at a time following immunization since today's commercial vaccine products are smooth and easy on the system. Some horses are known to be sensitive to immune stimulation and so should receive a nonsteroidal anti-inflammatory drug (NSAID) at the same time a vaccine is given (see p. 442). If a horse is headed for competition, follow guidelines for medication withdrawal when administering nonsteroidal anti-inflammatory medications (NSAIDs) prior to an event.

Brand Inspection

In the western United States, a brand inspection is required for horses moving distances greater than 75 miles. Check with the state brand inspector about local laws pertaining to traveling away from home with a horse. A permanent brand inspection card can be issued that is legal for a horse's lifetime unless he is sold to a new owner. Each time a horse is purchased, a new brand inspection must be obtained by providing proof of transfer of ownership.

The Value of Blood Tests

Blood tests are useful as screening devices and can add invaluable information to a physical exam. Caution should be taken to not overinterpret blood test results.

COGGINS TEST

One disease that needs to be screened in every horse is *Equine Infectious Anemia* (EIA—see p. 241). A negative Coggins test is required for interstate travel and for health certificates to many in-state events. Usually, this test is done annually, and a negative Coggins test should also be required for any newcomer to a farm, and for a potential horse purchase.

Testing Procedures for EIA

By 1972, a reliable testing procedure for Equine Infectious Anemia was developed by LeRoy Coggins, which relies on testing a blood sample collected from a horse. Because the Coggins test is so sensitive and specific, with less than 5 percent error, it has been used as a standard for control of interstate movement of horses. This test identifies inapparent carriers that are able to transmit the disease via flies to uninfected horses. An asymptomatic carrier could suffer a relapse or an acute episode brought on by stress-related transport, and this would ensure high enough levels of virus circulating in the bloodstream.

There are presently two methods to identify the presence of EIA virus antibodies in a sample of blood:

- *Agar-gel-immunodiffusion* (AGID): the AGID test will not detect an infected horse prior to antibody production, but by 42 days post-infection, antibodies will be present in the blood.
- C-ELISA (*Competitive Enzyme-Linked Immunosorbent Assay*) and the SA-ELISA test (*Synthetic Antigen* ELISA): this is a rapid test only requiring incubation of 2 hours instead of the 24-hour incubation time for the AGID Coggins test.

Foals born to EIA positive mares will be serologically positive until 6 to 9 months of age. For this reason, Coggins tests are not performed on foals less than 6 months of age.

COMPLETE BLOOD COUNT

A *complete blood count* (CBC) measures a horse's *white blood cell* (WBC) and *red blood cell* (RBC) mass. White blood cells are responsible for fighting infections, and the numbers of circulating WBCs and the types of these cells distributed in the blood profile alert of bacterial or viral problems, or ongoing stress factors.

The RBC count gives a glimpse at whether or not a horse is anemic. *Anemia* affects a horse's performance because less oxygen is carried through the tissues by the red blood cells to support metabolism of working muscles. If a horse has an excessively low RBC or low hemoglobin, there is a concern about low-grade chronic infection, or gastrointestinal ulcers.

CHEMISTRY PANEL

A *chemistry panel* gives information about electrolyte levels, muscle enzymes, and kidney and liver function. Enzymes are continuously released into the circulation as cells age and die, and there is a normal range predicted for horses. Even if chemistry values do not fall in the out-of-normal range, this does exclude a structural problem. As an example, kidney enzymes do not elevate until at least two-thirds of kidney tissues experience significant damage. As another example, the body compensates well for losses of electrolytes during exercise; although electrolyte imbalances occur within the cells, the problems may not be immediately evident in the serum.

On the other hand, liver enzymes are much more sensitive to abnormalities, and liver enzyme levels will rise with even minor damage. Similarly, we can review muscle enzyme values and look for early indications of recent muscular damage. Since episodes of *myositis* or *tying-up syndrome* (see p. 166) trigger release of muscle-specific enzymes, this information is important to performance capabilities of an athletic horse.

Another chemistry test often used in a working horse is that of *lactate testing* (see p. 152). Measuring lactate in the bloodstream is useful to compare fitness development of a horse to himself over time, but has been shown to be a poor predictor of athletic capability. As a value measured one time only, it is meaningless. This test is best performed during or immediately after exercise, and is often used with performance evaluation of a horse on a treadmill. Fit horses do metabolize lactate more quickly than less fit individuals. Heart rate, speed, and the distance a horse is asked to work while on a treadmill must be kept constant when evaluating lactate and comparing it from one test to the next. In this manner, it is used to track a horse's conditioning progress.

DRUG TESTING PROFILE

A *drug testing profile* uncovers minute quantities of drugs and medications circulating in the blood. Anti-inflammatory drugs disguise musculoskeletal problems, and tranquilizers often mask behavioral issues. The use of urine allows more sensitive screening for drugs, but blood is also useful. Drug tests are moderately expensive, but if there is any concern about the integrity of a seller, it is prudent to pursue a drug test.

Quarantine

The best means of controlling the spread of infectious disease is by quarantining a newcomer away from other horses for two to three weeks. Some viral infections take weeks to incubate to the point that a horse shows symptoms of disease. Disease is transmitted not just by direct contact, but also by physical vehicles (*fomites*) such as buckets, rakes, clothing, and hands. Quarantine should be pursued diligently: this means no shared feed tubs, no shared water buckets, no shared brushes or manure rakes. A quarantined horse should be removed as far as possible from other horses, and should not share a common fence line for the duration of the quarantine.

MONITORING A NEW HORSE

For at least the first week, a new arrival should be monitored closely for any sign of illness. A daily record log should be kept about a new horse's activity, appetite, water intake, rectal temperature, and bowel movements (see *Appendix A*, p. 567). Take a temperature reading once or twice a day. A normal horse's temperature should be less than 101° F (38° C). Check for discharge from eyes or nose, and listen for a cough. Observe how much the horse is eating, how much manure he is producing, and if possible, measure his water intake. An idle horse in the winter may drink between 5 and 10 gallons of water per day, while in the summer he may double that intake. Check that manure is moist and of normal consistency and amount. Most horses defecate between 8 to 12 piles in a 24-hour period.

Observe the horse's attitude. A horse moved to a new environment is generally quizzical about the goings-on around him. He should be interested in investigating everything and should demonstrate good energy. He should be hungry, and drink well. He should produce plenty of manure, and make an ample number of urine spots. Keep a written log of these observations to track concrete data; this allows for an objective opinion on how well the new horse is making the adjustment. The most astute observer may detect mild disease symptoms before the horse advances to a very sick state.

Good Hygiene

Hygienic management strategies are essential in keeping disease transfer on a farm to a minimum in any herd operation. It is best to handle unknown or sick horses last in the roster of chore duties. This prevents the carrying of potentially contaminated material on shoes or body to resident horses on a farm. If there is any concern at all about the health of a horse, change clothing and shoes before interacting with other horses. Use separate feed and water containers, and minimize sharing of tack, blankets, and grooming supplies as much as possible. Bridles and bits should not be used interchangeably between horses.

Internal Parasites and Control

A key feature of equine health management is effective control of internal parasites (*endoparasites*). Horses continually reinfect themselves with parasites while eating on ground contaminated with manure. Given the opportunity, most horses will defecate in an area separate from their feed supply. Heavily populated pastures do not provide horses enough space to separate a pasture into *roughs* (ungrazed grass around feces) and *lawns* (grazing area). In temperate, humid climates, such parasites proliferate year round; in harsher climates with winter temperatures, there is a period of months where the eggs lie dormant in the environment and so the risk of re-infection is lessened during that time. Twice-weekly removal of feces from pastures or corrals is an effective method of parasite control, especially when coupled with dewormer treatment at intervals of 4 to 8 weeks (fig. 15.1).

The Effect of Internal Parasites on Performance

Horses on an excellent preventive management program don't tend to die of parasite infection anymore as in decades past. However, even if visible problems are not appreciated, internal parasites have known impacts on a horse's performance. Internal parasites cause their damage as they migrate through the body, affecting the lungs, liver, and gastrointestinal tract in their travels. Intestinal worms sap nutrients from a horse and create problems like weight loss, colic, low energy and overall poor performance.

A typical presentation of a horse with obvious signs of parasitism reveals a potbelly, a poor, brittle hair coat, and significant weight loss. Subtle signs may be detectable with careful review of a horse's behavior and demeanor. A horse's attitude and performance may seem flatter than normal; he tries to put out, but doesn't exhibit his usual exuberance. In most cases, there may be no outward indication of a problem. But, a horse is not able to

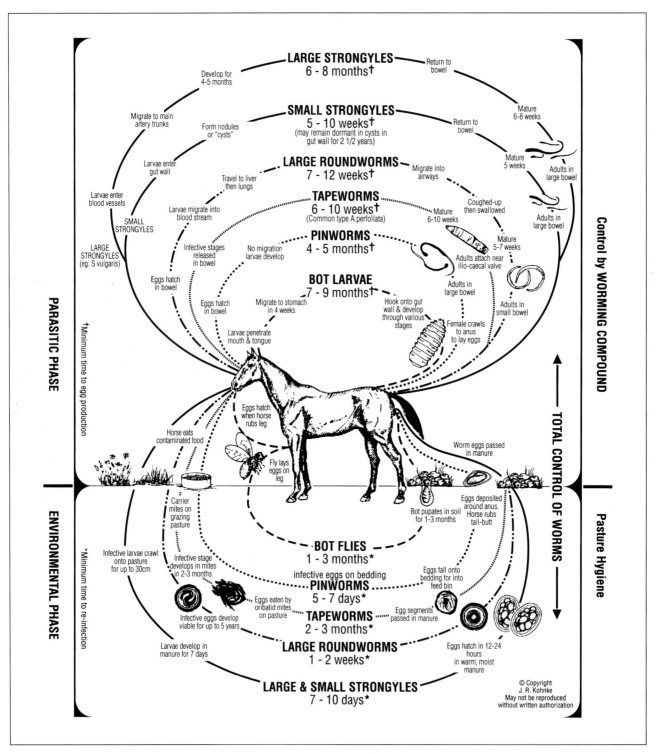

15.1 *The Life Cycles of Common Horse Parasites:* One of the basic principles in managing parasite larval infection is cleaning paddocks and pastures twice daily to minimize ingestion of infective larvae. Large and small strongyles can be infective as early as four days into the developmental phase so weekly manure removal is not sufficient as sometimes thought.

give his best performance, and you may not even realize that this is the case. Other things to look for in the horse:

- Tires easily
- Loses interest in his food
- Won't gain weight even with good quality feed available at all times
- Experiences occasional bouts of mild colic
- Periods of intermittent diarrhea, or loose stool
- Hair coat doesn't shine or is delayed in its winter shedding
- Lacking luster in appearance and posture

Parasitic invasion compromises a horse's ability to obtain sufficient nutrients from the feed. This has a critical impact on a horse's energy and performance. Parasitic migration can create enough minor damage to stimulate low-grade but chronic bleeding within organs, or intestinal ulcers. Chronic blood loss causes anemia and makes a horse less resistant to viral and bacterial infection.

Types of Internal Parasites

In general, horses obtain infective *larvae* through contaminated feed or water, manure eating *(coprophagy)*, or contaminated pastures. Adult worms are rarely seen in the feces unless a horse is severely parasitized. The various egg stages of the worms can only be viewed through the microscope.

LARGE STRONGYLES OR BLOODWORMS

One common internal parasite is the *large strongyle*. The three most common species of large strongyles affecting the horse are *Strongylus vulgaris, Strongylus equinus,* and *Strongylus edentatus.*

Clinical signs of strongyle infestation include:

- Diarrhea
- Colic
- Weight loss
- Poor hair coat
- Unthriftiness, depression, poor appetite, or dullness
- Anemia, resulting in reduced athletic performance or growth
- Changes in intestinal movement resulting in impactions, intestinal twists, or death
- Obstruction of the blood vessels, leading to death

SMALL STRONGYLES

Small strongyles are recognized as an important problem in horses, particularly as they have evolved unique strategies in maintaining themselves in their world. Small strongyles are resistant to cold and dry environments, yet more importantly, once within the horse they either develop rapidly (within two months) to adult stages, or they encyst within the wall of the large intestine. In an *encysted* state, they remain arrested in their development, only to become active up to two years later. While in the encysted state, they are unaffected by deworming products. It is difficult to diagnose infection with encysted forms since very few eggs would be present in a fecal sample (photo 15.2).

Damage to the intestinal wall may contribute to colic signs, especially as the larvae emerge from their cysts during winter and spring. Other clinical signs associated with the emergence of encysted small strongyles include fever, lack of appetite, weight loss or failure to gain, diarrhea, delayed shedding, and even intestinal ulcers. The younger the horse,

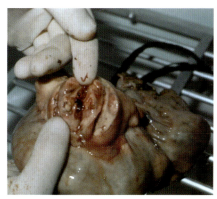

15.2 *Strongyle larvae can encyst themselves in the intestinal wall, creating an abscess. Related inflammation causes digestive disturbances, malabsorption, diarrhea, or colic. Photo: David Varra, DVM.*

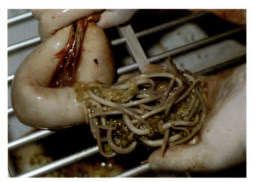

15.3 *Adult Ascarid worms can create a life-threatening impaction in the small intestines.* Photo: David Varra, DVM.

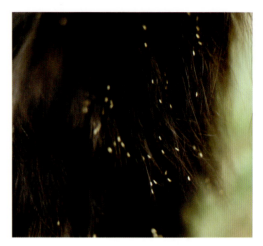

15.4 *Bot eggs are visible on the hairs of the legs where they are accessible to the horse's mouth when he scratches his face on his lower limbs.*

the more affected it is by encysted larvae due to a less developed immune response. Yet, both young and mature horses may carry encysted larvae with them to a clean pasture situation despite having been regularly dewormed. Eventually, the encysted larvae become egg-laying adults and infect a "clean" pasture, perpetuating the cycle.

ASCARIDS

Ascarids, known as roundworms, are especially a problem in horses less than 2 years of age, but can adversely affect any age horse if larvae are abundant in the environment (photo 15.3). Ascarid eggs are extremely resistant to environmental conditions and persist in the environment for years. Once infective ascarid larvae are ingested, the journey through the body begins in the small intestine, and continues through the circulatory system reaching the liver, heart, and the lungs. In the lungs, its migration sets up conditions to create a chronic cough, bronchitis, or pneumonia. In the small intestines, egg-laying adults may accumulate in sufficient numbers to compete with their host for nutrients, or may amass in a tangle to create an intestinal obstruction.

STOMACH WORMS

Bots

Bot "worms" are not actually worms at all, but are the larvae of the bot fly, *Gastrophilus* sp. (all species of the genus, *Gastrophilus*). The bot fly lays its eggs on the leg and chest hairs. When the horse licks or rubs the hairs, the eggs are transferred to the horse's mouth. Unhatched bot eggs can survive for up to six months on the hairs (photo 15.4).

Once in the mouth, hatched larvae burrow into the tongue and tissues of the mouth and esophagus. While in the mouth tissues, the bot larvae may cause pain with chewing, or may impede swallowing because of throat swelling. After about three weeks, the larvae travel to the stomach. The larvae attach to the stomach lining, and can cause ulcers, food impaction, colic, or *peritonitis,* which is inflammation of the abdominal wall (photos 15.5 A & B). Although rare, the stomach may rupture and cause death. Bot larvae require about ten months to develop once they enter the mouth.

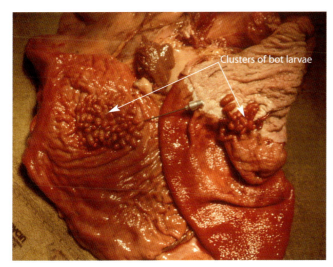
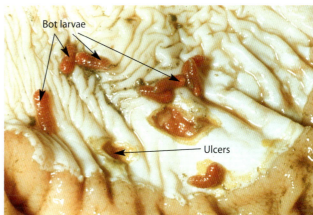

15.5 A & B *Bot larvae attach themselves to the stomach lining in clusters. When these larvae release from the intestinal wall, they leave behind erosions and ulcerated craters.* Photo: David Varra, DVM.

Certain species of bot larvae attach to the rectum as they pass to the anus. Their presence causes irritation and tail rubbing, and is often mistaken for *pinworm* infestation (see below).

Habronema

Stomach worms, *Habronema* spp. pass their eggs through the feces, and then fly larvae ingest the eggs. The horse either ingests the fly larvae and stomach worm egg, or infected adult flies deposit their larvae around the mouth and lips of the horse. From there they pass directly into the stomach and develop to the egg-laying stage, repeating the cycle. Larvae in the stomach may stimulate an immune response, forming large, tumorous masses. Although these disappear once the larvae are gone, areas of glandular stomach tissue are replaced with scar tissue.

Summer Sores

The most significant damage caused by the *Habronema* sp. is *summer sores*. If a horse's skin is broken from a wound or abrasion, flies feeding on the injury may infect it with *Habronema* larvae. The larvae do not grow or develop in the wound, but they cause a pronounced tissue response, resulting in a non-healing, persistent sore that is easily invaded by bacteria (see p. 388). Deworming a horse kills the larvae, reducing the horse's chances of contracting this parasite.

Trichostrongylus axei

Another stomach worm is *Trichostrongylus axei*, a common parasite of cattle and other ruminants. Horses infected by this worm exhibit a loss in condition, with diarrhea and/or constipation, protein loss, and anemia. A chronic inflammatory response develops in the stomach.

PINWORMS

Pinworms, or *Oxyuris equi* are ingested from feed contaminated with manure to develop in the cecum (part of the large intestine). Then, a fertilized, adult female enters the rectum, passes through the anus, and deposits her eggs around the anus and/or vulva. These eggs drop

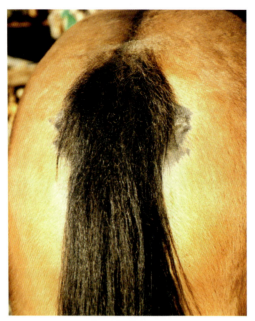

15.6 *Pinworms cause irritation of the anus as they exit the rectum. This causes a horse to rub his buttocks beneath the tail, as seen here.*

onto the ground or food (that has been placed on the ground), repeating the process. An affected horse itches and rubs the tailhead (top of the tail) with an associated loss of hair (photo 15.6 and see photo 13.31, p. 379). Pinworm eggs are not normally seen in the feces, but are obtained by pressing cellophane tape against the anus.

INTESTINAL THREADWORMS

Intestinal threadworms, *Strongyloides westeri*, are primarily a problem in foals and have been implicated in foal diarrhea and *scours*. The infective stage of the larvae is passed through the mare's milk, or penetrates the skin. As with ascarids, immunity to infection increases with age; by 4 to 5 months of age, foals are resistant to infection. Because of the association of foal scours with the life cycle of this parasite, deworming of scouring foals is recommended.

LUNGWORMS

Although their natural host is the donkey, *lungworms* can infect horses. Usually, donkeys do not show clinical problems, but will pass larvae in their feces. Horses pastured with donkeys are at high risk of infection, but it is also possible for horse-to-horse transmission to occur. Associated problems due to lungworms include a chronic cough, pneumonia, and pleuritis.

TAPEWORMS

Tapeworms have surfaced as a problem in all parts of the United States, particularly the eastern and southeastern states. Removal of competing parasites by dewormers may allow tapeworms to assume an abnormal growth rate. East of the Mississippi River, 62 to 96 percent of horses are infected with tapeworms, while west of the Mississippi River, 12 to 60 percent of horses are infected. The life cycle of tapeworms depends on a mite, which the horse ingests while eating pasture or hay.

Potentially, tapeworms pull nutrient reserves away from a horse. With chronic irritation to the small intestine, intestinal erosions may develop, or the tapes create an obstruction or cause an *intussusception* (piece of small intestine telescopes inside the cecum) necessitating surgical correction of an extremely painful and life-threatening colic. Eighty-one percent of colic due to an intussusception and 22 percent of spasmodic colic episodes are attributable to heavy infection with tapeworms. Tapeworms can also lead to impaction colic of the cecum. A blood test can identify the extent of tapeworm infection whereas a fecal analysis yields information only 3 percent of the time.

Preventive Management for Parasite Control

By minimizing an internal parasite burden in the horse, health and performance flourish, and gastrointestinal disturbances are averted.

Controlling internal parasites with dewormers is an essential part of management, but should be combined with intelligent husbandry.

HERD MANAGEMENT

Introducing New Animals to a Herd
New individuals should not be introduced to the herd immediately, but should be isolated. If there is no history of parasite control, deworm new arrivals 2 or 3 times, at 3 to 4 week intervals before allowing them to join the herd. Fewer eggs shed in the feces means less parasite contamination and less likelihood of reinfection. This practice protects those horses that have received excellent deworming management from reinfection. If absolute quarantine is difficult to manage on a farm, refrain from turning the horse into common pastures for at least 4 to 10 days as it will take that long for a horse to stop shedding parasite eggs once dewormed.

Concurrent Deworming Schedules
All members of a herd should be dewormed at the same time. If only a small percentage of a herd is dewormed, untreated horses continue to excrete eggs in their feces, recontaminating not only themselves, but the treated horses as well.

Monitoring with Fecal Analysis
To monitor effectiveness of a parasite control program for most internal parasites other than tapeworm infestation, compare a fecal sample analysis before deworming treatment with a fecal sample obtained 2 to 3 weeks following treatment. Have your veterinarian run an annual or biannual fecal exam to check for the presence and quantity of parasite eggs. The test is relatively inexpensive and yields valuable information. Fecal analysis by a veterinarian allows close monitoring of a parasite load within a horse, and observations of hair coat, body condition, weight gain, attitude, and performance provide other clues. A veterinary exam may reveal other metabolic, nutritional, or dental problems contributing to a horse's unthrifty health. Not all illness can be blamed entirely on worms.

There are many reasons why a fecal exam may show eggs in the sample, including the fact that some parasites have developed resistance to dewormer products. Ideally, it is best to run a fecal exam on at least 20 percent of the horses in a herd as some horses have marked differences in their immune system, with certain individuals shedding elevated numbers of parasite eggs. Identification of shedders enables application of a more aggressive deworming program for those individuals. Parasites such as the ascarids may produce 100,000 eggs per day, while large strongyles may only produce 5,000 eggs per day. Once the presence of eggs has been identified in a fecal sample, a tailored program can be discussed with a veterinarian as to appropriate medications to administer, and the frequency.

Natural Immunity
Normally over time, a healthy horse develops some degree of immunity to certain parasites, and can fend off massive infestation. The body's immune system recognizes the parasite's proteins (*antigens*) as foreign and launches an immune attack by forming antibodies. Dewormer efficacy of 100 percent may not be advantageous, because it eliminates the source of the antigens. Then, a horse's uneducated immune system cannot defend against future parasite infection.

Foals and young horses under 2 years of age that have not yet developed immunity may succumb to overwhelming parasite loads by ascarids or large strongyles if not regularly dewormed.

ENVIRONMENTAL MANAGEMENT
Parasite control methods diminish the number of infective larvae available to a horse. Twice-

weekly removal of manure from pasture and corrals is an effective method to remove parasite larvae before they become infective.

Contaminated forage results in reinfection with worm larvae. Careful pasture management prevents overgrazing that would otherwise encourage manure deposits to outstrip available forage. Chain dragging a pasture spreads the manure and prevents overgrazing of certain areas, while also breaking parasite life cycles. If economically feasible, mechanical removal of feces by pasture vacuums provides excellent parasite control. Harrowing spreads the larvae throughout the grazing area, damaging forage; therefore, it is not advised.

Collected manure should be composted before spreading it on a pasture. Heat within the compost pile kills infective larvae and prevents pasture contamination when the compost is spread on the pasture.

DEWORMING PRODUCTS

The pressures of urban living have promoted intensive research over the last decade into newer, more efficient, and safer dewormers in the form of pastes, powders, liquids, and pellets. Deworming medications are the other ingredient to a comprehensive parasite management program. In these days of concentrated housing where horses are at continual risk of reinfecting themselves, they should be dewormed at least every 6 to 8 weeks. Deworming at this interval interrupts the damaging life cycle of internal parasites.

Ideally, aggressive deworming programs of monthly treatments between April and October (in average United States climatic conditions) will kill most internal parasites. During the winter, due to dormancy and reduced maturation of worms in the body, deworming every 2 months is usually sufficient (see "recommended Deworming Schedules," p. 468).

Dewormer Classification

There are many anti-parasite products available on the market today for a horse. The objective is to limit the parasite burden of a horse by reducing the number of infective larvae (fig. 15.7). The chemical arsenal revolves around use of different classes of dewormers:

- *Benzimidazoles*: oxibendazole, oxfendazole, mebendazole, fenbendazole, thiabendazole, cambendazole
- *Pyrantel pamoate* (Strongid®), which comes in pellets, pastes, and liquid
- *Avermectins*: ivermectin (Eqvalan® or Zimecterin®) or moxidectin (Quest®)
- *Praziquantel* (targets tapeworms)
- *Organophosphates*: dichlorvos or trichlorfon (targets bots)
- *Piperazine* (only effective against ascarids)
- *Combination products* (such as ivermectin plus praziquantel)

Each drug kills intestinal worms by a different mechanism of action; for example, ivermectin interferes with neuromuscular coordination of the worm, causing a flaccid paralysis. Pyrantel also interferes with neuromuscular activity, but causes a spastic paralysis of the worm. Benzimidazoles interfere with energy metabolism so the worms die of starvation.

Daily Pyrantel Pellets

A formulation of *pyrantel* (Strongid®-C) is available as a pelleted alfalfa feed. A measured volume of these pellets fed each day to a horse kills ingested worm larvae before they reach migratory or invasive stages. Before beginning a course of such treatment, deworm the horse in a standard manner with a paste formula.

Use of this pelleted formulation of dewormer requires conscientious management. Horses on this plan must receive it daily according to manufacturer's recommendations,

INTERNAL PARASITES AND DEWORMER MEDICATION

Internal parasite	Dewormer product	Comments
Small strongyles (Cyathostomes)	Fenbendazole daily for 5 consecutive days or moxidectin	Moxidectin must be given with caution at exact body weight and should not be used in thin or debilitated horses
Large strongyles	Ivermectin or moxidectin or fenbendazole daily for 5 consecutive days	
Ascarids	Ivermectin or moxidectin or fenbendazole daily for 5 consecutive days	Piperazine not as effective as other dewormers listed here
Tapeworms	Praziquantel or pyrantel pamoate	Pyrantel pamoate must be given at double or triple dose to be effective
Bots	Ivermectin	Deworming for bots can be done twice a year, in summer and winter; best results are achieved in midwinter. Use of ivermectin is far safer than using an organophosphate so the latter is not used any more against bots
Lungworms	Ivermectin	
Threadworms (*Strongyloides westeri*)	Fenbendazole daily for 5 consecutive days or oxibendazole or ivermectin or moxidectin	This is particularly important to use in a pregnant mare prior to foaling and to use on mare and foal during lactation
Pinworms	Ivermectin or moxidectin or pyrantel pamoate or oxibendazole or fenbendazole	
Habronema	Ivermectin	Treatment will address skin lesions (summer sores)
Onchocerca cervicalis (see p. 385)	Ivermectin	This only kills microfilaria in the skin and not the adult stages so may need to deworm at regular intervals to eliminate
Eye worms (see p. 376)	Fenbendazole daily for 5 consecutive days	

15.7

or else some larval forms can slip by and invade the deeper tissues or blood vessels. There, they remain unaffected by the daily medication.

An advantage to continual daily feeding of pyrantel pellets is the prevention of intense infection from living in a highly contaminated environment. Overstocked and overgrazed pastures, confinement with horses that receive inadequate deworming, or location on a farm that has previously experienced poor parasite management are high risk factors that create problems for any horse. When feeding daily dewormer, a dose of ivermectin is used midsummer and midwinter to kill bots. There is no reason to use paste dewormers on a regular basis when feeding daily dewormer.

Efficacy of Dewormers

Another important characteristic of dewormers is described as *efficacy*, which is the effectiveness in achieving the desired result (greater than 85 percent kill of a particular parasite). Product labels advise of parasite targets.

RECOMMENDED DEWORMING SCHEDULES

Different climatic conditions dictate how a management program should be approached. For instance, in the northern United States, peak strongyle egg counts occur in the spring and summer with release of larvae from the intestinal walls. There is vast contamination of pastures and corrals at this time of year. Moisture and warm temperatures speed larval development into an infective stage.

Infective larvae are at their peak between April and October when temperatures range between 45 to 100° F (7 to 38° C). They can survive freezing temperatures, emerging in the spring with warmth and moisture.

In southern climates, warm and moist environmental conditions encourage persistent development of infective larvae year-round. Overcrowding or excessively unsanitary conditions may also require the deworming schedule to be increased. Each horse's immune response is different. A sick or unthrifty horse may have trouble ridding his body of parasites even with the aid of dewormers, especially if he is continuously re-exposed to infective larvae in mounds of uncollected manure.

Interval Deworming Strategy

Implementing an *interval* deworming strategy deworms horses at certain intervals throughout the year. In parts of the United States with year-round temperate climates, horses are constantly exposed to parasitic infection. It may be necessary to deworm some horses monthly; at the very least, deworming frequency is administered every 2 months throughout the United States. However, it is possible that horses that are only dewormed bi-monthly sustain migratory damage within intestinal blood vessels, the intestinal wall, liver, or in the lungs despite the absence of egg-laying adults. In warmer climates, more frequent interval deworming (every 30 days) may improve health and performance during active parasite seasons.

Rotation of deworming products allows overlap of strengths of different drug types to make up for weaknesses of other drugs that are less effective against certain parasite species; this reduces the chance that one type of worm builds to extreme proportions. There are three possibilities for rotational deworming:

- No rotation, i.e. continue with the same product year after year
- Slow rotation, i.e. switch drug classes once a year
- Rapid rotation, i.e. switch drug classes every few months

There is controversy over which strategy creates the most likely chance of emergence of resistant strains of parasites. Recent information suggests that a "no-rotational" method such as seen with intense use of ivermectin in sheep is contributing to the emergence of worm species that are becoming resistant to this drug. It would be possible, then, that equine parasite populations may also develop resistance if exposed to only one drug type for prolonged periods, the essence of a "no-rotation" strategy. Also, using only one product for long durations allows the overgrowth of parasites that remain unaffected by a certain drug.

At this time, no conclusions have been reached as to which is better, a slow rotation or a rapid rotation. A debate favoring the "slow rotation" as being better argues that "rapid rotation" encourages simultaneous development of resistance to multiple drugs. However, the general consensus is that some form of rotation is a more reliable treatment strategy for horses than no rotation at all. Of greater importance than which strategy is used to deworm is that of proper dosing, ensuring that a sufficient amount is given and that your horse doesn't spit it out. Underdosing selects for parasitic resistance (see p. 471).

Ivermectin should be incorporated into the program at least twice a year to control bots and migrating large strongyles. Using ivermectin as an exclusive product time after time also has a deleterious impact on the environment as this drug is excreted relatively unchanged in the feces. Ivermectin kills beneficial organisms in the environment that are responsible for cycling soil nutrients and degrading organic materials like manure.

Seasonal Deworming Strategy

Another philosophy recommends a seasonal strategy for deworming in an attempt to cut down costs, particularly in large populations of horses. Use of a seasonal method of deworming attempts to coincide the time of peak egg production with administration of deworming medications so adult parasites are killed prior to contaminating the environment with eggs. This strategy would reduce transmission potential within a herd although not necessarily eliminating parasites entirely from the horse or the environment.

In the frost-belt northern states, peak egg counts occur in spring and summer, so horses should be dewormed every 6 weeks during spring, summer, and fall but not during the winter months. In the southern United States, egg counts peak during autumn and winter, so these would be the seasons to institute parasite control based on a seasonal strategy; deworming would be suspended during the summer. It is thought that intense summer heat may kill larvae since environmental warmth causes them to be quite active with the chance to exhaust their nutrient supply. In hot and dry climates, like the southwestern United States, eggs and larvae are rapidly killed by ultraviolet and drying in a summer environment.

The only problem with a seasonal deworming approach is that it does not address migrational larvae that escape being killed and so remain within a horse, nor does it address larvae that remain dormant in the environment and then suddenly become active. For example, ascarids go dormant if the temperature drops below 50° F (10° C), while still remaining viable. A series of unusually warm days in winter in a northern climate could precipitate reinfection with previously dormant larvae yet no deworming treatment would be administered during this time.

Continuous Feeding Strategy

A different approach to deworming involves daily feeding of products such as Strongid®-C (pyrantel tartrate) to obliterate development of the parasites once the horse ingests the eggs. Strongid®-C kills larvae including large and small strongyles, thereby preventing migration to the intestinal wall where they would mature into egg-laying adults. By stopping damage incurred to the intestinal wall, Strongid®-C minimizes intestinal scarring that may interfere with efficiency in assimilating nutrients. This parasite control measure often improves the vitality of unthrifty horses; with improved feed efficiency, a hard-keeper may put on weight. Also, chronic colic that occurs with larval migration may be averted using continuous feed dewormer. In northern climates, it is especially beneficial to use continuous, daily dewormer during warm, temperate months, namely March through October, when there is the greatest likelihood of transmission. The use of this strategy is effective for individual horses that live in a herd with others that do not receive sufficient deworming treatments.

There is also an argument against the use of this continuous, dewormer strategy: feeding it year-round may reduce a horse's natural immune response by removing larval migration that normally stimulates a horse's immune system. There is also some argument that feeding continuous low-level doses of dewormer may potentially generate drug resistance within a population of parasites. Limiting the number of months a horse is fed daily dewormer to the seasonal time of active parasite transmission addresses these concerns. Not only is the cost of parasite control reduced by feeding the product only 6 to 8 months of the year, but also time off from the dewormer allows horses to experience a relatively minor degree of larval migration sufficient enough to maintain an active immune response.

This strategy is implemented by giving a full dose of dewormer paste the day prior to initiating feeding of the continuous deworming medication. Whether a horse is maintained year-round on daily dewormer or given some months off treatment, it is important to give ivermectin in mid-summer and mid-winter to kill bots and any migrating larvae that may have "slipped" through the cracks, especially if an owner misses a day of medication. In addition to having no effect on bots, pyrantel tartrate will not kill encysted small strongyle larvae. There is thought that it will manage tapeworms to some degree.

ADMINISTERING DEWORMERS

The individual horse, management and hygiene practices, and expertise at handling and restraining a horse determine how consistently a deworming task is performed. The method (paste, drench, oral spray applicator) by which a dewormer is given is not nearly as important as the frequency, the drug used, and the assurance that the entire dose is received. If uncertain, discuss with your veterinarian as to what is best for your horse.

Effective Deworming Technique

Dosage

Effective deworming depends on knowledge of body weight. Read package inserts about the toxic levels particular to a drug. Adjust upward of suspected weight, but stay out of the toxic range. A wide therapeutic index indicates the safety margin that protects a horse from toxic levels, yet is a strong enough dose to kill the parasite. Some products are particularly lenient in the safety margin while others must be administered at an exact, correct dose, particularly for mares and foals. If in doubt, consult a veterinarian about what amount and which product to use.

Paste Dewormers

If a paste dewormer is correctly administered, it is absorbed in the stomach and alters biochemical pathways necessary for parasite survival with no adverse effects on the host horse. There is no reason to deworm on an empty stomach as was done in the old days. In fact, feeding enhances absorption of a drug from the stomach.

When paste is administered, be sure all food is out of the mouth, then place the syringe on the back of the tongue. Hold the horse's head up and gently massage the tongue while depressing the plunger. Paste deworming should be executed with confidence, and with certainty that the horse receives the correct amount of drug. If a horse is particularly fractious, it is best to have your veterinarian perform the necessary task or administer dewormer in the feed.

Powder or Liquid Dewormers

If dewormers are given in powder or liquid form in feed, the total dose must be consumed within eight hours to be effective. It is ineffective if feed spills from a bucket, food is spit or dribbled onto the ground, or if the medication is pushed to the side. Oral medication mixed with molasses or corn syrup into a small amount of grain or bran improves chances of consumption of the entire dose. Watch the horse eat to be confident of success, or aware of failure.

Timing with Feed or Exercise

Administer a paste dewormer when a horse is at rest or completely cooled out following exercise. Best absorption of the product occurs when blood flow to the gut is optimal so it is ill-advised to deworm a horse just prior to or immediately following rigorous exercise. Deworming around feeding time delivers deworming medication to the intestines when blood flow is most active with digestive processes. Today's commercial deworming products are safe and there is no reason to "rest" a horse for days following deworming. Allow a few days following deworming before transporting a horse.

Ineffective Deworming Technique

Deworming failure occurs if an inappropriate dose is given, or if a horse does not actually receive all, or any, of the medication. A common error with paste dewormers occurs when a horse suddenly moves as the plunger is depressed, and part of the medication shoots out of the side of the mouth. Ensure that a horse's mouth is clean at the time of administration so the entire dose is swallowed and none is spit out along with residual feed from his mouth. A drink of water immediately after deworming may cause medication loss.

Although an owner may deworm every two months with an approved product, a horse may still show obvious signs of parasitism: poor hair coat, potbelly, and unthriftiness. A horse may fail to gain weight, or performance may suffer. These problems often disappear within weeks of a proper deworming in which an adequate dose is given and received by the horse.

Irregular Intervals

A problem arises when horses are dewormed at irregular or infrequent intervals and subsequently may have a large parasite load residing in the bowel. Some deworming products (benzimadazoles) kill endoparasites by interfering with energy metabolism to slowly starve the parasite, while others (avermectins) disrupt the nervous control of muscular activity, in effect paralyzing them. With a large load of adult worms in the bowel, there is the potential to develop an impaction as they amass in the gut as they die. In instances where the dewormers kill the parasites rapidly, the possibility exists for an immune reaction to the rapid and massive parasite death. The safest approach to avoid these situations is to implement consistent anti-parasite control management throughout a horse's lifetime: administer dewormer at least every 6 to 8 weeks at the recommended dose per body weight of horse.

Underdosing Causes Drug Resistance

Consistent underdosing can lead to larger problems than not deworming at all. Constant exposure to doses not large enough to kill, but large enough to stress the worm promotes the worm's drug resistance. When finally exposed to adequate levels of a drug, resistance capabilities prevent the worm from dying. Moreover, the parasites pass genetic resistance to larval offspring. Despite deworming, a horse could retain an overwhelming parasite load.

Allergic Reaction

When a horse with an overwhelming infection is dewormed, the destruction and breakdown of the worm expose the horse to foreign proteins. This exposure can result in an allergic reaction, or severe inflammation in the intestine where the parasite attaches, causing edema and thickening of the intestine. These reactions decrease absorption of nutrients and fluids, and may be

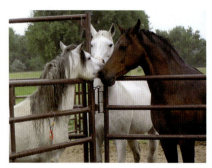

15.8 *Upon introduction of a new horse to a herd following quarantine, the new horse can be located in a paddock with a common fence line to others. This allows the horses to meet over the fence, and to establish a pecking order without the fighting and kicking that can occur with direct contact. Photo: Cathy Bender.*

accompanied by transient diarrhea. An overwhelming parasite infection produces a similar response, resulting in chronic diarrhea or colic.

The Meaning of Stress

Stress is defined as "the adverse effects in the environment or management system, which force changes in an animal's physiology or behavior to avoid physiological malfunction, thus assisting the animal in coping with his environment." So, stress is, in fact, a *normal* response to change. And, a reasonable amount of stress stimulates a horse to respond favorably to changes in routine. The body responds to stress by secreting increased levels of *cortisol* hormones that enable the animal to cope. But as with anything, too much is not a good thing.

Some horses may be emotionally stable, able to cope with new surroundings, showing no signs of stress. However, even an emotionally stable horse that has been hauled a long distance may experience transport stress, making him susceptible to disease (see p. 478). Stress suppresses the immune system, and even a seemingly healthy horse may fall prey to viral attack. Horses that have been shipped on commercial transport vans are particularly susceptible to falling ill after transport; they have been exposed to a diverse array of microorganisms that live in the vans, having been brought there by horses from all over the nation.

Not only does stress create the potential for a horse to become sick, but it also upsets the digestive system potentially leading to diarrhea, dehydration, an impaction, or colic. Also, a new horse often receives a different diet from what he is used to, including a new source of hay and water. Any change in dietary routines predisposes a horse to colic. Isolation of a horse allows monitoring of feed and water intake, frequency of bowel movements, and consistency of manure (see p. 458).

Psychological Stress

HERD INSTINCT

Under natural, free-ranging conditions, horses spend approximately 60 percent of their time grazing, preferably with the herd. Not only does frequent grazing satisfy a physiological need for roughage and a psychological need for chewing fiber, but grazing also involves a fair amount of wandering exercise during the course of a day.

As herd animals, horses enjoy the company of other horses. Grooming behavior, frolic, and play are just a few examples of social interactions between individuals within a herd. Horses like to touch, smell, and taste each other. A pecking order, or social hierarchy, is established through social interplay as each horse assumes a comfortable and secure social position within the herd.

SOCIAL ACCLIMATION

Another element in individual mental health is a horse's establishment of his place within a social hierarchy. Upon introduction of a new horse to a herd following quarantine, the new horse can be moved to his own paddock with a common fence line that is shared with others (photo 15.8). In this way, horses can meet over a fence and establish a pecking order without any horse being cornered, chased, or kicked. Disputes can be worked out over the fence with less risk of injury.

After several days, a new horse may be turned out with others after feeding time. Do this during the daytime when a horse's vision is at its best. Introduce a new horse to the herd when someone will be around to supervise should something go amuck. Make sure the meeting occurs in a large area where the newcomer can find refuge without being trapped in a corner, a loafing shed, or a stall.

A horse might first be turned into a pasture alone to learn location of fences and ditches and obstacles before being chased by others, or walk him around the entire perimeter so he knows the boundaries. It is worth the extra time to walk him around a fence perimeter in both directions to see the boundaries out of "both" eyes. Show him ditches and any other obstacles so he doesn't encounter them unexpectedly while at full gallop. Then add one other horse at a time, so a newcomer can "bond" without interrupting established relationships. These strategies make the transition as easy and as safe as possible.

To reduce feed competition in a herd situation, the use of a nose feedbag containing a specific grain ration allows a horse to eat his specified amount without interference from others. He can take his time chewing, and obtain every morsel. This strategy allows a hard-keeper to remain in a herd without having to separate him for every meal. Horses are happier with companionship and turnout than if confined to a stall or small paddock to eat.

ISOLATION AND CONFINEMENT

Psychological stress is imposed when a horse is removed from social interaction and isolated from others. Physiologic stress also occurs when a horse loses access to grazing and movement by being locked in a box stall. Limited land resources, attendance at horse shows or race events, or layup for an injury often finds horses confined to a small paddock, run, or stall. Stalls are a practical means of housing a large number of horses in a limited space, maximizing use of land and pasture resources. At horse shows and racetracks, a stall is usually the sole facility in which a horse is kept during his stay.

There are other circumstances, other than lack of acreage, which may cause a horse to be confined indoors. Stalls provide shelter from wind and cold, rain, or snow. Stalling a horse out of the sun also prevents sun-bleach of a sleek and lustrous hair coat, giving a competitive advantage in the show ring.

If a horse suffers from a musculoskeletal injury requiring confinement for a lengthy period, a stall is instrumental in ensuring rest. A stall restricts movement, so bandages or limb casts stay clean and dry, hastening the healing process.

Some horses tend to self-destruct if left to run loose in a pasture or paddock. Nervous horses may unceasingly gallop a fence line, risking strain and exhaustion. Mares in heat, or hormone-driven stallions may injure themselves or other horses during disputes across a pasture fence. Individuals that are too aggressive in the herd must be kept separate from other horses. For nervous or combative horses, housing within the quieting confines of a stall may prevent unnecessary mishaps. Dim indoor lighting and seclusion calms belligerent or nervous behavior.

Still other reasons require confinement of horses. A horse requiring a special diet can be fed without competition from a herd. Stalling a mare under lights during late winter or early spring hastens the onset of estrus so she can be bred earlier in the season. A mare due to foal is brought into a large foaling stall to provide a clean and sheltered environment that is easily monitored and safe from predators or dominant herd horses.

A confined horse becomes dependent upon humans for feed, exercise, and companionship.

Food may show up regularly two or more times a day, and in some cases free-choice hay is available at all times. Yet, exercise and human companionship is only forthcoming for an hour or two a day. Too much nutrition can lead to obesity (see p. 350). For horses permanently stalled, 22 to 24 hours a day is a long time in which to do nothing, day after day.

A lucky few have a door or window that opens to the outside, to stick a head out the opening, and look at the world around them. Visual stimuli and sunlight are welcome diversions from overwhelming boredom. Horses provided with free-choice hay have the luxury of fulfilling a ravishing need to chew fiber. Yet, because a horse can only consume around 2 percent of his body weight each day, he can only eat so much before becoming full. There is a lot of time leftover for "hanging out" with no way to vent pent-up energy.

Some stalled horses may have no window or door through which to gaze upon the outside world. Metal bars or mesh fencing may enclose a belligerent horse or a stallion to prevent him hanging his head into the barn aisle. Such horses experience no stimuli, no physical contact, and little or no exercise. Under such conditions, what do horses do?

STEREOTYPIC BEHAVIORS

Not all horses fare well in restrictive confinement. Removing a horse from a natural habitat in which he can roam, graze, and interact within a herd is a notable form of stress. A *stereotypic behavior* is one that develops as a result of stress, often related to confinement. A horse will embark on a repetitive habit that has no functional value to the horse's well-being and such stereotypic behavior is unresponsive to training. Once a behavioral pattern emerges, it is difficult to break the habit. If a problem is recognized in its beginning stages, immediate measures can be taken to alter a horse's environment. Initially, an unhappy horse may exhibit subtle behavioral changes while being saddled or ridden, or he may display uncharacteristic aggressive tendencies toward other horses or people. Ground manners may change, for example a horse may present his rear end as a person enters the stall, or he may lay ears back in agitation. To a sensitive owner, such warning signals may be glaringly obvious, but the reason behind them can remain elusive.

Start by asking what has changed in a horse's routine, including:

- Has the horse been moved from a paddock to a stall?
- Is the horse stalled in a different location from before?
- Has a buddy horse left the premises, or a new arrival moved in to an adjacent area?
- Have new employees assumed cleaning and feeding chores in the barn?
- Have feeding times been changed?
- Is the food quality different?
- Is it breeding season, a time that hormonally alters the behavior of mares and stallions?
- Have exercise levels changed?

If a horse could talk, he might say what is bugging him. In his simple way, a horse communicates distress by body language and mood.

Wood Chewing and Cribbing

Horses have a natural urge to chew. Wood chewers eat the insides of wooden stalls or fence rails in an insatiable demand for fiber. This behavior may also be due to boredom or a lack of minerals. Splinters can lodge in a horse's mouth when he consumes wood. On a rare occasion, a swallowed splinter can lodge in the throat, or irritate or puncture an intestine, with serious consequences. Good quality pasture or access to free-choice hay and salt help prevent wood chewing so a confined horse may need to be turned out.

Boredom may also spur a horse to latch his teeth onto an edge of the stall, a water container, or a feed bucket, contract his neck, pull back, and vocalize with a grunt. This behavior is referred to as *cribbing*. It is speculated that cribbing activates narcotic receptors within the central nervous system, causing an addiction. Wear of the teeth may identify a horse that has been a cribber for a long time: the upper, front incisors are excessively worn (see photos 11.13 A & B in chapter 11, *The Digestive System: The Oral Cavity, Dental Care, and the Intestinal Tract,* p. 289). A cribbing horse may also be a hard keeper because he turns away from food to nurture his habit. Small amounts of hay fed frequently may control cribbing, as might alternative strategies that offer more exercise and/or free time outside.

Cribbing is destructive to a facility, creating wear on fences and objects. It is also likely that other horses housed with a cribber may start the habit, as well. A cribbing strap or a muzzle are devices useful for deterring this behavior. Exercise and turnout are helpful in curbing the habit in its early stages. Electrifying fence lines prevents a horse from using the fences as a cribbing device. Surgery is available, but has inconsistent results.

Abnormal Movement

Other stereotypical vices are based on weird movement behavior, such as pacing, or weaving back and forth while standing in one place, remindful of the rocking motion used to calm an infant. Some horses dig holes of considerable depth in their stalls, while others kick at the walls with front or hind limbs, or both.

Stall-Kicking

A destructive vice is the habit of kicking the sides of a stall or run. Not only does damage to the facility cost money to repair, but a horse can also inflict serious damage upon himself. Splintered wooden walls and doors, doors separated from door posts, bent metal components, and razor sharp edges result from damage to the structural integrity of the stall; these pose hazards to a horse's vulnerable legs and face. Weakening of a wooden structure by continual kicking allows a solid impact to blow it apart, with a limb shooting through splintered wood. Serious lacerations can result.

Limb trauma related to kicking or pawing at walls can strain or sprain ligaments, tendons, or muscles. Areas like the front of the carpus (knee), fetlock, or back of the hock are particularly vulnerable to bruising and abrasion. *Capped hocks* or *hygromas* of the carpus (see p. 114) are caused by continuous trauma to bursal sacs underlying superficial tendons. Such blemishes are usually only of cosmetic significance, but if repeatedly aggravated, can develop into functional problems to impede performance.

Bruised muscle or connective tissue may develop serum or blood pockets, or an overwhelming inflammatory response known as *cellulitis*, which is accompanied by intense pain and swelling in the affected limb (see p. 438). Powerful impacts to the bottom of a foot as a horse kicks at a rigid wall can injure the coffin bone inside the hoof, even to the point of fracture.

Anxiety and Frustration

Frustration at restriction of movement creates anxiety, leading to displacement activities like pawing and kicking. Transfer of pent-up energy also assumes the form of kicking or striking out at confining walls. If a horse sees other horses running at play, frustration intensifies because the horse cannot join the frolicking herd.

Feeding Time

Some horses anticipate arrival of breakfast or dinner as soon as the feeding person is spotted near the barn. A horse displays an eager appetite by striking on a wall or door with his leg. What may start out as a small signal of impatience can escalate into an irrepressible habit.

Horses fed concentrated feed pellets as a substitution for hay spend less than an hour or two a day eating the entire daily quota. In a range habitat, a horse grazes intermittently for about 16 hours a day; feeding habits of a stalled horse on a pelleted diet contrast greatly. Boredom may be expressed initially as banging on the sides of the stall to get attention, or simply to have something to do. This type of problem may be resolved by feeding grass hay to accommodate a need to chew roughage throughout the day.

Space and Relationships

Some horses are territorial about their space, and may be particular about an adjacent neighbor. Once pleasant relationships are established between horses, try to house them side by side. Keeping buddies in sight of each other reduces stress. Although they are unable to make physical contact, the visible presence of a buddy has a strong calming influence.

Isolation Stress

Horses thrive with physical contact. A companionable horse that cannot nuzzle or smell a neighbor through a door or over a partition may strike at the walls in frustration. Isolation for a normally social animal is a cause of anxiety. Individuals craving contact or companionship may relax with the introduction of a goat or chicken that lives in the stall with the horse. Herd relationships and bonding are established between a horse and any living creature. All it takes is a little imagination, and finding a suitable animal.

Loners

Certain horses prefer to live by themselves, perhaps because that is how they were raised and they are used to it. If an adjacent horse reaches toward the stall of a "loner," the loner horse may feel his space has been violated. In frustration and territorial intent, a loner horse kicks and strikes at an offending neighbor even if a friendly horse only glances his way.

New Surroundings

If a horse is moved to a new barn or is stabled at horse shows, not only are the surroundings new and different, but so are the other horses housed next to and across from him. Not all horse personalities get along in enforced conditions, and the only separation may be a wooden partition with mesh fencing at the top. Feeling trapped and enclosed, a horse exhibits stress by striking at or kicking out at a neighbor. Walls of the stall take the brunt of the blows, but this activity may be the start of a persistent habit when a horse returns home.

Mares in heat, or stallions stalled next to stallions or cycling mares may pound on the walls from a breeding-related or physical dispute.

Protection for Stall Kickers

Boots and Padding

Methods to protect a horse from wreaking physical self-damage from stall-kicking include armoring him with hock boots, fetlock boots, shin boots, or knee pads to protect these areas from trauma. Vinyl-covered foam padding on walls and doors reduces abrasions and trauma caused by striking a surface. Continual upkeep of padding is time-consuming and costly. Lining a stall with straw bales reduces the impact of hoof blows, but further limits the internal space within a stall, increasing a sense of claustrophobia and restriction of movement.

Kick Chains

Sometimes success is achieved by applying kick chains to a hind leg so that every time a horse attempts to kick, he gets whacked in the leg by the chain. This terminates that particular behavior in many cases.

RELIEF FROM BOREDOM

Toys
Toys in a stall relieve boredom and help prevent many stall-related, stereotypic behaviors. Rubber or plastic balls hanging from the rafters give a horse something to bang or chew on without risk of injury. Gallon water jugs or commercially available hanging plastic "apples" and "carrots" also serve as playthings for bored or restless horses.

Self-Exercise
Pacing, weaving, kicking, and pawing are all manifestations of a need to move. A horse that is stalled for most of the day should be allowed daily self-exercise in a large turnout area or paddock. If turnout is not an option, then a stalled horse should be put on a "hot-walker" or hand-walked for at least an hour per day. Stopping to allow grazing of fresh grass is also a mental benefit.

Performance Exercise
A performance horse should be conditioned appropriately for his particular event. However, calm, easy riding substituted periodically for intense training relieves stress. A horse that associates riding with mental and/or physical pressure is likely to manifest his stress in odd ways, sometimes in a behavioral and sometimes in a disease state.

CHANGING THE ENVIRONMENT

Outdoor Stabling
Along with exercise, perhaps the best cure for an anxious horse exhibiting stress or stall-related stereotypic behavior is to move him outdoors. If possible, enlarge the spatial dimensions of an outdoor paddock relative to the previous size of his stall. Outside fence panels are used to restrict the area of movement if a horse is recuperating from an injury. Fresh air and sunshine, long-distance views, and seeing other horses significantly calm a horse. Removing the restrictive walls of a stall also removes a rigid surface for a horse to kick.

Adjusting for Personality Conflicts
A horse's anxieties can be further reduced by recognition of personality conflicts between horses, and physically relocating horses until proper relationships are established. It is also important to monitor how stable employees interact with a horse. This interaction may be difficult to evaluate unless a trainer arrives unannounced at the barn in time to watch reactions from the relationship. A horse may dislike a specific handler, groom, feed personnel, or helper. Anticipation at having to interact with a disliked person adds to a horse's stress level, with abnormal behaviors surfacing from underlying tension.

Changing Handlers or Location
If a previously well-adjusted horse starts demonstrating stereotypic or adverse behaviors, it may be time to consider changing handlers or location. Possibly there is no specific reason for a horse's neurotic behavior other than a dislike of the surroundings or discomfort with a farm's routine. Before entirely moving a horse off the property, it is worthwhile to move a distressed horse to different spots on a property in an attempt to rule out certain neighboring animals, visual stimuli, noises, and physical locations.

Sometimes, no matter where a horse is located on a particular farm, he remains stressed and unhappy. As soon as he is moved to a different facility, or to a new geographical location, he resumes the calm and quiet behavior for which he is known. Many of us can commiserate with specific geographical preferences, having encountered an uncomfortable situation at one time or another. People exhibit spatial preferences; some people elect to sit on an aisle or in the back of a crowded auditorium, while others thrive in a crowd. In working environments, some people prefer a secluded cubbyhole, while others desire to be in the middle of the hubbub.

Horses are no different in seeking spatial arrangements to suit individual temperaments. Yet, their choices are limited by human arrangements of a limited land resource. By eliminating a natural, free-ranging habitat, people remove a horse's ability to seek his place in a geographical and social context. Placing walls around his restless spirit, and curbing his eating behavior to suit human schedules reshape a horse's mental and physical state into something different from his natural predisposition.

Even within a restricted urban environment, horse owners should listen to the messages a horse conveys through his manners and actions. Fine-tuning an environment and eliminating stresses channel a horse's energies into more useful applications than stereotypic behaviors. Powers of concentration and learning abilities are improved in a happy horse, enabling him to give splendidly in athletic performance.

Transport Stress

One of the many givens in sport horse performance is that a horse will have to travel a distance to an event, sometimes for many days across the country in a horse trailer or van, or by air to an overseas event. The stress of such transport has far-reaching effects on many systems of the horse's body, most notably the immune and endocrine systems.

There are two features that should be considered when evaluating the risk factors associated with transporting a horse to and from an event. One is the effect that transport will have on performance once the horse has arrived at the event, while the other is the probability of developing respiratory disease (*shipping fever*) or colic. A multitude of transport stress studies have given a fair glimpse into the cumulative effects of horse transport. It is thought that transport in a horse trailer is equivalent to a horse walking for the duration of the trip. Studies have delved into the abilities of a horse to cope and how body changes related to stress affect an ability to perform.

Environmental Stress

Besides being removed from his familiar environment and friends back on the farm, a traveling horse withstands a barrage of new and different stimuli. Environmental considerations that take their toll on a horse in the trailer or van during traveling include the following (photo 15.9):

- Air quality
- Ambient temperature
- Ventilation
- Head position
- Noise
- Vibration and oscillation
- Body orientation

AMBIENT TEMPERATURE

In a perfect equine world, the ambient temperature ranges between 30 to 75° F (-1 to 24° C) and the air is still. During some long-distance transport situations, the temperature may fall below 30° F (-1° C). Then, the food energy consumed must be reassigned to produce additional metabolic heat to help a horse maintain his body temperature. For every 10° F (1.5° C) drop in environmental temperature, a horse needs 15 to 20 percent more calories. If a horse is clipped, or is unable to find shelter from wind or rain, his caloric requirements many increase by as much as 80 percent. This isn't likely to be the kind of weather a horse experiences inside a trailer, but it may well be what is encountered upon arrival at his destination. Such chilling temperatures may be a departure from the environment created inside the walls of the horse trailer.

During summer travel, heat is likely to be the more concerning feature of the environment. As so often occurs within a closed horse trailer, ambient temperature elevates between 75 to 90° F (24 to 32° C). Inside the trailer, the ambient temperature may be at least 10 to 15° F (6 to 9° C) greater than the outside temperature, thus subjecting a horse to significant heat stress. This heat, especially in the presence of high humidity, causes a horse to sweat. The respiratory rate may elevate to help rid the body of heat. Appetite diminishes, while the need for water increases. With this in mind, water should be offered every 4 to 6 hours during transport. When possible, driving should be done at night during adverse summer weather conditions.

AIR QUALITY

Since the state of the respiratory tract has a lot to do with how well a horse is able to perform, it is noteworthy that long-distance transport may exert deleterious effects on the respiratory tract (see chapter 10, *Respiratory Conditioning and Health*, p. 258). Numerous studies have indicated that the longer a horse spends in transport, the greater risk he has for developing a respiratory infection. This is a result of many variables.

Irritants to the Respiratory Lining

With increased travel time, levels of ammonia from urine and fecal accumulation markedly increase. Exhaust fumes from the truck may accumulate within the trailer if not vented in the correct direction. Similarly, the numbers of

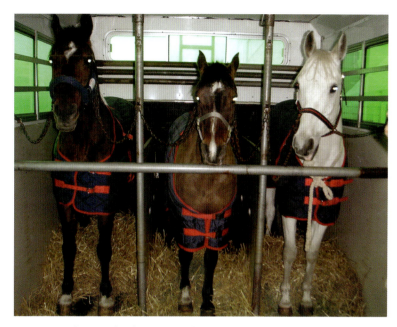

15.9 *Long distance hauling, particularly when there are several horses on the trailer, promotes an environment rich in bacteria, fungi, and ammonia fumes, all of which create significant health challenges to the respiratory system and immune function. The tight quarters, as seen here with several horses in a small space, amplifies these environmental challenges. Urine and manure excretions stirred up by moving feet contribute to airway irritation.*

bacteria and fungal spores increase. The more horses in the trailer, the greater these risk factors become because of more shared air, greater urine and fecal output, and more airborne particulates suspended in the breathed air.

While all these factors cause air quality to deteriorate over time within the trailer, they additionally deter normal clearance mechanisms within the trachea and lungs, particularly that of the *mucociliary escalator* lining the upper airways (see p. 255). This "escalator" is important for cleansing the lungs of foreign debris and microorganisms. The airways are lined with tiny cilia, like moving "hairs," that "sweep" debris and foreign matter out of the airways. Normal secretion of a mucous coating keeps the airways moist, and binds debris as it is moved upward and out of the airways. The horse then swallows this material or coughs it out to cleanse large numbers of particles from the lower airways. If the mucociliary escalator is not at optimal function, then the airways are at risk for invasion by naturally occurring opportunists in the pharynx, and in particular *Streptoccocus zooepidemicus*. Bacteria that seed the lungs may originate from common residents in the pharynx and tonsils. Poor air quality contributes to debilitating a horse's natural defense mechanisms against invasion by bacteria, molds, or viruses. The deeper the bacteria are allowed to invade into the respiratory tract, the greater the risk in developing disease.

Over 52 percent of *shipping fever* related illness, such as *pleuropneumonia*, becomes apparent after a horse arrives at his destination. High temperature and humidity promote bacterial and fungal growth, increasing exposure of the lungs to microbes. Coupling these factors with a suppressed immune system due to stress develops a situation ripe for disease, particularly of the respiratory tract.

Decreased Humidity

Under certain weather conditions, transport over long periods may be associated with decreased humidity within the trailer thus drying out the mucous lining of the airways; the mucociliary escalator is further assaulted and injured from doing its protective job. In addition, under normal circumstances lung *macrophages* (a form of white blood cell) control bacterial invasion by binding and then ingesting the invader. Cortisol hormones, which are released in times of stress, not only negatively influence the entire immune system of the horse, but also directly and adversely affect the functional response of macrophages to defeat bacteria. This has important ramifications if a horse with a pre-existing respiratory condition is hauled a distance to an event.

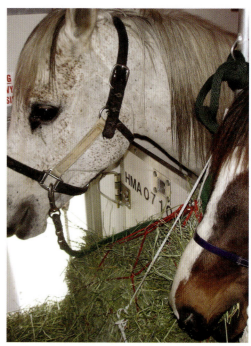

15.10 *While in a trailer, a horse's head is in an upright position that precludes clearance of debris from the airways. Particulate matter and dust from hay contribute to airway irritation. As these horses pull hay from the hay net, dust litters the air directly in front of their faces, causing them to inhale debris.*

Head Position

Most horses are tied in a trailer or are positioned such that the head is restrained in an upright position (photo 15.10). For respiratory-tract clearance, horses should not be tied with their heads up high. An elevated head position negatively affects the mucociliary clearance within the trachea. With this in mind, it is important to unload a horse at rest stops so he can drop his head down to drain any accumulated material from the airways.

Hay bags can be hung so a horse lowers his head to feed, allowing small particles to fall downward, away from his airways. Common sense dictates that hay bags or nets not be hung so low that he can entangle a leg.

Dust-Free Feed

Mangers in the trailer should be cleaned of stale hay and dust, and resupplied with fresh, non-dusty hay. Providing vacuum-cleaned hay further decreases fungal spores circulating in a trailer. Feeding hay in the trailer has been implicated in adding to airborne particulate matter that assaults the airways. Hay in the manger or hay hung in a net may shower the lungs with dust, mold spores, and bacteria. Wetting the hay may limit these particles to a more reasonable level.

Bedding

Bedding the trailer with straw significantly increases the risk factors of poor quality air in a trailer. Straw contains abundant mold spores and bacteria, so it is better to use paper or wood shavings.

Ventilation

An excellent strategy to combat climbing levels of airborne pathogens within a trailer is to promptly clean the trailer floor of manure and urine-soaked bedding at each rest stop. In addition, open the rear doors of the trailer to gain greater ventilation than achieved with only opening windows and vents. Any technique that encourages free flow of air through the trailer is an advantage to a traveling horse.

Avoid long delays at international border crossings, ferry connections, or at refueling stops. The longer a horse is kept in a small, enclosed space with limited air circulation, the more the temperature and humidity rise, and the greater the exposure to microorganisms that challenge the respiratory tract.

IMMUNE FUNCTION

Not only does air quality have an effect on a horse's ability to stave off disease, but also his current vaccination status is important in the face of long-distance transport. Whether he encounters new horses in the trailer or upon arrival at an event, such mixing of horses from other areas increases the likelihood of exposure to unfamiliar viral strains. Others may carry and shed disease although not being overtly sick themselves. Damage incurred to the airways during transport, as well as the current vaccine status of each horse will influence the probability of contracting disease. Compromising the immune system by increased bacterial numbers, reduced lung clearance mechanisms, increased levels of circulating cortisol, and exhaust fumes and ammonia elevations within the trailer have a combined effect on the overall immune function of a traveling horse. It is known that diminished immune function persists for one week following transport of 36 hours.

Immune Suppression of Cortisol

Increased production of steroid hormones, like cortisol, is a common response to fear or stress. However, cortisol has an adverse impact on the immune system. During a short trip, the cortisol response is minimal, but cortisol levels rise with longer transport, because of increased stress. Transportation within a short distance causes little change in a horse's immune status; when horses travel long distances, the immune system is compromised.

Cortisol reaches its peak within the first 5 hours of transport, with cortisol levels declining during later travel hours. This suggests that either horses become accustomed to the sensation of movement and noise, or they exhaust their hormonal supply so that less cortisol is released into the bloodstream. Onset of disease seems to correlate with what might be interpreted as a "failure to adapt" to transport. Horses that develop a fever have a corresponding increase in concentration of cortisol hormones in the blood. As long ago as 1917 it was recognized in army remount horses that rectal temperature should be monitored twice a day, before, during, and following transport. This remains a sound management practice.

Respiratory disease is associated with two prior events: 1) prolonged transport; and 2) strenuous exercise. Both these situations result in an increase release of cortisol in the horse. The longer the transport duration, the greater the risk of developing associated disease. Travel times of distances that require less than 12 hours to traverse greatly reduce the probability of developing transport-associated respiratory disease.

Studies have suggested that the use of vitamin C supplementation during and following transport may improve a horse's immune function. Recommendations propose feeding 5 to 10 grams twice daily of ascorbic acid (commercially available in powder form), and also supplementing with B vitamins (found in 1 to 2 tablespoons per day of Brewer's yeast) and adding 4000 to 6000 international units (IU) of vitamin E (commercially available in powder form) per day during travel.

Unnecessary Antibiotics

It used to be standard practice to give a horse a one-time injection of procaine penicillin just before shipping. This practice encourages development of bacterial resistance to antibiotics. A single injection does not instill a high blood level of antibiotic, nor does it persist long enough to effectively kill bacteria. There is no value in a single injection, and this practice should be discontinued.

Resist the impulse to start a horse on a preventive course of antibiotics before long-distance travel. The problem that most commonly confronts traveling horses stems from respiratory viruses for which there are no direct treatments. Once a viral infection is identified and diagnosed, a course of antibiotics may prevent bacterial infections that lead to pneumonia.

BEHAVIORAL ADAPTATIONS

In addition to the environmental features a horse encounters in his transport environment, other individualized responses to transport stress dictate how easy or how difficult it will be for a horse to adapt to his experience. Some horses experience anxiety with hauling, and this exacerbates the expenditure of energy. Others are herd-bound and do not do well with social isolation. A travel companion can offset this level of anxiety.

Companionship

A horse might settle into a better routine if accompanied by a calm equine companion that is experienced in such trips. The more times a horse undergoes an experience, provided he has not been alarmed or frightened, the more he becomes conditioned to traveling, and the less stress response he feels or exhibits. The immune system functions more efficiently, and is more capable of warding off the challenge of infection.

Effect of Driver Skills

The skill of the driver has a lot to do with how well a horse will weather the stress of hauling. Sudden starts and stops, abrupt turns, ever-changing acceleration and deceleration puts an added load on any horse traveling in the back of the trailer. These may seem like minor inconsistencies but when added up over the course of many hours of driving will have a great impact on the accumulated fatigue the horse may feel.

Vehicle Vibration

Most hauling vehicles have vibrations that exceed allowable vehicle vibrations for humans. This amplifies muscular fatigue required for balancing and counteracting the acceleration and deceleration. Traveling on freeways imposes the least vibration or oscillation on a horse, while using secondary roads imposes the most. Thick bedding and mats on the trailer floor help to slightly diminish road vibration and heat. Measures of heart rate and respiratory rate while a trailer is in motion suggest that vibrations and oscillations are significant stressors to a horse. These can be addressed by ensuring the best in trailer suspension equipment, using quality tires properly sized for the hauling vehicle, and by applying careful driving techniques. Riding in the back of a horse trailer allows one to appreciate how madly fatiguing it can be for long periods of time, particularly with a poor driver at the wheel.

Body Orientation

Muscular effort is required to retain balance while in motion. On journeys farther than 20 miles, analysis of blood samples shows an increase in muscle enzymes, reflecting the physical work that is required by a horse to maintain balance. Many studies have been done to evaluate the effect of body orientation as a stressor of the horse. The conclusion is that whether a horse faces forward or backward is not as profound an effect as once believed. Given a choice, most horses choose to face backward while in motion, but then turn frontward when the trailer has stopped or as it makes sharp turns. Nonetheless, body orientation is not a significant stressor, and most horses deal with whichever position they must travel with little concern.

MUSCULAR FATIGUE

A horse hauled in a trailer experiences the same degree of muscular work as he would if he had walked the distance. It makes sense, then, that attendant muscle fatigue will have a great impact on athletic performance. It is a good idea to stop frequently at rest areas, let the horse out to move around a bit, get some fresh air, and to put his head down to clear his airways. He'll be more comfortable urinating on still ground. He'll be more likely to take a good long drink of fresh, cool water when he can get his head down into a bucket. A horse can be seen to visibly relax as he puts his feet on solid ground for even a brief time. If nothing else, stop the trailer, open the back doors for ventilation, and take a 10 or 15 minute rest break every 4 hours or so. While on the road and once you have arrived at the destination, carefully monitor each horse's attitude, degree of mental calm, appetite, thirst, urination, and manure output.

PARTICULAR STRESS FEATURES OF A TRAVELING HORSE

As horses cross time zones on their travels, it is possible they experience upsets to their circadian rhythms much as people experience jet lag. Routines are changed; daily activity has little familiarity to normal. This creates an added stress on a horse. Appetite diminishes, leading to reduction in energy intake. In addition, horses traveling for 24 hours on the road in hot conditions decrease water intake by as much as 50 percent of normal despite being unloaded and offered water at 4-hour intervals. In one study, horses traveling 300 miles suffered 3 percent dehydration by the time of arrival at their destination.

Body Weight

Body weight is one determining value of how dehydrated a horse may be, but it must be taken into account that with diminished appetite there will be less intestinal fill (and weight) that compounds the body-weight loss. After 24 hours of transport, one study indicated the horses lost 6 percent of their body weight. Within 3 hours following rest and access to free-choice water, body-weight losses were only decreased by 2.4 percent. Yet at 24 hours following transport and recovery, body weight was still 3 percent (33 pounds) less than weight prior to transit. These results are similar to 4 percent body-weight losses found in horses transported commercially to slaughter after hauling 6 to 30 hours during summer conditions.

Dehydration Effects of Travel

Comparison of travel times and relative weight loss of a horse revealed the following:

Travel Time (hours)	Weight Loss (%)
2.5	1.1 – 1.6
4.5 – 6.5	1.0 – 1.9
41	3.5
60	5.2

On average, horses transported long distances will lose approximately 0.5 percent body weight per hour. This is a combination of food and water losses. It is known that even mild dehydration of 2 to 3 percent will affect performance. Horses that have lost 2½ percent of their body weight post-transit often do not recover until 2 to 3 days following transport. This has overwhelming repercussions for a competition horse, particularly one engaged in protracted exercise. If arriving at an event on the eve of a competition, there aren't many hours to rest tired muscles and replenish food and water deficits.

Horses that develop shipping fever lose about 51 pounds in transit. The correlation of weight loss with development of infection is significant. Weighing horses before and after a long trip is useful for deciding if preventive care should be initiated.

Heart Rate as Stress Indicator

Examination of the degree of stress a horse undergoes with transport uses heart rate and plasma cortisol concentrations as useful indices of stress. Heart rate elevates with stress or anxiety, pain, or illness (see "Normal Physiological Parameters," *Appendix A*, p. 567).

White Blood Cell Count

White blood cell counts are elevated after the first 3 hours of transport and remain elevated after a 24-hour recovery period. Study results (A.V. Rodier and C.L. Stull, University of California, Davis) demonstrate that "commercial transportation under hot environmental conditions elicits responses indicative of dehydration, muscle metabolism alterations, and possibly immune system compromise. While the responses of dehydration and muscle indices showed significant elevations with transportation, these parameters declined to pre-transit levels within 24 hours. However, the effects of cortisol may have affected energy metabolism and the immune system with elevated responses of white blood cells and glucose after 24 hours of recovery. This indicated that full recovery was not completed after 24 hours, thus the horse may be susceptible to disease challenges, and energy availability for performance may be altered."

Biorhythm

Studies in humans suggest that athletic exercise performed at an optimal time of day for that individual may improve performance by as much as 10 percent. In later afternoon, body temperature is higher and so muscle and joint flexibility are improved, as is nerve conduction velocity. On the other side of the coin when trying to relate this human response to horses, higher body temperature at that time of day may make a horse less tolerant of environmental heat stress.

Protective Bandages

SHIPPING BOOTS

Leg wraps and shipping equipment are useful to protect against trailer-inflicted injuries. No matter how well a horse loads or rides, accidents can happen. A scrambling, adjacent horse could step on a horse, or a horse can inflict self-injury in the trailer. Loading and unloading is the most dangerous time for legs. Trailer wraps provide a barrier between metal and flesh, and ground and flesh, particularly for a fractious, resistant horse. Ramps, or damp footing also create peril for legs; shipping boots provide limb protection (photo 15.11).

Shipping boots should cover the heel bulbs and pasterns, as well as the cannon bone region. Commercial, fleece-lined shipping boots with Velcro closures take only moments to apply. Cotton quilting, disposable diapers, or cotton pads are also useful when secured with polo wraps, track bandages, or ace bandages applied with correct tension.

HEAD BUMPER AND TAIL WRAP

A head bumper protects the poll of a fractious horse in case he rears up and hits his head on the edge or top of the trailer.

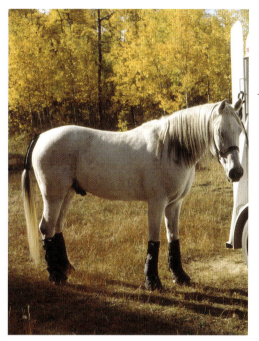

15.11 *The use of commercial shipping boots is a smart strategy to protect a horse's lower limbs from injury.*

A tail wrap or commercial neoprene tail bandage prevents abrasion at the dock of the tail. Another way to protect the tail from rubbing on the door or butt bar is to secure thick foam padding over the butt chain. Place a horse's tail inside the trailer so it is not hanging loose where it could hook on a protrusion, frightening and seriously injuring a horse.

The Eyes: A Horse's View of the World 16

Mental Perception

A horse's mental perception of the world around him and his responses to his environment have everything to do with optimal performance. "Mental conditioning" encompasses a feeling of trust between horse and rider, and this trust is built upon time and experience. As a horse moves under saddle, a rider has to trust that the horse won't suddenly leap out from beneath him, or bolt, buck, spin, or rear due to behavioral or fear factors. When a horse is asked to negotiate an obstacle or a tricky patch of ground, he should do what is asked at the moment asked. This willingness to obey relies a lot on a horse's trust in the rider as well as his mental perception of potential safety or danger. A horse may refuse to do a requested task because of lack of skill and confidence, but there are times when a rider just isn't clear about how a horse perceives the terrain or situation surrounding him. A rider might give mixed messages to a mount, and so a horse performs badly.

Similarly, a rider might request a horse to maneuver in a tricky situation. To the rider, the exercise may seem obvious and straightforward, but given the limitations of equine vision an obstacle may appear to the horse as a trap. This misunderstanding makes the situation potentially dangerous for both horse and rider. Often, the best way out of an untenable situation is to give a horse freedom of his head and body to negotiate what only he can feel beneath his feet. Putting him into dangerous positions with no options is self-defeating to both horse and rider. A horse may extract himself from that position by sheer will and determination, but in the process, the rider loses a measure of a horse's trust. A horse that says, "No, this isn't safe so consider another option, please" is one to respect. A dangerous horse may be one that "obediently" saunters into no-man's-land on blind faith. All does not appear equal in the eyes of the beholder, considering the differences between horse and human perceptions.

Spooky Behavior

How many times have you chided a horse for spooking at an innocuous rock, or for balking at an obstacle for no apparent reason? A horse exhibits such behaviors for the same reasons that he startles when someone walks quietly up behind him in the field and he doesn't notice until the last moment. Just as it seems his fleeing form will vanish to the far end of the pasture, he turns, blows, and stares from

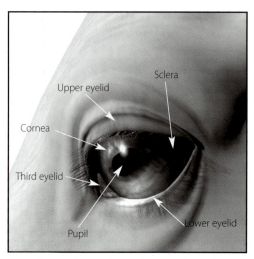

16.1 *External anatomy of the eye.*

Anatomy and Function of the Equine Eye

To understand the differences between the world as seen by humans, and the world that a horse sees requires a view of the way the brain acquires the input of images, and how the eye gathers light (figs. 16.1 and 16.2).

Pupil

Muscles that control the opening of the *pupil* respond involuntarily to the intensity of light passing through the eye. Like a diaphragm in a camera lens, the pupil dilates to allow maximum entry of light in dim conditions, and contracts to exclude excess brightness that may injure retinal-photoreceptor tissue in the back of the eye. An equine pupil is able to dilate more than six times that of a human in dim light.

Corpora Nigra

At the top surface of the *uveal* tissues that comprise the pupil, lie structures called the *corpora nigra*. These are visible as a couple of globular, darkly pigmented bodies located at the uppermost border of the pupil (photo 16.3). By protruding over the pupil when it is constricted in bright light conditions, corpora nigra assist in further occluding the central area of the pupil, acting like a "visor" to reduce glare in bright-light conditions.

The corpora nigra are normal structures in all horse eyes. Should corpora nigra develop to an excessively large size, they could interfere with a horse's vision when the pupil is contracted in bright sunlight. Although this is an uncommon problem, it could compromise a horse's field of vision, causing a horse to display shying behavior.

a safe distance, smelling and looking to see what monster alarmed him.

Animal behavior is predicated upon how they view the world, which senses are most operational, along with experiences gained through a lifetime. As humans peering out at the world around us, we take a lot for granted. Even people who need glasses to correct eyesight visually enjoy a world of fantastic depth and complexity. While standing on a mountain peak casting a gaze into an endless valley, a human can pick out objects far in the distance and visually resolve them into a definite form.

Human eyes are set close together centrally on the head. This allows for *binocular vision*: images from each eye superimpose perfectly on one another. This "message" is relayed to the brain so that the information is not interpreted as confusing double-vision. As riders upon a horse's back, the entire world around us is perceived as a clear picture, with objects assuming definite form and sense. What is it that a horse sees that causes him to swivel his neck and head in question, or to spook at fantasy monsters?

Retina

As light rays pass through the eye, they converge on the back of the eye on the *retina*, a light-sensitive tissue that converts light rays into nerve impulses and relays these to the brain through the optic nerve. Nerve receptors (*rods* and *cones*) comprising the retina are stimulated by light. Rods are most used for dim light conditions, while cones are mostly activated by bright light. A horse has nine to twenty times more rods than humans, allowing him to see far better than humans in dim light.

Tapetum

The retina, as a transparent surface, loses some light absorption as it passes through the eye. Lost light is incapable of stimulating the retina. Many animals have a physiologic mechanism to reflect "lost" light back to retinal receptors. Such ability relies on a hyper-reflective surface called the *tapetum lucidum*. Any light the retina does not recapture from tapetal reflection passes out of the eye. This is seen to us as the familiar bright eye glow of cats or deer as their eyes light up in a car's headlights at night. Illuminating a horse's eyes at night with a flashlight also produces a tapetal reflection.

By providing a second pass at photoreceptors of the retina, the tapetum achieves better vision for a horse in dim light. However, the tapetum also scatters some of the light, thereby reducing a horse's visual acuity.

Cornea and Lens

For light to reach the retina, it must pass through the foremost portions of the eye, including the *cornea* and the *lens*. As light travels through a homogeneous medium like air, light rays travel in a straight line at a uniform velocity. If light rays fall on a different medium, like water or the lens of the eye,

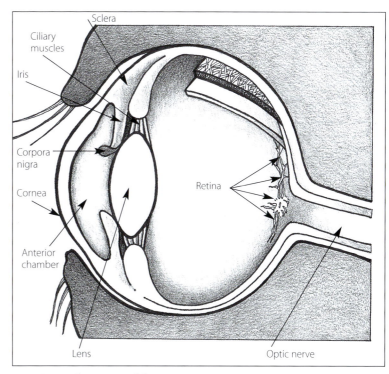

16.2 *Internal anatomy of the eye.*

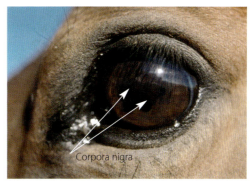

16.3 *The corpora nigra are normal structures in a horse's eyes, and are visible as globular, darkly pigmented bodies at the upper edge of the pupil.*

some light rays are reflected while other rays travel in a different direction and at a different velocity through the second medium. This is called *refraction*. It is the phenomenon experienced when viewing fish under water. The denser the medium, the more the light is bent and slowed, giving it a greater *index of refraction* than what is seen in a rarer (thinner) medium. With aging of the human eye, for example, the crystalline lens loses its resiliency and becomes denser.

As light passes through an eye, the biconvex surface of the transparent lens converges refracted rays to a point beyond. What the retina receives is information that produces a blurred impression of the image. The human lens changes its shape to appropriately bend the light rays to "focus" them into a sharp image. *Ciliary muscles* attaching to the lens capsule with *suspensory ligaments* achieve subtle alterations in lens thickness. Contraction of ciliary muscles releases tension on the suspensory ligaments; the lens thickens and changes focus for close vision. Relaxation of the muscle fibers enhances distant vision.

Such a phenomenon in people is called *accommodation*, or the ability to view objects at different distances with equal clarity. Humans are able to accommodate and focus on objects without moving the head. With aging, the suspensory ligaments are less responsive so bifocal glasses are needed for humans to accommodate near and far. For horses, the lens does not change shape as generously as it does in other species, but a horse is endowed with a long, flexible neck that elevates, lowers, or rotates the head for rapid focus adjustment of the eyes.

In people and most mammals, the retina that captures focused light has a uniform concave curve; light passed to it is received at similar focal lengths across the retina. Research (Australia) has discovered that a horse's retina is the same distance from the lens in all areas except the peripheral regions where the retina is closer to the lens. An area of the retina referred to as the *visual streak* enables a horse to see a narrow but clear panoramic view.

Third Eyelid

Horses have an additional protective barrier, the *third eyelid*, which passively sweeps across the eye like a squeegee to remove debris. It is also called the *nictitating membrane*. When the eye is open, this membrane is retracted back into the inner corner of the eye, its leading edge barely visible. Non-pigmented nictitating membranes are susceptible to *squamous cell carcinoma* (see p. 399).

A Horse's Focus and Perception

A horse raises his head to best focus on far away objects. By lowering the head, nearby objects are better focused. With each change in head position, the focal length of a horse's eyes is adjusted to form a sharp picture on the retina.

A horse's eyes are set on the sides of his head, allowing him to experience a more panoramic view than people (fig. 16.4). Each eye sees separate things at the same time. The panoramic field of a horse encompasses 330 to 350 degrees. (A cat only enjoys a panoramic view of 5 to 20 degrees because his eyes are centrally located on his face.) With very slight movements of the head, a horse is able to see just about everything around him, except for an area directly behind him that is obscured by his hindquarters. So, when negotiating obstacles, a rock, bush, or tree located directly behind a horse is invisible.

A horse's binocular field of view is limited to between 30 and 70 degrees, providing him with very poor depth perception or evaluation of position. The best binocular field for a horse is viewed down his nose rather than straight ahead. With head down, the binocular field is aimed toward the ground for grazing while the monocular fields from each single eye are able to scan the sideways environment in search of danger. When a horse raises his head with nose pointing forward, both eyes are used to scan the horizon, giving the horse the best possible binocular field. With head raised, lateral vision is at a minimum, but in this position, a horse sees well in front of himself and blind spots are eliminated. Elevation of the head enables a horse to focus on something that startles him or that poses a perceived danger.

One blind spot of a horse lies directly in front of him, encompassing an area comparable to the width of a horse. When a horse is "on the bit" with his head and nose in a vertical position, he is unable to see what is directly in front of him. Such a head position requires a horse to rely fully on his rider for navigation. When ridden in collected gaits, a horse's head is held in a stationary position and in a more erect manner than a horse would carry it, if given normal freedom. In the dressage arena or when showing in equitation classes, a lack of panoramic perception does not compromise a horse's safety, especially when rails or walls confine the limits of a horse's athletic world. Yet with head and neck so restricted, a horse may have difficulty compensating for changes in terrain on the trail or on a cross-country course. Allowing a horse more freedom with his neck and head while negotiating trails, cutting cows, or while jumping gives a horse better vision and elicits more confidence and ability. By rotating the head a bit to either side, a horse is able to amplify his visual perception to the side and immediately behind him.

Besides the blind spots directly in front of and behind his own body, a horse cannot see directly beneath his nose. A horse is unable to distinguish anything placed less than four feet in front of him, including what he eats. For food discrimination, he relies on keen senses of smell and taste. But for negotiating obstacles, he relies upon his vision. As a horse approaches a jump or a tree-fall across a trail, he must have had a good view and measure of the obstacle before it is directly upon him. If he can't see it from afar, an obstacle may scare him and cause

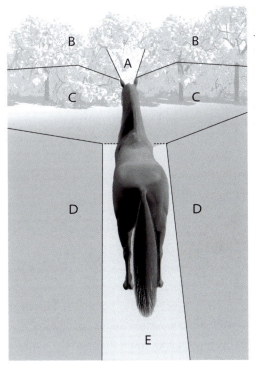

16.4 *Perception and field of vision as seen by a horse standing at rest: blind area (A); both eyes looking forward (B); lateral vision (C); rear vision (D); blind area (E).*

him to balk when asked to proceed forward. If it is a jump that comes upon him suddenly, he may refuse, run-out, or attempt a dangerous leap that could result in a fall.

In addition to the fact that a horse cannot see less than four feet in front of him, his face and nose obscure his line of sight. A horse cannot clearly see objects above the level of his eyes, so he may raise his head to get a better look. This poses a compromise in vision since a horse that holds his head high cannot see the ground in front of him.

Because equine eyes are set out to the side, one eye may see an object before the other does. Accordingly, when the other eye catches on the object, even a stationary rock may seem to "jump" at the horse. (Rapid blinking of your alternate eyes simulates such a "jumping" image, as a horse would see it.)

Imagine what a horse must see when a bright, white rock suddenly appears around the bend in the trail. This explains why there seem to be fantasy monsters lurking behind a rock or a tree, or why a piece of plastic becomes an object of terror. Survival instincts tell horses to stay clear of such dangers; this results in reactive shying at inconvenient times. Man has developed blinders to prevent a horse from being distracted by movements around him so he better concentrates on where he is going.

Color Vision

Horses do seem to be able to discriminate colors, but not quite as specifically as humans. A horse is best able to discriminate blues and reds from greys, but is not as good at discriminating greens or yellows from greys.

How to Apply Vision Principles to Riding

One of the more challenging things a horse person has to accomplish is to encourage a horse to concentrate on the task at hand. Not only do distractions confuse a horse from his job, but also as his head, eyes, and ears swivel around to look to the side, he does not see in front of him. Such lapse in attention results in jerky and weaving movement, and a horse may lose concentration and fail to negotiate a tricky section of terrain. As he throws his head in the air to "look" at his world from another vantage; he may knock down or trip over an obstacle that normally he would have stepped over gracefully. Or, he may balk and stop, or altogether spin away, returning in the direction from which he came. He may trip and stumble, putting him at risk of injury from a misstep. In varied equine sport disciplines, lapses in attention could cause a horse to lose a selected cow, refuse a jump, or slow down in speed; in effect, he loses the winning edge.

By holding the biologic phenomenon of the equine eye in our minds, we can better predict what might startle or scare our mounts. Providing good experiences boosts a horse's confidence, and builds a horse's trust in his rider. "Listening" to a horse's body posture tells volumes of information about his insecurities. By looking at the world through a horse-eye view, quirks of equine behavior become more understandable and more predictable. Many images that a horse perceives as confused and jumbled can be translated for him with a simple word or a steadying hand on his neck, turning it into a non-frightening situation. A scary rock or puddle, an alarming jump, or distracting crowds may melt into obscurity with steadying pressure of a rider's legs, seat, and hands to focus a horse's attention on the task at hand.

Eye Injuries

Abnormal Ocular Discharge

Ocular discharge accompanies many conditions of eye inflammation or injury. It may be clear and watery, or thick and yellow. Glands (*meibomian*) located within the eyelid produce tears, which are distributed across the eye by blinking. Normally, tears are removed through the *nasolacrimal duct*. Its openings (*puncta*) are located near the inside lower corner of each eye, and each duct courses through the facial bones to exit in the *nares* (the pair of openings of the nose). A horse with excessive tear production may have both a runny eye and nose. Eye inflammation from a painful condition elicits abundant tear production, referred to as *epiphora* (photo 16.5). Rose-bengal is a pink dye that is useful to evaluate devitalization of corneal epithelium related to problems with tear film production or from fungal infection.

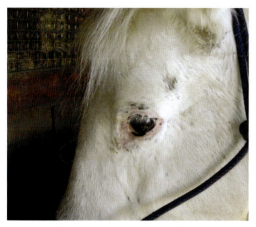

16.5 *Discharge (or weeping) from the eye is referred to as epiphora, and this is a common finding with any eye inflammation or blockage of the nasolacrimal duct. What is usually noted is matting of the fur and/or loss of hair at the corner of the eye.*

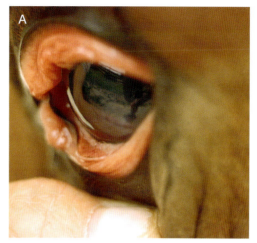

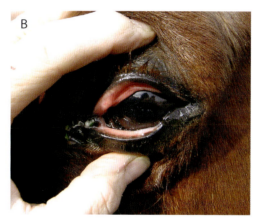

16.6 A & B *The upper and lower eyelids are lined with a highly vascularized tissue called the conjunctiva. Any irritation to the eye often results in swelling and reddening of this tissue, referred to as conjunctivitis, as seen here in both pictures.*

BLOCKAGE OF THE NASOLACRIMAL DUCT

Sometimes, the nasolacrimal duct is blocked to tear flow so tears leak from the corner of the eye, leaving a streaking stain down the face. It is valuable for a veterinarian to check the *patency* (opening) of the duct by evaluating the passage of yellow-green flourescein dye from the eye to the nose, or by passing a small tube into the nasal opening, and gently flushing fluid through by syringe pressure to see if it discharges into the eye. Duct blockage occurs following infection or longstanding inflammation that creates scarring at some point along its length. A previous laceration near the puncta may result in scarring and obliteration of the opening. Neoplasia also causes mechanical obstruction of a duct, as can a foreign body or parasite.

Conjunctivitis

The lining of the upper and lower eyelids is a highly vascularized tissue referred to as *conjunctiva*. When the eye experiences irritation of any kind, the conjunctiva quickly reacts by swelling and turning pink: *conjunctivitis* (photo 16.6 A & B). Usually this is accompanied by an ocular discharge.

Injury to the lid or *globe* (eyeball) creates inflammation of surrounding tissues, including the conjunctiva. It is common for flies feeding on secretions at the corners of the eye to cause conjunctivitis. A horse that constantly rubs his eyes (from flies or allergies) may also develop conjunctivitis. Other irritants that cause conjunctival swelling include fumes from ammonia created by urine, or from smoke. Allergies, dust, or mold also can be causes of conjunctivitis.

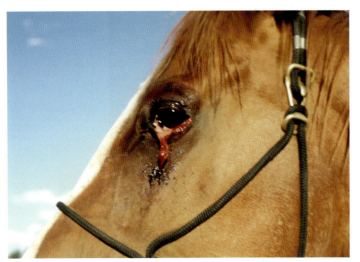

16.7 *Horses are known for catching their face on sharp objects or experiencing blunt trauma of the face and eyes. It is common to see an eyelid snag result in a dramatic injury like this. It is important to surgically repair any eyelid injury to maintain tear gland function, hydration of the eye, and protection of the eye from the elements.*

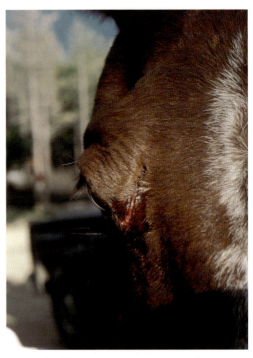

16.8 *This horse has a puncture wound very near the eye, and although the eye is not seemingly involved in this skin injury, immediate veterinary evaluation will ensure that the eye itself has not been harmed. Cold packs applied to the wound help contain swelling and provide relief.*

Eyelid Trauma

A horse's eyelids are prone to trauma whenever the face contacts an immovable object. It is common to see small or large portions of an eyelid torn, split, or hanging (photo 16.7). The eyelids have a tremendous blood supply so have great healing capacity if sewn back together. At the time of the initial injury cold or warm compresses can be applied until veterinary help arrives (photo 16.8). If there is a time delay, topical antibiotic ointment may keep the tissues moist so they are more amenable to suture repair.

Corneal Ulcer or Laceration

A common injury to a horse's eye is that of a scratch or abrasion on the cornea. Damage to corneal epithelium may result from abrasion from coarse hay, a tree branch, a whip, or a rope. Treated fences or posts may cause chemical burn of the cornea.

Tissues around and within an injured eye may swell, making the eye appear red and inflamed (photo 16.9). A scratch on the eye doesn't feel much different to a horse than it does for a person with a piece of dirt in an eye. There will be epiphora, sometimes clear, sometimes yellowish depending on the extent of an injury. The degree of discomfort a horse experiences, and a potential for serious eye damage warrants calling for immediate veterinary attention for any eye ailment. A veterinarian will anesthetize the eye to look for a foreign body and then determine the extent of the injury. Even a seemingly mild eye injury could turn into a serious problem.

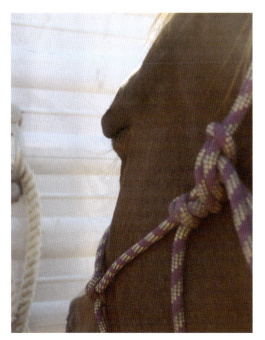

16.9 *Swelling and pain are usually associated with eye trauma and/or corneal ulceration. An affected horse is reluctant to open his eye, and at times the swelling may preclude him from doing so.*

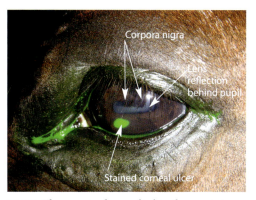

16.10 *Flourescein dye applied to the eye stains an area of ulceration a green color to outline the extent and depth of the corneal erosion. The blue seen above the corneal ulcer is a reflection off the lens behind the pupil. This is normal in all horse eyes. Just at the top margin of the blue color is a normal-appearing corpora nigra.*

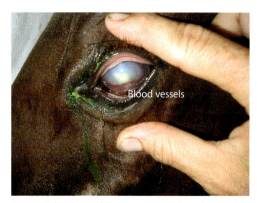

16.11 *Blood vessels migrate from the edge of the eye toward an ulcer that has been present for at least 3 to 5 days. This vascular supply is ancillary to healing, and will retract and dissipate once the ulcer has healed. In this photo, you can see a line of blood vessels along the entire bottom margin of the eye. The blue hue to the rest of the eye is due to corneal edema from inflammation, and is hazier and occupies the entire eye, as compared to the normal blue-opaque view of the lens through a normal pupil as seen in photo 16.10.*

Flourescein dye adheres to any break or scratch in the corneal epithelium, its green marker pinpointing the dimensions of a corneal ulcer (photo 16.10). An ulcer may be visible without dye by shining a penlight across the globe and looking for a ripple or irregularity on the surface. The cornea is usually a smooth, intact surface. An ulcer that has been present for a few days may have blood vessels migrating from the edge of the eye toward the ulcer. These vessels appear 3 to 6 days following injury, migrating at a rate of about 1 mm per day. A cloudy appearance also develops locally to the ulcer as a result of *corneal edema* (photo 16.11). Pain associated with a corneal ulcer often causes spasm of the ciliary muscles resulting in a constricted pupil that stays closed even in dark surroundings.

Contaminating bacteria or fungi have the potential to create an eroding ulcer of the cornea that could threaten loss of vision, or loss of the eye. Rapid veterinary intervention shortens healing time, and returns an eye to function as quickly as possible. An important treatment objective is to diminish associated pain and improve a horse's comfort level.

EYE IRRIGATION

Upon discovery of an eye injury, it is helpful to irrigate the eye with saline solution. Saline solution products are found on the supermarket shelf in the contact-lens-cleaning section. Or, mixing ½ tablespoon of salt in a quart of water makes an appropriate solution. A gentle stream of saline fluid squirted into an eye may loosen a piece of adhered hay or flush away a trapped piece of debris.

TYPES OF EYE MEDICATION

When medicating a horse's eye with topical antibiotics, only use products specifically intended for use in the eye! An ointment is preferable to drops as it has a longer contact time with the tissue, it provides a lubricating layer, it acts as a barrier against microbes, and less is lost through the nasolacrimal duct. Until a veterinarian has diagnosed the nature of the problem, do *not* use any eye ointment that contains a corticosteroid, such as hydrocortisone, dexamethasone, or some other "-sone" listed on the label, as this may worsen ulceration of the cornea. Broad-spectrum antibacterial eye ointments or drops, *without* steroids, can be applied every 2 to 3 hours to give relief. Human *ophthalmic lubricating ointments* (LacriLube®) are useful to maintain moistness in the eye; these are also found in the supermarket. General wound medications should never be used in the eye; their pH is not formulated for the eye and so could cause a "chemical burn" and pain.

Application of Eye Medication

When medicating an eye with ointment or drops, place the flat of your hand (the hand holding the tube of medicine) against the horse's face, and gently pull apart his eyelids with the thumb and index finger of your other hand. Lay a thin bead of ointment or a few drops of medication along the lower lid. As the horse closes his eyelids, the medication will coat the entire globe of the eye and provide relief. Resting the medicating hand on a horse's face allows the hand to follow him if he moves. In this way, there is less chance of poking him in the eye with the tip of a medication tube.

If an eye is badly damaged and the globe itself appears punctured, cover the eye with a bandage until help arrives. Apply a moistened, soft material (a Kotex pad or dampened gauze sponge as examples) over the eye, and bandage this into place with Elastikon® or Vetrap®. The top of women's pantyhose is useful to secure a bandage in place: cut off the legs and pull the top of the stocking over the horse's head, then cut holes out for the ears. An alternative would be to cut up a T-shirt to make it into an eye compress that is duct taped into place. A compress bandage keeps the eye tissues moist, blocks the eye from sun and wind, and maintains it as uncontaminated from debris as possible until a veterinarian can arrive.

Managing a Painful Eye

Any condition of the eye is likely to cause pain and discomfort for a horse. Eye inflammation responds well to nonsteroidal anti-inflammatory drugs (NSAIDs) given systemically, and to topical treatment with lubricating medications chosen specifically for each individual case by a veterinarian. Sometimes it is necessary to dilate the eye with topical *atropine* to relieve painful ciliary spasms. Placing a fly mask, or a mask with an eyecup on a horse during daylight hours relieves ultraviolet glare and insect irritation (photo 16.12). The use of fans in stalls reduces pestering by insects. Careful screening of the property with removal of sharp or blunt protrusions protects against lacerations and injury, and restricts a horse with an injury from scratching and causing additional damage. Care should be taken to protect a horse's eyes during restraint procedures.

Common Eye Diseases

Equine Recurrent Uveitis

A common ailment of the equine eye is *equine recurrent uveitis* (ERU) also known as *anterior uveitis*, *moon blindness*, or *periodic ophthalmia* (photo 16.13). This syndrome is one of the most common causes of blindness in horses. It is thought that almost all Appaloosa horses will develop this syndrome by the end of their lives, but any breed may be affected. It is estimated that 8 to 25 percent of horses in the United States have ERU.

CAUSES OF ERU

Uveitis describes inflammation and reactivity within the *uveal* tissues that make up the pupil. ERU is considered to be an immune-mediated disease related to irritation by foreign proteins such as viral or bacterial organisms that set off an inflammatory response within the eye. Examples include:

- *Leptospirosis infection* (identified in 26 to 70 percent of cases)
- *Onchocerciasis* (see p. 385)
- *Influenza virus* (see p. 267)
- *Herpesvirus* (see p. 270)
- *Septicemia* (from bacterial infection)
- *Streptococcal infection*
- *Lyme disease* (see p. 136)

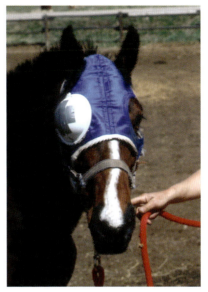

16.12 *When a horse has a painful eye, a patch or eyecup can be secured on a face mask to block sunlight.*

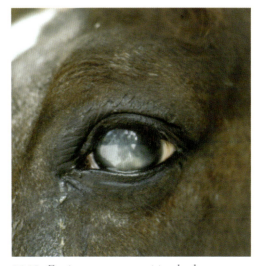

16.13 *Equine recurrent uveitis, also known as anterior uveitis, periodic ophthalmia, or moon blindness, is a common cause of blindness in horses, particularly in Appaloosa breeds. This eye has a glassy look due to an internal cataract that occurred from chronic and repeated bouts of inflammation. The horse's visual acuity is markedly restricted because of the opaqueness of the lens that limits his ability to resolve images.*

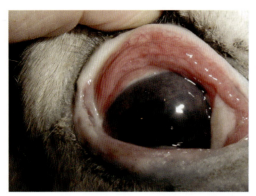

16.14 *Conjunctivitis and swelling are hallmarks of a horse with anterior uveitis due to diffuse inflammation of the eye.*

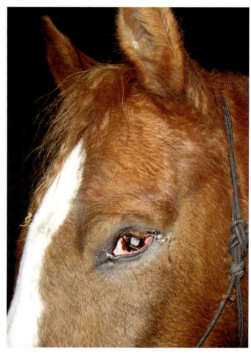

16.15 *Chronic inflammation or a traumatic injury may cause the eye globe, also referred to as the eyeball, to shrink in size and dimension to form a phthisis bulbi, as seen here. The eyeball loses its internal fluid and much like a grape shrinking into a raisin, the eye itself withers inside its bony orbit. Usually, this is not painful, but the horse has no vision in this eye.*

Physical injury to an eye from blunt trauma or a penetrating wound is a very common cause of uveal inflammation.

CLINICAL SIGNS OF ERU

A horse affected with ERU usually exhibits active signs of inflammation: the conjunctiva appears red and irritated, the upper eyelid appears swollen, there is a watery discharge from the corner of the eye, and the horse is extremely sensitive to bright light, preferring to squint or keep the eye closed when outside (photo 16.14 and see photo 16.9, p. 495). Inflammation and swelling within the uveal structures may elicit a corneal ulcer. Corneal edema that coincides with an ulcer makes the eye appear cloudy. A painful eye will have a constricted (*miotic*) pupil that will not dilate in subdued light.

Such painful uveitis episodes occur intermittently, with in-between periods of the eye (or eyes) appearing relatively normal. In some cases, a horse may have a subclinical attack that goes unnoticed by an owner, yet creates damage within the eye. Repeated incidents of inflammation form adhesions (*synechia*) between the uveal tissues and the lens. Eventually, a cataract may be evident, or an owner may notice the horse has vision problems or may be blind. In advanced cases, the eye shrinks in size and dimension, known as *phthisis bulbi* (photo 16.15).

MANAGEMENT OF ERU

A fly mask is useful for reducing ultraviolet glare that causes discomfort to horses with ERU. Efforts should be made to reduce insects and environmental dust, and to use quality bedding. Vaccination programs should be kept up-to-date, especially against respiratory viruses.

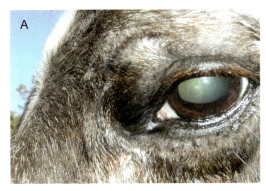 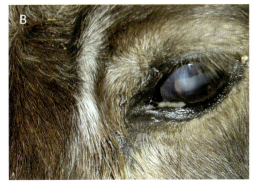

16.16 A & B *A cataract eventually develops as a result of scar tissue adhesions in the eye subsequent to prolonged, chronic inflammation from anterior uveitis. The lens appears opaque as it does in these two examples.*

Some affected horses need to be maintained on anti-inflammatory medications, both topical and systemic. The use of aspirin therapy works to minimize the frequency of episodes in many cases.

Cataract

Typically, the lens of a horse is a transparent flexible disc through which light easily passes. Damage to the lens that results in opacity of the lens fibers is called a *cataract* (photos 16.16 A & B). Eye inflammation, particularly from recurrent equine uveitis, can lead to progressive lens disease and eventual cataract development. (There is a congenital form of cataract that is present in the neonate.) The extent of lens damage can be assessed with diagnostic ultrasound of the eye.

Eye Tumors

Tissues of and surrounding the eyes tend to have a disproportionate incidence of cancer in the horse. Common tumors are *melanoma* in grey horses, and *squamous cell carcinoma* (SCC) in individuals that lack pigment in the lid margins (photos 16.17 A & B, and see

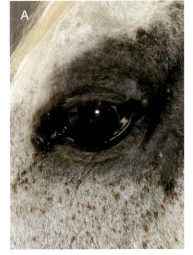 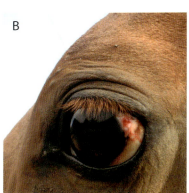

16.17 A & B *Common tumors around the eye include melanoma (A), and squamous cell carcinoma (B). In (A), the horse's skin around the eye is infiltrated with many melanomas.*

chapter 13, *The Skin as an Organ*, p. 397 and p. 399). Solar radiation and ultraviolet increase a horse's susceptibility to this cancer. The third eyelid, eyelids, and conjunctiva are common locations for development of SCC. Breeds most affected with SCC include Appaloosas, Paints, some draft breeds, and white or palomino horses. Single or multiple sarcoid tumors, although generally benign, also invade the lids or skin in proximity to the eye.

Anterior Segment Dysgenesis

Anterior segment dysgenesis (ASD) is a congenital disorder associated with chocolate-colored Rocky Mountain Horses. Many portions of the eye are affected, with the potential to develop a "pop-eye" appearance because of a slanted cornea, cataracts or lens subluxation, and retinal disease. This problem is linked to the silver dapple gene in this breed, which is passed to chocolate and chestnut-colored genes. Because chocolate with a flaxen mane is a popular coloration of the Rocky Mountain Horse, selective breeding favors this coat variation. Subsequently, there are increasing numbers of horses carrying the genetic code for this eye disease. The Rocky Mountain Horse Association is making efforts to identify horses carrying this gene in order to eliminate its continuance. Other horses, including miniature breeds that have this coat and mane combination, also have the potential for ASD.

Blindness

Blindness in the horse may occur following:

- Blunt head trauma with damage to the optic nerve
- Chronic inflammatory conditions of the eye, e.g. ERU
- Cataract
- Equine protozoal myelitis (see p. 510)
- ASD in the Rocky Mountain Horse
- Pituitary enlargement from Cushing's or an abscess
- Equine herpesvirus, neurologic form (see p. 508)

Common causes of blunt trauma that affect vision include flipping over backward or rearing up and hitting a solid object. Such an incident may fracture the base of the skull in a critical area related to vision, the *optic chiasm*, resulting in permanent blindness. Never leave a horse untended on cross-ties as traumatic injuries occur in cross-tie accidents. Other injuries related to falling are sport-related or may occur when loose in the pasture. Running headlong into an obstacle also creates sufficient impact to injure the optic nerve and cause retinal detachment.

TESTING FOR BLINDNESS

A blind horse has tremendous capabilities to compensate for his disability. Without putting a horse through a battery of tests, it is sometimes difficult to determine the extent of his vision deficit. Vision testing can be accomplished in a variety of ways. One crude method for testing whether or not a horse can see involves checking the *menace response*. Rapid movement of a hand toward a horse's eye should elicit a natural response to move away from the implied "menace." Care must be taken not to create air turbulence with a hand, as a horse that feels air current will move, whether he sees or not. Similarly, the hand should not contact a horse's face. Not all horses will move away when so menaced, so the absence of response does not necessarily imply that the horse has vision problems.

Another vision-testing technique entails applying a blindfold to each eye individually and then asking a horse to navigate through an obstacle course that requires visual assessment of the environment. Using ground poles, negotiating around barrels, or turning sharply into a doorway are suggested obstacles that test a horse's visual perception.

The Neurologic System in Health and Disease

Nervous System Function

Cranial Nerves

The cranial nerves control many nerve functions of the head. Some examples of cranial nerve function include:

- The ability to use the lips to grab food (*prehension*)
- Tone of the lips and tongue
- Ability to chew and swallow
- Tone of the eyelids
- Normal eye reflexes such as blinking and movements of the eyes
- Facial skin sensation
- Ear tone and movement
- Sense of smell
- Sense of hearing
- Sense of sight

Balance and Proprioception

The *vestibular system* coordinates orientation of the horse's torso, legs, and eyes relative to the position and movements of his head. Neurologic function of the vestibular system determines how well a horse is able to balance at rest, backing, in motion, and along irregular terrain or negotiating obstacles. Recognition of limb position and placement (*proprioception*) are part of the ability to retain balance, and coordinate appropriate limb movements. The ability of a horse to retain his balance when pushed or with specific positioning of the head and neck is an important normal vestibular response.

Strength and Posture

Neuromuscular strength is important for a horse to retain his balance. Strength of the limbs can be assessed by comparing each limb to its opposite. Positions of the torso and posture of each limb reveal problems with symmetry in stance or in movement.

Testing for Neurologic Function

MENTATION

A horse's alertness and response to external stimuli (*mentation*) give one a sense of how he responds to his environment. A normal horse should be bright and alert and interested in his surroundings, not depressed or apathetic.

CRANIAL NERVE FUNCTION

A horse should be offered food and examined for his ability to grab food, chew, and swallow while eating. Test the "menace response" by waving a hand gently toward each eye and noting if the horse blinks or moves away from the oncoming hand. Shining a bright light into each eye and observing if the pupils constrict down in response can measure pupillary response. Vision is evaluated using a blindfold test over each individual eye, with the horse asked to negotiate around and over obstacles of which he is not familiar (see p. 500). The ears, eyelids, and lips should be examined for symmetry. Notice should be taken of a head tilt that might indicate ear infection or traumatic or infectious involvement of bones of the inner ear (see p. 514).

GAIT EVALUATION

A normal horse is able to walk, trot, canter, and gallop with no indication of deficit or faltering. A horse should be observed at free movement in an arena or the paddock. In subtle cases, a horse may be asked to perform under saddle or in his specified sport. A horse that is neurologically unstable should never be ridden, for safety reasons.

A weak limb often has a longer stride length than normal, and a more pronounced arc to the limb lift. Neurologic deficits are "irregularly irregular" whereas lameness related to a musculoskeletal problem often shows up as a gait abnormality that is "regularly irregular." Signs of abnormal neurologic deficits include:

- *Ataxia* (loss of coordination—photo 17.1)
- Weakness (*paresis*) including knuckling, stumbling, or buckling
- *Circumduction* (wide, outward limb excursion) of a rear limb when moved on a tight circle
- Spastic limb movement

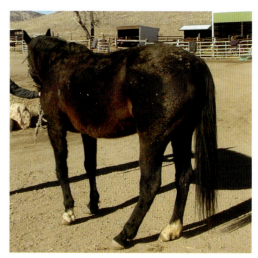

17.1 *This horse has a severe neurologic problem that has made her uncoordinated and ataxic. You can see her haunches listing to the right, while she keeps them thrust out to the left to try to maintain her stance and keep herself upright. When she is asked to walk, she is crooked and unstable, repeatedly losing her balance and almost falling down. A complete neurologic exam identified her as a horse with cervical stenosis, or Wobbler syndrome (see p. 517).*

- Difficulty backing, either refusal to do so, tilting, or backing with a base-wide positioning of the rear legs
- Muscle atrophy
- Loss of sensation
- Abnormal limb placement (*proprioceptive deficits*—photo 17.2)
- Toe dragging

OBSTACLE TESTING

Some neurologic deficits become more apparent when a horse is asked to negotiate a driveway curb or a pole set on the ground, when asked to back, when asked to circle tightly, or when asked to negotiate an uphill or downhill incline, or across a slope. When a horse is moved across or up an incline or is

The Neurologic System in Health and Disease

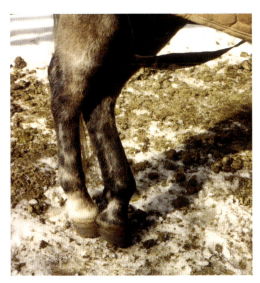

17.2 *When a hind limb is placed over the front of the opposite hind limb, a horse's normal response is to quickly return it to a normal position. This horse, afflicted with severe neurologic disease, was unable to comprehend that his rear limb was placed in an abnormal position, and so the limb remained as you see for an extended time of many minutes. This is referred to as a loss of proprioception, or loss of the ability to acknowledge placement of the legs at rest or when moving.*

asked to step over a pole or curb, the sensory input from the hooves and joints differs in every limb as to its position in space. Under these conditions, a horse with proprioceptive deficits will exhibit an exaggerated loss of coordination or may drag one or more limbs.

Positional problems may become apparent if a horse's head and neck are held in an elevated position, particularly if asked to go uphill. Blindfold testing is useful to identify deficits of the vestibular system, in which visual cues and nervous system reflexes interact to provide coordination and stability.

STRENGTH AND PROPRIOCEPTION

Moving a horse forward and then asking for an abrupt stop is a telling test as to the extent of a horse's coordination and placement of limbs.

A *sway test* is useful to determine neuromuscular strength and whether a horse is able to adjust his limb positioning when attempts are made to push him off balance. Abrupt pressure is applied from the side on the shoulder and hip, both at rest and when walking. A normal horse is able to resist losing his balance when pushed in this manner. A horse with neurologic weakness and/or proprioceptive deficits loses his balance and falls away from the push.

Similarly, a *tail-pull test* attempts to pull a horse sideways off balance with a firm pull on the tail. Pulling on the halter and tail at the same time also tests strength of a horse to resist unbalance.

Holding one forelimb off the ground evaluates how long a horse is able to stand on the opposite limb. Weakness may be evident by trembling of the limb, or by a horse losing his balance. If a horse is cooperative, an attempt can be made to hold up a limb while the examiner's shoulder pushes the horse to require him to "hop" to the side.

Pressure over the back and sacrum should cause a normal horse to reflexively arch his back upward. A horse with a neurologic deficit may not resist the pressure and if weak enough, may buckle in his rear limbs

A normal horse has good anal sphincter and tail tone. Touching the anus should elicit instant contraction of the anus and many horses will also clamp the tail in response. The tail should resist sideways or up-and-down pull; limpness and lack of response to manipulation of the tail or anus are signs of a neurologic deficit.

Infectious Neurologic Diseases

Viral Infection

WEST NILE VIRUS

What started out as a small outbreak of an encephalitis virus in the summer of 1999 extended its geographic bounds to reach coast to coast in the continental United States by 2003. The disease known as *West Nile virus* (WNV) is recognized for its inflammatory effects on the brain and neurologic system of humans and horses. Characteristics of WNV are similar in presentation to the effects seen with other equine encephalitis viruses (see p. 508). Birds are also affected by this virus, some dying as a result. Birds serve as carriers for the virus: mosquitoes feed on birds and then mosquitoes transmit the virus to infect a person or a horse with their bites. The mosquito is a necessary vector to transmit West Nile viral infection to horses and humans. Humans and horses are considered *dead-end hosts*, meaning that a horse cannot pass the virus (via mosquitoes) to another horse or to a human, nor can a human pass the virus to another human or horse.

Exposure to mosquito bites potentially infects any mammal, but this disease mostly manifests in birds, horses, and humans. The highest-risk months for contracting the virus are late summer and early autumn. With the disappearance of mosquitoes in winter, the disease vanishes until it again emerges in late summer.

Many horses demonstrate antibodies to the virus indicating exposure, but do not exhibit any clinical signs, while others demonstrate various degrees of neurologic disease. In both clinical trial studies and in natural settings, 10 percent of horses exposed to the virus will evidence signs of disease. One-third of horses that contract the disease will die or need to be euthanized. Every state is different in the numbers of horses that become exposed to the virus. This is due to variations in climate, topography, species of birds, and species of mosquitoes.

Confusing Diagnosis

Clinical signs seen with WNV infection include:

- Depression or listlessness in 50 percent
- Weakness, particularly in the rear quarters in 86 percent
- Fever in 32 percent
- Ataxia (loss of coordination), symmetrical (same on one side of the body as the other), in 94 percent
- Muscle *fasciculations* (tremors) in 50 percent
- Cranial nerve deficits in 43 percent
- Recumbency (lying down) in 45 percent
- Seizures in 3 percent.

When muscle fasciculations are seen in the face or muzzle, the probability that a horse is infected with WNV is 92 percent (spasms of the facial muscles and a noticeably tense expression of the lips and muzzle—photo 17.3); fasciculations in the head, neck, and shoulders correlates with WNV infection 90 percent of the time; and fasciculations of the head and neck only correlate with WNV infection about 84 percent of the time.

Some horses also demonstrate increased skin sensitivity (*hyperesthesia*) and react inappropriately to being touched, often becoming belligerent. Other signs consistent with an encephalitic virus may include head tilt, circling, twitching, hyperexcitability, paralysis, coma, convulsions, and death. When fever occurs, it develops several weeks prior to central nervous system signs caused by WNV;

fever is not typically present during the time that obvious neurologic symptoms appear. In a horse showing neurologic signs, other diseases that attack the central nervous system should be considered as well as suspecting WNV. These include: rabies, botulism, *Eastern* or *Western encephalitis* (also known as *sleeping sickness*), or *equine protozoal myelitis*, (EPM—see p. 510).

Monitoring for Disease

Each state has implemented excellent surveillance strategies to monitor the prevalence and presence of the virus. Crows are particularly sensitive to the deadly effects of this virus, as are pheasants. Dead birds are collected and tested; mosquitoes are collected and tested; live sentinel birds (chicken flocks) are tested. Chickens contract a short-term version of the virus without showing any obvious clinical signs. Following examination of an animal with suspicious neurologic signs, a local veterinarian will then report the findings to the state veterinarian's office. Blood tests on a suspect horse confirm the presence of circulating antibodies that indicate exposure to the disease.

Treatment with Serum Antibodies

An antibody serum product (West Nile Virus Antibody® by Novartis) has been conditionally approved to treat horses with West Nile virus. Unlike vaccinations, which challenge the immune system to respond to the presence of a foreign protein (virus), this antibody serum product contains preformed antibodies specifically targeted to neutralize the virus. A horse receiving this product is provided immediate protection against the disease. Yet, since an antibody does not stimulate a horse's immune response, the duration of protection lasts only up to 21 days. Use of this product is appropriate in two situations:

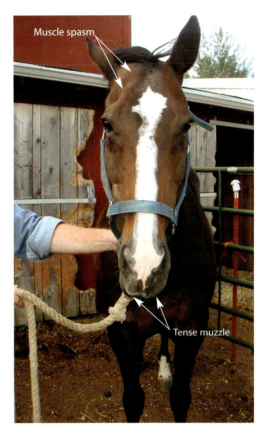

17.3 *West Nile virus elicits a variety of neurologic signs, one classic being that of facial muscle spasms, tics, or tremors. The right temple on this horse (the left of the photo) is tense and in spasm, while the horse's left temple is normal. He also displays a noticeably tense muzzle.*

- In the face of an acute infection
- If a horse has been exposed and is in imminent danger of infection before he is able to develop his own antibody protection as a normal response to a vaccine series

Hyperimmune Plasma

Another conditionally approved product that has been used to treat West Nile virus is that of *hyperimmune plasma* (HiGamm-Equi® by Lake Immunogenics) such as is used to treat failure of passive transfer in foals. The plasma is obtained from horses that have been hyper-vaccinated against West Nile virus and so have developed an exceptional antibody response. The plasma is a frozen product that is thawed and then given intravenously by a veterinarian. When given to a sick individual, antibodies already present in the plasma help to eliminate circulating virus in a sick horse's bloodstream. Best results are achieved when hyperimmune plasma is given to sick foals, or to a sick adult that has not yet become recumbent.

Other Treatment Options

The basic tenet of treatment for a horse afflicted with West Nile virus is to support the horse with hydration, energy, and comfort. Practitioners throughout the country have tried every reasonable medicine to shorten the duration of clinical signs, but in the end, it appears that time coupled with a horse's immune response and a lot of luck are the most important ingredients for success. No harm has been seen with various treatment efforts. Options that may have some benefit include the use of anti-inflammatory drugs such as corticosteroids, NSAIDs, or DMSO given systemically. Supportive care with intravenous fluids is necessary in recumbent horses or those not hydrating themselves. Bladder catheterization and/or bowel evacuation are important for affected horses that lose the ability to urinate or defecate. *Gentamycin*, although an antibiotic, has purported antiviral characteristics, and *interferon* has also been advocated as a useful antiviral agent.

Licensed Vaccines

Due to the concern over the lethal effects of this virus, a killed-virus vaccine (Innovator® by Ft. Dodge Animal Health) has received full licensing for use in horses. Vaccination protocol requires two intramuscular doses spaced 3 to 6 weeks apart to initiate immunity, and then yearly boosters just prior to the expected time of exposure risk. In high-risk areas and/or in horses that are highly stressed, it is suggested to boost the vaccine at 4 to 5 month intervals.

Vaccination of foals born to unvaccinated mares should begin at 2 months of age, boosted in 3 to 6 weeks, and a third booster given at 6 months. For foals born to mares immunized against WNV, vaccination should begin at age 3 to 4 months, followed by two additional boosters at 3 to 6 week intervals. Boosters in following years should follow the same protocol as for adult horses.

A genetically engineered vaccine (Recombitek® by Merial Labs) has also been developed to stimulate immunity. This is called a *recombinant DNA vaccine* that uses non-pathogenic canarypox virus that does not replicate or disseminate throughout the body. Using live-replicating canarypox virus as a vector, the vaccine delivers genes of the disease into the cells. There, an expression of targeted antigen, specifically of West Nile virus, is presented to the immune system in a way that closely resembles natural infection. This stimulates a horse immunized with this product to generate an "authentic" protective response. This vaccine stimulates both arms of the immune system to give the most complete protection possible against viral infection.

Vaccination protocol of the primary series of the recombinant product calls for a first injection, followed by a second dose 4 to 6 weeks later. Immunity is achieved 2 weeks following the second dose of vaccine. A booster should be given annually prior to the onset of mosquito season. Of horses receiving the initial series of two, the duration of immunity appears to be one year. Of horses in the clinical trial studies, 90 percent were protected against disease at 26 days after receiving only a single injection.

Results of Failure to Vaccinate

Studies have indicated that the greatest numbers of WNV cases occur in horses that did not receive any vaccine, making a convincing argument that the vaccine is highly effective in preventing *viremia* (presence of virus in the bloodstream). (A horse that is exposed but does not develop viremia does not demonstrate neurologic symptoms.) The killed virus vaccine (Innovator®) is reported to provide protection in 95 percent of horses. Of those horses that did contract the disease in spite of vaccination, 94 percent survived. Mortality is 14 percent in horses that only receive one vaccine of the two-dose series, whereas in nonimmunized horses, mortality is about 30 percent.

Post-Infection Follow-Up

For safety reasons for both horse and rider, it is important to have a veterinarian thoroughly assess neurologic function prior to riding a horse that had been previously stricken with West Nile virus. Of horses affected by West Nile virus, 40 percent retain some residual deficits, such as fatigue, gait-instability issues (stumbling, tripping, weakness), and muscle atrophy. Also, some demonstrate indications of memory loss, like not being able to remember the location of a door; some have vision problems. The most common deficit seen is that of a change in attitude with accompanying behavioral changes. Of horses that contract the disease and recover, 62 percent have been evaluated as fully capable of returning to work. All those who recover fully are horses that received full or partial immunization with the vaccine series.

From 9 to 15 percent of horses previously infected with West Nile virus suffer a relapse between 2 weeks to 5 months following illness, in spite of having seemingly recovered. All horses that relapsed were those that had not received vaccination against the disease.

Prevention and Mosquito Control

Implementation of mosquito control strategies is highly successful in minimizing the risk of viral infection. Coupling such strategies with immunization yields the best results in preventing infection. Consider ways to eliminate breeding and presence of mosquitoes. Stagnant water that stands for four days allows mosquito larvae to hatch. Limit water reservoirs by clearing property of vesicles that can fill with even small amounts of water. Some items are not obvious at first thought: flower pots, bird baths, rain gutters, wading pools, wheelbarrows, stock tanks, clogged roof gutters, discarded tires, swimming-pool covers, boat covers, discarded cans, or paint buckets. More obvious sites of water collection point to ditches, creeks, or ponds. Chlorine in swimming pools kills the larvae, but a swimming pool cover and other sites of standing water are more difficult to control. Routine cleaning of all containers of free-standing water minimizes their attraction as breeding sites for mosquitoes. Stock tanks should be cleaned monthly (or more often) to remove algae and debris. Aerate ornamental pools or stock them with fish that eat insect larvae. Turn over open containers so water cannot accumulate, or drill holes in container bottoms so water drains through.

On property with bodies of freestanding or slow moving water, additional strategies will need to be incorporated. Flysheets and leg nets limit the exposed surface area of a horse's body to mosquito bites, but cannot cover all a horse. Insect repellents should be used, but be cautious in assuming that mosquito repellents are a first defense in control. It is difficult to cover all a horse's body parts sufficiently, the repellents maintain only a limited duration of protection, and rain, or sweat, or rolling in the dirt removes them from a horse's fur. *Permethrin*-containing repellents are safe for use in horses and offer some protection against mosquitoes. The use of screened barns keeps mosquitoes away from horses during feeding times. It is difficult to know which species of mosquitoes are active to transmit the virus and each has a different feeding habit. Some feed during the daytime, while others feed only at dawn or dusk. This makes it difficult to predict which portion of the day to leave horses in the barn. Mosquitoes do lurk in corners and cracks in the barn. Spray these areas with insecticides to minimize this possibility. The use of fans to keep air moving in the stalls may deter attempts by mosquitoes to land and feed on horses (see p. 382).

EQUINE ENCEPHALITIS OR ENCEPHALOMYELITIS

Three forms of *equine encephalitis* may occur within the United States: *Eastern* (EEE), *Western* (WEE), or *Venezuelan* (VEE). Equine encephalitis is also referred to as *sleeping sickness*. Encephalitis virus is transmitted to horses or people in a similar fashion to West Nile Virus: the infection is harbored in birds and spread to mosquitoes that then infect horses or people. Both horses and people are dead-end hosts and cannot transmit virus to other horses or people, or to birds or mosquitoes.

Typically, Eastern encephalitis occurs along the eastern seaboard, while Western encephalitis shows up in the western part of the United States. The Venezuelan form is a disease mostly of Central or South America and is intermittently present in southern border states like Texas and New Mexico.

Clinical Signs of Encephalitis

Initially, an affected horse appears stiff, lethargic, off feed, and has a fever. Progressive clinical signs of equine encephalitis include those associated with central nervous system disease: depression, erratic behavior such as irritability or aggressiveness, muscular weakness, increased skin sensitivity (hyperesthesia), cranial nerve deficits that interfere with obtaining (*prehension*) and chewing of food, pressing the head into a wall or corner, loss of coordination, compulsive walking, paddling with limbs, and circling. Some affected horses are sensitive to light and sound, while others become blind. Encephalitis usually is fatal within 3 days of recognition of the first clinical signs, particularly if infected with EEE; recumbency and seizures usually precede death. EEE is most fatal, with death in 75 to 90 percent of infected horses. Although not as fatal a disease, mortality associated with WEE ranges from 19 to 50 percent.

Prevention

As with WNV, prevention relies on good immunization policies at least once or twice a year in mosquito-infested areas following an initial primary series of two injections. Control relies on aggressive attempts to prevent mosquito exposure and by mosquito eradication measures as described for WNV above.

EQUINE HERPESVIRUS, NEUROLOGIC FORM

Equine herpesvirus or *rhinopneumonitis* exists as several strains: EHV-1, EHV-2, EHV-3 (*coital exanthema*—see p. 536), and EHV-4. Although EHV-4 is the common form of viral respiratory disease related to equine herpesvirus (see p. 270), the neurologic strain (EHV-1) attacks the central nervous system in horses, and additionally causes respiratory disease and a potential to abortion. A horse will exhibit signs of respiratory infection 3 to 6 days following exposure of the EHV-1 virus; respiratory signs occur 7 to 10 days prior to the sudden onset of clinical neurologic signs. The virus is most transmissible to others during the period of fever and respiratory signs, with shedding from the respiratory tract lasting up to 2 weeks. As is common with herpesvirus infection in all animals, a horse may seem to recover from illness yet the virus may lie dormant for a time (*latency*) with a stress situation (transport, illness, performance) reactivating an infection.

Clinical Signs

Neurologic equine herpes infection mimics many other neurologic diseases; however, there are some specific characteristics that rate a high index of suspicion. Within a week prior to demonstrating neurologic symptoms, an infected horse develops a fever, appetite diminishes, and often a respiratory infection (with a watery nasal discharge and a cough) is evident. Within the central nervous system, blood vessel damage results in cellular death of neurons, with variable neurologic deficits related to specific areas of damage. An affected horse is overtaken suddenly with ascending paralysis that usually peaks to its worst state within 2 to 3 days of onset. Commonly seen clinical neurologic signs of paralytic rhinopneumonitis include poor tail tone along with fecal incontinence and urinary leakage due to partial or complete bladder paralysis. The hind limbs become weak or hind limb coordination falters, called ataxia, usually in a symmetrical fashion. Many horses afflicted with paralytic rhinopneumonitis go down and remain recumbent, the effects of the infection lasting for 3 weeks or more. An affected horse may become recumbent, with subsequent self-inflicted bodily trauma from attempts to rise. On rare occasions, there are associated lesions in the eyes, including blindness (see p. 500). Mortality occurs in about 25 percent, however, those horses that recover have a very good prognosis for return to function.

Prevention and Control

Vaccine is not currently available to protect against infection by the neurologic form of herpesvirus in horses. Spread of EHV-1 is through inhalation or ingestion of contaminated secretions or blood from infected horses. Efforts of control should be aggressive if the disease is confirmed on a farm so that the least number of herd members become infected. (See chapter 15, *Preventive and Mental Horse Health*, p. 458.)

- Strict segregation for 21 days: intermingling of horses should be halted, and groups of horses should remain where they are without introduction of new members or movement of individuals about a farm into other groups.
- Sick horses should be isolated and quarantined immediately for at least 3 weeks; *at least* 35 feet, and preferably further, should separate sick horses from those as yet unaffected.
- No horse should leave the property until 21 days after there is no longer evidence of active infection.

A mixture of 10 parts water to 1 part bleach is useful for cleaning contaminated stabling and equipment.

RABIES

Rabies is a serious neurologic viral disease that can affect horses, with the dangerous potential to infect humans handling an infected horse. A horse contracts rabies through saliva from the bite of rabid animals, like bats, skunks, raccoons, and fox, as examples. Incubation from the time of the bite to evidence of clinical signs may take as few as 9 days and as long as a year.

Clinical signs often are not typical for those seen in rabid carnivores: some horses may become aggressive, but more commonly, an affected horse is depressed and quiet rather than manic. A number of other signs occur, including loss of tail and anal sphincter tone (as seen with equine herpesvirus), increased skin sensitivity (as seen with equine encephalitis or WNV), self-mutilation, and lameness, or ataxia (as seen with West Nile virus, encephalitis, or EPM—see p. 510). The disease progresses rapidly to death within 5 to 10 days of onset of clinical signs.

Vaccination is available for horses to minimize the risk of rabies. In high-risk areas, horses should be vaccinated annually.

Parasitic Migration

EQUINE PROTOZOAL MYELITIS

Equine protozoal myelitis or *myeloencephalitis*, also known as EPM, is caused by a protozoan parasite, *Sarcocystis neurona* that finds its way to the central nervous system, namely the spinal cord. A similar organism that infects birds, *Sarcocystis falcatula*, has been implicated as a possible culprit, and new studies implicate *Neospora hughesi*, a protozoan infection in dogs, to be another possible infectious agent. To date, EPM remains confined to horses in the United States.

A carnivore that ingests sarcocyst-infected flesh of an intermediate host then becomes the carrier for *sporocysts* to pass in the feces. One known carrier of the organism is the opossum. Recent information suggests that striped skunks, nine-banded armadillos, sea otters, and domestic cats (especially those with compromised immune systems) may play a vector role as intermediate hosts. Opossums eating parasite-infected skunk or armadillo meat may become infected. Regardless of which scavenger carries the organism in its feces, a horse ingests feed or water that has been contaminated with infected feces; from the intestinal tract the parasite migrates to the central nervous system. Horses are considered "aberrant dead-end hosts" and cannot pass infection to other horses or animals.

Clinical Signs

EPM challenges veterinary diagnostic skills by presenting obscure signs that are consistent only in their inconsistency. Symptoms are elusive in this insidious disease until it has progressed for some time. All symptoms are related either to direct nerve damage or as a consequence of inflammation of the nerves caused by presence of the parasite. Swelling or death of nerve tissue elicits varying clinical responses. Signs vary depending on the location of spinal cord damage; this accounts for the asymmetrical appearance of muscle groups that have partially lost normal nerve signals for maintaining muscle tone and development. At first, a horse may demonstrate an odd characteristic to his hind limb gait, or it may appear that certain muscle groups seem less developed or atrophied as compared to muscles on the other side. This is most visibly appreciated in the hip muscles or shoulder muscles, or a horse's topline musculature appears asymmetrical. In some cases, a horse begins making respiratory noise related to nerve dysfunction of the laryngeal cartilage.

Damage within the spinal cord creates a "classic" problem in the horse, referred to as the "Three 'A'" appearance: asymmetric ataxia with focal muscle atrophy. As described, muscle atrophy is a prominent feature of this disease (photos 17.4 A & B). In addition, this description paints a picture of a horse that has lost coordination (ataxia), with one side worse than the other (asymmetrical). Problems generally show up in the rear legs, but may initially begin as behavioral issues with a horse stopping or running out at fences, refusing to perform lateral work, or seeming clumsy or lazy. Loss of coordination may begin as a general weakness, with a horse collapsing behind, or having difficulty backing up. Anxiety caused by feeling out of control may cause some horses to react dramatically to being asked to perform precision tasks, while others simply quit their jobs. Behavioral changes also accompany EPM, with some normally placid horses becoming aggressive.

Confusion with Other Problems

Part of the challenge of diagnosing EPM is that the variety of problems it creates are confused with common abnormalities found in just about any horse. In about 10 percent of horses affected by EPM, the cranial nerves may also

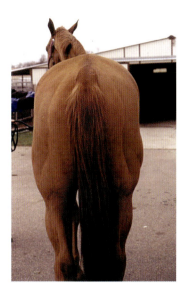 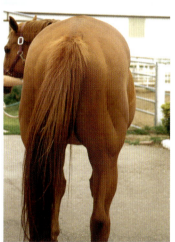

17.4 A & B *This horse first presented with behavioral changes and gait abnormalities, but he also exhibited other hallmark signs of equine protozoal myelitis: asymmetric ataxia and atrophy, as seen here with atrophy of his left hip (A). Following three months of EPM medication, he recovered some muscle tone and bulk to his left hip, although there remains some degree of permanent atrophy (B). His behavior and performance improved, and he returned to use as a safe riding horse although no longer able to compete at high levels of performance.*

be affected leading to abnormalities in the airways such as "roaring" (*laryngeal hemiplegia*—see p. 258) or *dorsal displacement of the soft palate* (see p. 259). In other cases, damage to nerve supply of muscles, tendons, or ligaments may cause lameness problems that delay an actual diagnosis. Some horses may show very subtle signs early on, with the disease never worsening beyond subtle performance issues.

Any oddity in gait may surface subsequent to infection with EPM. Examples include upward fixation of the patella resulting from weakness of affected quadriceps muscles (see p. 118), or back pain that develops as a consequence of persistent asymmetry in the gait of the rear limbs. A horse may experience tying-up syndrome due to loss of functional muscle fiber contraction (see p. 166). Or, a horse expresses behavioral problems secondary to effects of the protozoa on the brainstem or due to anxiety or pain related to gait instability or discomfort. More mildly affected horses may simply change their working attitude, while others react with more obvious problems such as throwing the head, refusing fences, carrying the head high, falling on the forehand, or reducing stride length, especially at a gallop. Not all horses change their behavior. A well-trained dressage horse, for example, may seemingly lose his strength in certain exercises, but a strong rider can "hold" the horse together in collected work. Yet, if left to his own devices the horse will demonstrate a gait irregularity.

In addition to obscure lameness or behavioral problems, EPM can mimic other neurologic syndromes, such as spinal tumors or abscesses, *equine herpesvirus myelitis* (neurologic rhinopneumonitis—see p. 508), *equine motor neuron disease,* or Wobbler syndrome (*cervical stenotic myelopathy*—see p. 517). Because of the dangers inherent in riding a horse with known neuromuscular instability, it is important to track down the source of the problem so a proper diagnosis can be established, and appropriate treatment initiated if possible.

How is EPM Diagnosed?

Failing identification of a clear-cut clinical picture that is consistent with the "Three 'As'" of asymmetric ataxia with muscle atrophy, other measures can be taken to confirm a diagnosis of EPM.

Blood-Testing for EPM

A blood test is a noninvasive means of screening for EPM. If a horse tests positive to a blood test, that only means that the horse has been exposed to the parasite and has mounted an immune response to it, yet is not necessarily affected by clinical disease as a result. A negative blood test indicates that the horse has never "seen" the protozoa in his system, so any performance issues or neurologic abnormalities should be examined with another cause in mind.

In spite of attempts to screen for EPM with blood and spinal-fluid testing at the time of a prepurchase exam, there is limited value in using these tests on neurologically normal horses.

Spinal Tap

In horses demonstrating abnormal neurologic signs, achieving a definitive diagnosis of EPM requires a more invasive diagnostic procedure: a spinal tap to harvest a sample of *cerebrospinal fluid* (CSF). This technique proceeds relatively uneventfully in most cases, but risks are involved. The procedure is done with the horse standing under sedation. A 6-inch needle is inserted into the lumbosacral joint space to the depth of the spinal canal. Even with meticulous technique, a horse may jump suddenly, bolt, or fall down when the needle is inserted into the correct site.

Biochemical analysis of the CSF yields valuable information. The *Western blot assay* detects the presence of antibodies to the parasite. Finding EPM antibodies in the CSF with this test indicates the presence of an active infection, provided the CSF sample was *not* contaminated with blood. Any blood contamination may result in a false positive. Another testing process, the *DNA polymerase chain reaction* (PCR) test, directly detects presence of the parasite and does not rely on the horse having mounted an immune response to the parasite. However specific this test may be, it is not as sensitive as once thought because the parasite is typically located in nervous tissue rather than floating freely in the cerebrospinal fluid. When a horse's immune response is actively functioning, it is difficult to detect parasite DNA in the CSF. In addition, other inflammatory elements (total protein and albumin quotient, white blood cells, and immunoglobulin levels) are examined in blood and CSF to help corroborate a diagnosis.

Trial by Treatment

Another means of "diagnosing" EPM is by instituting treatment and observing if signs abate. Some response may be appreciated within a few weeks, but full treatment requires at least a couple of months to eliminate the disease. Treatment is relatively harmless in most instances, albeit expensive.

Treatment Options for EPM

Treatment is deemed successful if a horse clinically improves at least one grade (on a scale of 0 to 5) within 3 months following treatment or the Western blot test of spinal fluid converts to negative. "Successful" treatment occurs in 60 to 81 percent of cases. Bear in mind that improving a Grade 4 horse one grade to Grade 3 may still render a horse unfit for riding and unsafe to have around.

Previously used medications to treat this disease included oral *pyrimethamine* given once daily and *sulfadiazine* administered twice daily. At least 4 months of treatment is necessary with this approach to ensure parasitic kill, and in many cases even prolonged treatment cannot clear the parasite from the central nervous system. Relapses are common. Side effects of this medication occur, such as worsened inflammation within the spinal cord during treatment as the parasites die off, and anemia from bone marrow suppression.

One medication that is currently approved by the FDA in treatment of EPM for horses is *ponazuril* (Marquis® by Bayer Animal Health), an anti-protozoal oral paste that is used once daily. (It is recommended to double the label dose and administer for 28 days, or it should be given at the label dose for 60 days.) The active ingredient, ponazuril, is able to penetrate the blood-brain barrier. It reaches therapeutic levels within the central nervous system to target the parasite at its source and attack it at many stages of its life cycle. Treatment with ponazuril achieves 62 percent success rate, with 30 percent returning to their original level of performance. Some horses in the initial studies did relapse following the 28 days of treatment, indicating that a longer course of therapy may be necessary. Some horses continued to improve following cessation of treatment. It has also been recommended to follow up ponazuril treatment with sulfadiazine for another month. The medication is meant to clear the horse of the parasite but it cannot repair pre-existing damage to the spinal cord and nerves that developed prior to treatment. Other than occasional instances of loose feces or loss of appetite, the drug has been demonstrated to be safe. No studies as yet have determined its safety in breeding or pregnant animals.

Another approved anti-protozoal medication for treatment of EPM is *nitazoxanide*. In pilot studies, this medication improved 70 percent within 3 months, with 11 percent making a full recovery. It is recommended to add corn oil to the diet to increase absorption of this drug. Label instructions should be followed closely and each horse monitored carefully.

Vitamin E supplementation at doses of 6000 to 8000 IU/day is speculated as being helpful to manage many neurologic conditions.

Vaccination and Control

A conditionally licensed vaccine (Ft. Dodge Laboratories) targeting EPM is available for horses. Its efficacy is questionable at this time.

The most effective management strategy that one can use to control the disease is to keep scavengers (opossums, raccoons, skunks) away from food and water sources as best as possible. Secure lids on grain bins, and clean up spilled feed to limit attraction of scavengers. Heat-treated complete feed is also available to minimize risk of ingestion of sporocyte-contaminated feces.

Even when stalls are not in use, close stall doors so varmints cannot enter to contaminate the area with feces. Normal disinfectants are incapable of inactivating the infective sporocysts; however, steam-cleaning at temperatures of 140° F (60° C) for 1 minute will do so. Fencing is available to keep opossums off horse property. Dispose of dead raccoon, skunk, or cat carcasses so opossums cannot eat infected meat. Minimize stressors on at-risk horses: pregnancy, transport, competition, and treatment of lameness issues with corticosteroids are examples of instances that reduce a horse's native immune system.

PARASITE DAMAGE

Fly warbles (*Hypoderma* spp.) can also create neurologic problems if these parasites follow an aberrant migration path to the brain spinal cord instead of a normal exit from the back muscles (see p. 380).

Bacterial Infection

TETANUS

Tetanus is caused by *Clostridium tetani*, which are bacteria found in the soil and in the gastrointestinal tract (see chapter 14, *Equine First Aid, Medication, and Restraint*, p. 422). These bacteria thrive in anaerobic conditions, lacking in oxygen, such as found in a deep, penetrating

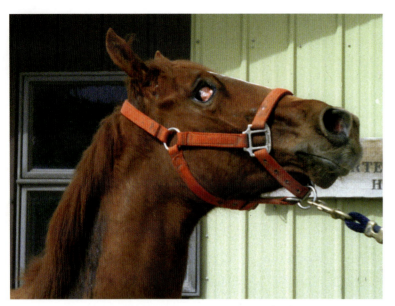

17.5 *This horse shows classic signs of tetanus: rigid facial muscles, prolapse of the third eyelid, and nostrils that remain flared due to tetanic muscle spasms. Photo: Ray Randall, DVM.*

wound. A wound provides entry of the spores of *Clostridium tetani*, which then proliferate to produce exotoxins. The exotoxin reaches the brain through the bloodstream, or migrates up peripheral nerves to the central nervous system. It slows normal nerve transmission by preventing release of a chemical neurotransmitter, *acetylcholine,* and by preventing release of an inhibitory transmitter, *glycine,* at the neuron. A wound may occur 2 to 30 days prior to the onset of clinical signs. Once clinical signs appear, the disease progresses rapidly within just a few days.

Symptoms begin in the head and forequarters, as uncontrolled, skeletal-muscle spasms resulting in "lockjaw." The horse may experience an increased heart rate or heart arrhythmia. Facial muscles become rigid. An affected horse cannot acquire, chew, or swallow food. Nostrils flare, the third eyelid descends over the eye, and the ears remain rigid and upright due to persistent spasms of the facial muscles (photo 17.5). As exotoxin progressively paralyzes the body, the horse assumes a stiff "sawhorse" stance with legs extended in a rigid position. If the horse goes down, he is unable to rise due to the rigidity of legs and neck. An afflicted animal is hypersensitive to noise and other external stimuli and is overly sensitive to being touched. Rapid paralysis descends from head to toe. Eventually, paralysis of the diaphragm or complications of aspiration pneumonia cause a horse to suffocate. Or, the horse may succumb to dehydration or malnutrition because spasms of the muscles of chewing and swallowing preclude drinking or eating. The disease is fatal 50 to 80 percent of the time.

A toxoid vaccination is available as prevention against this disease. Following an initial immunization series of 2 injections spaced 4 weeks apart, every horse should receive an annual booster of tetanus toxoid; this is normally given along with "spring" shots. The vaccine should be boosted again if the horse experiences a deep wound 8 to 12 months from the time of the last vaccination (see p. 422).

Neurologic Irritation or Compression

Ear Inflammation

OTITIS MEDIA-INTERNA

Infection of the middle ear creates an inflammatory response in the inner ear structures. Or, trauma to the head or a chronic ear infection may cause fracture of tiny bones adjacent to the ear structures, which then creates damage to a few of the cranial nerves. In any of these situations, a horse may develop *otitis media-interna*. This syndrome may go unrecognized initially but subtle behavioral changes may warrant further investigation. An affected horse might toss his head, rub his ears, chew more vigorously than usual on the bit, or may be resistant to having one or both ears handled. As an ear infection progresses, more overt neurologic signs become evident:

- Facial paralysis with lip, ear, and/or eyelid droop (photo 17.6)
- Head tilt (photo 17.7)
- Corneal ulcer due to dry eye from inability to blink (see p. 494)
- *Nystagmus* (horizontal involuntary movement of the eye)
- Circling
- Ataxia with falling

Treatment with anti-inflammatory medication and antibiotics can lead to successful resolution in mild to moderate cases. Fractured bones within the head carry a less favorable prognosis.

Tick Paralysis

On occasion, a tick may attach itself to a horse, and a neurotoxin in its saliva is injected into the horse. This neurotoxin causes an ascending paralysis that begins with neurologic weakness and paralysis in the hind end, and gradually moves forward until the diaphragm is paralyzed, causing death. The paralysis is dose-dependent, and so small or very young horses are more often affected. If such an event occurs, conduct a careful search for an imbedded tick; removal of the tick, including all its head parts, will elicit rapid resolution of the paralysis (see "Ticks," Chapter 13, *The Skin as an Organ*, p. 387).

Headshaking

Headshaking is considered to be a concern when a horse incessantly and violently shakes his head or sneezes in the absence of obvious external stimuli. A horse afflicted with head-

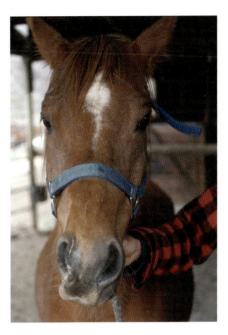

17.6 *Facial paralysis is often implicated in cases of inner ear infection. The muzzle of this horse is pulled away from the affected left ear. This is as a result of the paralysis of the left side of the face and increased tone on the right.*

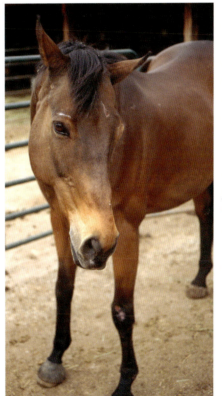

17.7 *A head tilt and drooping ear are also signs of an inner ear infection, along with facial paralysis. Abrasions on this horse's knee and head are a result of ataxia and incoordination that caused him to have difficulty standing and to fall down. Aggressive medical treatment of his inner ear infection for several months returned him to about 80 percent normal. Some cases require surgical intervention for best results.*

shaking may swing the head in a horizontal, vertical, or circular motion, but most often the motion is vertical. Some horses attempt to rub their faces on any available surface. Some persistently snort or sneeze, and twitch their lips. Most affected horses exhibit two or three of these symptoms. Exercise often (41 percent of the time) sets off such an attack of headshaking, as can sunlight or insects. Headshaking is a problem that renders a horse difficult to ride. Signs of the problem tend to be seasonal in occurrence, being present mostly in spring, summer, and tapering off in the fall.

There are many possible reasons as to why a horse steadily shakes his head. One theory suggests that *photic* headshaking may be triggered by exposure to light that activates the facial sensory nerve (the *infraorbital* branch) of the *trigeminal nerve*. Another theory suggests that headshaking may be associated with nerve pain (*neuralgia*) in the trigeminal nerve as it crosses the face. The horse may feel sensations of burning, itching, tingling, or electric-shock-like irritation in the nerve.

Many disease processes may elicit an inflammatory response that a horse finds extremely irritating. It is difficult to pin down the exact cause in most cases. Of 60 possible cited causes, common examples include:

- Ear ticks or mites (see chapter 13, *The Skin as an Organ*, p. 387)
- Guttural pouch infection (see p. 277)
- Eye irritation or vision problems (see chapter 16, *The Eyes*, p. 492)
- Otitis media-interna (see p. 514)
- Dental issues or mouth pain (see p. 284)
- Bitting issues (see p. 253)
- Previous facial or muzzle trauma
- Back pain and/or poor saddle fit (see chapter 8, *The Horse's Back*, p. 203)
- Neck pain
- Equine protozoal myelitis (EPM—p. 510)
- Equine herpesvirus (EHV-1—p. 508)
- Allergic rhinitis
- Seasonal or photic headshaking associated with lengthening daylight hours or exposure to sunlight
- Trigeminal nerve pain

Strategies to manage headshaking behavior:

- Muzzle nets (Equilibrium Products) that cover the top half of the muzzle provide relief in up to 33 percent of cases by suppressing headshaking much in the same way as when we apply finger pressure to our nose to prevent a sneeze.
- Stall confinement out of direct sunlight can help.
- Facemasks block some ultraviolet light in cases of photic headshaking improving 52 percent of cases.
- Medication such as *cyproheptidine* gives relief in 70 percent, and *carbamazine* yields an 80 percent success rate.
- Neurectomy of the infraorbital nerve has had limited success and is fraught with complications such as painful neuromas and self-trauma.
- At the time of writing, research is evaluating the use of drugs like *fluphenazine* or *capsacin* in managing headshaking.

Horner's Syndrome

Horner's syndrome is the name attributed to a collection of neurologic signs that include drooping (*ptosis*) of the upper eyelid, constriction (*miosis*) of one or both pupils of the eye, and protrusion of the third eyelid or *enophthalamus* (recession of the eyeball within the orbit). Sweat glands on the side of an affected nerve may also be damaged such that spontaneous sweating is seen along the neck or head. This can be a consequence of trauma to nerves surrounding the local area of an IM or IV injection. (Localized damage to muscles of the neck or hip can also result in such spontaneous sweating near an old area of injury.)

Horner's syndrome results from nerve damage in specific locations, such as:

- The spine at the level of the first-through-third thoracic vertebrae (T1–3)
- The brachial nerve plexus in the armpit
- A space-occupying problem in the neck or around the throatlatch area
- A fracture of the lower skull
- An abscess behind the eye
- A guttural pouch infection

EPM may elicit Horner's-like symptoms, but other neurologic deficits, like ataxia, would also be present.

Cervical Vertebral Malformation aka Wobbler Syndrome

Cervical vertebral malformation (CVM), also known as *Wobbler syndrome,* is caused by compression of the spinal cord due to *stenosis* (narrowing) of the cervical canal of the spinal column. One cause of stenosis may be related to abnormal development of the articular processes of one or more spinal vertebrae of the neck. This may occur as an inherited trait or may be due to *osteochondrosis* of the vertebrae as part of the Developmental Orthopedic Disease (DOD). (See chapter 5, *Joints,* p. 131.) Stenosis of the vertebral channel places damaging pressure on the spinal cord, resulting in serious neurologic deficits. Neurologic signs related to spinal-cord compression may be intermittent at first.

Problems typically appear in horses less than 2 or 3 years of age. Rapidly growing horses, particularly those receiving rich nutrition, seem to be most affected. A "wobbler" demonstrates ataxia and weakness of all four limbs, with gait abnormalities most noticeable in the rear limbs (see photo 17.1, p. 502). The front limbs demonstrate weakness and stumbling, whereas the rear limbs are usually ataxic. Spastic gait movement is common. There may be signs of excess wear of the toes, particularly in front, due to toe-dragging. Muscle wasting is evident in some cases. Head and neck positioning may elicit or worsen ataxia and lack of proprioception, as will circling or negotiation of a hill.

In older horses, a wobbler condition may develop secondary to osteoarthritis of vertebral processes that results in narrowing of the spinal canal. In some cases, the spinal canal may have been somewhat restricted in dimension, but it is not until osteoarthritic impingement occurs that an older horse begins to show neurologic signs. Although 35 percent of mature horses have been identified with cervical spinal arthritis, only 1 in 35 will be afflicted with neurologic abnormalities related to spinal-cord impingement.

Diagnosis is based on clinical presentation, radiographic (X-ray) exam of the neck, and *myelogram* (injection of dye into the spinal column followed by radiographic evaluation) under general anesthesia. Treatment is best managed with surgery to stabilize the vertebrae, although in many cases, neurologic deficits are only improved one grade (out of five). If a young horse is treated quickly enough, 80 percent achieve some improvement, and reports claim that 63 percent improve sufficiently to continue athletic pursuits. There are safety and ethical ramifications to riding any horse with neurologic deficits, and these must be considered.

Equine Motor Neuron Disease

Equine motor neuron disease (EMND) has been identified only relatively recently, since the

1990s. It has been linked to a deficiency of vitamin E in the diet. It is seen in horses that have been stabled at the same location for at least 1½ years, with either minimal or no access to pasture, and fed only a diet of grass hay. Signs associated with EMND include muscle weakness, trembling, shifting of weight in the rear limbs, and muscle atrophy. Muscle wasting is most obvious over the back, neck, and upper limb muscles. Ataxia is not a feature of this disease as it is in many other neurologic syndromes. An affected horse loses weight and body condition in spite of a hearty appetite. Some horses with EMND tend to lie down more than normal. Many are extremely sensitive to touch (*hyperesthesia*). The tailhead tends to be carried in a somewhat elevated position, in contrast to the head and neck, which seem to be carried lower than normal. Persistent elevation of the tailhead is due to atrophy and contraction of the muscles of the tail head.

The disease appears to be progressive, with more noticeable deterioration over time. About 30 to 40 percent of affected horses demonstrate a brown, streaking discoloration (*lipopigment deposition*) in the retina of the eyes. Diagnosis is confirmed via a biopsy of the spinal accessory nerve or of the dorsal sacrocaudal muscle over the tailhead, and also by use of *electromyography*, which detects nerve activity in muscles.

Treatment is achieved with provision of daily supplemental vitamin E (10,000 IU twice a day) along with quality pasture and alfalfa hay, both of which are high in vitamin E. About 40 percent of cases will continue to deteriorate and end up being euthanized, while 40 percent will improve over 4 to 6 weeks once supplemented with vitamin E and moved to a different environment with access to pasture. The remaining 20 percent retain permanent muscle atrophy. Prevention is dependent upon access to green forage or daily supplementation (6000 to 8000 IU) of vitamin E in high-risk locations.

Shivers

Shivers is a neuromuscular disorder often found concurrent with *equine polysaccharide storage myopathy* (see chapter 4, *Muscle Endurance*, p. 172). A horse affected by shivers demonstrates muscular weakness, trembling, and abnormal limb action that typically appear in the rear limbs. With disease progression, there is generalized muscle atrophy, and abnormal limb action affects the front limbs, as well. Draft horses and Warmbloods seem most affected, although shivers has also been identified in Quarter Horses, Thoroughbreds, Arabians, and Morgans. It has been reported that 80 percent of shivers cases occur in stallions or geldings.

At first impression, the gait abnormality resembles stringhalt (see p. 524) or upward fixation of the patella (see p. 118). However, the limb aberration is seen mostly in the initial steps of walk, just before the horse stops, and if the horse is backed-up or circled tightly. When a horse with shivers advances an affected rear limb, the leg is flexed abnormally high and the limb moved away from the midline (*adduction*). This posture persists for several seconds. Abnormal limb movement occurs sporadically rather than with every step as seen with stringhalt. The tail of a horse with shivers is elevated for the duration of abnormal limb flexion; there is concurrent quivering of the tail and/or muscles of the hind leg. A farrier may first note a mild case as persistent tremors in a horse's limb when held up for shoeing.

Cold weather, anxiety, and restriction of exercise amplify shivers signs. The syndrome is a progressive degeneration; it may take 10 years to manifest severe signs following recognition of an initial gait abnormality. Dietary management of EPSSM (high fat, and low starch, low sugar diet) can yield improvement, and may slow the progression of the shivers condition.

Polyneuritis Equi

Polyneuritis equi, or PNE, previously referred to as *cauda equina*, is a neurologic condition not commonly seen in horses. It is thought that the nervous system is affected by an immune reaction concurrent with viral inflammation.

An affected horse is afflicted with paralysis and loss of sensation of the tail and anal sphincter as well as other cranial nerve and peripheral nerve deficits. Acute onset exhibits itself as extreme sensitivity around the anus and/or head, causing a horse to rub or chew his tail. Then, as the disease progresses to a chronic form, the horse is affected with paralysis of the tail, anus, rectum, penis, and bladder. Urine incontinence results from loss of bladder tone; colic may result from an inability to defecate. There is often muscle atrophy of the hip muscles, and some ataxia, and other gait abnormalities. Cranial nerve signs may appear in horses with head involvement. Usually, there is evidence of profound muscle wasting as the disease progresses.

There is no known treatment for PNE other than to address the symptoms and prevent colic from fecal retention, or urinary tract infection from distention of the bladder.

Narcolepsy

NORMAL SLEEP PATTERNS

Normal sleep patterns of horses include periods of slow-wave sleep (SWS) and rapid eye movement sleep (REM). Most horses normally sleep an average of 3 to 5 hours per day, but REM sleep only occurs for, at most, 1 hour a day. A horse must lie down on his side (lateral recumbency) to achieve REM sleep. SWS can occur with a horse in a standing position, head down, legs locked. A horse sleeping in SWS may also lie down resting on his sternum, with his legs tucked beneath him.

ABNORMAL SLEEP

Narcolepsy is a sleep disorder that is characterized by excessive sleepiness and a sudden onset of REM sleep. A standing horse may lower his head and suddenly buckle for no apparent reason, having dozed off without warning. An affected horse usually catches himself before falling; it is common to see chronic abrasions and thickened skin on the front of the fetlocks and/or carpal joints (knees) in narcoleptic horses. Usually, such episodes are intermittent and occur while a horse is being groomed or saddled, or is standing relaxed in the stall or paddock.

The cause of narcolepsy seems to be a result of abnormal biochemical-neurotransmitter signals in the brain. Adult-onset narcolepsy occurs in horses more than 2 years of age. Generally, narcolepsy is inconvenient to a horse owner but does not preclude athletic pursuits. Caution should be taken to keep a relaxed horse in an "awake" state, and to take care about where a horse is tied so if he starts to fall, minimal injury is incurred. On a rare occasion, narcoleptic collapse may occur in a horse while he is ridden, but this is the exception rather than the rule. Such an unusual case poses a hazard to safety and that horse should not be ridden.

Sleep Deprivation

At times, behavioral, social, or pain-related conditions may cause a horse to be incapable of normal sleep cycles or an inability to lie down to achieve REM sleep. An affected horse may have a sudden attack of extreme muscular weakness (*cataplexy*) that causes him to appear to fall. Such horses are considered "narcoleptic" although in fact, their problem is not one of a biochemical-neurotransmitter abnormality, but rather is a problem of sleep deprivation and exhaustion. Examples of conditions that might interfere with a horse's normal sleep include:

- Fear, as for example, loud noises, fireworks, new environment
- Stress
- Transport
- Social isolation or separation anxiety
- Herd aggression or bullying
- Arthritis or musculoskeletal injury that prevents a horse from lying down
- Colic conditions that make it painful to stay on the ground
- Lung or abdominal infection that makes it painful to lie down

DIFFERENTIAL DIAGNOSIS OF NARCOLEPSY

Sudden collapse with or without loss of consciousness may occur due to a variety of reasons, including:

- *Syncope* (fainting spell)
- Cardiovascular collapse from heart problems
- Equine protozoal myelitis (EPM—see p. 510)
- Seizures
- Botulism (see p. 525)
- Tying-up syndrome (see p. 166)
- Hyperkalemic periodic paralysis (HYPP—see p. 176)

Diagnostic workup with a thorough clinical examination, echocardiography, electrocardiography, and blood tests is important to rule out such other medical issues.

Syncope

A horse may collapse suddenly due to an episode of *syncope*, which is like a fainting spell. Rapid elevation of a horse's head and neck with flexion of the poll may precipitate such an event. Such evasion postures may be elicited by deworming procedures, during dental procedures, or even when an intravenous injection is administered and a horse tries to move away. It is postulated that elevation of the head activates *baroreceptors* in the head that are acutely sensitive to postural changes. Such a positional change stimulates reflex activity of the *vagus nerve* with the result that blood pressure lowers rapidly and the horse loses consciousness and so, faints.

Seizures

A horse that is experiencing seizure behavior will collapse suddenly, but unlike the collapse seen with narcolepsy, a seizuring horse will have spasms of the jaw and facial muscles, and the spine arches in rigid contraction (*opisthotonus*) during the seizure episode.

Seizures usually appear after several seconds of warning (*pre-ictal*) as an observable behavioral or postural change.

Neurologic Trauma

The Fallen Horse

There are many ways a horse can fall. He may be running and suddenly slip or trip. He can get tangled in a jump or come off it wrong. He might attempt to jump a fence and end up flipping over it instead. He can rear up and fall over; this is a common accident seen with securing a horse in crossties. He can slip on a longe line and hit the ground hard on his side.

One minute he's on his feet, and then suddenly, without warning, he's down. In many cases, a fallen horse jumps up, shakes himself off, and goes on, seemingly unharmed. But, when 1000 pounds or more of horseflesh hits the ground, it is not unusual for something to go wrong. In the worst cases, damage is done to the spine or the head, the exact degree of injury being dependent upon how the horse lands. Only half the time is the fall actually observed.

RISK ACTIVITIES

A horse can fall under any conditions, at play in the pasture or at work in training or competition. Jumping horses may have the most risk in falling, but other sport horses also can hit the ground with a simple misstep. Polo ponies crashing into one another or in a tight turn are prone to falling. A trail horse can step onto an unstable piece of ground or tangle in a branch or bush and go down. Just about any athletic endeavor is fraught with perils, particularly if the horse isn't paying attention or if the footing or terrain is hazardous.

WHAT TO DO IF A HORSE HAS FALLEN

Whenever a horse is known to have fallen, have a vet come at once and evaluate the damages. Don't ride the horse until there is assurance that he has not suffered any neurologic injury. Sometimes all that is evident are some nicks and scrapes and bruises, and nothing more. Sometimes there are obvious signs of trauma related to neurologic problems such as a head tilt, dropped ear, or an unsteady gait. The look in a horse's eyes gives information as to the seriousness of mental change, or pain. A veterinarian will examine all body parts and check for more significant injuries. Anti-inflammatory medication is administered to minimize the effects of the trauma. There may be areas that will benefit from ice packs to reduce the effects of the initial damage.

A complete physical exam by a veterinarian evaluates heart, breathing, and gut sounds. The musculoskeletal system will be examined and palpated to check for injury. Finger probing will evaluate for pain over the ribs, spine, or back, and along each limb. The interior of the eyes will be examined with an ophthalmoscope to identify if there has been any injury to the optic nerve. Cranial nerves will be evaluated to ensure proper function. Coordination will be observed at all gaits, backing, and turning, and on an incline when possible. Establishment of baseline parameters enables monitoring over the next several days and rapid recognition of an abnormality.

SWISS STUDY

A study was made of 100 neurologic cases that entered the Veterinary Teaching Hospital at the University of Zurich through December 1997. Trauma was determined in 22 of them. Of 12 horses that were observed to have fallen, 9 showed immediate neurologic deficits, one demonstrated problems between 6 to 12 hours later, and two of the horses showed clinical signs more than 2 months following the incident.

One-third of the horses that experienced spinal trauma were recumbent; the others were ataxic to varying degrees. Those horses that improved immediately with treatment or within 6 weeks of initiating treatment had a good prognosis. The recumbent horses were all euthanized due to lack of response or continued deterioration. Horses don't do well when they are unable to rise. After a few days, there is the potential for serious, life-threatening complications:

- Muscle compression and damage, and myoglobin release
- Kidney failure from myoglobin release
- Lung congestion and pneumonia

If a horse remains down for too long, he may never be able to rise. It is always best to find a sling to support the horse off the ground, and failing that, the horse should be rolled consistently to the opposite side every 2 to 4 hours to relieve pressure on the muscles and lungs on each side (photo 17.8).

This study yields some insightful information about trauma as related to falls. Information that is not available includes the number of cases of horse falls in which a horse gets up and

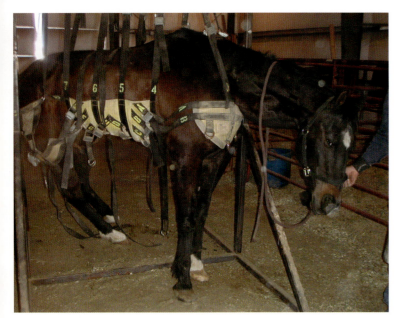

17.8 A recumbent horse that is unable to rise can suffer damage to his muscles or lungs from lying on his side for extended time with the weight of his body mass bearing down and obstructing circulation in these organs. As seen here, the horse is lifted from the ground and the sling suspends him to "stand" in a more natural position. A sling is important to support a recumbent horse and enable circulation in the limbs and ample expansion of his lungs.

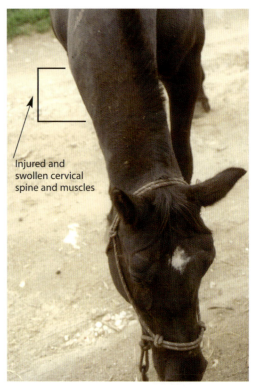

Injured and swollen cervical spine and muscles

17.9 This horse suffered a significant injury to her cervical spine, causing her head and neck to remain in this position until pain and swelling were under better control.

carries on as if nothing has happened, or the number of cases in which a horse falls or flips, breaks his neck, and dies instantly. None of these occurrences were reported to be included as part of the statistics. The Swiss study reviews potential areas of injury that are at risk from the brute weight of a horse falling on himself.

Spinal Trauma or Vertebral Fracture

The most common area of injury in a fall is the *cervical* spine as a horse often falls on his flexed neck. More than half the cases of spinal trauma incurred injury to the cervical spine (photo 17.9). Other horses injured the *thoracic* or *lumbar* spines, depending on how they landed.

A horse that is recumbent has a poor prognosis. Recumbency is often related to lesions found in the caudal cervical or thoracic spine. Horses that injure the more cranial part of the cervical spine are usually able to stand, although with some degree of ataxia and unsteadiness.

There are instances where a horse may have fallen and is seemingly fine until months or years later. At that time, neurologic deficits start to develop, commonly due to degenerative arthritis within the spinal column that is secondary to trauma incurred in the original fall.

Head Trauma

A horse that hits his head or is kicked in the

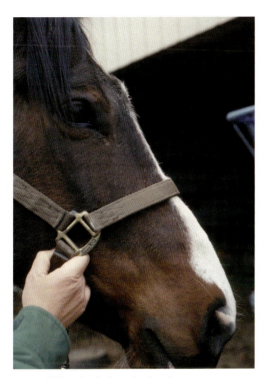

17.10 *When kicked in the head, it is not uncommon for a horse to suffer a skull fracture into the sinus, as seen here. Often, these heal with only a cosmetic concern, but on occasion, surgical intervention is necessary to align the bones for healing, and so there is no impediment to air flow through the sinus.*

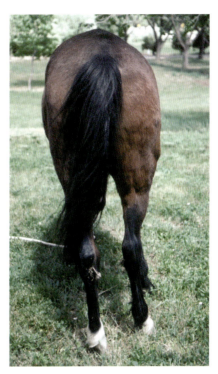

17-.11 *Muscle asymmetry and atrophy as visible on this horse's right hip area point to previous trauma and/or pelvic or spinal injury. The reason for this asymmetric appearance should be evaluated carefully in considering if this horse is safe to ride.*

head can injure it in many ways (photo 17.10). Most often a horse hits his poll or the base of the skull, particularly in cases where the horse rears and flips over backward. A horse may become stuporous or depressed, even lapsing into a coma. There may be loss of cranial nerve function, including vision. There are varying degrees of disturbed limb function relative to where a lesion is located in the brain. Loss of equilibrium may occur with fractures of small bones (*temporohyoid bones*) near the ear. Some signs of head trauma are subtle and may pass unrecognized. Some are hard to miss, especially for an owner who is sensitive to a horse's demeanor and personality.

Body Trauma

Not all injuries related to a fall result in neurologic problems. Many instances result in musculoskeletal injury such as a fractured shoulder, a "knocked-down" hip (photo 17.11), a cracked rib, or muscle strain. Leg injuries are more obvious to discern but sometimes injury to the back is not revealed until a horse is returned to work under saddle or asked for a high level of performance. On an odd occasion, a horse that hits the ground hard on his side might experience bruising of the internal organs, setting him off his feed for some days. Other times, some serious injury may become apparent with the development of muscle atrophy.

BEFORE THE FALL

Not all cases of injury are clear-cut. There are as many variations on the theme of what can go wrong as there are ways to fall and land. Not all injuries are incurred when a horse hits the ground, but rather they occur as the horse attempts to stay on his feet, or as a result of what caused the horse to fall in the first place. Examples of these might be hyperextension of a joint, tendon, or ligament, or a limb fracture.

PREVENTION

No one wants to witness a horse falling, nor does anyone want to be on a horse that is falling. Other than a freak accident, there are ways to minimize the chances of this occurring. Besides owning a horse with good athletic ability, some applied strategies might help a horse stay on his feet:

- Make sure the feet are trimmed and shod on a regular basis with attention paid to preventing the toes from growing too long ("backing up" the toes).
- Have a vet review a horse's movement a couple times a year to check for musculoskeletal pain or subtle lameness that could result in a misstep.
- Condition a horse to the intended athletic tasks so he is fit for the job and not prone to fatigue during exercise.
- Don't cross-tie a horse, and especially don't cross-tie one and leave him unattended.
- Be cautious in turning horses out when the ground is slippery with mud or ice.
- Ensure sturdiness of fences and build them at heights that will deter a horse from considering trying to jump over them.
- Pasture compatible horses together to minimize the chance that one might be run into or over a fence.
- Remove obstacles from pastures when possible.
- Fence-out farm equipment, gullies or ravines from the vicinity of horses.
- Lead a horse through an unfamiliar property in both directions before turning him loose to show him fence lines, ditches, and obstacles.
- When in the saddle, ensure that a horse's attention is focused at all times.

Sweeny

Damage to the *suprascapular* nerve can create a condition of muscle atrophy known as *sweeny*. The suprascapular nerve controls nerve function of the muscle belly that lies in front of the spine of the scapula (shoulder blade). A direct blow may injure this nerve where it passes across the lower part of the shoulder near the shoulder joint. It may also be injured if a horse slips and falls, thereby stretching the nerve.

The most noticeable indication of sweeny is that of muscle atrophy; however, because the muscles of the shoulder are what support movement of the shoulder, then a horse with weak or atrophied shoulder muscles will tend to *abduct* (position away from the body) the shoulder joint when bearing weight on the limb.

Therapy is aimed at reducing inflammation to the nerve with ice and anti-inflammatory medications. The use of electrostimulation may maintain some tonus activity in the muscle belly while waiting for the nerve to recover. A horse that does not make steady recovery within a couple of months may be a candidate for surgical decompression of the suprascapular nerve.

Stringhalt

There are multiple types of *stringhalt*, some related to plant ingestion, others related to trauma or irritation of a nerve. Horses affected by stringhalt have an involuntary flexion of one or both hind limbs. This high-stepping limb movement is best seen at a walk. There may be associated muscle atrophy of the hindquarters.

ACQUIRED STRINGHALT

This syndrome (found mostly in Australia but also in the Pacific Northwest) is due to ingestion of false dandelion or flatweed (*Hypochaeris radicata*), especially following drought conditions. The plant may affect about 15 percent of horses in a herd. Most of these cases resolve spontaneously once the plant is eliminated from a horse's access, although complete recovery may take from 2 weeks up to 2 years (see *Appendix C,* p. 571).

TRAUMATIC STRINGHALT

Another cause of stringhalt may be related to trauma or compression of a nerve at a trauma site. Some cases may be a result of damage to entrapment of the *obturator nerve* in the hip region. The spastic, exaggerated limb movement may be related to lack of coordination of nerve impulses regulating excursion of the stifle. Other cases may be related to irritation or scar-tissue adhesions following trauma in the upper region of the rear cannon bone or hock.

Nutrition-Related Neurologic Disease

Botulism

An oxygen-deficient environment encourages growth of bacteria called *Clostridium botulinum*, of the same family of germs that creates tetanus. *Clostridium botulinum* produces spores and a powerful toxin that affects the neuromuscular system. The syndrome it produces is more commonly known as *botulism*, rapidly fatal to man and horses. It is also referred to as *shaker foal syndrome* in foals or *forage poisoning* in adult horses.

There are several different forms of the botulism toxin that affect horses. Around the mid-Atlantic seaboard and Kentucky, the organism exists in the soils producing a Type B toxin. In Florida and in parts of California, poisoning has been attributed to the Type C toxin.

Horses are extremely susceptible to the *Clostridium botulinum* toxin; compared to a mouse, a horse is 10,000 times more sensitive. The same dose administered without effect to a small rodent is enough to kill a 1000-pound horse.

HOW IS A HORSE INFECTED?

There are three possible ways for a foal or a horse to contract the syndrome. The most common route of infection is referred to as a *toxicoinfectious* form, with the horse or foal ingesting spores that live in the soil. About 18 percent of soils in the United States contain these spores. Once in the intestinal tract, the spores vegetate and the bacteria proliferate, ultimately generating the lethal toxin. Some predisposing irritation in the horse's intestinal lining allows *Clostridium botulinum* bacteria to grow. In foals, stomach ulcers seem to be the most likely suspect areas where bacteria set up housekeeping. Ulcers may develop because of too rich a diet (either from a mare's milk or supplemental feed), subsequent to stress, or in an area of the bowel that has been irritated by sand ingestion or parasites. Youngsters, generally between 2 to 8 weeks old are most at risk. Foals taste and lick everything, including the ground. The spores are ingested, and the organisms then colonize the gastrointestinal tract to quickly produce a sick foal.

A second form of infection occurs when the toxin is already preformed in the environment, and a horse or foal eats it directly from contaminated feed. (This is similar to the crisis encountered by humans eating contaminated canned goods.) Feed that is contaminated with putrefied remains, or water that has been contaminated with animal remains are possible sources of infection for adult horses, hence the term "forage poisoning." A warm, moist environment allows plant or animal matter to decompose rapidly. A decomposing animal, such as a rodent or bird that inadvertently got bound in the baler is one source of contamination of horse feed. Decomposing plant matter (including hay or grain) is another source of the organism and subsequent elaboration of toxin. Any feed that shows signs of mold encourages an environment that is favorable for botulism. This applies not only to baled hay or grain, but also to silage or feed bagged in plastic. In situations of feed contamination, more than one animal is often affected.

Although infrequent, a deep wound can also be a source of local production of toxin. A deep wound that has been infected with *Clostridium botulinum* may contain the right conditions conducive to growth of the bacteria, namely an anaerobic tissue environment coupled with the presence of this organism. Such a situation occurs in a traumatic wound from an infected umbilical cord, or at a castration site.

SIGNS OF BOTULISM

The progression of signs seen with botulism is initially confusing because the horse looks fine and is alert and hungry, at first. He has no fever, and continues to eat and drink. However, he doesn't chew or swallow normally due the neurologic involvement of facial muscles. Saliva may drool from his nose or mouth. An affected horse may display a stiff or shuffling gait as the muscles weaken. Flank and shoulder muscles tremble. (When botulism poisoning is seen in a foal, it is called shaker foal sydrome because of the intensity of shaking and tremoring of his muscles.) Often, the horse has poor tone of the tail, tongue, and eyelids. The pupils may dilate. As *flaccid paralysis* progresses, the horse's muscles become weak, and he has difficulty staying on his feet. And, as respiratory muscles become more involved, an affected horse is labored in his breathing or may pant. Eventually, generalized muscle weakness causes recumbency, with the potential for respiratory paralysis and death. The more toxin the horse has within his body, the more profound the signs and the more quickly the syndrome progresses. Without treatment, rapidly affected horses or foals die within 48 hours.

Toxin Effects

The toxin that is elaborated by the *Clostridium botulinum* organism interferes with calcium utilization in the body in such a way that an insufficient amount of the neurotransmitter, *acetylcholine*, is released at the neuromuscular junction. This chemical is responsible for firing of the nerves to make muscles work and move. The toxin creates a situation comparable to what would happen if nerves were surgically cut at many locations at once. First affected are the muscles of the face and head that control chewing or swallowing. Eyelid tone diminishes, and facial muscles lose their tight appearance. Eventually, all skeletal muscle and respiratory muscles are affected. The central nervous system is not affected; on initial appearance the horse seems alert with no signs other than those related to progressive, generalized muscle weakness.

The more slowly the syndrome develops, the greater the chance for recovery. A horse that reaches a critical stage in the disease may be treated aggressively with antitoxin and antibiotics and recover; however, reduced nerve function to the muscles will cause them to atrophy, at least for a time. Wasted muscle mass can eventually recover to normal provided the toxin is arrested early enough with treatment.

TREATMENT

It may be difficult to differentiate beginning signs of botulism from a variety of other neuromuscular syndromes. The key to successful treatment is quick recognition of the poisoning. There is an antitoxin on the market available to combat the Type B toxin. Prior to the availability of this toxin, survival from the disease approached 10 percent at best. Now, more than 70 percent of affected horses have a fair chance at surviving if antitoxin is given early in the course of disease. By binding to circulating toxin, the antitoxin blocks further effects of toxin but cannot reverse damage already done. Any toxin already attached to the neuromuscular junction continues to create clinical symptoms, and these must run their course.

An affected horse should be kept quiet so as not to further stress the muscles and use up limited supplies of neurotransmitter. Antibiotics combat poisoning by killing *Clostridial* organisms within the intestinal tract so no further toxin is produced. Supportive care, such as feeding through a nasogastric tube or providing mechanical ventilation, allows a horse to weather through the worst of a crisis. Intravenous fluids treat dehydration that develops with impairment of swallowing. Other problems associated with the illness also need to be addressed. Stalls should be deeply bedded to prevent skin sores from forming while a horse is recumbent. Muscle massage helps maintain circulation in the muscles of a down horse.

PREVENTION OF BOTULISM

The prevalence of this form of poisoning in areas of high foal production in Kentucky and along the Atlantic seaboard stimulated the development of a vaccine against the Type B toxin. Unfortunately, Type B toxoid has limited cross-protection against the Type C strain of toxin; currently there is no vaccine available for Type C botulism.

Vaccination protocol calls for 3 doses of *Clostridium botulinum* Type B toxoid given at 1-month intervals. Boosters are repeated annually. Pregnant mares are vaccinated 1 month prior to foaling so the colostrum contains antibodies to the botulism organism to protect the foal in his first few months. Vaccinate horses that live in a high-risk area for botulism, as well as horses that will be transported to those areas of concern.

Moldy Corn Poisoning

Also known as *encephalomalacia* or *blind staggers*, this disease is associated with consumption of corn that has been contaminated by the fungus, *Fusarium moniliforms*, which elaborates toxins. This fungus thrives on corn plants that have been stressed by drought, disease, or insects prior to harvest. High humidity and moisture encourage proliferation of the mold. Exposure to high doses over a short period of time results in liver toxicity, while low doses ingested over a longer time (3 to 4 weeks) result in brain damage, or encephalomalacia. Clinical signs include decreased appetite, behavioral changes such as depression, anxiety, or hyperexcitability, and neurologic signs such as circling, blindness, difficulty chewing or swallowing, muscle tremors, ataxia, recumbency, and eventually coma. Depending on the amount of toxin ingested, moldy corn poisoning takes 7 to 75 days before the horse demonstrates clinical signs; once signs are seen, death occurs within 2 to 3 days.

Toxic Plants That Affect the Nervous System

SORGHUM-SUDAN GRASS

Neurologic deficits related to ingestion of *sorghum-sudan grass* are similar to signs seen with *polyneuritis equi*, described on p. 519. Sorghum species, including Sudan grass, create problems of the urinary tract and kidneys with the horse dribbling urine and becoming unstable and weak in the rear legs. This plant has a cyanide-like substance that accumulates during stress conditions of drought or freezing, or during periods of rapid growth. The toxin elicits degeneration of nerves supplying the urinary bladder and rear quarters. Muscles around the anal region relax, the penis protrudes, tail tone weakens, and the bladder loses tone and the horse may develop a bladder or kidney infection as a result. Hind limb ataxia and weakness develop as well as a classic sign of this toxicity: "bunny hopping," in which the horse lifts both hind limbs off the ground simultaneously.

LOCOWEED

Many of the plants that cause nervous system disorders have an alkaloid as their toxic principle. Locoweeds (*Astragalus* spp. and *Oxytropis* spp.) are familiar plants that create such toxicity. An affected horse is referred to as being "loco." Typically, horses won't eat this plant unless other forage becomes scarce. Some horses become addicted to locoweed, and if enough plant material (30 percent of a horse's body weight) is ingested over weeks or months, a horse's temperament may change. There may be spells of unpredictable and dangerous behavior followed by progressive deterioration in coordination and mental alertness. Visual impairment is a common symptom, as is difficulty in eating and drinking. The brain and spinal cord slowly degenerate and unless a horse is removed early enough from access to the plant, the ailment becomes irreversible.

LUPINE AND LARKSPUR

Lupine (*Lupinus argenteus*) also contains alkaloids that cause a horse to act nervous, froth at the mouth, or go into convulsions. Just as lupine is found both in the wild and as an ornamental, larkspur (*Delphinium* spp.) is found in both environments. Larkspur exerts central nervous system effects of muscle twitching, excess salivation, collapse, convulsions, or respiratory failure.

YELLOW STAR THISTLE AND RUSSIAN KNAPWEED

Yellow star thistle (*Centaurea solstitialis*) and a close relative, Russian knapweed (*Acroptilon repens*), are plants that initiate degeneration of the brain tissue to produce *nigropallidal encephalomalacia*. Distinctive symptoms include difficulty taking in and chewing food or swallowing water due to paralysis of the tongue and chewing muscles. The facial and lip muscles become overly tonic and rigid, the horse assuming a fixed stare. A horse suffering from toxicity is depressed and may also demonstrate muscle tremors, wander aimlessly, and may be ataxic. An affected horse usually dies of starvation. Despite the spiny nature of the thistles, horses seek them out; over time the effects become evident. Neurologic damage is irreversible.

BRACKEN FERN AND HORSETAIL

When other forage is scarce, horses may consume bracken fern (*Pterydium aquilinium*). Long-term (30 to 60 days) consumption of this plant destroys an important vitamin called *thiamine* (vitamin B1). Thiamine deficiency leads to brain degeneration, with an affected horse showing signs of depression, lack of appetite, weight loss, muscle tremors, and incoordination. An affected horse often stands with a base-wide stance, and his back may be arched. If treated with thiamine supplementation before a horse becomes recumbent, death may be averted. Horsetail (*Equisetum* spp.) has similar thiamine destruction effects as bracken fern, but generally a horse's appetite remains, although poisoning effects become dangerously progressive due to thiamine deficiency. Horsetail is also fairly unpalatable so a horse is less likely to consume it, unless it ends up baled in the hay.

NIGHTSHADE

An unusual toxic reaction has been known to occur in horses eating silverleaf nightshade (*Solanum eleagnifolium*) in conjunction with being dewormed with ivermectin. Ingestion of this plant in hay or pasture amplifies the amount of ivermectin that is absorbed by the brain tissues, resulting in toxic levels. Affected horses show neurologic signs such as drooping lips and ears, drooling, incoordination, head pressing, and depression. Clinical signs occur within 24 hours of medication with ivermectin. The most effective treatment is to immediately remove the plant from the diet.

MALLOW

Ingestion of the mallow plant (*Malva* spp.) may cause a syndrome of muscle tremors similar in appearance to "shivers."

LATHYRISM

Seeds of singletary pea (*Lathyrus hirsutus*) eaten over weeks or months induce a stringhalt-like syndrome with partial paralysis of the hind legs. An early sign is suspected when the horse stands with his hind limbs forward beneath his body. Removal of the plant from the diet allows recovery.

MILKWEED

Usually horses find western-whorled milkweed (*Asclepias* spp.) to be bitter and unpalatable although it may inadvertently be eaten if baled with hay. Clinical signs vary, including: loss of coordination, muscle tremors, depression, gastrointestinal-tract irritation, respiratory problems, convulsions, or death.

WATER HEMLOCK

Water hemlock (*Cicuta maculata*) is known for its potent poisoning effects, particularly when rootstock is consumed. If enough of the plant is eaten, convulsion, respiratory failure, and death may occur within 30 minutes. If a horse survives beyond 6 hours, he is likely to recover with no ill effects.

For a complete description and explanation of plants that are toxic in horses see *Appendix C*, p. 571, and a *A Guide to Plant Poisoning of Animals in North America* by Anthony P. Knight (Teton New Media, 2001).

Reproductive Strategies and Health   18

Promoting Genetic Improvement

Only with conscientious recognition of undesirable traits, and a concerted effort to eradicate these characteristics will a breeder promote continued improvement of horses. Discuss suspected flaws with a veterinarian and other breeders. Be hypercritical of a mare. Before breeding, carefully assess the contribution a mare or stallion can make to the horse population. Breeding a horse that is crippled due to conformational defects does little to improve the equine world at large and may produce a foal with similar problems (photo 18.1).

Breeding an excellent mare to a poor stallion, or vice versa, is a bad investment. It is best not to cut corners by diluting good stock. The initial cost of breeding a mare is only a small part of raising a foal to performance age. Select an excellent stallion and an excellent mare to ensure improvement of the genetic pool. Analyze the performance of the sire and his offspring, and the mare and her offspring. Critically evaluate compatibility of conformational aspects between stallion and mare.

Scientific Interference

The days of spontaneously breeding a mare in a whimsical moment have vanished, as quality

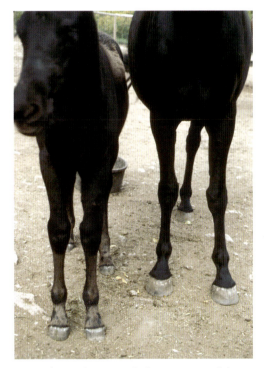

18.1 *The conformational characteristics of the mare contribute 50 percent to the genetic makeup of a foal, so be selective when choosing her. This Morgan foal has inherited the relatively straight legs, ample joints, and solid feet from her dam, as well as her black coloration. If you look very carefully, you might notice that the mare's left front limb rotates outward very slightly from the carpus (knee), and so does the foal's left front limb. Inheritance of specific genetic characteristics cannot be controlled, but a breeder can be selective about what traits to attempt to propagate.*

stallions and mares must schedule time for propagation of the species. With human interference and manipulation of reproductively less efficient animals, we may, in fact, perpetuate the necessity of scientific manipulation. Mother Nature no longer selects for reproductively sound horses that breed and foal without human assistance. Many other variables arise as we breed for athletic performance and beauty, and remove the natural selection process for reproductive efficiency. A poorly conformed, slanting vagina (see p. 545), urine pooling (see p. 547), or an infected uterus (see p. 548) often are medically or surgically repaired. These conformational problems are genetically passed to a foal, allowing continued propagation of problems that would have been selected away in the gene pool.

Breeding Evaluation

Besides careful consideration of the contributions that a stallion or a mare may make to the gene pool, both genders should undergo a thorough reproductive exam to ensure a sound return on the investment involved in getting a mare in foal.

The Stallion

A breeding stallion has a unique role in the breeding world. Not only is it possible to ride him as a performance horse, but his genetic characteristics also may be passed on to future generations without significant interruption of a competition schedule. Because of his lasting influence to a genetic line, a stringent selection process should be applied to selecting a stallion. Both a potential stallion owner and broodmare owner should seek the best complement of mare and stallion.

A stallion's disposition and temperament are vital to the enjoyment of a stallion and his progeny. A bad-tempered stallion is hazardous to his handlers, to farm personnel, and to broodmares (photo 18.2). Bad disposition is potentially passed to a foal. It is wise to geld a dangerous stallion rather than risk passing poor temperament to future offspring.

Before investing in a breeding stallion, evaluate the stallion's performance results. If he has progeny old enough to compete, track their performance results, both successes and failures. Examine offspring to see if the desired characteristics are passed to succeeding generations. Pedigree may suggest potential, but recent generations of offspring prove, or disprove the athletic value of a specific genetic line.

When considering a stallion, match him to a mare with a complementary body type and conformational strengths. Find a stallion with similar desirable characteristics to reinforce them in a foal, and with characteristics that improve or correct weak components of a mare. If a mare has too many faults, consider breeding a different mare rather than risk perpetuation of conformational defects in the offspring. A mare or stallion that has been retired due to lameness caused by conformational problems should not be considered as a breeding prospect. There is no sense in breeding a mare or stallion only to create a foal with similar unsoundness.

Breeding Performance

Not only do good looks, strong conformation, and an impressive athletic record make a stallion excellent for propagating these desirable traits, but also he must be able to perform his duties as a breeding horse. To adequately evaluate a stallion's reproductive capacity, his semen should be collected and analyzed. In the process of collecting semen, information is also gained regarding a stallion's libido and breeding behavior. Subsequent to previous bad experiences, the breeding process may intimi-

Reproductive Strategies and Health

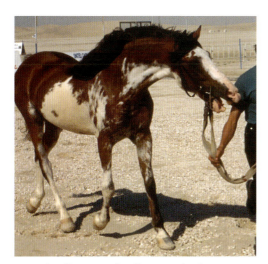

18.2 *An ill-tempered stallion can be dangerous to people, and may pass this disposition to the foal. The stallion here is expressing mild aggression by nipping at his handler's arm and posturing while being led.*

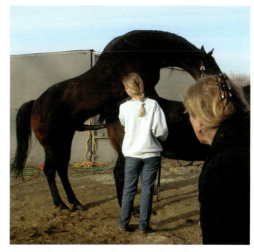

18.3 *A breeding stallion must be able to rise on his hind legs to mount a mare or a phantom breeding dummy. Age-related or degenerative musculoskeletal conditions may make it difficult for him to breed unless the breeding shed has an area with a ramped pit that places the mare below the stallion.*

date a stallion, whether he is bred by *live cover* or is collected in an *artificial vagina* (AV). It is valuable to discover if a stallion is aggressive and difficult to handle when presented with a mare in heat, or if he has trouble attaining and holding an erection, mounting a mare or dummy, or achieving ejaculation. However, it is premature to make too many assumptions about the performance of an inexperienced stallion in his first attempts.

A breeding stallion must be able to rise on his hind legs to mount a mare or a phantom breeding dummy (photo 18.3). Some breeding sheds create special facilities to place a mare in a low point on the ground to allow an arthritic stallion easier access to her. Such management considerations by a breeding farm are as important as the overall health of the stallion because they ensure the success of live coverage.

Stallion management is fairly straightforward as it relates to incorporating breeding into a competitive riding schedule. Horses are usually retained as intact stallions in order to propagate favorable genetic characteristics. But, some stallion owners like to ride and be around a stallion and have little interest in breeding. With the use of chilled and frozen semen in today's reproductive arsenal, breeding of a stallion takes little away from his competitive obligations. Once a stallion has been booked, a stallion owner only needs to know the day that semen is required, and then the stallion is collected, the semen shipped, and the stallion returns immediately to life as usual.

STALLION APPRAISAL FOR A MARE OWNER

Before embarking on the fine details of breeding a mare, first investigate the background of a chosen stallion. When possible, look at his offspring to see if his get are as anticipated. Is he registered and is he licensed for breeding so a future foal can be registered? Inquire as to how good his conception rates are with transported semen. There's no sense breeding to a stallion with poor semen quality, as this becomes an expensive exercise in frustration. Talk to the stallion manager and obtain percentages of settled mares and live foals produced by a stallion. Discuss shipped-semen fertility with the stallion's veterinarian, if possible. Confirm how far in advance a stallion farm must be notified prior to a request for semen collection, and how late into the season they are willing to breed in the event that multiple attempts are needed to settle a mare. (For discussion on live cover versus artificial insemination, see p. 550.)

BOOKING TO A STALLION

Long before it is time to breed a mare, arrangements should be made with the stallion manager to "book" the mare in time for the breeding season ahead. A stallion can only breed so many mares each season, especially if he is involved in a show or performance schedule. To avoid profound disappointment at finding a stallion's bookings filled, plan as much as a year in advance.

THE BREEDING CONTRACT

Usually, a written contract is executed between stallion breeder and mare owner. Read the contract thoroughly; make sure all wording is understandable. Discussion of mare care and liability for veterinary services while a mare is at the breeding farm should be included in the contract to avoid misunderstandings. Determine if the stud fee includes semen collection charges if transported semen is to be used. If not, veterinary expenses can add up if a stallion must be collected repeatedly for a mare that fails to conceive on the first cycle she is bred.

Many stud farms require a uterine biopsy, bacterial culture, and cytology (cellular evaluation) of the mare's uterus before entering into a breeding contract. The costs of a pre-breeding evaluation for a mare must be further considered when determining the financial feasibility of breeding a mare. Most stud fees include a *live foal guarantee* (LFG), meaning that if a mare fails to conceive, aborts, or gives birth to a dead foal, the mare owner is not liable to pay the stud fee or is promised a breeding the following season at no charge. Review the contract for a clause stating a live foal guarantee to avoid loss of the stud fee and related expenses should something go wrong.

TEASING PROGRAMS

No matter whether a mare is to be bred by live cover, or inseminated with shipped semen or with semen freshly collected from a stallion on the property, find a reputable breeding facility that manages a competent breeding operation. Valuable time is lost without proper *teasing* techniques, teasing frequency, and record-keeping. Interview a stallion manager about the farm's record-keeping and inquire if there is a consistent daily teasing program to detect when a mare is in heat. A significant cause of "infertility" is management's failure to identify if a mare is in *estrus* and ready for breeding. An excellent teasing program is a key to success so a breeder can identify when a mare is in heat. This may be difficult in some mares with "silent" heats that refuse to show to any stallion or show to only one particular stallion. In these cases, daily rectal palpation and ultrasound exams may be necessary to identify breeding time. Careful attention to teasing records also minimizes the number of times a stallion is required to inseminate a mare. The fewer times he must breed her or be collected reduces the chances for injury and infection, and increases the number of mares he can breed in a season.

General Physical Exam

A thorough exam evaluates soundness of a stallion's breeding capabilities. A breeding exam begins with a thorough history and general physical examination of a stallion's overall health. Deworming and vaccination schedules are reviewed, and prior experience or problems associated with breeding are discussed. A complete history of medical or surgical events should be disclosed to determine if a past problem is injurious to a stallion's career as a breeding horse.

A breeding stallion should be in good flesh, neither too fat nor too thin. His teeth should be fully checked for problems that may interfere with continuing good condition. His heart and lungs should be examined at rest and with exercise to detect abnormality. A broodmare owner with the intent of using a stallion at stud also should carefully critique a stallion's straightness of limbs, size and health of feet, and general body proportions to determine if the stallion will complement the mare. The stallion contributes half the genetic information; therefore, his defects can be passed on to offspring.

MAINTAINING STALLION HEALTH

A breeding stallion is a performance horse that can continue in his duties well into his twenties if he is properly cared for and conditioned. An idle stallion becomes obese and unhealthy, and is prone to laminitis, colic, and heart failure. A stallion's body condition score should be carefully monitored to ensure the quality of his diet (see p. 345). A stallion that is exercised regularly has greater longevity in the breeding sheds. Turning a stallion into a paddock or pasture each day is good for his mental health, but forced exercise for 30 to 60 minutes a day is required to keep him fit and in prime metabolic condition.

HERITABLE ABNORMALITIES

It is important to identify the existence of undesirable, heritable traits such as a retained testicle (*cryptorchidism*), scrotal or umbilical hernia, parrot mouth (see p. 12 and photo 11.11, p. 287), eye cataracts (see p. 499), or *combined immunodeficiency disease* (CID), a fatal disease of Arabians. These abnormalities are passed down in a genetic link, and the presence of one or more of such heritable traits renders a stallion unsuitable for breeding. Similarly, HYPP (see p. 176) and HERDA (see p. 392) are genetically linked diseases to be avoided.

Other syndromes that are not entirely linked to genetics but may have a heritable tendency are developmental abnormalities such as angular-limb deformities (see p. 22), osteochondrosis (OCD—see p. 133), or cervical spinal malformation or Wobbler syndrome (see p. 517). Ascertain if a stallion has a history of such problems in his lineage or in his get. Investigate soundness problems that have developed in a stallion or his offspring. Identify conformational abnormalities that interfere with continual soundness, like too long a pastern slope (see p. 26), or post-legged hindquarters (see p. 33). A mare contributes half of the genetic information to the foal; therefore, not all problems can be traced exclusively to a stallion.

Reproductive Exam

Examination of both the internal and external genital structures is an important part of a stallion's breeding exam (fig. 18.4). The prepuce is checked for injury, scars, or tumors. Both testicles are measured with calipers across the widest part of the scrotum, and their consistency is determined by manual palpation.

THE TESTICLES

The *testicles* should feel firm, whereas a soft, mushy, or hard consistency may indicate degen-

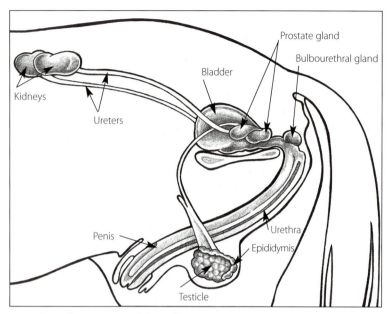

18.4 *Reproductive tract of the stallion.*

THE PENIS

After a stallion is lightly teased, his *penis* is examined for skin lesions consistent with melanoma, squamous cell carcinoma, sarcoids, or warts (see "Skin Growths," p. 392), or summer sores (see p. 388). Evidence of inflammation around the urethra may signal a mild infection or a venereal disease.

VENEREAL DISEASE

EIA and EVA

As part of a general physical exam, the stallion should be blood tested for *equine infectious anemia* (EIA—see p. 241) and *equine viral arteritis* (EVA—see p. 556). Both viral diseases are potentially passed as a venereal infection to a mare. EVA can be passed to other mares by the respiratory route. Not all stallions shed EVA virus in their semen, but the semen should be evaluated as this virus can cause abortion. Any mare to be bred to a stallion that has tested positive for EVA should be vaccinated before breeding.

Coital Exanthema

Another viral venereal disease is called *equine herpesvirus* (EHV-3) or *equine coital exanthma*. This may be identified as vesicular lesions on the penis and prepuce of a stallion or on the vaginal lining of a mare. Similar vesicles or ulcers may be present in the mouth. The virus is highly infectious, passed through live cover or by physical contact transfer by fomites (see p. 458) or insects. Stallions or mares may be asymptomatic carriers, but horses with active herpes lesions should not be bred by live coverage, although the virus does not interfere with conception rates.

Contagious Equine Metritis

A stallion that is imported into the United States from Europe must be quarantined for *contagious equine metritis* (CEM), a bacterial

eration or disease. A rectal exam or internal ultrasound exam evaluates the health of the internal genital glands.

Testicular size is highly correlated to the amount of sperm output, which determines fertility. Although a young colt may begin producing viable semen by 13 months of age, most stallions are not purposely put to stud until they are 2 to 3 years old. Testicles of a stallion at that age should each measure 5 centimeters or more in width. Size of the testicles depends on the age of a stallion, with maximum size attained by 6 years of age. Testicular size is heritable; if a stallion has undersized testicles, not only is he potentially a poor sperm producer, but small testicles could also be passed on as an undesirable trait. Size of the testicles does decrease with a horse in training, the stress of competition (especially racing), and with medication such as anabolic steroids.

infection caused by *Taylorella equigenitalis*. A stallion carries the bacteria only as a surface contaminant on his penis, whereas infection of a mare persists in her reproductive tract. A stallion's immune system does not respond to the disease by building antibodies that circulate in the blood. Therefore, blood-testing a stallion for exposure to the bacteria does not identify a carrier stallion. The only way to determine CEM infection is by taking repeated *bacterial cultures* swabbed directly from the penis.

Bacterial Culture

Both before and after ejaculation, a bacterial culture is taken by gently inserting a cotton swab into the urethra. Then the swab is taken to a lab, which can determine the presence of other bacterial organisms that may be transferred from a stallion to a mare through the semen. Some bacteria may cause a serious enough uterine infection to prevent conception or induce spontaneous abortion.

SEMEN EVALUATION

Semen is evaluated for its quality by collecting samples on successive days until semen quality has stabilized. Evaluating semen in this manner gives a realistic picture of how much sperm a stallion can produce, its color and structure, and how vital the sperm.

Color

The color of the semen is examined for blood (*hemospermia*) or urine; either substance damages fertility by killing sperm cells.

Motility

One of the most important aspects of semen fertility is the *motility* (movement) of the sperm. Activity of each sperm and its propensity to swim in a forward direction is referred to as *progressive motility*. A drop of semen is placed on a warm slide and examined under a microscope immediately after collection to determine the percent of sperm that are motile compared to those that are inactive. An ideal sample for shipped, cooled semen has over 80 percent of sperm showing active progressive motility, but greater than 50 percent motility may be considered acceptable for live cover or for artificial insemination of the mare at the site of semen collection. Raw semen of fertile stallions retains at least 10 percent motility for 6 hours. If semen motility diminishes to less than 10 percent within 2 hours, conception rates are poor.

Structure

The structure (*morphology*) of individual sperm cells is important to their effective motility. Sperm with defective tails are unable to swim forward, and may travel in circles or in reverse. The head of a sperm must be perfect since the *acrosome* of the head eventually penetrates the egg. Even if a sperm is able to swim to its destination, a defective acrosome would prevent it from fertilizing the egg. Preferably more than 60 percent of the sperm cells should be normal with less than 10 percent showing major structural defects.

Concentration

The *concentration* of sperm is important to a stallion's fertility. This figure is obtained by a *spectrophotometer* that counts the total number of sperm cells in a measured sample. The minimum concentration necessary to ensure conception of a mare is estimated at 500 million sperm cells (5×10^8) per dose for immediate insemination on the farm or if shipped.

Other Factors Affecting Fertility

Stress Level

Stress of competition reduces the fertility of a stallion and has a marked effect on his breeding performance. This should be considered if a mare is booked to a stallion that is actively campaigning between breeding dates. Semen that had ample potency on collection may be infertile at insemination twelve or more hours later. This is particularly significant if semen is to be transported long distances. A letdown period of several days may be necessary to improve a stallion's chance for conception.

Semen Extenders

Semen extenders provide sperm with adequate energy and nutrients so are a vital aspect of the longevity of shipped semen. An extender must be matched for compatibility with each stallion's semen. An ideal semen extender increases conception rates of mares receiving transported semen.

Season

The season a stallion is bred also affects his fertility. April through August is the normal breeding season in the Northern Hemisphere. These summer months offer the optimum fertile period for breeding, not only for a stallion, but also for a mare.

SIRING RECORDS

The potency of a stallion with a past breeding history can be put to the test by examining his siring records. This is particularly helpful when selecting a stallion for transported semen, as the costs of semen collection, air transport, and insemination will escalate with each estrous cycle a mare does not conceive. If a stallion has a history of standing to stud, it is possible to categorize him as a satisfactory, questionable, or unsatisfactory breeder.

Satisfactory Breeder

A satisfactory breeder achieves at least a 75 percent conception rate during a single breeding season. A satisfactory breeder can potentially accommodate a large booking for the season if the season is extended from mid-February to mid-August, and the mares are presented to him at staggered cycles. It is possible for a fertile stallion to be booked to as many as 45 mares for natural cover, or to 125 mares for artificial insemination if his semen quality is consistent throughout the breeding months.

Questionable Breeder

A stallion would fall into the questionable category if he has problems with libido, ineffective ejaculation, or if his semen quality is marginal.

Unsatisfactory Breeder

An unsatisfactory breeder is a stallion that has poor semen quality leading to low fertility. A stallion with heritable defects or venereal disease is excluded as breeding stock, and by definition is unsatisfactory.

The Mare

Reproductive Cycle

A mare is *seasonally polyestrus*, meaning that she cycles many times during the breeding season. Her optimal fertile period is between April and August (in the Northern Hemisphere), although many mares are bred earlier. Most mares stop cycling in the winter months (*anestrus*) between November and February. In February and March, she enters a *transitional period*. Pituitary hormones controlling the reproductive cycle respond to longer daylight hours, stimulating activity of the ovaries to start producing *follicles* (egg sacks) that eventually mature (fig. 18.5). Rupture of a mature follicle releases an egg for potential fertilization.

During the transitional period, estrous cycles are erratic, and may be prolonged without the production of an actual egg. Normally, during April through August, a mare cycles every 21 days, with visible signs of *estrus* (winking of the vulva, tail lifting, or frequent urinations) present for about 5 days.

Nature protects the survival of the species by maximizing fertility of both the mare and the stallion during the warmer times of the year. Then, a gestation period of 11 months allows a foal to be born into a welcoming and nutrient-rich environment for both mare and foal. By evaluating a mare's reproductive capabilities, health problems may be addressed and resolved before the breeding season. Each time a mare is bred, there is a risk of injury or uterine infection. If fertility is coordinated with the proposed breeding date she will become pregnant with fewer breedings, thereby minimizing infection risk.

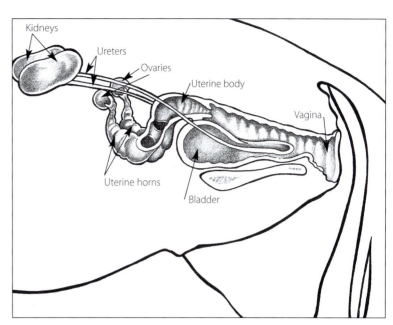

18.5 *Reproductive tract of the mare.*

HORMONAL MANIPULATION

Techniques to synchronize follicle maturation with a proposed breeding date include use of specific hormones or hormonal analogs, such as *progesterone*, *prostaglandins*, or *human chorionic gonadotropin* (HCG). Hormonal manipulation of a mare is not practical until her ovaries are active and cycling.

If she is in the quiescent, winter anestrus period, or just entering the transitional period around February or March, hormonal drug therapy may be ineffective in coordinating the timing for breeding. Only 20 to 30 percent of mares cycle and ovulate at regular intervals during February and March, whereas over 80 percent do so by April or May.

ARTIFICIAL LIGHTING

Manipulation of natural hormonal surges with artificial lighting can advance the erratic two-month transitional period to encourage mares to cycle earlier in the year. Photoreceptors of the eyes detect light, which sends a message to the *pineal gland* located behind the *hypothalamus* in the brain. The pineal gland releases *melatonin* when the days are short, and this suppresses hormonal activity of the reproductive system. With increasing daylight hours, a "message" is created that inhibits release of melatonin. Longer daylight hours of spring can be mimicked using artificial lighting. In response, the hypothalamus produces *gonadotropin-releasing hormone* (GnRH—see p. 541) to stimulate the pituitary gland to release hormones that activate a mare's ovaries (or a stallion's testes). (A horse will produce this as a normal hormone, but there are exogenous injectable or pelleted forms that are administered IV or subcutaneously to control timing of breeding.) Activity within the ovaries causes follicles to form, mature, and ovulate. Each estrous cycle reoccurs approximately every three weeks to provide a breeder with many opportunities to get a mare in foal.

Lighting Recommendations

For this method to work best, 16 hours of "daylight" is required. The type of light is not as important as the number of hours a mare is exposed to it. Incandescent, fluorescent, mercury vapor, and tungsten lights are all successful in stimulating a mare's reproductive activity. It is necessary to provide 2 months of lengthened daylight to enhance ovarian activity; within 60 days, follicles mature and ovulate. To maximize the use of artificial lighting, start a mare under lights on the first day of December when an anticipated breeding is planned around the first day of March.

Lights should be turned on from 4:30 P.M. until 11:00 P.M. This schedule ensures a total of 16 hours of both natural and artificial light. As an energy-saving alternative, studies indicate that 1 to 2 hours of artificial light applied 8 to 10 hours after sunset may be sufficient to stimulate the pineal gland. Using this strategy, turning the lights on from 1:00 A.M. to 4:00 A.M. hastens the transitional period.

A 200-watt incandescent bulb, or two 40-watt fluorescent bulbs are placed 10 feet above a mare in a 12 by 12 foot stall. There should be enough light to read a newspaper in the stall at eye level with a mare. The mare should not be able to remove her head from the light source; otherwise the pineal gland is not stimulated by light. The brighter the light, the sooner a mare will ovulate, up to a point. Once a mare has ovulated with this strategy early in the season, maintain her under lights to stimulate hormonal activity until springtime is normally underway.

Blanketing and Food

A mare that is put under lights is also stimulated to shed her winter coat. In a cold climate, premature shedding requires blanketing and shelter. A mare may require extra food to maintain good body condition. If an early breeding schedule is implemented in colder climates, indoor housing must be available to a mare foaling in January, February, or March to avoid climatic stress on a foal.

PREVENTIVE MEDICINE

A preventive medicine program, if not already in place, should be instituted before breeding. This program includes:

- Deworming on a regular schedule with products approved for pregnant mares
- *Rhinopneumonitis* vaccine administered in advance of breeding, and boosted at 5, 7, and 9 months of pregnancy to reduce risk of viral abortion
- Regular *encephalitis* (EEE and WEE), *West Nile*, *tetanus*, and *influenza* boosters at appropriate intervals

Estrous Behavior

PERFORMANCE ASPECTS OF RIDING A MARE

Some incidents leading to poor performance can occur due to a mare's estrous cycle. Despite fairly imperceptible and mellow heat cycles, mares often urinate small amounts frequently when in heat. It is possible that by voiding the bladder more often and by being slightly more anxious due to hormonal influences, hydration deficits may develop of her own making. When housed in proximity to a stallion (or a "desirable" gelding), some mares expend a lot of energy stimulating his interest instead of spending needed time to eat, drink, and relax. Although a stallion (or gelding) may not be equally interested in soliciting a mare's attention, she might spend most of her time weaving in front of the fence showing off for him, and not drinking much. Some owners have misinterpreted a mare's anxiety as being elicited by excitement of an event rather than recognizing it as a stallion's (or gelding's) influence that distracts the mare from taking care of herself.

Another note of interest involves a specific occurrence that happens during a heat cycle: ovulation. Painful colic symptoms in mares sometimes occur related to rupture of a follicle off an ovary during ovulation. The symptoms are transient (usually less than several hours), and on rectal palpation, sensitive mares may nearly buckle when the affected ovary is gently touched. Ovulation has been known to induce transient, but severe colic pain. It is often difficult for an owner to discern if colic symptoms are related to ovulation or to more significant intestinal issues that require treatment.

The other tendency that has been noted in nervous fillies/mares particularly at Thoroughbred racetracks is the predisposition to develop muscle cramping related to recurrent exertional rhabdomyolysis (RER—see p. 166). Such cases of myositis may be related to a heritable tendency of abnormal muscle metabolism or equine polysaccharide storage myopathy (EPSSM—see p. 172). Any management strategies that diminish stress and excitement do have a favorable effect on reducing the incidence of RER. Although no correlation has been drawn between plasma progesterone activity and abnormal muscle enzymes with exercise, the incidence of RER has been noted to decrease when mares are placed on progesterone therapy.

HORMONAL CONTROL OF ESTROUS BEHAVIOR

Treatment with hormones during a competitive season is an acceptable method of removing "mare-ish" behavior that makes a female horse irritable, cranky, and unwilling to work when asked.

Altrenogest

Currently, only one product is approved to suppress estrus in horses: a dose of 1 ml per 110 pounds of body weight of *altrenogest* (Regumate®) is top-dressed over a mare's feed each day to inhibit heat cycles. Altrenogest is a form of progesterone that shuts down the activity on the ovaries so a mare won't come into heat until she stops ingesting it. There are other injectable forms of progesterone, but Regumate® is the easiest to give (see below). It is possible that some mares on altrenogest may continue to cycle and ovulate without outward signs of estrus.

Many competitive associations have specific rulings on the use of certain medications during competition, so make sure there is approval for use of altrenogest for your intended sport. However, even some organizations that profess a "no tolerance" policy on any drugs or medications will permit the use of Regumate® to control estrous behavior in mares.

Progesterone is readily absorbed through human skin. This can wreak havoc on normal hormonal cycles of women, causing uterine bleeding, missed or delayed periods, and mood swings. There are easy ways to handle Regumate® without posing a human hazard. One means is to wear latex or rubber gloves when pulling a dose into a syringe to squirt onto the grain. Another simple method is to obtain a box of 10 cc blood-collection tubes ("red tops") from a vet, and while wearing gloves, fill all 100 tubes with a daily dose of Regumate® to provide more than a three-month supply of daily dosings. At feeding time, flip off the red-top lid and pour the medication into the feed without having any of the liquid contact human skin. The tubes can be refilled for another round. There are also commercial spray applicators that deliver a measured dose from a bottle to squirt on the food or in a mare's mouth. Normally, altrenogest is used from March or April through September or October, as most mares in the Northern Hemisphere shut down their active heat cycles from November through February.

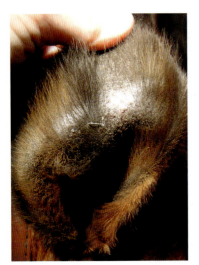

18.6 *In addition to hormonal therapy to manage estrous behavior, there are reports that insertion of a staple in an important acupuncture point in the inner ear can control or eliminate estrous cycles for a time.*

GnRH

Use of *gonadotropin-releasing hormone* (GnRH) has been attempted to suppress reproductive activity in mares. Immunization with this material is safe and reversible, potentially resulting in estrus suppression for 25 to 30 weeks. However, the results are not as predictable or as controllable as found with use of altrenogest.

One GnRH product, deslorelin (Ovuplant®), is used to stimulate ovulation (see p. 539). It comes in the form of a pellet that is injected under the skin. If the pellet is not removed within 48 hours following ovulation, it may suppress subsequent follicular growth in many mares, resulting in delay in return to estrus. In some cases, a mare may not return to estrus for up to a year unless the implant is removed immediately following ovulation.

Cattle Implants

An implant of a combination of progesterone and *estradiol* (Synovex®) has been attempted to control estrous behavior. In cattle, these implants slowly release hormones over a period of 3 to 5 months. However, studies in horses were not able to demonstrate inhibition of ovarian activity or suppression of estrus in those receiving implants. Cattle implants may not provide sufficient levels of progesterone and the release rate may be too slow to modify estrous behavior in mares.

MECHANICAL CONTROL OF ESTROUS BEHAVIOR

One strategy that has been tried with some success is the insertion of a 35 mm glass ball (marble) into the uterus to prevent estrous cycling. A sterile glass ball is inserted through the cervix into the uterus within 24 hours following ovulation. This method has achieved successful suppression of estrus for about 3 months in roughly 40 percent of attempts. The glass ball is not typically detrimental to the *endometrium* (uterine lining) and its removal is usually fairly straightforward, with no interference in future conception. It is recommended to remove the glass ball in the autumn to minimize the risk of uterine infection.

ACUPUNCTURE CONTROL OF ESTROUS BEHAVIOR

It may be possible to use acupuncture to control estrous behavior. Acupuncture sessions often need to be repeated just prior to a mare's expected estrous cycle, but in some instances this is an effective alternative to hormonal therapy. One specific ear point is alleged as useful acupuncture control by inserting a surgical staple for a longer lasting effect (photo 18.6).

HERBAL OPTIONS TO ELIMINATE ESTROUS BEHAVIOR

Herbal strategies of feeding *valerian root* (*Valeriana officinalis*) or *chaste tree berries* (*Vitex agnus castus*) have been tried to calm a mare and to alter ovarian function. To date, these products have not been tested scientifically, so beneficial effects are not known. In addition, many competitive organizations (as for example, USEF and FEI) forbid the use of many herbal or natural products as these may affect performance.

SURGICAL OPTIONS TO ELIMINATE ESTROUS BEHAVIOR

Removal of a mare's ovaries (*ovariectomy*) is a surgical option provided there is no intent to use her as a future broodmare, as this procedure is irreversible. The availability of laparascopic instruments allows a surgeon to make a small incision in the flank, look inside with fiber-optic equipment, find the ovaries, and remove them from the abdomen. The horse only needs to be confined for a week, and then is returned back to work. Complications, such as hemorrhage and infection can arise, but this is a relatively safe procedure. Some mares continue to display elements of "mare" behavior due to continued secretion of hormonal precursors from the adrenal glands.

Abnormal Estrous Cycles

PERFORMANCE-RELATED

Often, the stress of intense competition temporarily alters normal reproductive cycling. Some mares stop cycling altogether, or may display erratic heat cycles.

ANABOLIC STEROIDS

Anabolic steroids are sometimes used to "improve" a horse's body condition, growth, and muscling. Anabolic steroids have adverse effects on a mare's endocrine system. A mare that is influenced by the male sex hormone properties of these drugs has inconsistent or absent estrous cycles. If given repetitively, anabolic steroids can cause a mare to display stallion-like behavior. Once administration of the drug is stopped, the effects are reversible but may require several months for a mare to return to normal estrous cycles.

PAIN

A horse that suffers from a serious injury that involves intense pain may have difficulty cycling or conceiving. Pain interferes with hormone production and may interrupt a normal estrous cycle (see p. 544).

Mare Pre-Breeding Exam

PREPARING FOR BREEDING

A mare is a project to manage when considering breeding her in conjunction with using her athletic abilities in the best performance years of her life. The time between impregnation to weaning takes well over a year in a mare's life, this having considerable impact on her conditioning and fitness. During at least half of this period, the latter trimester of pregnancy and while a foal is by her side, she cannot be maintained in steady work.

When the decision is made to breed, it should be noted that a mare cannot be removed from rigorous athletics and be expected to conceive immediately. If a mare is engaged in competitive athletics or on a show circuit, she should be rested from work at least two months before breeding. This "let-down" period reduces her stress load and allows her reproductive pattern to settle into a regular cycling interval. Over several months her psychological state also adjusts to a relaxed environment.

Once a chosen stallion has been proven to have fertility capabilities based on his reproductive exam and conception rate, it is time to carefully scrutinize a mare's capabilities to settle and carry a foal to term. Before starting down the path of artificial insemination or natural cover, have a pre-breeding veterinary exam done on a mare to evaluate uterine health and ovarian activity. Ensuring the reproductive health of a mare from the onset avoids wasted time during the crucial period of a breeding season, as well as unnecessary and repeated expenses that result in frustration and financial loss. A veterinary pre-breeding examination may detect external and internal abnormalities of a mare that can lead to reproductive failure.

GENERAL PHYSICAL EXAM

A general physical exam is performed to ensure health of the heart and lungs, and soundness of limbs and feet. Heart murmurs or arrhythmias reduce metabolic efficiency. Chronic lung disease interferes with the oxygen supply important to placental and fetal health. A chronic cough from obstructive pulmonary disease (*heaves*) can cause enough straining to develop a "windsucking" vagina (*pneumovagina*) that pulls bacteria inward, resulting in inflammation or infection of the uterus.

Evaluation of hair coat bloom and quality denotes the success of parasite control programs, and hormonal regularity. A rough coat may reflect internal health problems or an intestinal parasite load. A mare that is late in shedding her winter coat may also lack an appropriate hormonal response to the longer daylight hours of breeding season.

Severe, chronic pain caused by arthritis, laminitis, or other limb problems may stress a mare sufficiently to reduce her chances not only of conception but also of carrying a foal to term. A mare with chronic laminitis poses an added reproductive risk. If a laminitic mare has difficulty with birthing or develops a uterine infection (*metritis*) after foaling, she is at risk of worsened laminitis due to absorption of bacterial endotoxins into the bloodstream.

Weight Concerns

As an athletic mare is pulled from performance, she may be too thin to encourage normal reproductive cycling. Without good dental care, a mare may be unable to meet nutritional needs important to maintaining pregnancy, fetal development, and lactation. Body condition is examined during a pre-breeding exam so that appropriate nutritional adjustments can be discussed. Once athletic activity is minimized, she should begin to gain weight. A slow, controlled weight-gain program (*flushing*) can be implemented 1 to 2 months before the breeding season. Mares that are on a steady weight-gain program before the breeding period attain estrus one month sooner than mares that are not gaining weight. A fit, breeding mare has a thin layer of flesh covering her ribs so they are not visible but can be felt as the hand is run lightly across the ribs, and a body condition score of 5 (see p. 346).

A halter horse pulled from the show circuit may have the opposite problem from the athlete: she may be too fat. Obesity is detrimental to conception and reproductive health; however, a malnourished horse is also at risk for infertility. High-energy rations should be removed from the diet of a halter horse intended for breeding and the halter mare should be fed a balanced maintenance diet with ample roughage and minimal grain. (For more discussion on body condition and dietary management, refer to chapter 12, *The Digestive System: Nutritional Management*, p. 345.)

Maturity

A mare should not be bred until she is sexually and skeletally mature to prevent additional stresses and demands on her own growing body. The period of greatest fetal demand occurs in the last trimester (8 to 11 months) of pregnancy. A mare should not be bred any earlier than 3 years of age. A mare bred at that time approaches her fourth year before a foal taxes her system with rapid developmental growth and the subsequent energy demands of lactation.

EXTERNAL EXAM OF A MARE'S REPRODUCTIVE SYSTEM

A common reason for failure to conceive, or for early embryonic death, is infection of the uterus (*metritis*). The unique anatomy of the *perineum* (the area around the anus and vulva) provides the first line of defense in protecting the uterus from bacterial invasion.

The Perineum

A normal mare has a vertical vulva with full *labia* (lips of the vulva) that are tightly aligned in a snug fit so that neither air nor feces can enter the vagina. In a normal mare, about 80

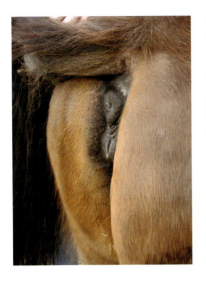 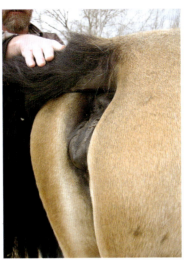

18.7 A & B *Normal alignment of the lips of the vulva renders them slightly forward of the anus (A). Consequently, fecal matter falls away during defecation rather than draining into the vagina where it can create a vaginal and/or uterine infection that affects fertility. A "tipped vagina" occurs when the perineum is sunken in with the anus positioned in front of the vulvar lips; this allows persistent fecal contamination of the vagina and uterus (B).*

percent of the vulva is positioned below the pelvic brim, with the anus positioned very slightly behind or directly above the vulva so feces do not fall onto the labia. Melanoma and squamous cell carcinoma are common cancers found in the perineal area (see "Skin Growths," p. 392). Their presence should be noted, along with identification of any hindrance they may pose to breeding or foaling.

Tipped Vagina

Another barrier to uterine contamination is the *vestibular seal* created by the back portion of the vagina, the hymen if present, and the pelvic floor. In a mare with a *tipped vagina*, the labia sit high above the pelvic brim, the anus is pulled forward, and the vulva tilts horizontally such that constrictor muscles of the vulva and vestibule cannot prevent contamination of the reproductive tract (photos 18.7 A & B). With the vagina tipped forward and the anus recessed inward, feces fall directly onto the labia. The labia may gap, and then "windsucking" (see p. 544) pulls air and feces into the reproductive tract. To check for windsucking, place the flat surface of the hands on each labial lip, and gently part them. In a windsucking mare, air is aspirated into the vulva as the labia are manually parted, resulting in a sucking sound. In many older mares, or in very thin horses, the position of anus and vulva is abnormally altered due to loss of muscle tone. A mare with a tipped vulva is also prone to developing urine pooling (see p. 547). Not only does a tipped vulva develop from age-related conformational changes or severe weight loss, but it may also be caused by an inherited defect, evident at birth. Such fillies should be identified early so corrections can be made to enhance their future fertility. Conformation is heritable, and undesirable traits may be passed down from mare to foal. Normally, Mother Nature accounts for this problem by rendering poorly conformed mares unbreedable, but surgical techniques enable continued fertility and breeding of these mares.

Caslick's Surgery

Contamination to the reproductive tract may result in infertility from infection and subsequent scarring of the uterus. Following breeding and conception, a mare with a for-

18.8 *A Caslick's surgical procedure sutures together the vaginal lips to prevent feces from draining into the vagina and uterus. An opening is left at the bottom end of the vulva to allow unobstructed urination. A Caslick's should be opened at least two weeks prior to the anticipated foaling date.*

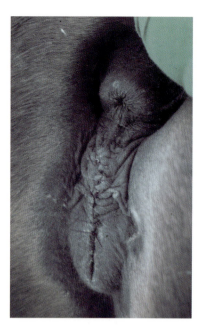

ward-tipped vagina can have a Caslick's surgery (*episioplasty*) performed by a veterinarian. This surgery closes the lips of the vulva to prevent contamination (photo 18.8). Local anesthetic is placed along the borders of the vulva, tissue is trimmed away, and the two "lips" are sutured together to join as they heal, allowing sufficient space at the bottom for normal urination. Several weeks before foaling, the Caslick's must be opened to allow normal birth of a foal without tearing.

Third Degree Perineal Laceration

On occasion, a foal is delivered with an improperly aligned leg, which tears the perineum, referred to as *third degree perineal laceration*. With this condition, torn flesh between the rectum and the vagina allows feces to fall directly into the vagina. These mares should have the perineum reconstructed well ahead of the next breeding time to adequately clear a uterine infection from the system. This requires three phases of surgical repair; up to a year of healing time is necessary before breeding the mare again.

Udder Evaluation

In a pre-breeding evaluation, the udder is examined for abnormalities in size or consistency, tumors or scar tissue, or evidence of previous or current *mastitis* (inflammation of the udder). The thighs and underside of the tail are also examined for evidence of abnormal vaginal discharge.

INTERNAL EXAM OF A MARE'S REPRODUCTIVE SYSTEM

Rectal and Ultrasound Exam

Once a mare's overall body health and external genitals have been thoroughly evaluated, examination of the internal reproductive tract can begin. Initially, a *rectal examination* is performed with a veterinarian inserting an arm covered by a lubricated, plastic sleeve into the rectum. The veterinarian manually palpates the ovaries, uterus, and cervix to assess general health, activity, and abnormalities. An *ultrasound examination* adds to the thoroughness of the internal rectal exam: an ultrasound probe is carried into the rectum to provide visualization of all structures of the reproductive tract (photo 18.9). Size of the ovaries is determined, while the amount of follicular activity present on each ovary ascertains if a mare is currently cycling. The tone and size of the uterus and cervix establish if fluid, air, tumors or abscesses, adhesions, or scar tissue are present, all of which are significant findings. A flaccid and doughy-feeling uterus may signal infection within, or abnormal endocrine function. The presence, location, and size of *uterine cysts* are recorded from the ultrasound imaging. Cysts often resemble an embryo, thereby confusing a diagnosis of pregnancy or twins on ultrasound exam, and in some cases, cysts may interfere with conception.

Reproductive Strategies and Health

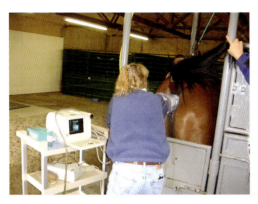

18.9 *Ultrasound of the mare is an important tool in evaluating the stage and development of follicles on the ovaries to accurately predict timing of breeding.*

Maiden Mare

A *maiden* mare is a mare of any age that has never been exposed to semen. Once she has been "bred," whether she conceives or not, she is no longer a maiden. An untouched uterus is typically a sterile environment provided that conformational abnormalities do not exist that might cause uterine inflammation or infection. A maiden mare should be examined rectally and with ultrasound to determine if all appropriate reproductive "equipment" is present; that is, two ovaries, a cervix, and a normal-shaped and positioned uterus (see fig. 18.5, p. 539). On rare occasions, abnormalities such as lack of an ovary, tumor of an ovary, or a split cervix may be found.

In a maiden mare, a reproductive exam often stops after rectal palpation, ultrasound, and vaginal exam. There is no reason to assume any possible uterine infection unless conformation of the vulva appears suspect, or if vaginal inflammation or urine pooling has been confirmed. For a mare that has been bred, with or without conception, or for a poorly conformed maiden mare, the pre-breeding exam uses all available diagnostic tests.

Vaginal Exam

After thoroughly washing the perineum and wrapping the tail to prevent pulling debris inward, the next step is a *vaginal speculum exam* (photo 18.10) to visually inspect the vagina for:

- Inflammation
- Congestion
- Abnormal discharge
- Tearing of the vagina or vulva from prior births
- Cervical lacerations or adhesions

The color and moistness of mucous membranes within the vagina reflect vaginal health and endocrine function. Air bubbles may indicate chronic windsucking, while a collection of fluid on the vaginal floor warns of other serious problems, such as infection or urine pooling.

The cervix is the third barrier to uterine contamination, and its integrity is important to reproductive health. In a maiden mare, a hymen may be present, and can be broken down at this time. Blood is spermicidal and interferes with semen fertility; therefore, it is best to open the hymen before breeding.

Urine Pooling

An important cause of infertility is a syndrome known as *urine pooling (vesiculo-vaginal reflux)* on the floor of the vagina. Urine is not only spermicidal, but it is an irritant that causes inflammation of the vagina *(vaginitis)*, inflammation of the cervix *(cervicitis)*, and inflammation of the uterus *(metritis)* with subsequent infertility. If urine is not entirely voided clear of the reproductive tract, small, residual amounts drain forward to collect on the vaginal floor. A veterinarian can see the urine by shining a flashlight into the vagina with a speculum in place. Suspect fluid can be analyzed biochemically to confirm that it is urine.

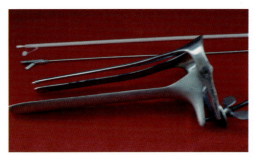

18.10 *A vaginal speculum is inserted into the vagina to allow visualization of the vaginal lining and the cervix. With a flashlight, the examiner can see if the mare has an inflammatory condition of the vagina, if she is subject to urine pooling, or if there is abnormal discharge from the uterus draining through the cervix. Adhesions, scar tissue, and cysts in the vagina can also be visualized with this procedure.*

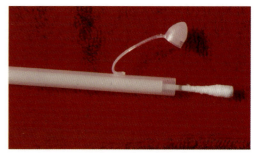

18.11 *A long, guarded culture swab is inserted through the cervix and into the uterus. Once in the uterus, the swab is pushed forward to pop open the protective cap, and rotating the swab for about 30 seconds collects uterine fluid and cells. Then the swab is pulled back into its plastic sheath, and the sample is submitted to the lab for bacterial culture and examination of a cellular smear.*

A mare with a tipped vulva is particularly susceptible to urine pooling (see photo 18.7 B, p. 545). With normal vulvar conformation, entry into the vagina requires an upward path, ensuring that urine is drained down and out. A tipped vulva directs the entry downward so urine tends to flow into the vagina. Urine pooling occasionally occurs during estrus when the reproductive tract relaxes, or if a Caslick's surgery is improperly sewn.

To correct urine pooling, *urethral extension surgery* "builds" a urethral tunnel from pre-existing shelves of tissue within the vagina. Urine travels outward through the tunnel, and cannot collect within the vaginal cavern. In one study, this surgery resulted in a conception rate of 92 percent of mares with previous urine pooling, and 65 percent carried foals to term.

Bacterial Culture of the Uterus

A bacterial culture is obtained directly from the uterus to determine presence of infection of the uterine lining. A very long cotton swab is passed through the cervix, guarded in a plastic sheath (photo 18.11). A protective cap on the end of the sheath is pushed open once in the uterus, and uterine secretions soak into the swab for 30 seconds. The swab is pulled back into its sterile protective sheath and removed from the reproductive tract. The sample is sent to the lab to be checked for bacterial growth over the next 48 hours. If bacterial growth does occur, the lab can determine the antibiotic to which the bacteria is susceptible.

Effectiveness of Bacterial Culture

By itself, bacterial culture of the uterus has a poor correlation with the presence of actual disease. It has been demonstrated that as many as 61 percent of mares do not show significant bacterial growth on culture in spite of having an active uterine infection. Other mares may have non-harmful bacteria resident in the uterus, with no accompanying disease. Bacteria are detected in the uterine lining of 80 percent of mares up to 3 days after breeding, and up to 30 days after foaling. A normal mare's immune system quickly clears them from the reproductive system.

Reproductive Strategies and Health

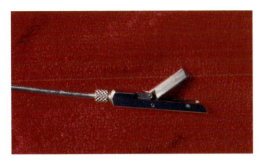

18.12 *An extended, stainless steel uterine biopsy tool is inserted through the cervix into the uterus to collect a tissue sample for cellular examination. Here you can see the open jaws of the biopsy instrument. These will close and bite into the uterine lining to retrieve a tissue sample. A mare does not have nerve endings in her endometrial lining, so is unaware of any sensation when the sample is taken.*

However, bacterial culture and antibiotic sensitivity testing of the superficial uterine lining is helpful in confirming other diagnostic findings, such as:

- An abnormal-feeling uterus
- Presence of fluid or urine pooling
- Continued infertility
- Results from uterine biopsies and *cytology* (cellular evaluation)

Specific bacteria, such a *beta-hemolytic Streptococci*, *Klebsiella*, *Pseudomonas*, *E coli*, and yeasts, are significant if found on the culture. An infected uterus needs to be treated with local antibiotics and/or systemic antibiotics before breeding.

Cytology Evaluation of the Uterus

The swab that is used to gather secretions from the uterus also collects cells from the uterine lining; these cells are used to make a *cytology* sample. The cotton swab is rolled onto a glass slide, and the cells are stained for examination under a microscope in the lab for inflammatory cells, debris, or bacteria. The presence of specific inflammatory cells provides warning signals about the duration and severity of an infection.

Uterine Biopsy

The most informative diagnostic tool for analyzing the viability, health, and structure of the equine uterus is the *uterine biopsy*. A special instrument is inserted through the cervix into the uterus, and its movable jaws are closed to tear off a "tag" of tissue (photo 18.12). The uterine lining of the mare, unlike humans, has no nerve endings; therefore a horse does not feel the tug or tearing of tissue as the biopsy sample is taken. At the lab, the sample is prepared for examination under a microscope. A random sample of the uterus provides adequate information about overall uterine health.

Biopsy Evaluation with the Kenney Classification System

Often, infertility is caused by uterine infections in the deep tissue layers. These can only be inspected by biopsy of the tissue. Microscopic evaluation identifies infection, inflammation, or scarring (*fibrosis*) of the glands that support uterine nutrition. There is a direct correlation of biopsy findings with fertility, which makes this procedure an invaluable diagnostic tool. A Kenney classification system categorizes the degree of uterine pathology, or disease, and predicts a mare's chance of reproductive success.

- *Grade I Uterus*: Grade I uterus has at least an 80 percent chance of conception, with minimal or no pathological changes (infection, inflammation, or gland scarring) present in the endometrium.
- *Grade II Uterus*: Grade II describes moderately severe inflammation and gland scarring that interferes with the ability of

the endometrium to adequately support a foal to term. *Grade II A* uterus is associated with a 50 to 80 percent chance of success of maintaining a pregnancy. A mare with this classification has a reasonably good possibility for return to Grade I status with appropriate treatment. *Grade II B* uterus has more widespread abnormalities in the endometrium, and will have limited success (10 to 50 percent) of carrying a foal to term.

- *Grade III Uterus*: Grade III classification is the most severe, with irreversible, widespread inflammatory changes and periglandular scarring, providing less than a 10 percent chance of conception and carrying a foal to term. Widespread scarring in the uterus decreases uterine motility during a critical period when normal motility is essential for continued pregnancy.

With diminished uterine motility, an embryo may not migrate throughout the uterus during days 5 to 15 after conception. *Embryonic migration* stimulates chemical signals that block the release of *prostaglandins* from the uterus. Without embryonic migration, release of prostaglandins causes a premature reduction of progesterone, a hormone that is necessary for maintaining early pregnancy. The embryo often does not survive. Extensive scarring of the uterus, and particularly of the glandular areas, also reduces nutrient supplies essential to support a developing embryo.

Fiber-Optic Exam of the Uterus or Vagina

Evaluation and surgical removal of *uterine cysts* is facilitated with the use of a fiber-optic instrument (*endoscope*) inserted into the uterus.

The Breeding Process

NATURAL COVER OR ARTIFICIAL INSEMINATION

An accomplished mare makes a worthy broodmare to maintain excellent performance characteristics. If a local stallion is appealing and natural (live) cover is an option, then logistics are easier to arrange by delivering the mare to the stallion's farm. However, shopping for a quality stallion often turns up attractive candidates living in far-away corners of the United States. The days of hauling a mare long distances for breeding have been replaced with the use of *shipped semen* (photo 18.13). Now, a mare can remain safely at home, available for riding and companionship.

The dream of breeding to a quality stallion far from home no longer poses an obstacle with today's technology in the world of *artificial insemination,* known as AI. With a good team working alongside a mare, the possibilities are endless. Semen can even be shipped from other countries. Artificial insemination may be used on mares at the breeding farm, or for mares living long distances from a stallion. Costs incurred by using artificial insemination include semen collection and transport of cooled or frozen semen to the mare at home, along with veterinary fees to collect the stallion and to evaluate and inseminate the mare.

For long-distance breeding methods with AI or for embryo transfer, plan ahead to work out problems such as airline schedules, show schedules, or synchronizing ovulation for embryo transfer candidates. Check with the breed registry to confirm that methods other than live cover are permitted so a foal may be registered. (The Thoroughbred registry still does not permit artificial insemination.)

DETECTING ESTRUS

An essential part of the breeding process is the

ability to recognize when a mare is in heat. Not all mares are obvious about this, and unless a tease gelding (or mare) or a stallion is available, this can be the hardest part of the entire project. To compound matters, not all mares show to just *any* stallion. Just like people, there has got to be a basic attraction, but fortunately, mares tend to be far less picky than people.

Some mares are easy to read; they beome temperamental, and show obvious signs of estrus like "winking" the lips of the vulva, and they squat and urinate small amounts frequently (photos 18.14 and 18.15). The lips of the vulva may be caked with urine from frequent urinations, and the tail and lower legs are often soiled and smell of urine when in heat (photo 18.16). Some mares back up to a fence and rub their hind end, or they throw their haunches in front of every gelding in sight, making their desires plain to read. However, there are the silent types, that don't declare their interest. These mares are generally the easiest to ride and compete because they keep their minds on their job. To breed a mare of this nature makes it more challenging to determine when she is in heat.

Those mares with "silent" heats can be placed on a hormonal program to synchronize her heat cycle to a specified time. She can be given a daily dose of progesterone (Regumate®) for 10 to 14 days, and then would receive a prostaglandin (Estrumate®) injection to bring her into heat within 3 to 7 days. This is also an advantageous strategy if the selected stallion is involved with a busy competitive schedule during the breeding season. Then, breeding can be timed for when he is conveniently available for semen collection, and when it is most opportune to have the mare bred.

THE BREEDING

Once a mare is seen to be in heat, the project begins. First, the vet is notified and an ultra-

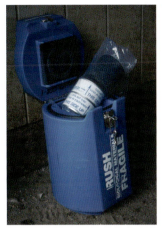

18.13 *An Equitainer™ is only one of many containers that are used for shipping cooled semen. The semen is placed atop coolant inside an insulated area, and this keeps semen at a specific temperature for up to 36 hours while it is shipped by air.*

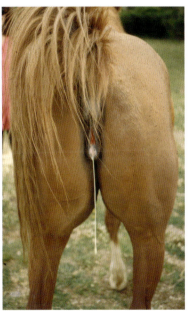

18.14 *This mare is demonstrating the hallmark signs of estrus. She is urinating frequent and small amounts, winking her clitoris with each expression of urine, and standing with legs spread and tail raised.*

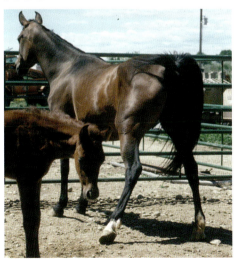

18.15 *This mare is in heat, evident by repeated behavior of squatting and urinating, with her tail held to the side.*

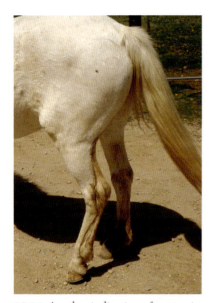

18.16 *Another indication of a mare in estrus is the soiling of her hind legs with frequent expressions of urine that mix with dirt. You will notice a urine-laden odor to the limbs, as well.*

sound exam starts to track the development of one or more active follicles on the ovaries (see photo 18.9, p. 547). By bouncing sound waves at the ovaries with an ultrasound probe inserted into the rectum, a visual image appears on the computer screen to show the exact dimensions of each follicle. This allows a reasonable estimation of the appropriate time to breed. Serial exams are performed daily, and sometimes twice a day, to determine when a follicle reaches a size of 30 mm or more. This is the minimum size most follicles reach before they are ripe enough to ovulate. Some grow as large as 60 mm before they are ready to ovulate. On rectal exam, a veterinarian can also manually feel the consistency of a ripening follicle: a firm follicle is likely still in developmental stages; if it is softening, it is more likely to rupture soon. Once a follicle reaches at least 30 to 35 mm and begins to soften, semen will be ordered, assuming all other parts of the reproductive organs (uterus and cervix) are also responding to the influence of estrous hormones. These structures are also evaluated with ultrasound at the time of the rectal exam.

To ensure availability of the semen, it is a prudent to give a stallion manager advance warning to expect a call for an order in the next few days. Then, when the semen order is placed, it is collected immediately, shipped overnight, and the mare is inseminated the following day. The veterinarian usually gives an injection of human chorionic gonadotropin (HCG) at the time the semen is ordered or implants the mare with GnRH (Ovuplant®) analog 24 hours prior to ordering semen (see p. 542). These strategies stimulate the final development and rupture of the egg from the follicle within 24 to 48 hours, to synchronize with insemination. A mare's ovaries should be followed through ultrasound to ensure ovulation; if the follicle remains, she may need to be rebred about 36 hours after the first breeding. It is helpful also to track whether a second follicle develops concurrent with the first so careful monitoring for twins can be done at the pregnancy check. Good quality semen generally lives up to 48 hours in a mare's reproductive tract. Ideally, semen should be present in the reproductive tract about 12 hours prior to ovulation; however, mares do conceive successfully even if bred within 8 to 12 hours following ovulation.

PREGNANCY CHECK

Between 12 to 16 days following insemination or natural cover, a recently bred mare is ultrasounded for the presence or absence of an embryo (photos 18.17 A & B). This is an opportune time to check for twins, which can be managed by manual crushing of one of the embryos (photo 18.18). Otherwise, a mare often loses them both, or in the worst case both embryos continue to develop, ultimately resulting in abortion, death of one or both foals, or of the mare due to a dangerous delivery.

If a mare is found to be "empty" (not pregnant) at the time of this initial ultrasound exam, the breeding process can begin again about 18 days following her ovulation. Most mares cycle every 18 to 21 days, and remain in heat for a range of 3 to 7 days, with a 5-day heat being common.

The Details of Artificial Insemination

THE EXPENSE OF AI

Artificial insemination has associated expenses. First off, there is the stud fee, including a non-refundable booking fee of several-hundred dollars. A stallion contract stipulates which of the first and/or subsequent semen collections will be covered as part of the stud fee. Sometimes, a mare owner receives one breeding cycle of stallion collection with the stud fee, and usually this only entitles a mare owner to receive a single semen package for that one cycle. Subsequent breedings mean more out-of-pocket expenses for a mare owner, ranging from $250 to $500 each time for stallion handling, collection, and laboratory fees.

There is also the overnight-shipping fee for the special container that maintains semen in a cooled state. This usually runs $40 to $60 each shipment, as it must arrive to the mare as quickly as possible. The stallion farm will require prompt return of this container so it can be used for shipping semen elsewhere. This generally costs $15 for a two-day shipping return. A container deposit (around $250) is required, an expense to be refunded later.

Fees on the mare end range from $250 to $500 each cycle depending on the number of ultrasound exams required, and how many farm trips a vet must make. If hormones (altrenogest and prostaglandin) are needed to regulate the timing of the mare's cycle or to synchronize one or more mares, plan on at least another $75 to $100 per horse.

Assuming a mare settles (is impregnated), there are fees associated with blood typing of both her and her foal. Many breed registries also require registration fees. Plan on an additional $100 to $150 to secure the paperwork that results in legal registration of a foal.

The overall financial outlay for getting a mare in foal over and above the stud fee, if all goes well, may only be several hundred dollars but typically ranges between $1,000 to $1,500 in cases that don't settle the first time.

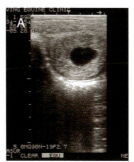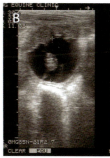

18.17 A & B *Ultrasound of an embryo at 15 days (A) and 23 days (B). At 15 days, the embryonic vesicle is round and well circumscribed. At 23 days, the vesicle is more irregular in shape, and the heart can be seen to beat.*

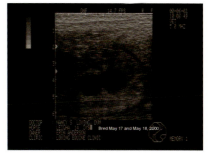

18.18 *Twins at day 14 as seen on diagnostic ultrasound. These two embryonic vesicles are bumped up against each other, and must be separated before a veterinarian crushes one to reduce the pregnancy to a singleton. This is done by manual massage of the uterus with an arm in the rectum, or by waiting a few hours when the embryos migrate through the uterus and are likely to move away from each other. After day 16, the embryo(s) adhere to the uterine wall and the opportunity for manual crushing is lessened.*

THE RELATIVE VALUE OF AI

There are many benefits from using AI as a breeding tool:

- Tapping into a broader gene pool than what is locally available

- Minimized risk of injury to breed with AI as compared to live cover by a stallion
- Minimized risk of uterine infection with artificial insemination that is done in as sterile a manner as possible
- Reduced post-breeding reaction to semen that occurs with live cover so less uterine fluid and edema develop that might prevent successful conception
- Mare accessible to ride at home since semen is sent to the farm
- Eliminates the cost of transport of a mare to the breeding farm, including time off from a job, and the cost of wear-and-tear on a transport vehicle
- Eliminates the cost of *mare care* at a breeding farm, which can range from $5 to $30 per day
- Minimizes the stress on a mare created by transport to a new geographical location and housing in an unfamiliar environment with different handlers, feed, and daily routine

Veterinary care of a mare during the breeding process is of paramount importance. Coupling the expertise of a competent vet on the mare's end with good fertility of both mare and stallion provides a success rate of AI as high as 85 to 90 percent. Considering the averages for live cover run 60 to 65 percent, it is possible to improve a mare's statistical chances of getting pregnant by using AI.

There are also downsides to using artificial insemination:

- More creative management is necessary for heat detection.
- Nights, weekends, and holidays may interfere with timing of ovulation and semen collection, unless a dedicated veterinarian is available to work those times to track a mare's estrous cycle, and to breed when she is ready.
- Someone needs to be available to assist a vet in daily exams of a mare, or the mare may need to be taken into a veterinary clinic for the duration of her heat cycle.
- There will be added expenses for veterinary management of the stallion on his end and the mare on her end.

THE MARE WITH A FOAL BY HER SIDE

The other aspect of AI on a mare with a foal by her side is that conception rates with AI on the first foal heat are poor relative to live cover. So, it is best to allow a mare to cycle through that "nine-day" heat and then breed on the following heat cycle. However, AI lets an owner keep a mare and foal on the farm to enjoy the first few months of a foal's life while also minimizing the risks incurred with transporting a neonate to strange territory.

BREEDING SEVERAL MARES AT ONCE

It is common practice to collect semen from a stallion on the premises, and having synchronized several mares to the same estrous cycle, all the mares can be bred at the same time. Not only does a stallion have to perform as stud fewer times to breed all the mares, but this facilitates management eleven months later when it is time to monitor the mares for foaling.

FROZEN SEMEN

Frozen semen adds a different spin on the process of AI since timing of breeding no longer needs to be synchronized with availability of the stallion. Frozen semen does not have the success rate of chilled semen, and more diligent ultrasound exams must follow follicular growth. Due to the difficulty in getting a mare to settle (50 to 60 percent success) with frozen semen, it is important to ensure there is a "live foal guarantee" clause in the breeding contract. Not all stallion semen freezes well, in spite of great care taken during the thaw cycle prior to insemination.

EMBRYO TRANSFER

Another more involved and expensive option for breeding is *embryo transfer* (ET). In this process, a mare is bred, but then the embryo is flushed from the mare's uterus seven days following ovulation. The recovered embryo is then surgically transplanted into a surrogate mare's uterus to bring to term. This may cost at least $5,000, but the advantage is that it maintains a mare in competitive condition without losing eleven months of pregnancy plus the months required to raise the foal to weaning age.

In addition, the ET process allows harvest of multiple embryos during a breeding season. In a good year, three or four offspring from a similar or different matings may be obtained during a season. Those in the breeding business or those with an exceptional combination of a mare and stallion may find this strategy to be a worthwhile investment, but not all breed registries will allow ET.

Reproductive Diseases and Problems

Granulosa Cell Tumor

A *granulosa cell tumor* is a common problem seen in mares, usually affecting only one ovary. An affected mare demonstrates stallion-like behavior and unusual aggression. This "tumor" of the ovary causes it to enlarge significantly in size; this is easily identified with rectal palpation or ultrasound exam (photo 18.19). Although considered a tumor, this is a benign condition without malignancy as seen with cancer; rather, the ovary enlarges because it is filled with multiple small cysts. Hormonal overactivity by an abnormal ovary causes the other to regress in size and function.

Blood tests to measure testosterone, inhibin, and progesterone confirm the presence of an ovarian tumor. Elevations in testosterone explain stallion-like behavior, which is exhibited in about 60 percent of mares with a granulosa cell tumor. Treatment relies on surgical removal of the abnormal ovary. This should restore follicular function of the temporarily dormant ovary that remains, although it may take as long as eight months for normal ovarian function to return.

Mare Reproductive Loss Syndrome

During the seasons of 2001 and 2002, an epidemic abortion storm ran through central Kentucky and neighboring states. It was estimated that 9 percent of the foal crop loss in 2001 and 26 percent of that in 2002 was a result of *mare reproductive loss syndrome* (MRLS).

Ongoing research is attempting to isolate the exact course of this crisis, but current theory is that eastern tent caterpillars are much of the cause. Previous theories speculated that *mycotoxin* (toxin created by molds) in pasture, or *cyanide* from cherry trees might be the inciting cause. Some molds in the presence of *frass* (caterpillar excrement) may play a role in causing the onset of unilateral blindness and pericarditis found to occur in adult animals. However, mycotoxin has been ruled out as a potential cause of the abortion storm. Cyanide from cherry trees no longer seems to be implicated. Currently, investigation continues into bacteria that may be associated with MLRS.

Equine Viral Arteritis

The process of breeding a mare is a step-wise adventure. There is the decision as to which stallion to use, whether to transport the mare to the breeding farm for live cover or to go the route of using shipped semen. Then, there is the checking for pregnancy and the waiting for a lengthy gestation. Each step is fraught with

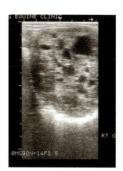

18.19 *An ovary that is affected with a granulosa cell tumor has multiple, loculated follicles, and an enlarged size as seen on diagnostic ultrasound. An affected mare displays stallion-like behavior and aggression.*

obstacles, some a matter of logistics and finances, others due to invisible problems. One consideration must also be about microbes that lurk in the background, waiting to abort a much-anticipated foal. One such microbe is the virus known as *equine viral arteritis* (EVA), which has made a significant impact on the equine-breeding industry since the 1980s. With increased opportunities to breed mares by using chilled or frozen semen, the chances of spreading this viral disease are on the rise, not just within this country but between nations. Although EVA makes its most devastating impact on breeding farms, it can infect horses of all ages and breeds.

DISEASE BY EQUINE VIRAL ARTERITIS VIRUS

The EVA virus in its most innocuous form invades the respiratory tract to create general influenza-like symptoms such as fever, reduced appetite, depression, nasal discharge, and weepy eyes. But, unlike many other infectious viral diseases in horses, one notable symptom of EVA is pronounced swelling of the limbs, and occasionally swelling of the sheath or udder. A skin rash may also accompany this disease. In foals, the respiratory form may complicate into life-threatening pneumonia. And, in mares, the most heartbreaking result of infection with EVA is abortion.

Mature, non-pregnant horses recover well from EVA infection, with no other ill effects. The only medical treatment necessary may be supportive care to ensure that the horse eats and drinks, and whatever treatment is necessary to keep a horse comfortable from the effects of the virus. Because EVA appears a lot like other viral respiratory infections, it is not readily identified without blood-testing specifically for this virus.

The virus is transferred from horse to horse through respiratory secretions, and can become rampant in horses that have congregated at an event such as a horse show, a racing meet, or a sales barn. Once exposed to the virus, a horse shows clinical signs within 1 to 2 weeks, and abortion occurs within 1 to 3 weeks of exposure at any stage in the pregnancy. The biggest concern about this disease lies in its ability to undermine the breeding industry since it is carried as a venereal disease and shed in the semen of infected stallions.

SHEDDING STALLIONS

A stallion can silently harbor this virus in his semen. The only means of identifying if a stallion is infected is to test for the disease. A mare owner should inquire if a stallion has been tested for EVA prior to breeding. The carrier rate among stallions that have blood-tested positive for the disease ranges from 30 to 60 percent with a mean carrier rate amongst all breeds of 43 percent. The prevalence of this disease seems to vary depending on breed. There is a 1 to 3 percent incidence of EVA in Arabians and Thoroughbreds, while Standardbreds are afflicted with as high as 70 to 80 percent of the stallions being carriers. The Gluck Equine Research Center in Kentucky is instrumental in screening all breeds of stallions for this disease. If a stallion tests negative for EVA antibodies in his blood, then he is not likely to carry the virus in his semen. The same is true if he has been vaccinated against EVA before being infected with the disease.

Once a stallion's semen has been infected with EVA, he harbors the virus in his accessory sex glands for years and it passes into his semen with each ejaculate. A stallion's fertility is not affected, but shed virus is able to survive cooling and freezing of infected semen, and has been known to remain infective in frozen semen for more than 15 years. Once a stallion has been infected, there is no cure; most times a stallion becomes a carrier for life, although an occasional stallion will clear the infection on his own. The focus on the carrier state lies solely with the stallions; mares, geldings, and sexually immature colts do not persistently carry the disease. Once recovered from viral effects, they are no longer communicable to others. A mare that has been infected with EVA-contaminated semen will develop protective immunity to the disease, and will clear the virus from the reproductive tract with no later threat of abortion related to EVA.

At this time, EVA is not a reportable disease in the United States, and there is no requirement for testing of shipped semen throughout the nation. It is recommended that semen coming into the USA from out of the country should be tested for EVA antibodies at a qualified testing laboratory. Currently there are no federal requirements that this be done. The only current "safeguard" against entry of EVA-infected semen is based on pre-export testing in the country of origin, which may or may not be reliable in its testing abilities. Because of the inadvertent danger of transmitting this disease at epidemic proportions throughout the horse population with the use of chilled and frozen semen, the American Horse Council (AHC) has urged the United States Department of Agriculture (USDA) to outline a protocol for limiting this risk. The protocol (http://www.nawpn.org) enables breeders to identify infected and shedding stallions and to take precautions in broodmares.

A vaccine used in prevention must be an approved and licensed modified live vaccine (Fort Dodge Laboratories). Before vaccinating any horse with the EVA viral vaccine, contact the state regulatory agency to confirm the appropriate protocol for this disease. Not all horses should be vaccinated against EVA unless they are at risk of being bred to EVA-shedding stallions. Many countries will not allow importation of any horse demonstrating EVA antibodies in the blood whether these

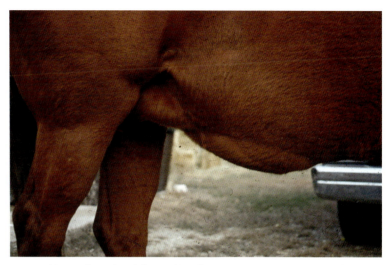

18.20 *Edema along the abdominal midline is common in a mare in her last trimester of pregnancy. This swelling is caused by compression of the lymphatic drainage as a result of the weight of the foal. Pasture exercise alleviates this edema to some degree.*

were induced by vaccine or natural infection. A competition horse that has the possibility of traveling abroad from the United States should be carefully considered when deciding whether to use this horse as a breeding prospect, or not. It is important to have documentation of a serologically negative blood test prior to vaccination in order to prove a horse did not develop EVA antibodies due to natural exposure.

Foaling and Complications

In the weeks or days prior to foaling, it is common for a mare to develop swelling along the midline of the belly due to edema related to the weight of the fetus in the abdomen (photo 18.20). Her udder will gradually enlarge for up to a month before parturition. Globules of milk colostrum will form a wax at the end of the nipples, usually within 72 hours of foaling (photos 18.21 A & B). She should not be leaking any colostrum until the birth of the foal.

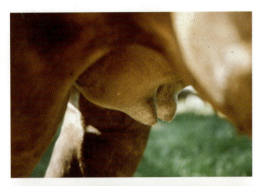
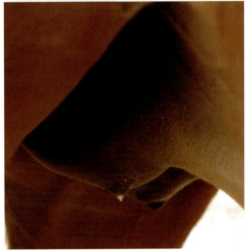

18.21 A & B *Udder edema and waxing of the nipples alert an owner that the mare is likely to foal within a few days.*

For a mare, the birth of her foal is an explosive process, in the best of circumstances requiring less than half an hour from the time her water breaks to the time the foal has been propelled through the birth canal into a less protective world (photo 18.22). The first few hours after birth are a critical period for both mare and foal. In a wilder existence a pregnant mare would attempt to find a secluded place to lie down and have her foal, safe from predators. A newborn foal is a precocious creature, able to rise to his feet within hours of birth. The spindly limbs quickly gain enough coordination to flee predators, the foal a running shadow close on his mother's heels (photo 18.23). In the first hour or two before a foal rises on wobbly legs, mother and baby come to intimately know each other by taste and smell. A lasting, imprinted bond developed in those first hours enables the infant to recognize mother as his source of protection and food and to turn to her for example.

Usually the foaling process proceeds uneventfully; however, problems can arise both during and following birth. The variety of possible foaling complications is too numerous to discuss in full detail here, but the most common situations are discussed below.

FESCUE TOXICOSIS

Tall fescue is a common pasture and hay forage for horses throughout the United States and Canada. Fescue toxicity is caused by an *endophytic fungus* (*Neotyphodium* or *Acremonium*), which produces an ergot alkaloid. Fescue grass itself is not toxic, but rather it is the fungus that flourishes within the grass, and especially the seed heads. The fungus is not visible to the naked eye. Other similar alkaloids are generated from fungi, such as *Claviceps* spp. These infect oats, cereal rye grain, or Kentucky bluegrass. *Ergot alkaloids* exert detrimental effects on a pregnant mare and fetus by overly stimulating production of *dopamine*. Excess dopamine then inhibits *prolactin* secretion important to stimulating lactation and other signals that prepare a mare's body for birth.

Signs of Fescue Toxicity

Common signs of fescue endophyte toxicity include reproductive problems such as prolonged gestation of up to a month, lack of udder development, absence of milk production, abortion, thickened placenta, retained placenta, stillbirth or weak foal, and high rate of foal mortality. Clinical signs include *red bag*, in which the amniotic sac covering the foal is thickened and dark red; it does not break open at the time of foaling; without human intervention, a foal suffocates.

Prevention of Fescue Toxicity

In fescue areas known for endophyte infection, pregnant mares should

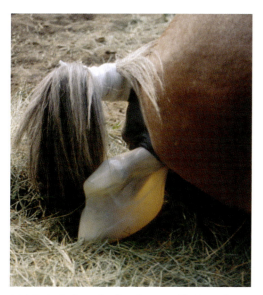

18.22 *At foaling, the first thing visible from the vulva should be the foal's front feet in the amniotic sac. This foal is in normal presentation, with the feet pointing down, indicating that his head and back are positioned parallel to the mare's backbone. In this presentation, the mare's pelvic shape most easily allows passage of the foal from the birth canal.*

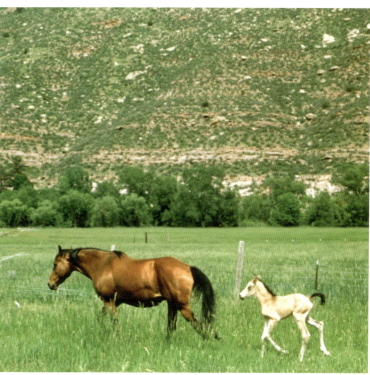

18.23 *A newborn foal is a precocious youngster, able to get up on his spindly legs within a couple of hours of birth. This genetically programmed ability enables a foal to follow close to his dam, and flee from predators that would lurk in a wild environment.*

be removed from this source of forage in the latter months of pregnancy, at least by day 300 of gestation, and preferably 3 months prior to foaling. Pastures can be mowed to eliminate infected seed heads.

Daily doses of oral *domperidone* can be given to mares in late gestation to counteract adverse responses to the fungus. Domperidone blocks the prolactin-depressing effects of ergot alkaloids. Domperidone therapy should be administered starting about 3 weeks prior to the anticipated foaling date.

DYSTOCIA

Once a mare's water breaks, the foal should be delivered from the birth canal within a short hour. Any time longer than this portends a problem and a veterinarian should be called. While waiting, it is sometimes helpful to get the mare up if she is down; this enables repositioning of a foal that is not progressing properly through the birth canal. If a vet is expected fairly soon, resist the attempt to insert a hand into the vagina to try to correct a foal that is incorrectly positioned. A veterinarian may

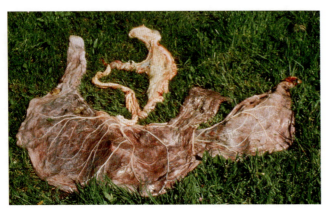

18.24 *When spread on the ground, a normal placenta (passed within an hour or two of foaling) assumes the shape of the uterus with its two horns, somewhat resembling a pair of billowy pantaloons. The color of the placenta also reveals information about its health and the health of the foal during the pregnancy. The placenta is examined carefully to make sure it is intact and that no portion has remained inside the mare, as retained pieces could potentially be life-threatening.*

suggest advice over the phone that includes attempting to reposition a leg that is caught over the foal's head, or to exert gentle downward traction to relieve a shoulder or hip lock. With veterinary advice, these things can be tried. Generally, the prudent course is to await professional help.

RETAINED FETAL MEMBRANES

By nature's curious design, it is during the first hour or two, while the foal is alternately resting and testing out his legs, that the mare will go through a period of cramping associated with expulsion of the *fetal membranes*, which include the *placenta* and *amnionic sac*. (The amnion encloaks the foal so it is passed immediately at birth, while the placenta is adhered to the uterine lining and so must loosen and pass after the foal and amnion have exited the birth canal.) She may repeatedly lie down and get up as uterine contractions grip her abdomen. It is important to identify if a mare's cramping is due to uterine contractions or due to intestinal colic pain. There is a high incidence of colic post-foaling in mares, and many times the colic problem requires surgery for correction. The loss of the space-occupying mass of the foal allows for intestinal displacements, particularly of the large colon. Persistent and unrelenting colic pain is cause for immediate veterinary intervention.

On average, fetal membranes are rapidly expelled within 15 to 60 minutes after birth of the foal, but this process could take up to 3 hours in a normal situation. It is common practice to call a veterinarian for a post-foaling exam at which time the expelled placenta is inspected to be sure it has passed in entirety. When spread on the ground, a normal placenta resembles a pair of billowy pantaloons, each "leg" representing one of the two uterine horns (photo 18.24). If all or any portion of the fetal membranes is retained for longer than 3 hours, this is considered a *retained placenta* and requires immediate veterinary attention (photo 18.25).

A retained placenta endangers a mare's health in several different ways. As it hangs partially in and partially out of the mare's uterus, it acts like a wick to draw contaminants into the reproductive tract. Retention of the placental tissue increases the potential for bacterial infection of the uterus. This poses an immediate threat to her health as well as potential reduction in future fertility. Bacterial overgrowth of the uterus accumulates toxins, which are picked up by the bloodstream from the inflamed uterus. The mare may become very sick, and she may develop crippling laminitis as a consequence (see p. 74).

A dangling placenta should never be removed manually. Not only can pulling on the retained placenta result in life-threatening uterine hemorrhage, but tugging on tightly adhered tissue may also tear the uterine lining.

Scar tissue repair of torn areas reduces a mare's fertility in succeeding breeding seasons. The weight of the membranes helps to loosen and detach them, so it is best not to cut them.

A mare that is agitated by the placenta knocking about her hocks might endanger a foal by kicking at the "alien" tissue or by startling and bolting over the foal. In this case, the amnion can be wadded into a plastic bag, leaving it to dangle about a foot from the vulva. The entire "package" of tissue can be tied to the tail with twine. Let a veterinarian deal with the problem by infusing the mare's uterus with antiseptic solutions and placing her on antibiotics and anti-inflammatory medication (see p. 442).

PASSIVE TRANSFER AND ANTIBODY PROTECTION

It is prudent to wash between a mare's udder and her rear end prior to the foal suckling. This minimizes the amount of environmental bacterial contaminants ingested by a foal. During the second stage of labor, the mare often defecates, soiling the hind end. As a foal seeks the udder following birth, he contacts these areas of fecal contamination. Cells that line the gut of the newborn foal do not selectively discriminate amongst large molecular weight materials and so are able to also absorb pathogenic bacteria in addition to protective *immunoglobulins* from the first milk, known as *colostrum*. Immediate disinfection of the stall following foaling also limits the numbers of bacteria a foal obtains through licking and tasting. Excellent hygiene goes a long ways to minimizing the risk of a septic foal.

A newborn foal should suckle within 2 hours of birth. It is important for a foal to ingest sufficient colostrum to obtain vital antibodies that help fend off disease until he is old enough to develop antibodies of his own. Protective antibodies are passed in the colostrum that is consumed in the first 6 to 12 hours following

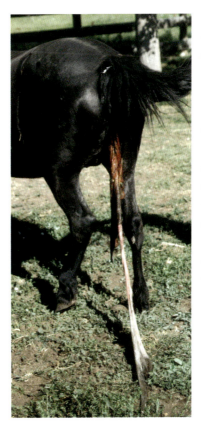

18.25 *Retained placental membranes, in whole or even as small pieces, pose a dangerous health situation. Here, the amniotic sac (the white tissue touching the ground) and placenta (pink above the amnion) are hanging out of the mare because the placenta is still adhered to the uterine lining and will not slip free. A retained placenta creates conditions for bacterial infection of the uterus with absorption of toxins from the uterus into the bloodstream; circulating toxins can elicit laminitis or septic shock. Uterine infection also reduces future fertility.*

birth. Following this time, "gut closure" of cells lining the intestinal tract render them incapable of absorbing the large protein molecules of colostrum. A foal should consume at least 1 to 2 quarts of colostrum in the initial hours. Eight hours following the first suckle, a blood sample may be taken from the foal to evaluate the level of immunoglobulin G, or IgG. This level should surpass 800 mg/dl. Any IgG value of less than 800 mg/dl or any foal born into an unsanitary environment (heavy manure contamination, soiled bedding, dirty stall or paddock) is cause for a plasma transfusion.

UMBILICAL PROBLEMS

Immediately following birth, it is recommended to disinfect the navel with a solution of *chlorhexidine* (Nolvasan®) prepared by mixing

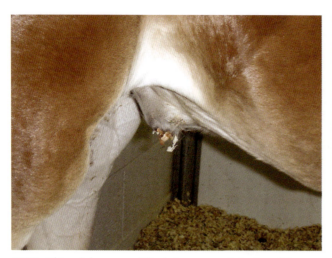

18.26 This colt has an umbilical abscess—an infection of the umbilical stump. Oozing from the end of the navel has caused shavings to stick to it. Swelling extends up into the belly wall, and an ascending infection can cause showering of bacteria through the body and a systemic septic infection and/or infection within the joints. An umbilical abscess is also called "navel ill."

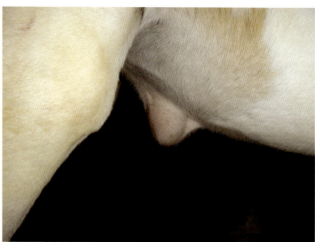

18.27 A swollen umbilicus that appears on first examination to be an umbilical abscess when, in fact, there is a herniation in the abdominal wall and intestines have slipped through the hernia to become incarcerated. If you can push upward on the swelling with a finger and the segment of bowel is returned to the abdomen to diminish the swelling, then that confirms the diagnosis. Ultrasound exam can differentiate between a hernia and abscess in confusing cases.

1 part of stock solution to 4 parts water to make a 0.5 percent solution. Not only does chlorhexidine exert an effective bacterial kill, it retains residual antibacterial activity that is not inactivated by organic material. This is the currently recommended navel dip rather than using *tamed iodine* or *tincture of iodine* preparations as advocated in years past. Iodine compounds are caustic and cause tissue death along with scabbing. Bacteria that collect beneath a scab can travel up the umbilical cord to create a systemic and potentially fatal *septicemia*. Also, sloughing of skin adjacent to the umbilicus can lead to the development of a *patent urachus* that causes urine to be continually excreted from the umbilical stump.

Umbilical Abscess

Umbilical infections, or "navel ill," are serious and life-threatening (photo 18.26). Not only can entry of bacteria through the umbilicus create a generalized septicemia, but these bacteria also can migrate to the joints causing severe degenerative joint disease that prevents a foal from becoming an athlete, should he survive. Despite diligent soaking of the navel in antiseptic solutions, it is important to monitor a foal's rectal temperature, his appetite, frequency and consistency of bowel movements, and alertness and activity. Not all umbilical infections present with an enlarged or abnormal appearing navel. Sometimes it is necessary to have a veterinarian ultrasound the umbilicus to detect an associated internal problem.

Umbilical Hernia

At birth a foal may have a defect in the abdominal wall along the midline of the belly around the umbilical stump, referred to as an *umbilical hernia* (photo 18.27). A one-to-two-finger-wide opening does not usually pose a problem, and many of these resolve as the foal grows. However, if the defect is more than two fingers wide, it is large enough for a loop of small intestine to slide into the hernial sac. By gently pushing on the swelling with a finger, you can usually push the bowel out of the hernia back into the abdomen. However, entrapment (*incarceration*) of a loop of bowel in the hernia creates the potential for the intestinal piece to lose its blood supply and strangulate. Such an event can be sudden in onset, accompanied by severe signs of colic pain. An umbilical hernia is easily corrected with surgery to prevent an acute crisis.

RUPTURED BLADDER

At birth, compression of a foal through the birth canal has the potential to rupture the foal's bladder. This problem is more common in male colts than in fillies. The colt may start out acting okay until a day or two has passed, at which time he shows signs of weakness and illness. Blood tests, a belly tap, and diagnostic ultrasound are used to confirm the presence of a ruptured bladder. This requires immediate surgical intervention and aggressive medical management to correct severe electrolyte imbalances associated with pooling of urine in the abdomen.

MECONIUM IMPACTION

At birth, a newborn foal eliminates his first feces, called *meconium*. This is waste material and debris that has accumulated in the lower intestines throughout the course of gestation. This feces appears like blackberry jam, dark brown or black in color, wadded together as fecal balls. Impaction with meconium can cause persistent rectal straining or colic signs. Meconium may be retained if there is insufficient ingestion of colostrum and dehydration, or because of compromising conditions at birth such as prematurity, dystocia, or oxygen deprivation. A commercially available Fleet® *enema* should be given following birth to assist a foal in eliminating this material. If a foal does not receive relief from an enema, then a veterinarian will need to be involved in resolving this condition.

DUMMY FOAL

The term "dummy foal" aptly describes the presentation of a foal suffering from *neonatal maladjustment syndrome*, or NMS. Usually this syndrome is a result of asphyxia at birth that occurred due to compromise of the placenta just prior to or during the birth process. Lack of oxygen causes the brain to swell as well as injuring other organ systems. These foals appear stupid, not able to figure out how to nurse, perhaps not even trying to nurse. Such a foal quickly runs out of energy and lapses into sleep, or may have seizures. It is prudent to summon veterinary help immediately if a foal appears slow to relate to the world around him. Some dummy foals may also be septic due to an infection attained in utero.

NEONATAL ISOERYTHROLYSIS

Neonatal isoerythrolysis (NI) occurs when a mare has produced antibodies against the red blood cells of her foal, and these antibodies are passed to the foal in the colostrum. The mare becomes sensitized to blood of the fetus that has an incompatible blood type inherited from the stallion. Usually, exposure of a mare to her foal's blood occurs during gestation as a result of a placental abnormality (*placentitis*), or due to a difficult birth. Sensitization also occurs subsequent to a mare having received a blood transfusion (or plasma contaminated with blood) at a previous time in her life. When her foal suckles, he consumes proteins from the colostrum that cross-react with his own blood, causing rapid breakdown of the foal's own red blood cells, and death. The solution to this problem depends on blood testing both mare and stallion prior to foaling. NI doesn't usually

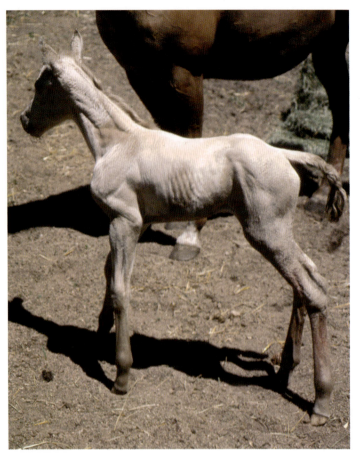

18.28 *Contracted tendons that buckle the legs of a neonate may make it difficult for him to follow the mare, or to stand and nurse. In the immediate days following birth, treatment with an intravenous injection of oxytetracycline often resolves mild to moderate flexural contracture.*

may be administered by bottle or stomach tube during the first hours, and then milk replacer supplemented to the foal while the mare's colostrum is milked out continually. Once the dam is producing regular milk, it is safe for the foal to suckle.

FLEXURAL LIMB DEFORMITY OR CONTRACTED TENDONS

One situation that is present at birth or develops over the first few days is that of *contracted tendons* (photo 18.28, and see chapter 7, *Strong Tendons and Ligaments,* p. 198). This develops at the pastern, the fetlock, or in the carpus (knee). It may be related to malposition of a foal in utero or due to ingestion of a toxic weed by the mare during pregnancy. Whether mild or severe, these buckled legs are often treatable with an intravenous injection of *oxytetracycline*. It is theorized that the oxytetracycline injection binds calcium and thereby initiates limb relaxation. It is best to contact a vet immediately for this therapy rather than waiting. Limb contracture typically worsens with time without therapy. Heavy bandaging or splinting the limbs also facilitates tendon relaxation. For those limbs that do not respond, surgery may be the only solution.

HOW DOES A SICK FOAL PRESENT?

A normal foal nurses frequently and vigorously, as often as 5 to 7 times each hour. He sleeps hard in between feedings and playtime, but is rambunctious in his play (photo 18.29). A normal foal is inquisitive and active, checking everything in his surroundings. When a foal is disinterested in what is going on around him, seems to sleep more often than not, is listless and quiet, then something is wrong. A sick foal can decline very quickly so any abnormality must be identified rapidly and veterinary care implemented immediately. A sick foal shows any or all of the following signs:

show up with the first foal, but may with subsequent pregnancies.

Identification of a potential problem allows nonstop monitoring of the mare so human intervention may be present at foaling. The foal will need to be separated completely from the dam for the first 24 to 48 hours and fed by bottle. Or, the foal can be with the dam but only if wearing a muzzle that prevents him from nursing the colostrum. Suitable colostrum

- Elevated rectal temperature above 102° F (39° C) occurs in half of sick foals
- Abnormally low rectal temperature less than 97° F (36° C)
- Diarrhea
- Lethargy or weakness
- Infrequent or absence of nursing: the mare's udder is distended or drips milk
- Sleeping more often than not
- Lack of interest in surroundings, little response to stimuli
- Swollen joint or joints, with or without lameness
- Swollen navel with or without discharge

A PREMATURE FOAL

It is important to identify a foal that may be born prematurely as he is highly susceptible to developing serious medical problems early on in all body systems. One cannot rely on the gestational age of a foal as insurance that a foal is ready for birth. Any foal born prior to 320 days gestation is not considered full-term. Any foal born after 320 days of gestation that has any of the following characteristics may still be considered premature:

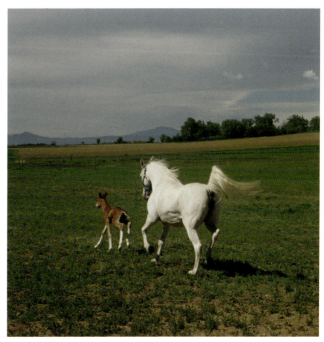

18.29 *A normal foal has abundant energy, and he nurses often, about 5 to 7 times per hour. He naps frequently also, but wakes up bright and alert, wanting to drink milk and then play. He is inquisitive and curious about everything in his surroundings.*

- Low birth weight (a neonate should weigh about 10 percent of the dam's weight: for example, a 1000-pound mare should have a 100-pound foal)
- Hair coat silky or short, especially on the rump
- Demonstrates muscle weakness, tendency to "flop," or unable to stand without getting stronger with time
- Inadequate or absent suckle reflex
- Thin skin
- Droopy lips and/or ears
- Domed forehead
- Bulging eyes
- Tendon laxity of the limbs
- Incomplete ossification of the carpal joints (knees) and hocks as seen on X-ray films

Appendix A

Normal Physiological Parameters

	NORMAL	RANGE
Rectal temperature, at rest, adult (F)	98 – 100.5	(97 – 101)
Rectal temperature, at rest, adult (C)	36 – 38	(36.1 – 38.3)
Rectal temperature, working, adult (F)	101 – 103	
Rectal temperature, working, adult (C)	38 – 39	
Heart rate, resting (beats per minute)	32 – 44	(24 – 48)
Respiratory rate, resting (breaths per min)	12 – 24	(8 – 28)
Mucous membrane color	pink	
Capillary refill time (seconds)	2	
Jugular refill time (seconds)	2 – 3	
Bowel movements (piles per day)	8 – 12	
Borborygmi (intestinal noise, each quadrant)	2 per minute	
Water intake (gallons per day)	5 – 20	
Urine output (liters per day)	1½ – 8	

Appendix B

Common Drug and Supply Names, Uses, and Actions

Many drugs are formulated as generic products although some may be best recognized by their proprietary names. Sampling for drug testing occurs at random at competitions. Some organizations, like the Fédération Equestre Internationale (FEI—www.horsesport.org) and the American Endurance Ride Conference (AERC—www.aerc.org) have strict "no-drug" policies, while others, such as the American Quarter Horse Association (AQHA—www.aqha.com), the United States Equestrian Federation (USEF—www.usef.org), and the racing industry limit use of drugs. To avoid legality issues, contact the applicable organization well in advance of an event.

DRUG (OR SUPPLY) NAME	BRAND NAME	ACTION OR USAGE
Acepromazine		Tranquilizer
Acetazolamide	Diamox®	Diuretic to manage HYPP
Albuterol		Bronchodilator
Aloe Vera		Topical cream
Alpha-tocopheryl	Vitamin E	Vitamin
Altrenogest	Regumate®	Progesterone/Hormone control
Aluminum hydroxide antacid	Maalox-TC®, Mylanta II®, Neigh-Lox®	Gastric ulcer treatment
Aluminum powder spray	Aluspray®	Wound protection
Anabolic steroid	Winstrol-V®, Equipoise®	Appetite and condition enhancer
Ascorbic acid	Vitamin C	Vitamin
Aspirin powder		Anterior uveitis treatment
Atropine		Pupil dilation
Betamethasone	Celestone®	Corticosteroid anti-inflammatory
Branched chain amino acids	BCAA®	Muscle endurance supplement
Butorphanol tartrate	Torbrugesic®	Analgesic
N-butylscopolammonium bromide	Buscopan®	Anti-spasmodic for colic
Cambendazole	Camvet®	Dewormer
Capsaicin	Capsacin®	Skin disorders, or headshaking treatment
Carbamazine		Headshaking treatment
Carnitine		Muscle supplement
Chlorhexidine	Nolvasan®	Antiseptic
Chondroitin sulfate		Joint supplement
Chorionic gonadotropin (HCG)		Managing ovulation
Chromium tripicolinate		Managing Cushing's or EMS
Cimetidine	Tagamet®	Anti-ulcer treatment, melanoma treatment
Cisplatinin		Cancer treatment
Clenbuterol	Ventipulmin®	Bronchodilator
Cloprostenol	Estrumate®	Managing ovulation
Clotrimazole	Lotrimin®	Skin fungal treatment
Conforming roll gauze	Kling®	Wound dressing

Drug	Brand	Use
Copper sulfate	Kopertox®	Hoof medication
Cyproheptadine		Managing Cushing's or headshaking
Dantrolene sodium	Dantrium®	Muscle relaxant
Deslorelin	Ovuplant®	Managing ovulation
Detomidine HCl	Dormosedan®	Sedative
Dexamethasone	Azium® or generic	Corticosteroid anti-inflammatory
Diazepam	Valium®	Sedative
Dichlorvos		Insecticide
Dimethyl Sulfoxide	Domoso®	Anti-oxidant, anti-inflammatory agent
Dinoprost	Lutalyse®	Managing ovulation
Dipyrone		Anti-spasmodic for colic
Domperidone	Equidone®	Stimulates lactation in fescue toxicosis
Doxycycline		Antibiotic
Epinephrine		Adrenalin
Erythropoietin	Epogen®	Blood booster
Estradiol cypionate	ECP®	Proposed treatment for upward fixation of the patella
Fenbendazole	Panacur®	Dewormer
5-Fluorouracil (5-FU)		Cancer treatment
Flunixin meglumine	Banamine®	Nonsteroidal anti-inflammatory drug
Fluphenazine		Behavior modifying psychotropic drug
Furosemide	Lasix®	Diuretic
Gentamycin sulfate	Gentocin®	Antibiotic
Glucosamine		Joint supplement
Glycine	DMG®	Muscle supplement
GnRH (gonatrotropin releasing hormone)	Ovuplant®	Managing ovulation
Griseofulvin	Fulvicin®	Anti-fungal
Hyaluronic acid or Hyaluronate sodium	Legend®, Hyalovet®, Hylartin-V®	Joint treatment
Hydrocortisone		Corticosteroid anti-inflammatory
Hydroxyzine		Anti-histamine
Hyperimmune plasma		Immune treatment
Interferon		Anti-viral treatment
Isoxsuprine HCl		Vasodilator
Ivermectin	Eqvalan®, Zimecterin®	Dewormer
Ketoprofen	Ketofen®	Nonsteroidal anti-inflammatory drug
Magnesium sulfate	Epsom salts	Poultice, anti-inflammation
Mebendazole	Telmintic®	Dewormer
Metamizole	Dipyrone®	Anti-spasmodic to treat colic
DL-Methionine		Hoof supplement
Methocarbamol	Robaxin®	Central-acting sedative
Methylprednisolone	Depo-Medrol®	Corticosteroid anti-inflammatory
Miconazole	Conofite®	Anti-fungal
Mineral oil		Grain overload treatment via stomach tube
Moxidectin	Quest®	Dewormer
Naproxen		Nonsteroidal anti-inflammatory drug
Nitazoxanide	Navigator®	EPM treatment
Nitrofurazone	Furacin®	Topical antibiotic
Nitroglycerin		Vasodilator

Non-adhesive sterile dressing	Telfa®, Surgipad®, ABD dressing®, Combine pad	Wound dressing
Omeprazole	Gastroguard®, Ulcerguard®	Anti-ulcer medication
Oxfendazole	Febantel®	Dewormer
Oxibendazole	Anthelcide-EQ®	Dewormer
Oxytetracycline		Antibiotic
Oxytocin		Hormone
Penicillin, procaine, or potassium		Antibiotic
Pentoxyfylline		Vasodilator
Pergolide		Cushing's treatment
Permethrin		Insecticide
Phenylbutazone		Nonsteroidal anti-inflammatory drug
Phenylephrine HCl		Treatment for nephrosplenic entrapment
Piperazine		Dewormer
Pitcher plant extract	Sarapin®	Treatment for back pain
Polymyxin B		Antibiotic to prevent endotoxin toxicity
Polysulfated glycosaminoglycan	Adequan®	Joint supplement
Ponazuril	Marquis®	EPM treatment
Povidone iodine	Betadine®, Betadyne®	Antiseptic
Praziquantel	Droncit®	Dewormer against tapeworms
Prednisone		Corticosteroid anti-inflammatory
Prednisolone		Corticosteroid anti-inflammatory
Prostaglandin F2 alpha	Estrumate®, Lutalyse®	Managing ovulation
Psyllium hydrophilic muciloid	Equi-Aid®, Sand-Lax®, Sand-Ex®	Managing sand colic
Pyrantel pamoate	Strongid®	Dewormer
Pyrantel tartrate	Strongid® C or C2X, Equi-Aid CW® or SW®	Dewormer
Pyrethrin		Insecticide
Pyrimethamine		EPM treatment
Ranitidine HCl		Anti-ulcer medication
Self-adherent flexible tape	Vetrap®, Flexus®, Medi-Rip®, Equisport®	Wound dressing
Self-adhesive stretch tape	Elastikon®, Elastoplast®	Wound dressing
Silver sulfadiazine	Silvadene®	Topical wound dressing
Sucralfate	Gastrafate®	Anti-ulcer medication
Sulfadiazine		EPM treatment
Sulfamethoxazole/Trimethoprim		Antibiotic
Tetracycline		Antibiotic
Tetrachlorvinphos	Equitrol®	Insecticide feed-through
Thiabendazole	Tresaderm®	Topical anti-fungal
Thiamine HCl		Vitamin
Tilurdonate	Skelid®	Navicular disease treatment
Tincture of iodine	Thrushbuster®	Hoof medication
Triamcinolone acetonide	Vetalog®	Corticosteroid anti-inflammatory
Triamcinolone ointment	Dermalone®, Panalog®, Animax®	Corticosteroid anti-inflammatory
Trichlorfon		Insecticide
Triple antibiotic	Neosporin®	Topical antibiotic
Tryptophan		Calming agent
Vitamin E/Selenium		Vitamin/mineral
Xylazine HCl		Sedative
Zinc oxide	Desitin®, Thuja zinc	Topical skin protectant

Appendix C

Common Toxic Plants

PLANT	LATIN NAME(S)	SYSTEM AFFECTED	CLINICAL SIGNS
Acorns (Oak)	*Quercus* spp.	Gastrointestinal	Abdominal pain Constipation Bloody diarrhea Severe weakness
Alsike clover	*Trifolium hybridum*	Skin Gastrointestinal	Photosensitivity Liver disease
Avocado leaves	*Persea americana*	Muscular Nervous Gastrointestinal	Swelling of head, tongue, cheeks, and throatlatch Facial pain Abdominal edema Depression Colic
Bindweed seeds	*Convolvulus arvensis*	Gastrointestinal	Colic
Black locust tree	*Robinia pseudoacacia*	Gastrointestinal Nervous Cardiovascular Respiratory Musculoskeletal	Diarrhea Depression Cardiovascular collapse Labored breathing Laminitis
Black walnut	*Juglans nigra*	Musculoskeletal	Laminitis
Bracken fern	*Pteridium aquilinum*	Nervous	Thiamine deficiency with depression, muscle tremors, incoordination
Buckeyes or horse chestnuts	*Aesculus* spp.	Nervous	Ataxia Muscle tremors Hyperexcitable or depressed
Buckwheat	*Fagopyrum esculentum*	Skin	Photosensitivity
Buttercup	*Ranunculaceae* spp.	Gastrointestinal	Mouth blisters Colic Diarrhea

Castor bean	*Ricinus* spp.	Gastrointestinal Nervous Cardiovascular Respiratory Musculoskeletal	Diarrhea Depression Cardiovascular collapse Labored breathing Laminitis
Chives		Gastrointestinal	Liver and kidney disease
Chokecherry	*Prunus* spp.	Cardiovascular	Respiratory distress Death from cyanide
Cocklebur	*Xanthium* spp.	Gastrointestinal	Liver disease
Curly dock	*Rumex crispus*	Cardiovascular	Kidney disease
Eggplant		Gastrointestinal	G-I irritation
False dandelion (flatweed)	*Hypochaeris radicata*	Musculoskeletal	Acquired stringhalt
Fescue endophyte fungus	*Neotyphodium* or *Acremonium*	Reproductive	Abortion Red bag birth Weak or dead foal No lactation
Groundsel	*Senecio* spp.	Skin	Photosensitivity
Gumweed	*Grindelia* spp.	Skin	Selenium toxicity indicator
Hoary asylum	*Berteroa incana*	Musculoskeletal Gastrointestinal	Laminitis, limb swelling Diarrhea and fever
Horsebrush	*Tetradymia* spp.	Skin	Photosensitivity
Horseradish		Gastrointestinal	Stomach irritation
Horsetail	*Equisetum* spp.	Nervous	Thiamine deficiency when used with ivermectin: depression, muscle tremors, incoordination
Houndstongue	*Cynoglossum* spp.	Skin Gastrointestinal	Photosensitivity Liver disease
Jimsonweed or thorn apple	*Datura stramonium*	Gastrointestinal Nervous	G-I irritation Depression
Kentucky coffee tree	*Gymnocladus dioicus*	Gastrointestinal Nervous	G-I irritation Depression of CNS
Leafy spurge	*Euphorbia esula*	Gastrointestinal	G-I irritation
Legumes (alfalfa, clover, pea)		Skin	Photosensitivity
Mallow	*Malva* spp.	Nervous	Muscle tremors/shivers
Mountain laurel	*Kalmia* spp.	Gastrointestinal	Abdominal pain Diarrhea Excessive salivation
Larkspur	*Delphinium* spp.	Nervous	Muscle twitching Excess salivation Collapse Convulsions Respiratory failure
Locoweed	*Astragalus* spp. and *Oxytropis* spp.	Nervous Ophthalmic	Depression Behavior changes Vision problems

Appendix C   573

Lupine	*Lupinus argenteus*	Nervous	Anxiety Excess salivation Convulsions
Mustard seed	*Brassica* spp.	Gastrointestinal	Colic
Nightshade	*Solanum eleagnifolium*	Gastrointestinal Nervous	G-I irritation Depression
Paintbrush	*Castileja* spp.	Skin	Selenium toxicity indicator
Persimmons	*Diospyros virginia*	Gastrointestinal	Impaction colic
Potatoes		Gastrointestinal	G-I irritation
Prince's plume	*Stanley pinnata*	Skin	Selenium toxicity indicator
Red maple	*Acer* spp.	Cardiovascular	Hemolytic anemia Death
Rhododendron	*Rhododendron* spp.	Gastrointestinal	Abdominal pain Diarrhea Excessive salivation
		Nervous Cardiovascular	Respiratory depression Sudden death
Russian knapweed	*Centaurea* spp.	Nervous	Brain degeneration Paralysis of tongue and chewing muscles
Singletary pea	*Lathyrus hirsutus*	Nervous	Partial paralysis of hind legs Stringhalt-like gait
Snakeweed	*Gutierrezia* spp.	Skin	Selenium toxicity indicator
Sorghum	*Sorghum* spp.	Urinary Musculoskeletal	Urine dribbling Weak in rear legs
St. Johnswort	*Hypericum perforatum*	Skin	Photosensitivity
Sudan grass	*Sorghum* spp.	Urinary Musculoskeletal	Urine dribbling Weak in rear legs
Tansy ragwort	*Senecio* spp.	Skin	Photosensitivity
Tomatoes		Gastrointestinal	G-I irritation
Vetch	*Astragalus* spp.	Skin	Photosensitivity Selenium toxicity indicator
Water hemlock	*Cicuta maculata*	Nervous	Convulsion Respiratory failure Death
Western-whorled milkweed	*Asclepias* spp.	Nervous	Depression Muscle tremors Incoordination
		Gastrointestinal Respiratory	G-I irritation Respiratory problems
Woody aster	*Xylorrhiza* spp.	Skin	Selenium toxicity indicator
Yellow star thistle	*Centaurea* spp.	Nervous	Brain degeneration Paralysis of tongue and chewing muscles
Yew (Japanese)	*Taxus cuspida*	Cardiovascular	Sudden death

Appendix D

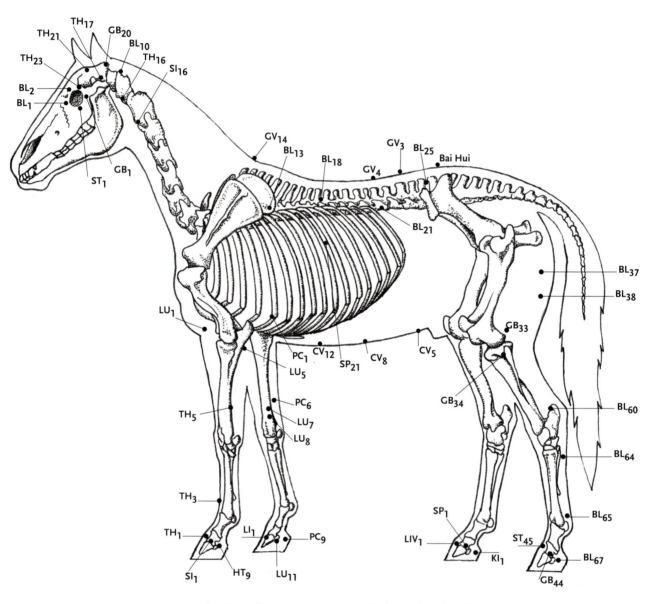

Commonly Used Acupuncture Points in the Horse

Bibliography

Adams, O.R. *Lameness in Horses.* Third Edition. Lea and Febiger, Philadelphia, 1979.

Alsup, E.M. "Dimethyl Sulfoxide." *Journal of the American Veterinary Medical Association,* Vol. 185, No. 9 (November 1984), pp. 1011–1014.

Antikatzides, T.G. "Soft Laser Treatment of Musculoskeletal and Other Disorders in the Equine Athlete." *Equine Practice,* Vol. 8, No. 2 (February 1986), pp. 24–29.

Asquith, R.L., E.L. Johnson, J. Kivepelto, and C. Depew. "Erroneous Weight Estimation of Horses." *Proceedings of the American Association of Equine Practitioners* (1990), pp. 599–607.

Austin, S.M., J.A. DiPietro, J.H. Foreman, G.J. Baker, and K.S. Todd. "Parascaris Equorum Infections in Horses." *Compendium on Continuing Education,* Vol. 12, No. 8 (August 1990), pp. 1110–1118.

Bain, F.T. "Hyperbaric Oxygen Therapy for Horses." *Journal of Equine Veterinary Science* (March 2003), Vol. 23, No.3, pp. 103–106.

Baker, D.J. "Rationale for the Use of Influenza Vaccines in Horses and the Importance of Antigenic Drift." *Equine Veterinary Journal,* Vol. 18, No. 2 (1986), pp. 93–96.

Balch, O.K., M.H. Ratzlaff, M.L. Hyde, and K.K. White. "Locomotor Effects of Hoof Angle and Mediolateral Balance of Horses Exercising on a High-Speed Treadmill: Preliminary Results." *Proceedings of the American Association of Equine Practitioners* (1991), pp. 687–705.

Banks, William J. *Applied Veterinary Histology.* Williams and Wilkins, Baltimore, 1981, pp. 245–261.

Barber, S.M. "Second Intention Wound Healing in the Horse: The Effect of Bandages and Topical Corticosteroids." *Proceedings of the American Association of Equine Practitioners* (1989), pp. 107–116.

Bareley P.L. " Studies with Equine Streptococci." *Aust.Vet. J.* 1942; 18: 189–194.

Baucus, K.L., S.L. Ralston, et al. "The Effect of Copper and Zinc Supplementation on Mineral Content of Mare's Milk." *Equine Veterinary Science,* Vol. 9, No. 4 (1989), pp. 206–209.

Baucus, K.L., E.L. Squires, S.L. Ralston, and A.0. McKinnon. "The Effect of Transportation Stress on Early Embryonic Death in Mares." *Proceedings of the Equine Nutrition and Physiology Symposium* (1987), pp. 657–662.

Baxter, G.M. "Equine Laminitis." *Equine Practice,* Vol. 14, No. 4 (April 1992), pp. 13–22.

Baxter, G.M. "Wound Healing and Delayed Wound Closure in the Lower Limb of the Horse." *Equine Practice,* Vol. 10, No. I (January 1988), pp. 23–31.

Bayly, W.M., H.D. Liggitt, L.J. Huston, and W.W. Laegreid. "Stress and Its Effect on Equine Pulmonary Mucosal Defenses." *Proceedings of the American Association of Equine Practitioners* (1986), pp. 253–262.

Beech, J. "Equine Muscle Disorders 2." *Equine Veterinary Education* (August 2000), pp. 281–286.

Beeman, M. "Conformation: The Relationship of Form to Function." *Quarter Horse Journal* Reprint.

Bennett, D. "Principles of Conformation Analysis." Selected Articles from *Equus* 117–177.

Bentz, B.G., Erkert, R.S., and Blaik, M.A. "Evaluation of Atrial Fibrillation in Horses." *Compendium of Continuing Education*, Vol. 24, No. 9 (Sept 2002), pp. 734–739.

Berry, D.B. 2nd, and Sullins, K.E. "Effects of Topical Application of Antimicrobials and Bandaging on Healing and Granulation Tissue Formation in Wounds of the Distal Aspect of the Limbs in Horses." *Am J Vet Res* 2003 Jan; 64(1): 88–92.

Bertone, J.J., J.L. Traub-Dargatz, R.W. Wrigley, D.G. Bennett, and R.J. Williams. "Diarrhea Associated With Sand in the Gastrointestinal Tract of Horses." *Journal of the American Veterinary Medical Association* (December 1988), Vol. 193, No. 11, pp. 1409–1412.

Blagburn, B.L., D.S. Lindsay, C.M. Hendrix, and J. Schumacher. "Pathogenesis, Treatment, and Control of Gastric Parasites in Horses." *Compendium Continuing Education,* Vol. 13, No. 5 (May 1991), pp. 850–857.

Boffi, F.M., Cittar, J., Balskus, G., Muriel, M., and Desmara, E. "Training-Induced Apoptosis in Skeletal Muscle." *Equine Vet J Supplement* 2002 September; (34): 276–8.

Booth, N.H. and L.E. McDonald, eds. *Veterinary Pharmacology and Therapeutics.* Fifth Edition. Iowa State University Press, Ames, 1982.

Bowker, R.M. "Contrasting Structural Morphologies of 'Good' and 'Bad' Footed Horses." *Proceedings of the American Association of Equine Practitioners* (2003), Vol. 49, pp. 180–209.

Bradley, R.E., T.J. Lane, R.F. Jochen, B.P. Seibert, and K.M. Newcomb, "Distribution and Frequency of Benzimidazole Resistance in Equine Small Strongyles." *Equine Practice,* Vol. 8, No. 2 (February 1986), pp. 7–11.

Brama, P.A., TeKoppele, J.M., Bank, R.A., Barneveld, A., and van Weeren, P.R.. "Development of Biochemical Heterogeneity of Articular Cartilage: Influences of Age and Exercise." *Equine Vet J* 2002 May; 34(3) : 265–9.

Bramlage, L. and Editorial Staff. "Surgical Repair of Bowed Tendons." *Thoroughbred Times* (February 1992), pp. 22–24.

Bramlage, L.R., N.W. Rantanen, R.L. Genovese, and L.E. Page. "Long-term Effects of Surgical Treatment of Superficial Flexor Tendinitis by Superior Check Desmototomy. " *Proceedings of the American Association of Equine Practitioners* (1988), pp. 655.

Bridges, C.H. and F.D. Harris. "Experimentally Induced Cartilaginous Fractures (Osteochondritis Dissecans) in Foals Fed Low-Copper Diets." *Journal of American Veterinary Medical Association,* Vol. 193, No. 2 (July 1988), pp. 215–221.

Brosnahan, M.M. and Paradis, M.R. "Assessment of Clinical Characteristics, Management Practices, and Activities of Geriatric Horses." *Journal of American Veterinary Medical Association,* Vol. 223, No. 1 (July 1, 2003), pp. 99–104.

Bryans, J.T. "Control of Equine Influenza." *Proceedings of the American Association of Equine Practitioners* (1980), pp. 279–285.

Buffa, E.A., et al. "Effect of Dietary Biotin Supplement on Equine Hoof Horn Growth Rate and Hardness." *Equine Veterinary Journal,* Vol. 24, No. 6 (1992), pp. 472–474.

Burch, G.E. "Transcutaneous Electrical Stimulation." *Equine Practice,* Vol. No. 9 (October 1985), pp. 6–11.

Byron, C.R., Orth, M.W., Venta, P.J., Lloyd, J.W., and Caron, J.P. "Influence of Glucosamine on Matrix Metalloproteinase Expression and Activity in Lipopolysaccharide-Stimulated Equine Chondrocytes." *Am J Vet Res.* 2003 Jun; 64 (6): 666–71.

Cantile, C., Del Piero, F., Di Guardo, G., and Arispici, M. "Pathologic and Immunohistochemical Findings in Naturally Occuring West Nile Virus Infection in Horses." *Vet Pathol* 2001 Jul; 38(4): 414–21.

Carleton, C.L. "Basic Techniques for Evaluating the Subfertile Mare." *Veterinary Medicine* (December 1988), pp. 1253–1261.

Carlson, G.P. "Medical Problems Associated With Protracted Heat and Work Stress in Horses." *Compendium on Continuing Education,* Vol. 7, No. 10 (October 1985), pp. 542–550.

Chanter, N., Newton, J.R., and Wood ,J.L.N. "Detection of Strangles Carriers." *Vet.Record* 1998; 142: 496.

Clabough, D. "Streptococcus Equi Infection in the Horse: A Review of Clinical and Immunological Considerations." *Equine Veterinary Science,* Vol. 7, No 5 (1987), pp. 279–283.

Clarke, A.F., T.M. Madelin, and R.G. Allpress. "The Relationship of Air Hygiene in Stables to Lower Airway Disease and Pharyngeal Lymphoid Hyperplasia in Two Groups of Thoroughbred Horses." *Equine Veterinary Journal,* Vol. 19, No. 6 (1987), pp. 524–530.

Clayton, H.M. "Comparison of the Stride of Trotting Horses Trimmed With Normal and a Broken-Back Hoof Axis." *Proceedings of the American Association of Equine Practitioners* (1988), pp. 289–298.

Clayton, H.M., et al. "Double-Blind Study of the Effects of an Oral Supplement Intended to Support Joint Health in Horses with Tarsal Degenerative Joint Disease." *Proceedings of the American Association of Equine Practitioners* (2002), Vol. 48, pp. 314–317.

Clayton, H.M. "Hock Motion." *Journal of Equine Veterinary Science* (August 2003), Vol. 23, No. 8, pp. 365–366.

Clayton, H.M. "Time-Motion Analysis in Equestrian Sports: The Grand Prix Dressage Test." *Proceedings of the American Association of Equine Practitioners* (1989), pp. 367–373.

Clayton, H.M. *Conditioning Sport Horses.* Sport Horse Publications, Saskatoon, Saskatchewan, Canada, 1991.

Coffman, J.R. "Muscle Fibers: Coupling and Contraction and Energy Metabolism." *Equine Sportsmedicine,* Vol. 3, No. 2 (1984), pp.1–3.

Coffman, J.R. "Stress and the Racehorse." *Equine Sportmedicine,* Vol. 3, No (1984), pp. 1, 7–8.

Colles, C.M. "A Technique for Assessing Hoof Function in the Horse." *Equine Veterinaty Journal,* Vol. 21, No. 1 (1989), pp. 17–22.

Colles, C.M. "The Relationship of Frog Pressure to Heel Expansion." *Equine Veterinary Journal,* Vol. 21, No. 1 (1989), pp. 13–16.

Collier, M., et al. "Electrostimulation of Bone Production in the Horse." *Proceedings of the American Association of Equine Practitioners* (1981), pp. 71–89.

Collins, L.G., and D.E. Tyler. "Phenylbutazone Toxicosis in the Horse: A Clinical Study." *Journal of the American Veterinary Medical Association,* Vol. 184, No. 6 (March 1984), pp. 699–703.

Colquhoun, K.M., et al. "Control of Breeding in the Mare." *Equine Veterinary Journal,* Vol. 19, No. 2 (1987), pp. 138–142.

Comben, N., Clark, R.J., and Sutherland, D.J. "Clinical Observations on the Response of Equine Hoof Defects to Dietary Supplementation with Biotin." *Vet Record* 1984 Dec 22–29; 115 (25–26): 642–645.

Cook, W.R. "Diagnosis and Grading of Hereditary Recurrent Laryngeal Neuropathy in the Horse." *Equine Veterinary Science,* Vol. 8, No. 6 (1988), pp. 431–455.

Cook, W.R. "Recent Observations on Recurrent Laryngeal Neuropathy in the Horse: Applications to Practice." *Proceedings of the American Association of Equine Practitioners* (1988), pp. 427–478.

Cook, W.R. "Some Observations on Form and Function of the Equine Upper Airway in Health and Disease: 1. The Pharynx." *Proceedings of the American Association of Equine Practitioners* (1981), pp. 355–391.

Cook, W.R. "Some Observations on Form and Function of the Equine Upper Airway in Health and Disease: 2. The Larynx." *Proceedings of the American Association of Equine Practitioners* (1981), pp. 393–451.

Cook, W.R. *Specifications for Speed in the Racehorse: The Airflow Factors.* The Russell Meerdink Company, Ltd., 1993.

Cook, W.R., et al. "Upper Air-way Obstruction (Possible Asphyxia) as the Possible Cause of Exercise-Induced Pulmonary Hemorrhage in the Horse: An Hypothesis." *Equine Veterinary Science,* Vol. 8, No. 1 (1988), pp. 11–26.

Cox, J.H. and R.M. DeBowes. "Colic-like Discomfort Associated With Ovulation in Two Mares." *Journal of the American Veterinary Medical Association,* Vol. 191, No. I I (December 1987), pp. 1451–1452.

Cox, J.H. and R.M. DeBowes. "Episodic Weakness Caused by Hyperkalemic Periodic Paralysis in Horses." *Compendium on Continuing Education,* Vol. 12, No. 1 (January 1990), pp. 83–88.

Crabill M.R., Honnas C.M., Taylor D.S., Schumacher J., Watkins J.P., Snyder J.R. Stringhalt Secondary to Trauma to the Dorsoproximal Region of the Metatarsus in Horses: 10 cases (1986-1991). *J Am Vet Med Assoc* 1994 Sept 15; 205 (6): 867–9.

Crawford, W.H., R. Vanderby, Jr., et al. "The Energy Absorption Capacity of Equine Support Bandages. " V C. 0. T., Vol. 1 (1990), pp. 2–9.

Crowe, O., Dyson, S.J., Wright, I.M., Schramme, M.C., Smith, R.W. "Treatment of 45 Cases of Chronic Hindlimb Proximal Suspensory Desmitis by Radial Extracorporeal Shockwave Therapy." *Proceedings of the American Association of Equine Practitioners* (2002), Vol. 48, pp. 322–325.

Crowell-Davis, S., W. Crowell-Davis, and A. Caudle. "Preventing Trailering Problems: Part II." *Equine Practice,* Vol. 9, No. I (January 1987), pp. 32–33.

Currey, J.D. "The Mechanical Consequences of Variations in the Mineral Content of Bone." *Journal of Biomechanics,* Vol. 2 (1969A), pp. 2–11.

Currey, J.D. "The Relationship Between Stiffness and the Mineral Content of Bone." *Journal of Biomechanics,* Vol. 2 (1969B), pp. 477–480.

Custalow, B. "Protein Requirements During Exercise in the Horse." *Equine Veterinary Science,* Vol. 11, No. 1 (1991), pp. 65–66.

Cymbaluk, N. "Water Balance of Horses Fed Various Diets. " *Equine Practice,* Vol. 11, No. 1 (1989), pp. 19–24.

Daft, B.M., Barr, B.C., Gardner, I.A., Read, D., Bell, W., Peyser, K.G., Ardans, A., Kinde, H., and Morrow, J.K. "Sensitivity and Specificity of Western Blot Testing of Cerebrospinal Fluid and Serum for Diagnosis of Equine Protozoal Myeloencephalitis in Horses With and Without Neurologic Abnormalities." *J Am Vet Med Assoc* 2002 Oct 1; 221 (7): 1007–13.

Davis, M.S., Lockard, A.J., Marlin, D.J., Freed, A.N. "Airway Cooling and Mucosal Injury During Cold Weather Exercise." *Equine Vet J Supplement* 2002 September; (34): 413–6.

Deeg, C.A., Ehrenhofer, M., Thurau, S.R., Reese, S., Wildner, G., Kaspers, B. "Immunopathology of Recurrent Uveitis in Spontaneously Diseased Horses." *Exp Eye Res* 2002 Aug; 75 (2): 127–33.

Del Piero, F., Wilkins, P.A., Dubovi, E.J., Biolatti, B., and Cantile, C. "Clinical, Pathologic, Immunohistochemical, and Virologic Findings of Eastern Equine Encephalomyelitis in Two Horses." *Vet Pathol* 2001 Jul; 38 (4): 451–6.

Denoix, J.M., Thibaud, D., and Riccio, B. "Tiludronate as a New Therapeutic Agent in the Treatment of Navicular Disease: A Double-Blind Placebo-Controlled Clinical Trial." *Equine Vet J.* 2003 June; 35 (4): 407–13.

Derksen, F.J., et al. "Chronic Obstructive Pulmonary Disease Roundtable Discussion." *Equine Practice,* Vol. 13, No. 5 (May 199 1), pp. 25–28. *Equine Practice,* Vol. 13, No. 7 (July/August 1991), pp. 15–19.

Derksen, F.J. "Physiology of Airflow in the Athletic Horse." *Proceedings of the American Association of Equine Practitioners* (1988), pp. 149–158.

DiPietro, J.A. and K.S. Todd. "Anthelmintics Used in Treatment of Parasitic Infections of Horses." *Equine Practice,* Vol. 11, No. 4 (April 1989), pp. 5–15.

DiPietro, J.A., T.R. Klei, and D.D. French. "Contemporary Topics in Equine Parasitology." *Compendium on Continuing Education,* Vol. 12, No. 5 (May 1990), pp. 713–720.

Divers, T.J. and D. Dreyfuss. "Evaluating the Horse With a Poor Racing Performance." *Veterinary Medicine* (May 1990), pp. 522, 529.

Divers, T.J., de Lahunta, A., Hintz, H.F., et al. "Equine Motor Neuron Disease." *Equine Veterinary Education* (April 2001), pp. 89–93.

Divers, T.J. et al. "Equine Motor Neuron Disease in 17 Horses (1990-1992). *Proceedings of the American Association of Equine Practitioners* (1992), pp. 553–554.

Divers, T.J. et al. "Equine Motor Neuron Disease: A Review of Clinical and Experimental Studies." *Proceedings of the American Association of Equine Practitioners* (2003), pp. 230–232.

Drudge, J.H. and E.T. Lyons. *Internal Parasites of Equids With Emphasis on Treatment and Control.* Hoechst-Roussel Agri-Vet Company, 1986.

Drudge, J.H. and E.T. Lyons. *Internal Parasites of Equids With Emphasis on Treatment and Control, Revised 1989.* Hoechst-Roussel Agri-Vet Company.

Drudge, J.H., E.T. Lyons, and S.C. Tolliver. "Strongyles–An Update." *Equine Practice*, Vol. 11, No. 4 (April 1989), pp. 43–49.

Duren, S., C. Wood, and S. Jackson. "Dietary Fat and the Racehorse." *Equine Veterinary Science*, Vol. 7, No. 6 (1987), pp. 396–397.

Dwyer, Roberta M. "The Practical Diagnosis and Treatment of Metabolic Conditions in Endurance Horses." *Equine Practice, Vol. 8*, No. 8 (September 1986), pp. 21–33.

Dyer, Robert M. "The Bovine Respiratory Disease Complex: A Complex Interaction of Host, Environmental, and Infectious Factors." *Compendium on Continuing Education, Vol.* 4, No. 7 (July 1982), pp. 296–307.

Dyson, S., and Murray, R. "Pain Associated With the Sacroiliac Joint Region: A Clinical Study of 74 Horses." *Equine Vet J* 2003 May; 35 (3): 240–5.

Editorial Staff. *Dynamics of Equine Athletic Performance. Proceedings of the Association of Equine Sports Medicine* (1985), Veterinary Learning Systems Co., Inc.

Editorial Staff. "Conformation." *Practical Horseman* (May 1992), pp. 54–60, 90–91.

Editorial Staff. "Round Table on Interval Training." *Thoroughbred Times* (February 1992), pp. 14–21.

Editorial Staff. *Proceedings of a Roundtable on Equine Influenza* (December 1987), Coopers Animal Health, Inc.

Editorial Staff. "Hyperkalemic Periodic Paralysis Presents Medical and Ethical Challenge." *Journal of the American Veterinary Medical Association*, Vol. 202, No. 8 (April 1993), pp. 1203–1209.

Edwards, Gladys Brown. *Anatomy and Conformation of the Horse.* Dreenan Press, Ltd., Croton-on-Hudson, New York, 1980.

England, J.J. "Veterinary Virology, Part II: Pathogenesis of Viral Infections." *Compendium on Continuing Education*, Vol. 6, No. 2 (February 1984), pp. 145–154.

Equine Respiratory Medicine and Surgery. *Equine Veterinary Journal*, Vol. 19 (September/ October 1987), No. 5.

Erickson, B.K., Erickson, H.H., and Coffman, J.R. "Exercise-Induced Pulmonary Hemorrhage During High Intensity Exercise: Potential Causes and the Role of Furosemide." *Proceedings of the American Association of Equine Practitioners* (1989), pp. 375–379.

Erickson H.H. A Review of Exercise-Induced Pulmonary Hemorrhage and New Concepts for Prevention. *Proceedings of the American Association of Equine Practitioners* (2000), Vol. 46, pp. 193–196.

Essen-Gustavsson, B., D. McMiken, et al]. "Muscular Adaptation of Horses During Intensive Training and Detraining." *Equine Veterinary Journal*, Vol. 21, No. 1 (1989), pp. 27–33.

Ewert, K.M., J.A. DiPietro, J.H. Foreman, and K.S. Todd. "Control Programs for Endoparasites in Horses." *Compendium on Continuing Education*, Vol. 13, No. 6 (June 1991), pp. 1012–1018.

Fadok, V.A. and P.C. Mullowney. "Dermatologic Diseases of Horses, Part 1: Parasitic Dermatoses of the Horse." *Compendium on Continuing Education*, Vol. 5, No. 11 (November 1983), pp. 615–622.

Feige, K., Furst, A., Kaser-Hotz, B., and Ossent, P. "Traumatic Injury to the Central Nervous System in Horses: Occurrence, Diagnosis, and Outcome." *Equine Veterinary Education* (August 2000), pp. 275–280.

Firshman, A.M, Valberg, S.J., Bender, J.B., and Finno, C.J. "Epidemiologic Characteristics and Management of Polysaccharide Storage Myopathy in Quarter Horses." *Am J Vet Res* 2003 Oct; 64(10): 1319–1327.

Fitzgerald, B. "Insulin Resistance and Inflammatory Challenges." *Equine Disease Quarterly* Jan 2004, vol 13, No. 1, pp. 3–4.

Foil, L.D. and C.S. Foil. "Arthropod Pests of Horses." *Compendium on Continuing Education*, Vol. 12, No. 5 (May 1990), pp. 723–730.

Foil, L.D. and C.S. Foil. "Dipteran Parasites of Horses." *Equine Practice,* Vol. 10, No. 4 (April 1988), pp. 21–38.

Foil, L.D., et al. "The Role of Horn Fly Feeding and the Management of Seasonal Equine Ventral Midline Dermatitis." *Equine Practice*, Vol. 12, No. 5 (May 1990), pp. 6–14.

Folsom, R.W., Littlefield-Chabaud, M.A., French, D.D., Pourciau, S.S., Mistric, L., and Horohov, D.W. "Exercise Alters the Immune Response to Equine Influenza Virus and Increases Susceptibility to Infection." *Equine Vet J* 2001 Nov; 33 (7): 664–9.

Fox, S.F. "Management of Thermal Burns-Part I." *Compendium on Continuing Education*, Vol. 7, No. 8 (August 1985), pp. 631–639.

Fox, S.F. "Management of Thermal Burns-Part 2." *Compendium on Continuing Education*, Vol. 8, No. 7 (July 1986), pp. 439–444.

Franklin, S.H., Naylor, J.R., and Lane, J.G. "Effect of dorsal displacement of the soft palate on ventilation and airflow during high-intensity exercise." *Equine Vet J Supplement* 2002 September; (34): 379–83.

Franklin, S.H., Naylor, J.R., and Lane, J.G. "The Effect of a Tongue-Tie in Horses with Dorsal Displacement of the Soft Palate." *Equine Vet J Supplement* 2002 September; 34): 430–3.

Frape, D.L. "Dietary Requirements and Athletic Performance of Horses." *Equine Veterinary Journal*, Vol. 20, No. 3 (1988), pp. 163–172.

Frazier, C. "Cardiac Recovery Index." *AERC Endurance News* (September 1992), pp. 4–6.

Frazier, D. "Equine Dietary Adaptation: Cardiac Recovery Index." *AERC Endurance News* (November 1992), pp. 10–15.

Fredriksson, G., H. Kindahl, and G. Stabenfeldt. "Endotoxin-Induced and Prostaglandin-Mediated Effects on Corpus Luteum Function in the Mare." *Theriogenology*, Vol. 25 (1986), pp. 309–316.

Freestone, J.F. and Carlson, G.P. "Muscle Disorders in the Horse: A Retrospective Study." *Equine Veterinary Journal*, Vol. 23, No. 2 (1991), pp. 86–90.

French, D.D. and Chapman, M.R. "Tapeworms of the Equine Gastrointestinal Tract." *Compendium on Continuing Education*, Vol. 14, No. 5 (May 1992), pp. 655–661.

French, D.D., Klei, T.R., and Hackett, G.E. "Equine Parasites: Dollars and Sense." *Equine Practice*, Vol. 10, No. 5 (May 1988), pp. 8–14.

Fricker C., Riek, W., and Hugelshofter, J. "A Model for Pathogenesis of Navicular Disease." *Equine Veterinary Journal*, Vol. 14 (1982), pp. 203–207.

Gach, J. "Trailer Studies Reveal Fewer Harmful Effects Than Expected." *Equus* 120 (1987), pp. 12–16.

Galey, F.D., Whiteley, H.E., Goetz, T.E., Kuenstler, A.R., Davis, C.A., and Beasley, V.R. "Black Walnut (Juglans Nigra) Toxicosis: A Model for Equine Laminitis." J Comp Pathology 1991; 104; 313–326.

Genetzky, R.M. "Chronic Obstructive Pulmonary Disease In Horses–Part 1 " *Compendium on Continuing Education*, Vol. 7, No. 7 (July 1985), pp. 407–414.

Gentry, L.R., Thompson, D.L., Fernandez, J.M., Smith, L.A., Horohov, D.W., and Leise, B.S. "Effects of Chromium Tripicolinate Supplementation on Plasma Hormone and Metabolite Concentrations and Immune Function in Adult Mares." *Journal of Equine Veterinary Science* 1999; 4: 259–265.

Geor, R.J., Ommundson, L., Fenton, G., and Pagan, J.D. "Effects of an External Nasal Strip and Furosemide on Pulmonary Haemorrhage in Thoroughbreds Following High-Intensity Exercise." Equine Vet J 2001 Nov; 33(6): 577–84.

Gerring, E.L. "All Wind and Water: Some Progress in the Study of Equine Gut Motility." *Equine Veterinary Journal*, Vol. 23, No. 2 (1991), pp. 81–85.

Getty, Robert, ed. *Sisson and Grossman's The Anatomy of the Domestic Animals.* Volume 1. WB Saunders Company, 1975.

Geyer, H. and Schulze, J. "The Long-Term Influence of Biotin Supplementation on Hoof Horn Quality in Horses." *Schweiz Arch Tierheilkd* 1994: 136 (4): 137–149.

Gibson, K.T. and Steel, C.M. "Conditions of the Suspensory Ligament Causing Lameness in Horses." *Equine Veterinary Education*, February 2001, pp. 50–64.

Gillespie, J.R. and Robinson, N.E., eds. *Equine Exercise Physiology 2*. ICEEP Publications, Davis, California, 1987.

Gillis, C. and Meagher, D. "Tendon Response to Training." *The Equine Athlete*, Vol. 4, No. 5 (September/ October 1991), pp. 26–27.

Ginther, O.J. *Reproductive Biology of the Mare.* McNaughton and Gunn, Inc., Ann Arbor, Michigan, 1979.

Glade, M.J. "Feeding Innovations for the Performance Horse." *Equine Veterinary Science*, Vol. 4, No. 4, pp. 165–166.

Gluck Equine Research and Service Report. "Mare Reproductive Loss Syndrome Update." Spring 2003, Vol. XVII, No. 1.

Goehring, L.S. and Oosterbaan, M.M. "The Mystery of Equine Herpes Myeloencephalopathy." *Equine Veterinary Education* (February 2001), pp. 53–59.

Goetz, T.E., Boulton, C.H., and Ogilvie, G.K. "Clinical Management of Progressive Multifocal Benign and Malignant Melanomas of Horses With Oral Cimetidine." *Proceedings of the American Association of Equine Practitioners* (1989), pp. 431–438.

Goetz T.E., Ogilvie, G.K., et al. "Cimetidine for Treatment of Melanomas in Three Horses." *Journal of the American Veterinary Medical Association*, Vol. 196, No. 3 (February 1990), pp. 449–452.

Goodman, N., et al. "An Equine Roundtable Discussion on Lameness." *Equine Practice, Vol.* 12, No. 8 (September 1990), pp. 28–33.

Goodrich, L.R., Moll, H.D., Crisman, M.V., Lessard, P., and Bigbie, R. " Effects of Equine Amnion on the Pinch Grafts of the Distal Limbs of Ponies. " *Am J Vet Res*, 61:326–29, 2000.

Gorham, S. and M. Robl. "Melanoma in the Gray Horse: The Darker Side of Equine Aging." *Veterinary Medicine* (May 1986), pp. 446–448.

Grant, B.D., L.J. Smith, et al. "Hill Training for High-Speed Performance Horses." *The Equine Athlete*, Vol. 1, No. I (December 1988), pp. 6–7, 15–16.

Graves M, Rashmir-Raven, A.M., and Black, S.S. "Clinical Snapshot, Ehlers-Danlos like syndrome in a Quarter Horse Gelding." *Compend Contin Educ Pract Vet* (2001) vol 23 (9) pp. 827–837.

Green, E., et al. "Endotoxemia Roundtable Discussion." *Equine Practice, Vol.* 14, No. 9 (October 1992), pp. 7–12. *Equine Practice, Vol.* 14, No. 10 (November/December 1992), pp. 13–18. *Equine Practice, Vol.* 15, No. I (January 1993), pp. 7–14.

Griffiths, I.R. "The Pathogenesis of Equine Laryngeal Hemiplegia." *Equine Veterinaty Journal, Vol.* 23, No. 2 (1991), pp. 75–76.

Hackett, G.E., Uhlinger, C., Mitchell, R., McCashin, F.B., and Conboy, S. "Continuous Deworming Programs: Roundtable Discussion." *Equine Practice, Vol.* 14, No. 7 (July/August 1992), pp. 13–18. *Equine Practice*, Vol. 14, No. 8 (September 1992), pp. 27–33.

Hahn, C.N. "Horner's Syndrome in Horses." *Equine Veterinary Education* (April 2003), pp. 111–117.

Halldordsottir, S. and Larsen, H.J. "An Epidemiological Study of Summer Eczema in Icelandic Horses in Nor-way." *Equine Veterinary Journal*, Vol. 23, No. 4 (1991), pp. 296–299.

Hamlen, H.J., Timoney, J.F., and Bell, R.J. "Epidemiologic and Immunologic Characteristics of *Streptococcus Equi* Infection in Foals." *Journal of American Veterinary Medical Association* 1994; 204 (5): 768–775.

Hamm, D. and E.W. Jones. "Intra-Articular and Intramuscular Treatment of Noninfectious Equine Arthritis (DJD) With Polysulfated Glycosaminoglycan (PSGAG)." Equine *Veterinary Science*, Vol. 8, No. 6 (1988), pp. 456–459.

Harkins, J.D. and S.G. Kamerling. "A Comparative Study of Interval and Conventional Training Methods in Thoroughbred Racehorses." *Equine Veterinary Science* (January/February 1990), pp. 45–51.

Harkins, J.D. and S.G. Kamerling. "Effects of Induced Alkalosis on Performance in Thoroughbreds During a 1600 Meter Race." *Equine Veterinary Journal*, Vol. 24, No. 2 (1992), pp. 94–98.

Harman, J. "Acupuncture for Horses." *AERC Endurance News* (August 1991), pp. 8–9.

Harman, A.M. Moore, S., Hoskins, R., and Keller, P. "Horse Vision and an Explanation for the Visual Behaviour Originally Explained by the 'Ramp Retina'." *Equine Veterinary Journal* 1999, Vol. 31, No. 5, pg. 384.

Harper, Frederick. "Control of the Broodmare's Reproductive Cycle." *Equine Veterinary Science*, Vol. 9, No. 2 (1989), pp. 112–115.

Harris, P. and D.H. Snow. "Plasma Potassium and Lactate Concentrations in Thoroughbred Horses During Exercise of Varying Intensity." *Equine Veterinaty Journal*, Vol. 23, No. 3 (1992), pp. 220–225.

Hassel, D.M., Schiffman, P.S., and Snyder, J.R. "Petrographic and Geochemic Evaluation of Equine Enteroliths." *Am J Vet Research* 2001 Mar; 62 (3): 350–358.

Hart, C. "Equine Conformation of the Top Endurance Athlete." *AERC Endurance News* (August 1990), pp. 10–11.

Hassel, D.M. "Enterolithiasis." *Clinical Techniques in Equine Practice*, Vo. 1, No. 3 (September 2002), pp. 143–147.

Hayes, Horace M. *Points of the Horse.* Arco Publishing Company, Inc., New York, 1969.

Haynes, P. "Obstructive Disease of the Upper Respiratory Tract: Current Thoughts on Diagnosis and Surgical Management." *Proceedings of the American Association of Equine Practitioners* (1986), pp. 283–290.

Helge, J.W., Watt, P.W., Richter, E.A., Rennie, M.J., and Kiens, B. "Fat utilization During Exercise: Adaptation to a Fat-Rich Diet Increases Utilization of Plasma Fatty Acids and Very Low Density Lipoprotein-Triacylglycerol in Humans." *J Physiol* 2001 Dec 15; 537 (Pt 3): 1009–20.

Henneke, D.R. "A Condition Score System for Horses." *Equine Practice, Vol.* 7, No. 8 (September 1985), pp. 13–15.

Herd, R.P. "Epidemiology and Control of Equine Strongylosis at Newmarket." *Equine Veterinary Journal*, Vol. 18, No. 6 (1986), pp. 447–452.

Herd, R.P. and A.A. Gabel, "Reduced Efficacy of Anthelmintics in Young Compared With Adult Horses." *Equine Veterinary Journal*, Vol. 22, No. 3 (1990), pp. 164–169.

Hickman, J. "Navicular Disease-What Are We Talking About?" *Equine Veterinary Journal*, Vol. 21, No. 6 (1989), pp. 395–398.

Hinchcliff, K.W., Lauderdale, M.A., Dutson, J., Geor, R.J., Lacombe, V.A., and Taylor, L.E. "High Intensity Exercise Conditioning Increases Accumulated Oxygen Deficit of Horses." *Equine Vet J* 2002 Jan; 34 (1): 9–16.

Hines, M.T., Schott, H.C., and Byrne, B.A. "Adult-Onset Narcolepsy in the Horse. *Proceedings of the American Association of Equine Practitioners* (1992), pp. 289–296.

Hintz, H.F. "Factors Which influence Developmental Orthopedic Disease." *Proceedings of the American Association of Equine Practitioners* (1988), pp. 159–162.

Hintz, H.F., et al. "Effects of Protein Levels on Endurance Horses." *Journal of Animal Science,* Vol. 51 (1980), p. 202.

Hintz, H.F. "Biotin." *Equine Practice,* Vol. 9, No. 9 (October 1987), pp. 4–5.

Hintz, H.F. "Effect of Diet on Copper Content of Milk. " *Equine Practice,* Vol. 9, No. 8 (1987), pp. 6–7.

Hintz, H.F. "Protein Needs of the Equine Athlete." *Equine Practice*, Vol. 8, No. 6 (1988), pp. 5–6.

Hintz, H.F. "Some Myths About Equine Nutrition." *Compendium on Continuing Education*, Vol. 12, No. 1 (1990), pp. 78–81.

Hintz, H.F. "The 1989 NRC Estimates of Protein Requirements." *Equine Practice*, Vol. 11, No. 10 (1989), pp. 5–6.

Hintz, H.F. "Weighing Horses." *Equine Practice*, Vol. 10, No. 8 (1988), pp. 10–11.

Hodgson, D.R. "Exertional Rhabdomyolysis." *Current Veterinary Therapy 2*, WB Saunders Co., Philadelphia, 1987, pp. 487–490.

Hodgson, D.R. "Myopathies in the Athletic Horse." *Compendium on Continuing Education*, Vol. 7, No. 10 (October 1985), pp. 551–556.

Holcombe, S., et al. "Effect of Commercially Available Nasal Strips on Airway Resistance in Exercising Horses." AJVR 2002; 63: 1101–1105.

Hommas, C.M., J. Schumacher, and P.W. Dean. "Laryngeal Hemiplegia in Horses: Diagnosis and Surgical Management." *Veterinary Medicine* (October 1985), pp. 752–763.

Houpt, K.A. "Thirst in Horses: The Physiological and Psychological Causes." *Equine Practice*, Vol. 9, No. 6 (June 1987), pp. 28–30.

Houston, C.S. *Going Higher. The Story of Man and Altitude*. Little, Brown, and Company, Boston, 1987.

Huddleston, A.L., P. Rockwell, D.N. Kulund, and R.B. Harrison. "Bone Mass in Life-Time Tennis Athletes." *Journal of the American Medical Association*, Vol. 244 (1980), pp. 1107–1109.

Hudson, J.M., Cohen, N.D., Gibbs, P.G., and Thompson JA. "Feeding Practices Associated With Colic in Horses." *J Am Vet Med Assoc* 2001 Nov 15; 219(10): 1419–25.

Hurtig, M.B., S.L. Green, H. Dobson, and J. Burton. "Defective Bone and Cartilage in Foals Fed a Low Copper Diet." *Proceedings of the American Association of Equine Practitioners* (1990), pp. 637–643.

Hustead, D. "Vaccines: What's Ahead?" *Large Animal Veterinarian* (March/April 1990), pp. 8–11, 36–37.

Ivers, T. "Osteochondrosis: Undernutrition or Overnutrition?" *Equine Practice*, Vol. 8, No. 8 (September 1986), pp. 15–19.

Ivers, T. "Cryotherapy: An In-Depth Study." *Equine Practice*, Vol. 9, No. 2 (February 1987), pp. 17–19.

Jeffcott, L.B. "Conditions Causing Thoracolumbar Pain and Dysfunction in Horses." *Proceedings of the American Association of Equine Practitioners* (1985), pp. 285–296.

Jeffcott, L.B. "Examination of a Horse with a Potential Back Problem." *Proceedings of the American Association of Equine Practitioners* (1985), pp. 271–284.

Jeffcott, L.B. "Osteochondrosis in the Horse-Searching for the Key to Pathogenesis." *Equine Veterinary Journal* (1991), Vol. 23, No. 5, pp. 331–338.

Jeffcott, L.G., and Clarke, A.F., eds. *Thermoregulatory Responses During Competitive Exercise in the Performance Horse*, Vols. I and II. *Equine Veterinary Journal Supplement 22*, July 1996.

Jeffcott, L.B. and Galin G. "The Sacroiliac Joint of the Horse and Chronic Changes Associated with Poor Competitive Performance." *Proceedings of the American Association of Equine Practitioners* (1985), pp. 335–351.

Jennings, S., T.N. Meacham, and AX Huff. "Management of the Brood Mare." *Equine Practice*, Vol. 9, No. 1 (January 1987), pp. 28–31.

Johnson, P.J. and Kellam, L.L "The Vestibular System. Part II:Differential Diagnosis." *Equine Veterinary Education* (June 2001), pp. 185–194.

Jones, W.E. "Muscular Causes of Exercise Intolerance." *Equine Veterinary Science* (1987), Vol. 7, No. 5, pp. 312–316.

Jones, W.E. *Equine Sports Medicine*. Lea and Febiger, Philadelphia, 1989.

Jones, W.E. *Sports Medicine for the Racehorse*. Second Edition. Veterinary Data, Wildomar, California, 1992.

Jones, W.E., ed. *Nutrition for the Equine Athlete*. Equine Sportsmedicine News, Wildomar, California, 1989.

Jorm L.R. Strangles in horse studs: Incidence, risk factors and effect on vaccination. Aust Vet J 1990: 67: 436–439.

Josseck, H., Zenker, W., and Geyer, H. "Hoof Horn Abnormalities in Lipizzaner Horses and the Effect of Dietary Biotin on Macroscopic Aspects of Hoof Horn Quality." *Equine Vet Journal* 1995 May, 27 (3): 174–182.

Kaneene, J.B., Miller, R., Ross, W.A., Gallagher, K., Marteniuk, J., and Rook, J. "Risk factors for colic in the Michigan (USA) Equine Population." *Prev Vet Med* 1997 Apr: 30 (1): 23–36.

Kempson, S.A. "Scanning Electron Microscope Observations of Hoof Horn from Horses with Brittle Feet. *Vet Record* 1987 Jun 13: 120 (24): 568–570.

Kiley-Worthington, M. "The Behavior of Horses in Relation to Management and Training-Towards Ethologically Sound Environments." *Equine Veterinary Science*, Vol. 10, No. 1 (1990), pp. 62–71.

Kindig, C. et al. "Efficacy of Nasal Strips and Furosemide in Mitigating EIPH in Thoroughbreds" *J. Appl Physiol* 91:1396–1400, 2001.

King, J.N. and E.L. Gerring. "The Action of Low Dose Endotoxin on Equine Bowel Motility." *Equine Veterinaty Journal,* Vol. 23, No. 1 (1991), pp. 11–17.

Knight, D.A., A.A. Gabel, et al. "Correlation of Dietary Mineral to Incidence and Severity of Metabolic Bone Disease in Ohio and Kentucky." *Proceedings of the American Association of Equine Practitioners* (1985), pp. 445–461.

Knight, D.A., A.A. Gabel, et al. "The Effects of Copper Supplementation on the Prevalence of Cartilage Lesions in Foals." *Equine Veterinary Journal,* Vol. 22, No. 6 (1990), pp. 426–432.

Knight, D.A., S.E. Weisbrode, L.M. Schmall, and A.A. Gabel. "Copper Supplementation and Cartilage Lesions in Foals." *Proceedings of the American Association of Equine Practitioners* (1988), pp. 191–194.

Kohnke, J. "Liquid Vitamin Supplements." *Equine Practice,* Vol. 8, No. 10 (1986), pp. 7–9.

Kohn C.W. and Fenner, W.R. "Equine Herpes Myeloencephalopathy." *Vet Clinics of North America: Equine Practice,* Vol 3:2 August 1987, pp. 405–419.

Kopp, K. "Do Horses Bend?" *Equus* 115, pp. 31–38, 110.

Koterba, A. and G.P. Carlson. "Acid-Base and Electrolyte Alterations in Horses With Exertional Rhabdomyolysis. *"Journal of the American Veterinary Medical Association,* Vol. 180, No. 3 (February 1982), pp. 303–306.

Kronfeld, D.S. "Equine Syndrome X, the Metabolic Disease, and Equine Grain-Associated Disorders: Nomenclature and Dietetics." Journal of Equine Veterinary Science (December 2003), Vol. 23, No. 12, pp. 567–569.

Kronfeld, D.S. "Symposium Sheds New Light on Equine Ventilatory Adaptations, Muscle Glycogen." *DVM Magazine* (September 1989), pp. 12,14.

Kronfeld, D.S. and S. Donoghue. "Metabolic Convergence in Developmental Orthopedic Disease." *Proceedings of the American Association of Equine Practitioners* (1988), pp. 195–202.

Kurcz, E.V., L.M. Lawrence, K.W. Kelley, and P.A. Miller. "The Effect of Intense Exercise on the Cell-Mediated Immune Response of Horses." *Equine Veterinary Science,* Vol. 8, No. 3 (1988), pp. 237–239.

Laegreid, W.W., L.J. Huston, R.J. Basaraba, and M.V. Crisman. "The Effects of Stress on Alveolar Macrophage Function in the Horse: An Overview." *Equine Practice,* Vol. 10, No. 9 (1988), pp. 9–16.

Landeau, L.J., D.J. Barrett, and S.C. Batterman. "Mechanical Properties of Equine Hooves." *American Journal of Veterinary Research,* 44 (January 1983), p. 100.

Lawrence, L.M., K.D. Bump, and D.G. McLaren. "Aerial Ammonia Levels in Horse Stalls." *Equine Practice,* Vol. 10, No. 10 (November/ December 1988), pp. 20–23.

Leadon, D.P., C. Frank, and W. Backhouse. "A Preliminary Report on Studies on Equine Transit Stress." *Equine Veterinary Science,* Vol. 9, No. 4 (1989), pp. 200–201.

Leadon, D.P. "A Summary of a Preliminary Report of an Investigation of Transit Stress in the Horse." *AESM Quarterly,* Vol. 3, No. 2 (1988), pp. 19–20.

Leadon, D.P., et al. "Environmental, Hematological and Blood Biochemical Changes in Equine Transit Stress." *Proceedings of the American Association of Equine Practitioners* (1990), pp. 485–490.

Lee, A.H., S.F. Swaim. "Granulation Tissue: How to Take Advantage of It in Management of Open Wounds." *Compendium on Continuing Education,* Vol. 10, No. 2 (February 1988), pp. 163–170.

Lee, A.H., S.F. Swaim, et al]. "Effects of Nonadherent Dressing Materials on the Healing of Open Wounds in Dogs." *Journal of the American Veterinary Medical Association,* Vol. 190, No. 4 (February 1987), pp. 416–422.

Lee, S. and C.L. Davidson. "The Role of Collagen in the Elastic Properties of Calcified Tissues." *Journal of Biomechanics*, Vol. 10 (1977), pp. 473–486.

Lees, M.J., P.B. Fretz, and K.A. Jacobs. "Factors Influencing Wound Healing: Lessons From Military Wound Management." *Compendium on Continuing Education,* Vol. 11, No. 7 (July 1989), pp. 850–855.

Lees, M.J., P.B. Fretz, J.V. Bailey, and K.A. Jacobs. "Second Intention Wound Healing." *Compendium on Continuing Education,* Vol. 11, No. 7 (July 1989), pp. 857–864.

Lekeux P, Art T. The respiratory system: anatomy, physiology, and adaptations to exercise and training. In: Hodgson DJ, Rose RJ, eds. *The Athletic Horse: Principles and Practice of Equine Sports Medicine.* Philadelphia: WB Saunders Co., 1994; 78–127.

Lentz L.R., Valberg S.J., Herold L.V., Onan G.W., Mickelson J.R., Gallant E.M. "Myoplasmic calcium regulation in myotubes from horses with recurrent exertional rhabdomyolysis." *Am J Vet Res* 2002 Dec; 63(12): 1724–31

Lerner, D.J. and McCracken, M.D. "Hyperelastosis Cutis in 2 Horses." *J of Equine Med and Surg*, 1978 (July/Aug) 2:350–352.

Liu, I.K.M. "Update on Respiratory Vaccines in the Horse." *Proceedings of the American Association of Equine Practitioners* (1986), pp. 277–282.

Lopez-Rivero, J.L., et al. "Comparative Study of Muscle Fiber Type Composition in the Middle Gluteal Muscle of Andalusian, Thoroughbred, and Arabian Horses." *Equine Sportsmedicine* (November/December 1989), pp. 337–340.

Lopez-Rivero, J.L., A.M. Diz, E. Aguera, and A.L. Serrano. "Endurance Training in Andalusian and Arabian Horses." *Equine Practice,* Vol. 15, No. 4 (April 1993), pp. 13–19.

Lopez-Rivero, J.L., et al. "Muscle Fiber Size in Horses." *The Equine Athlete,* Vol, 3, No. 2 (March /April 1990), pp. 1–11.

Lopez–Rivero, J.L., et al. "Muscle Fiber Type Composition in Untrained and Endurance-Trained Andalusian and Arab Horses." *Equine Veterinary Journal,* Vol. 23, No. 2 (1991), pp. 91–93.

Lorenzo-Figueras M, Merritt AM. "Effects of exercise on gastric volume and pH in the proximal portion of the stomach of horses." Am J Vet Res 2002 Nov; 63 (11): 1481–7.

MacFadden, K.E. and L.W. Pace. "Clinical Manifestations of Squamous Cell Carcinoma in Horses." *Compendium on Continuing Education,* Vol. 13, No. 4 (April 1991), pp. 669–676.

MacNamara, B., S. Bauer, and J. Lafe. "Endoscopic Evaluation of ExerciseInduced Pulmonary Hemorrhage and Chronic Obstructive Pulmonary Disease in Association With Poor Performance in Racing Standardbreds." *Journal of the American Veterinary Medical Association,* Vol. 196, No. 3 (February 1990), pp. 443–445.

Madigan, J.E. "Equine Granulocytic Ehrlichiosis: A Disease of Horses and Humans." *Proceedings of the American Association of Equine Practitioners* (1996), pp. 308–310.

Madigan, J.E., Valberg,S.J., Ragle, C., and Moody, J.L. "Muscle Spasms Associated with Ear Tick (*Otobius megnini*) Infestations in Five Horses." *Journal of the AmericanVeterinary Medical Association.* 1995, 207: 1,74–76.

Madigan, J.E. "Owner Survey of Headshaking in Horses." *Journal of American Veterinary Medical Association,* Vol. 219, No. 3 (August 1, 2001), pp. 334–337.

Madigan, J.E., Kortz G., Murphy, C. and Rodger, L. "Photic Headshaking in the Horse: 7 Cases." *Equine Veterinary Journal* 1995, 27 (4): 306–311.

Mair, T.S. and Edwards, G.B. "Strangulating Obstructions of the Small Intestine." *Equine Veterinary Education,* August 2003, pp. 244–250.

Mal, M.E., T.H. Friend, D.C. Lay, S.G. Vogelsang, and O.C. Jenkins. "Physiological Responses of Mares to Short Term Confinement and Social Isolation." *Equine Veterinary Science,* Vol. 11, No. 2 (1991), pp. 96–102.

Manning, T. and C. Sweeney. "Immune-Mediated Equine Skin Diseases." *Compendium on Continuing Education,* Vol. 8, No. 12 (December 1986), pp. 979–986.

Manohar, M., Hutchens, E., and Coney, E. "Pulmonary Haemodynamics in the Exercising Horse and Their Relationship to Exercise-Induced Pulmonary Haemorrhage." Br Vet J. 1993 Sep-Oct; 149 (5): 419–28.

Manohar, M. and Goetz, T. E. "Pulmonary Vascular Pressures of Strenuously Exercising Thoroughbreds During Intravenous Infusion of Nitroglycerin." *American Journal of Veterinary Research*, 60:1436–1440, 1999.

Martin, R.K., J.P. Albright, W.R. Clarke, and J.A. Niffenegger. "Load Carrying Effects on the Adult Beagle Tibia." *Medicine and Science in Sports and Exercise,* Vol. 13 (1981), pp. 343–349.

Mathews, K.A. and Binnington, A.G. "Sugar Treatment for Wounds." *Compendium of Continuing Education,* Vol 24, No. 1 (January 2002), pp. 41–49.

Mathews, K.A. and Binnington, A.G. "Wound Management Using Honey." *Compendium of Continuing Education,* Vol 24, No. 1 (January 2002), pp. 53–59.

Mayhew, I.G. "Neuroanatomical Localization of Lesions with Emphasis on the Spinal Cord." *Proceedings of the American Association of Equien Practitioners* (1993), pp. 101–105.

McCarthy, R.N. "The Effects of Exercise and Training on Bone." *Trail Blazer Magazine* (August/ September 1991), pp. 16–17.

McClure, S.R. and Merritt, D.K. "Extracorpoeral Shock-Wave Therapy for Equine Musculoskeletal Disorders." *Compendium of Continuing Education,* January 2003, pp. 68–70.

McCue, P.M. "Estrus Suppression in Performance Horses." *Journal of Equine Veterinary Science* (August 2003), Vol 23, No. 8, pp. 342–344.

Mcllwraith, C.W., ed. *AQHA Developmental Orthopedic Disease Symposium (1986),* Amarillo, Texas.

McMiken, D. "Muscle Fiber Types and Horse Performance." *Equine Practice,* Vol. 8, No. 3 (March 1986), pp. 6–14.

Melick, R.A. and D.R. Miller. "Variations of Tensile Strength in Human Cortical Bone With Age." *Clinical Science,* Vol. 30 (1966), pp. 243–248.

Mero, J.L. and Pool, R.R. "Twenty Cases of Degenerative Suspensory Ligament Desmitis in Peruvian Paso Horses." *Proceedings of the American Association of Equine Practitioners* (2002), Vol 48, pp. 329–334.

Meschter, C.L., et al. "The Effects of Phenylbutazone on the Intestinal Mucosa of the Horse: A Morphological, Ultrastructural, and Biochemical Study." *Equine Veterinary Journal,* Vol. 22, No. 4 (1990), pp. 255–263.

Meyers, M.C., G.D. Potter, et al. "Physiologic and Metabolic Response of Exercising Horses to Added Dietary Fat." *Equine Veterinary Science,* Vol. 9, No. 4 (1989), pp. 218–223.

Mills, D.S., Cook, S., Taylor, K., and Jones, B. "Analysis of the Variations in Clinical Signs Shown by 254 Cases of Equine Headshaking." Vet Rec 2002 Feb 23; 150 (8): 236–40.

Mills D.S., and Taylor, K. "Field study of the Efficacy of Three Types of Nose Net for the Treatment of Head Shaking in Horses." Vet Rec 2003 Jan 11; 152 (2): 41–4.

Minnick PD, Brown CM, Braselton WE, Meerdink GL, Slanker MR. "The Induction of Equine Laminitis With an Aqueous Extract of the Heartwood of Black Walnut (Juglans nigra). Veterinary and Human Toxicology 1987; 29: 230–233.

Morgan K, Funkquist P, Nyman G. "The Effect of Coat Clipping on Thermoregulation During Intense Exercise in Trotters." *Equine Vet J Suppl* 2002 Sep; (34): 564–7.

Moore, J.N. and D.D. Morris. "Endotoxemia and Septicemia in Horses: Experimental and Clinical Correlates." *Journal of the American Veterinary Medical Association*, Vol. 200, No. 12 (June 1992), pp. 1903–1914.

Morris, E.A. and H.J. Seeherman. "Clinical Evaluation of Poor Performance in the Racehorse: The Results of 275 Evaluations." *Equine Veterinary Journal*, Vol. 23, No. 3 (1991), pp. 169–174.

Morris, E.A., et al. "Scintigraphic Identification of Skeletal Muscle Damage in Horses 24 Hours After Strenuous Exercise." *Equine Veterinary Journal*, Vol. 23, No. 5 (1991), pp. 347–352.

Morris, E.A. and H.J. Seeherman. "Equisport: A Comprehensive Program for Clinical Evaluation of Poor Racing Performance." *Proceedings of the American Association of Equine Practitioners* (1989), pp. 385–397.

Morris, E.A. and H.J. Seeherman. "Evaluation of Upper Respiratory Tract Function During Strenuous Exercise in Racehorses." *Journal of the American Veterinary Medical Association*, Vol. 196, No. 3 (February 1990), pp. 431–438.

Morris, E.A. and H.J. Seeherman. "The Dynamic Evaluation of Upper Respiratory Function in the Exercising Horse." *Proceedings of the American Association of Equine Practitioners* (1988), pp. 159–165.

Mullowney, P.C. "Dermatologic Diseases of Horses, Part IV: Environmental, Congenital, and Neoplastic Diseases." *Compendium on Continuing Education*, Vol. 7, No. 1 (January 1985), pp. 22–32.

Mullowney, P.C. "Dermatologic Diseases of Horses, Part V: Allergic, Immune Mediated, and Miscellaneous Skin Diseases." *Compendium on Continuing Education*, Vol. 7, No. 4 (April 1985), pp. 217–228.

Munroe, G.A. "Cryosurgery in the Horse." *Equine Veterinary Journal*, Vol. 18, No. 1 (1986), pp. 14–17.

Murray, M.J. "Phenylbutazone Toxicity in a Horse." *Compendium on Continuing Education*, Vol. 7, No. 7 (July 1985), pp. 389–394.

Naylor, J.M., et al. "Familial Incidence of Hyperkalemic Periodic Paralysis in Quarter Horses." *Journal of the American Veterinary Medical Association*, Vol. 200, No. 3 (February 1992), pp. 340–343.

Neely, D.P., I.K.M. Liu, and R.B. Hillman. *Equine Reproduction*. Hoffman-La Roche, Inc., 1983.

Newton, S.A., Knottenbelt, D.C., and Eldridge, P.R. "Headshaking in Horses: Possible Aetiopathogenesis Suggested by the Results of Diagnostic Tests and Several Treatment Regimes Used in 20 Cases." Equine Vet J. 2000 May; 32 (3): 208–16.

Newton J.R. Wood J.L.N. Chanter N. "Long Term Carriage of Streptococcus Equi in Horses. Satellite article. Equine Vet. Edu. 1997; 9 (2): 98–102.

Newton, J.R., Wood, J.L.N., and Dunn M.N. " Naturally Occurring Persistent and Asymptomatic Infection of the Guttural Pouches of Horses with *Streptococcus Equi*." Vet.Record 1997; 140: 84–90.

Nilsson, B.E. and N.E. Westlin. "Bone Density in Athletes." *Clinical Orthopedics*, Vol. 77 (1971), pp. 179–182.

Nout, Y.S. and Reed, S.M. "Cervical Vertebral Stenotic Myelopathy." *Equine Veterinary Education*, August 2003, pp. 268–281.

Nunamaker, D.M. "On Bucked Shins." *Proceedings of the American Association of Equine Practitioners* (2002), pp. 76–89.

Oldham, S.L., G.D. Potter, et al. "Storage and Mobilization of Muscle Glycogen in Exercising Horses Fed a Fat- Supplemented Diet." *Equine Veterinary Science*, Vol. 10, No. 5 (1990), pp. 353–359.

O'Grady, S.E. and Poupard, D.A. "Physiologic Horseshoeing." *Journal of Equine Veterinary Science* (March 2003), Vol 23, No. 3, pp. 123–124.

O'Neill W, McKee S, Clarke AF. "Flaxseed (Linum usitatissimum) supplementation associated with reduced skin test lesional area in horses with Culicoides hypersensitivity." Can J Vet Res 2002 Oct; 66 (4): 272–7.

Parker, A.R. "Domperidone." *Compendium of Continuing Education*, October 2001, pp. 906–908.

Parraga, M.E., Spier, S.J., Thurmond, M., and Hirsh, D. "A Clinical Trial of Probiotic Administration for Prevention of Salmonella Shedding in the Postoperative Period in Horses with Colic." *J Vet Intern Med*. 1997 Jan–Feb; 11(1):36–41.

Pascoe, J.R., McCabe, A.E., Franti, C.E., and Arthur, R.M. "Efficacy of Furosemide in the Treatment of Exercise-Induced Pulmonary Hemorrhage in Thoroughbred Racehorses." Am J Vet Res. 1985 Sep; 46(9): 2000–2003.

Pascoe, J.R. "Exercise-Induced Pulmonary Hemorrhage." *Equine Veterinary Science*, Vol. 9, No. 4 (1989), pp. 198–200.

Pascoe J.R. "Exercise-induced Pulmonary Hemorrhage: A Unifying Concept." *Proceedings of the American Association of Equine Practitioners* (1996), Vol. 42, pp. 220–226.

Petrov R., MacDonald M.H., Tesch A.M., and Van Hoogmoed L.M. "Influence of Topically Applied Cold Treatment on Core Temperature and Cell Viability in Equine Superficial Digital Flexor Tendons." Am J Vet Res. 2003 Jul; 64 (7): 835–44.

Peyton, L.C. "Wound Healing in the Horse Part 2: Approach to the Treatment of Traumatic Wounds." *Compendium on Continuing Education*, Vol. 9, No. 2 (February 1987), pp. 191–200.

Peyton, L.C. "Wound Healing: The Management of Wounds and Blemishes in the Horse-Part I." *Compendium on Continuing Education*, Vol. 6, No. 2 (February 1984), pp. III–117.

Pinche C.A. "Clinical observations on an outbreak of strangles." Can. Vet. J. 1984; 25: 7–11.

Pirie RS, Collie DD, Dixon PM, McGorum BC. "Evaluation of Nebulised Hay Dust Suspensions (HDS) for the Diagnosis and Investigation of Heaves. 2: Effects of Inhaled HDS on Control and Heaves Horses." Equine Vet J 2002 Jul; 34 (4) : 337–42.

Piotrowski, G., M. Sullivan, and P. T. Colahan. "Geometric Properties of Equine Metacarpi." *Journal of Biomechanics*, Vol. 16 (1983), pp. 129–139.

Platt, D. "The Role of Oral Disease-Modifying Agents Glucosamine and Chondroitin Sulphate in the Management of Equine Degenerative Joint Disease." *Equine Veterinary Education*, August 2001, pp. 262–272.

Pollitt, C.C. *Equine Laminitis*. RIRDC, Kingston, Australia, Nov 2001.

Pollit, C.C., Kyaw-Tanner, M., French, K.R., Van Eps, A.W., Hendrikz, J.K, and Daradka, M. "Equine Laminitis." *Proceedings of the American Association of Equine Practitioners* (2003), Vol. 49, pp. 103–115.

Pollit, C.C. "Monitoring the Heart Rate of Endurance Horses." *Trail Blazer Magazine* (May 1992), pp. 16–17.

Pollit, C.C. "Monitoring the Heart Rate of Endurance Horses, Part 2." Trail *Blazer Magazine* (July/August 1992), pp. 8–11.

Pollit, C.C. "The Role of Arteriovenous Anastomoses in the Pathophysiology of Equine Laminitis." *Proceedings of the American Association of Equine Practitioners* (1991), pp. 711–719.

Pool, R.R. "Adaptations of Bones, Joints, and Attachments of the Limbs of the Horse in Response to Developmental and Infectious Diseases and to Biomechanical Forces Encountered in Athletic Performance." *Proceedings from the Denver Area Veterinary Medical Association Seminar* (January 1991).

Pool, R.R. "Developmental Orthopedic Disease in the Horse: Normal and Abnormal Bone Formation." *Proceedings of the American Association of Equine Practitioners* (1988), pp. 143–158.

Pool, R.R. "Pathophysiology of Athletic Injuries of the Horse: Bones, Joints, and Tendons." *AESM Quarterly*, Vol. 3, No. 2 (1988), pp. 23–29.

Pool, R.R. "Pathogenesis of Navicular Disease." *Proceedings of the American Association of Equine Practitioners* (1991), p. 709.

Porter, Mimi. "Physical Therapy for Equine Athletes." *AESM Quarterly*, Vol. 3, No. 3 (1988), pp. 40–43.

Porter, Mimi. "Techniques of Treatment." *Equine Veterinary Science* (March/ April 199 1), pp. 191–194.

Porter, Mimi. "Therapeutic Electricity." *Equine Veterinary Science* (January I February 1991), pp. 59–64.

Porter, Mimi. "Therapeutic Electricity: Physiological Effects." *Equine Veterinary Science* (March /April 199 1), pp. 133–140.

Porter, Mimi. "Therapeutic Ultrasound." *Equine Veterinary Science* (July/ August 1991), pp. 243–245.

Porter, Mimi. "Therapeutic Ultrasound." *Equine Veterinary Science* (September/October 1991), pp. 294–299.

Poulos, P.W., and M.F. Smith. "The Nature of Enlarged 'Vascular Channels' in the Navicular Bone of the Horse." *Veterinary Radiology* (1988), Vol. 29, pp. 60–64.

Powell, D., et al. "Rhinopneumonitis Roundtable Discussion." *Equine Practice*, Vol. 14, No. 4 (April 1992), pp. 8–12. *Equine Practice*, Vol. 14, No. 5 (May 1992), pp. 30–36. *Equine Practice*, Vol. 14, No. 6 (June 1992), pp. 17–20.

Power, H.T., Watrous, B.J., de Lahunta, A., "Facial and Vestibulocochlear Nerve Disease in Six Horses." *Journal of the American Veterinary Medical Association* 1983, 183: 10, 1076–1080.

Pratt, G.W. "An In Vivo Method of Ultrasonically Evaluating Bone Strength." *Proceedings of the American Association of Equine Practitioners* (1980), pp. 295–306.

Pratt, G.W. "The Response of Highly Stressed Bone in the Race Horse." *Proceedings of the American Association of Equine Practitioners* (1982), pp. 31–37.

Pugh, D.G. and J.T. Thompson. "Impaction Colics Attributed to Decreased Water Intake and Feeding Coastal Bermuda Grass Hay in a Boarding Stable." *Equine Practice*, Vol. 14, No. I (January 1992), pp. 9–14.

Rabin, D.S., N.W. Rantanen, et al. "The Clinical Use of Bone Strength Assessment in the Thoroughbred Race Horse." *Proceedings of the American Association of Equine Practitioners* (1983), pp. 343–351.

Ragle, C.A., Meagher, D.M., Schrader, J.L., and Honnas, C.M. "Abdominal Auscultation in the Detection of Experimentally Induced Gastrointestinal Sand Accumulation." *J Vet Intern Med* 1989 Jan–Mar; 3 (1) : 12–14.

Ragle, C.A., Meagher, D.M., Lacroix, C.A., and Honnas, C.M. "Surgical Treatment of Sand Colic: Results in 40 Horses." *Vet Surg* 1989 Jan–Feb; 18 (1): 48 –51.

Ralston, S.L. and K. Larson. "The Effect of Oral Electrolyte Supplementation During a 96 Kilometer Endurance Race for Horses." *Equine VeterinaryScience*, Vol. 9, No. 1, pp. 13–19.

Ralston, S.L. "Common Behavioral Problems of Horses." *Compendium on Continuing Education*, Vol. 4, No. 4 (April 1982), pp. 152–159.

Ralston, S.L. "Nutritional Management of Horses Competing in 160 Kilometer Races." *Cornell Vet*, Vol. 78, No. 1 (1988), pp. 53–61.

Ralston, S.L. "Patterns and Control of Food Intake in Domestic Animals." *Compendium on Continuing Education,* Vol. 6, No. 11 (1984), pp. 628–634

Reed, S.M., Savillle, J.A., and Schneider, R.K. "Neurologic Disease: Current Topics In-Depth." *Proceedings of the American Association of Equine Practitioners* (2003), pp. 243–256.

Reef, V.B., B.B. Martin, and A. Elser. "Types of Tendon and Ligament Injuries Detected With Diagnostic Ultrasound: Description and Follow-up." *Proceedings of the American Association of Equine Practitioners* (1988), pp. 245–248.

Reef, V.B., B.B. Martin, and K. Stebbins. "Comparison of Ultrasonographic, Gross, and Histologic Appearance of Tendon Injuries in Performance Horses." *Proceedings of the American Association of Equine Practitioners* (1989), p. 279.

Reilly, D.T. and A.H. Burstein. "The Mechanical Properties of Cortical Bone." *Journal of Bone and Joint Surgery,* Vol. 56A (1974), pp. 1001–1022.

Reilly, J.D., Martinelli, M.J., and Pollitt, C.C., and Green, R.E. *The Equine Hoof and Laminitis. Equine Veterinary Journal* Supplement 26, September 1998.

Reilly, J.D., Cottrell, D.F., Martin, R.J., and Cuddeford, D.J. "Effect of Supplementary Dietary Biotin on Hoof Growth And Hoof Growth Rate in Ponies: A Controlled Trial." *Equine Vet J Supplement* 1998 Sept; (26): 51–57.

Reinemeyer, C.R. "Anthelmintic Resistance in Horses." *Equine Veterinary Science,* Vol. 7, No. 6, pp. 390–391.

Reinemeyer, C.R., S.A. Smith, A.A. Gabel, and R.P. Herd. "Observations on the Population Dynamics of Five Cyathostome Nematode Species of Horses in Northern USA." *Equine Veterinary Journal,* Vol. 18, No. 2 (1986), pp. 121–124.

Reinemeyer, C.R. and J.E. Henton. "Observations on Equine Strongyle Control in Southern Temperate USA." *Equine Veterinary Journal,* Vol. 19, No. 6 (1987), pp. 505–508.

Richardson, D.W. "Pathophysiology of Degenerative Joint Disease." *Equine Veterinary Science,* Vol. 11, No. 3 (1990), pp. 156–157.

Ridgway, K.J. "Cardiac Recovery Index: Avoiding Inappropriate Utilization." *AERC Endurance News* (October 1991), pp. 5–7.

Ridgway, K.J. "Respiration as an Evaluation Parameter for Distance Riding." *AERC Endurance News* (October 1990), pp. 4–5.

Ridgway, K.J. "Exertional Myopathies. " *Proceedings of the American Association of Equine Practitioners* (1991), pp. 839–843.

Robb, E.J. and D.S. Kronfeld. "Dietary Sodium Bicarbonate as a Treatment for Exertional Rhabdomyolysis in a Horse." *Journal of the American Veterinary Medical Association,* Vol. 188, No. 6 (March 1986), pp. 602–607.

Robinson, N.E., editor. *Current Therapy in Equine Medicine 2,* WB Saunders Company, 1987.

Robinson, N.E., editor. *Current Therapy in Equine Medicine 5.* Saunders, 2003.

Robinson, N.E. and R. Wilson. "Airway Obstruction in the Horse." *Equine Veterinary Science,* Vol. 9, No. 3 (1989), pp. 155–160.

Robinson, N.E., et al. "Physiology of the Equine Respiratory Tract and Changes in Disease: The Role of Granulocytes." *Proceedings of the American Association of Equine Practitioners* (1984), pp. 253–261.

Robson P.J., Alston T.D., Myburgh K.H. "Prolonged suppression of the innate immune system in the horse following an 80 km endurance race." Equine Vet J 2003 Mar; 35 (2): 133–7.

Roche, J.F., L. Keenan, and D. Forde. "Some Factors Affecting Fertility of the Mare." *Equine Practice,* Vol. 9, No. 1 (January 1987), pp. 8–13.

Romeiser, K. "Tying-Up: Old Problem, New Twist." *Equus* 126, pp. 60–64, 128–129.

Rooney, J. "Passive Function of the Extensor Tendons of the Fore and Rear Limbs of the Horse." *Equine Veterinary Science,* Vol. 7, No. 1 (1987), pp. 29–30.

Rose, R.J. and D.R. Lloyd. "Sodium Bicarbonate: More Than Just a 'Milkshake'?" *Equine Veterinary Journal,* Vol. 24, No. 2 (1992), pp. 75–76.

Ross, M.W., Genovese, R.L., and Reef, V.B. "Curb: A Collection of Plantar Tarsal Soft Tissue Injuries." *Proceedings of the American Association of Equine Practitioners* (2002), pp. 337–342.

Ross, M.W. and Dyson, S.J., eds. *Diagnosis and Management of Lameness in the Horse."* Saunders, Philadelphia, 2003.

Rossano, M.G., Kaneene, J.B., Schott, H.C., Sheline, K.D., and Mansfield, L.S. "Assessing the Agreement of Western Blot Test Results for Paired Serum and Cerebrospinal Fluid Samples From Horses Tested for Antibodies to *Sarcocystis neurona.*" Vet Parasitol. 2003 Jul 29; 115 (3): 233–8.

Rubin, S.I. "Non-Steroidal Anti-Inflammatory Drugs, Prostaglandins, and the Kidney. " Journal *of the American Veterinary Medical Association,* Vol. 188, No. 9 (May 1986), pp. 1065–1068.

Rude, T.A. "Vaccines, Bacterins, Toxoids Can Cause Allergic Reactions." *DVM Magazine* (May 1989), pp. 42–44. Ruff, C.B. and W.C. Hayes. "Bone Mineral Content in the Lower Limb." *Journal of Bone and Joint Surgery,* Vol. 66A (1984), pp. 1024–1031.

Ruohoniemi, M., Kaikkonen, R., Raekallio, M., and Luukkanen, L. "Abdominal Radiography in Monitoring the Resolution of Sand Accumulations from the Large Colon of Horses Treated Medically." Equine Vet J 2001 Jan 33 (1): 59–64.

Ruggles, A.J. and M.W. Ross. "Medical and Surgical Management of Small Colon Impaction in Horses: 28 Cases (1984–1989)." *Journal of the American Veterinary Medical Association*, Vol. 199, No. 12 (December 1991), pp. 1762–1766.

Ruth, D.T. and B.J. Swites. "Comparison of the Effectiveness of Intra-Articular Hyaluronic Acid and Conventional Therapy for the Treatment of Naturally Occurring Arthritic Conditions in Horses." *Equine Practice*, Vol. 7, No. 9 (October 1985), pp. 25–29.

Schott II, H.C., D.R. Hodgson, J.R. Naylor, and W.M. Bayly. "Thermoregulation and Heat Exhaustion in the Exercising Horse." *Proceedings of the American Association of Equine Practitioners* (1990), pp. 505–513.

Schott II, H.C. "Aspects of Heat Production, Dissipation, and Exhaustion in the Exercising Horse." AERC *Endurance News* (November 1991), pp. 5–6.

Schroter R.C., Marlin D.J., Denny E. Exercise-induced pulmonary haemorrhage (EIPH) in horses results from locomotory impact induced trauma–a novel, unifying concept. Equine Vet J 1998; 30: 186–192.

Scott, J. and Butler, D. "Effect of Several Externally Applied Irritants on Hoof Growth." *American Farriers Journal* December 1980, p. 148.

Scott, B.D., G.D. Potter, et al. "Growth and Feed Utilization by Yearling Horses Fed Added Dietary Fat." *Equine Veterinary Science*, Vol. 9, No. 4 (1989), pp. 210–214.

Scraba, S.T. and O.J. Ginther. "Effects of Lighting Programs on Onset of the Ovulatory Season in Mares." *Theriogenology*, Vol. 24 (1985), pp. 667–679.

Serun G.S. Reactions to strangles vaccination. Aust Vet I. 1995; 72 (12): 480.

Severin, G.A. "Equine Ophthamology" *Proceedings of the American Association of Equine Practitioners* (1998), Vol. 44, pp. 105–124.

Shabpareh, V., E.L. Squires, V.M. Cook, and R. Cole. "An Alternative Artificial Lighting Regime to Hasten Onset of the Breeding Season in Mares." *Equine Practice*, Vol. 14, No. 2 (February 1992), pp. 24–27.

Shaw, K., et al. *Strongid® C: A Roundtable Discussion.*. Pfizer, Inc., 1990.

Shively, M.J. "Equine-English Dictionary: Part I-Standing Conformation." *Equine Practice*, Vol. 4, No. 5 (May 1982), pp. 10–20, 25–27.

Smith, C.A. "Electrolyte Imbalances and Metabolic Disturbances in Endurance Horses." *Compendium on Continuing Education*, Vol. 7, No. 10 (October 1985), pp. 575–584.

Smith, J.D., et al. "Exercise-Induced Pulmonary Hemorrhage Findings, A Workshop." *Equine Practice*, Vol. 14, No. I (January 1992), pp. 19–25. *Equine Practice*, Vol. 14, No. 2 (February 1992), pp. 9–15. *Equine Practice*, Vol. 14, No. 3 (March 1992), pp. 28–32.

Smith H. "Reaction to Strangles Vaccination." Short contributions. Aust. Vet J.1994; 71(8): 257–258.

Smith, M.J. "Electrical Stimulation for Relief of Musculoskeletal Pain." *The Physician and Sportsmedicine*, Vol. 11, No. 5 (May 1983), pp. 47–55.

Smith R.K., Birch H.L., Goodman S., Heinegard D., Goodship A.E. "The influence of ageing and exercise on tendon growth and degeneration-hypotheses for the initiation and prevention of strain-induced tendinopathies." Comp Biochem Physiol A Mol Integr Physiol 2002 Dec; 133(4): 1039–50.

Snook, C.S., Hyman, S.S., Del Piero, F., Palmer, J.E., Ostlund, E.N., Barr, B.S., Desrochers, A.M., and Reilly, L.K. "West Nile Virus Encephalomyelitis in Eight Horses." *J Am Vet Med Assoc* 2001 May 15; 218 (10): 1576–1579.

Snow, D.H. "Sweating and Anhidrosis." *Equine Sportmedicine*, Vol. 5, No. 2 (1986), pp. 4–5, 8.

Snow, V.E. and D.P. Birdsall. "Specific Parameters Used to Evaluate Hoof Balance and Support." *Proceedings of the American Association of Equine Practitioners* (1990), pp. 299–312.

Solomons, B. "Equine Cutis Hyperelastica." Equine Vet J, 16:541–542, 1984.

Specht, T.E. and P.T. Colahan. "Surgical Treatment of Sand Colic in Equids: 48 Cases (1978–1985)." *Journal of the American Veterinary Medical Association, Vol. 193*, No. 12 (December 1988), pp. 1560–1563.

Spier, S.J. "Current Facts About Hyperkalemic Periodic Paralysis (HYPP) Disease." *The Quarter Racing Journal* (April 1993), pp. 44–47.

Spier, S.J. "Use of Hyperimmune Plasma Containing Antibody to Gramnegative Core Antigens." *Proceedings of the American Association of Equine Practitioners* (1989), pp. 91–94.

Spier, S.J. and G.P. Carlson. "Hyperkalemic Periodic Paralysis in Certain Registered Quarter Horses." *The Quarter Horse Journal* (September 1992), pp. 68–69, 120.

Spier, S.J., G.P. Carlson, et al. "Genetic Study of Hyperkalemic Periodic Paralysis in Horses." *Journal of the American Veterinary Medical Association*, Vol. 202, No. 6 (March 1993), pp. 933–937.

Spier, S.J., G.P. Carlson, et al. "Hyperkalemic Periodic Paralysis in Horses." *Journal of the American Veterinary Medical Association*, Vol. 197, No. 8 (October 1990), pp. 1009–1016.

Stabenfeldt, G.H. and J.P. Hughes. "Clinical Aspects of Reproductive Endocrinology in the Horse." *Compendium on Continuing Education*, Vol. 9, No. 6 (June 1987), pp. 678–684.

Stashak, Ted S. *Adams' Lameness in Horses.* Fourth Edition. Lea and Febiger, Philadelphia, 1987.

Stull, C. "Muscles for Motion." *Equine Practice,* Vol. 8, No. 4 (April 1986), pp. 17–20.

Subcommittee on Horse Nutrition, Committee on Animal Nutrition, Board of Agriculture, National Research Council, *Nutrient Requirements of Horses.* Fifth Revised Edition. National Academy Press, Washington DC, 1989.

Sukanta, K., et al. Dutta, Ramesh Vemulapalli, and Biswajit Biswas "Association of Deficiency in Antibody Response to Vaccine and Heterogeneity of *Ehrlichia risticii* Strains with Potomac Horse Fever Vaccine Failure in Horses " *Journal of Clinical Microbiology,* February 1998, p. 506–512, Vol. 36, No. 2.

Sullins, K.E., S.M. Roberts, J.D. Lavach, G.A. Severin, and D. Lueker. "Equine Sarcoid." *Equine Practice,* Vol. 8, No. 4 (April 1986), pp. 21–27.

Swaim, S.F. and A.H. Lee. "Topical Wound Medications: A Review." *Journal of the American Veterinary Medical Association,* Vol. 190, No. 12 (June 1987), pp. 1588–1592.

Swaim, S.F. and D. Wilhalf. "The Physics, Physiology, and Chemistry of Bandaging Open Wounds." *Compendium on Continuing Education,* Vol. 7, No. 2 (February 1985), pp. 146–155.

Swann, P. *Racehorse Training and Feeding.* Racehorse Sportsmedicine and Scientific Conditioning, Australia, 1985.

Swann, P. *Racehorse Training and Sports Medicine.* Racehorse Sportsmedicine and Scientific Conditioning, Australia, 1988.

Sweeney C.R. Streptococcus equi infection in horses. Satellite article. *Equine Vet Educ.* 1996; 8 (6): 317–322.

Sweeney, C.R., C.E. Benson, et al. "Description of an Epizootic and Persistence of Streptococcus Equi Infections in Horses." *Journal of the American Veterinary Medical Association,* Vol. 194, No. 9 (1989), pp. 1281–1285.

Sweeney, C.R., C.E. Benson, et al. "Streptococcus Equi Infection in Horses Part 1." *Compendium on Continuing Education,* Vol. 9, No. 6 (June 1987), pp. 689–693.

Sweeney, C.R., C.E. Benson, et al. "Streptococcus Equi Infection in Horses Part 2. " *Compendium on Continuing Education,* Vol. 9, No. 8 (August 1987), pp. 845–851.

Sweeney, C.R., et al. "Equine Roundtable Discussion: Respiration." *Equine Practice* (May 1989), pp. 16–24. *Equine Practice* (June 1989), pp. 10–16. *Equine Practice* (July/August 1989), pp. 29–40.

Swenson, M.J., ed. *Dukes' Physiology of Domestic Animals.* Ninth Edition. Cornell University Press, 1977.

Tarwid, J.N., P.B. Fretz, and E.G. Clark. "Equine Sarcoids: A Study With Emphasis on Pathologic Diagnosis." *Compendium on Continuing Education, Vol.* 7, No. 5 (May 1985), pp. 293–300.

Templeton, J.W., R. Smith III, and L.G. Adams. "Natural Disease Resistance in Domestic Animals." *Journal of the American Veterinary Medical Association, Vol.* 192, No. 9 (May 1988), pp. 1306–1315.

Texas Veterinary Medical Association Annual Meeting. "Hyaluronic Acid Use in the Horse: A Roundtable Discussion." Schering Animal Health, February 1988.

The Veterinary Clinics of North America, Equine Practice, *Advanced Diagnostic Methods,* August 1991, Vol. 7, No. 2.

The Veterinary Clinics of North America, Equine Practice, *Back Problems,* April 1999, Vol. 15, No. 1.

The Veterinary Clinics of North America, Equine Practice, *Behavior,* December 1986, Vol. 2, No. 3.

The Veterinary Clinics of North America, Equine Practice. *Clinical Nutrition,* August 1990, Vol. 6, No. 2, pp. 281–293, 355–371, 393–418.

The Veterinary Clinics of North America, Equine Practice, *Clinical Pharmacology,* April 1987, Vol. 3, No. 1.

The Veterinary Clinics of North America, Equine Practice, *Emerging Infectious Diseases,* December 2000, Vol. 16, No. 3.

The Veterinary Clinics of North America, Equine Practice, *Endocrinology,* August 2002, Vol. 19, No. 1.

The Veterinary Clinics of North America, Equine Practice, *The Equine Foot,* April 1989, Vol. 5, No. 1, pp. 109–128.

The Veterinary Clinics of North America, Equine Practice, *Exercise Physiology,* December 1985, Vol. 1, No. 3.

The Veterinary Clinics of North America, Equine Practice, *Laminitis,* August 1999, Vol. 15, No. 2.

The Veterinary Clinics of North America, Equine Practice, *Management of Colic,* April 1988, Vol. 4, No. 1.

The Veterinary Clinics of North America, Equine Practice. *Neurologic Disease,* August 1987, Vol 3, No 2.

The Veterinary Clinics of North America, Equine Practice, *Parasitology,* August 1986, Vol. 2, No. 2.

The Veterinary Clinics of North America, Equine Practice, *Podiatry,* August 2003, Vol. 19, No. 2.

The Veterinary Clinics of North America, Equine Practice, *Racetrack Practice,* April 1990, Vol. 6, No. 1.

The Veterinary Clinics of North America, Equine Practice, *Reproduction,* August 1988, Vol. 4, No 2

The Veterinary Clinics of North America, Equine Practice, *Respiratory Diseases,* April 1991, Vol. 7, No. 1.

The Veterinary Clinics of North America, Equine Practice, *Respiratory Disease,* April 2003, Vol. 19, No. 1.

The Veterinary Clinics of North America, Equine Practice, *Selected Neurologic and Muscular Disease,* April 1997, Vol. 13, No. 1.

The Veterinary Clinics of North America, Equine Practice, *Stallion Management,* April 1992, Vol. 8, No. 1.

The Veterinary Clinics of North America, Equine Practice, *Therapeutics for Gastrointestinal Diseases,* December 2003, Vol. 19, No. 3.

The Veterinary Clinics of North America, Equine Practice, *Toxicology,* December 2001, Vol. 17, No. 3.

The Veterinary Clinics of North America, Equine Practice, *Wound Management,* December 1989, Vol. 5, No. 3.

Thomas, H.S. "Using A Twitch." *American Farriers Journal* (July/August 1989), pp. 28–30.

Thompson, K.N., J.P. Baker, and S.G. Jackson. "The Influence of High Dietary Intakes of Energy and Protein on Third Metacarpal Characteristics of Weanling Ponies." *Equine Veterinary Science, Vol.* 8, No. 5 (1988), pp. 391 394.

Thomson, J.R. and E.A. McPherson. "Chronic Obstructive Pulmonary Disease in the Horse." *Equine Practice,* Vol. 10, No. 7 (July/August 1988), pp. 31–36.

Timoney J.F. Artiushin S.C. Detection of streptococcus equi in equine nasal swabs and washes by ONA amplification. Short communication. Vet.Rec. 1997; 141: 446–447.

Timoney J.F. Equine Strangles: 1999. AAEP Proceedings. 1999; 31–37.

Timoney J.F. Umbach A. Boschwitz J.E. Streptococcus. equi susbsp. Equi expresses 2M-like proteins including a homologue of the variable M-like protective protein of sbsp. Zooepidemicus. Equine infection. Dis. 1990; 7: 189–193.

Tinker, M.K., White, N.A., Lessard, P., Thatcher, C.D., Pelzer, K.D., Davis, B., and Carmel, D.K. "Prospective Study of Equine Colic Risk Factors." *Equine Vet J* 1997 Nov, 29 (6): 454–458.

Tnibar MA. "Treatment of Upward Fixation of the Patella in the Horse: An Update." *Equine Veterinary Education*, October 2003, pp. 306–312.

Tnibar MA. "Medial Patellar Ligament Splitting for the Treatment of Upward Fixation of the Patella in 7 Equids." Vet Surg 2002 Sep-Oct; 31 (5): 462–7.

Todhunter, R.J. and G. Lust. "Pathophysiology of Synovitis: Clinical Signs and Examination in Horses." *Compendium on Continuing Education, Vol.* 12, No. 7 (July 1990), pp. 980–991.

Traub-Dargatz, J.L., J.J. Bertone, et al. "Chronic Flunixin Meglumine Therapy in Foals." *American Journal of Veterinary Research,* Vol. 49, No. 1 (January 1988), pp. 7–12.

Traub-Dargatz, J.L. "Non-Steroidal Anti-Inflammatory Drug-induced Ulcers." *Proceedings of the American Association of Equine Practitioners (1988) Association of Equine Practitioners* (1988), pp. 129–132.

Turner, A.S. "Local and Systemic Factors Affecting Wound Healing." *Proceedings of the American Association of Equine Practitioners* (1978), pp. 355–362.

Turner, A.S. and Tucker, C.M. "The Evaluation of Isoxsuprine Hydrochloride for the Treatment of Navicular Disease: A Double Blind Study." *Equine Veterinary Journal, Vol.* 21, No. 5 (1989), pp. 338–341.

Turner, T.A. "Hindlimb Muscle Strain as a Cause of Lameness in Horses." *Proceedings of the American Association of Equine Practitioners* (1989), pp. 281–290.

Turner, T.A. "Navicular Disease Management: Shoeing Principles." *Proceedings of the American Association of Equine Practitioners* (1986), pp. 625–633.

Turner, T.A. "Shoeing Principles for the Management of Navicular Disease in the Horse." *Journal of the American Veterinary Medical Association,* Vol. 189 (1986), pp. 298–301.

Turner, T.A., S.K. Kneller, R.R. Badertscher II, and J.L. Stowater. "Radiographic Changes in the Navicular Bones of Normal Horses." *Proceedings of the American Association of Equine Practitioners* (1986), pp. 309–314.

Turner, T.A., R.C. Purohit, and J.F. Fessler. "Thermography: A Review in Equine Medicine." *Compendium on Continuing Education,* Vol. 8, No. 11 (1986), pp. 855–861.

Turner, T.A., K. Wolfsdorf, and J. Jourdenais. "Effects of Heat, Cold, Biomagnets, and Ultrasound on Skin Circulation in the Horse." *Proceedings of the American Association of Equine Practitioners* (1991), pp. 249–257.

Turrel, J.M., S.M. Stover, and J. Gyorgyfalvy. "Iridium- 192 Interstitial Brachytherapy of Equine Sarcoid." *Veterinary Radiology,* Vol. 26, No. 1 (1985), pp. 20–24.

Uhlinger, C.A., and M. Kristula. "Effects of Alternation of Drug Classes on the Development of Oxibendazole Resistance in a Herd of Horses." *Journal of the American Veterinary Medical Association,* Vol. 201, No. I (July 1992), pp. 51–55.

Uhlinger, C.A. "Equine Small Strongyles: Epidemiology, Pathology, and Control." *Compendium on Continuing Education,* Vol. 13, No. 5 (May 1991), pp. 863–868.

Valberg, S. "Metabolic Response to Racing and Fiber Properties of Skeletal Muscle in Standardbred and Thoroughbred Horses." *Equine Veterinary Science, Vol.* 7, No. 1 (1987), pp. 6–12.

Valberg, S. "Myopathies Associated With *Streptococcal Equi* Infections in Horses." *Proceedings of the Association of Equine Practitioners* (1996), Vol. 42, pp. 292–293.

Valberg, S. "Tying-Up Syndrome in Horses." *Hoof Print* (September/ October 1991), pp. 35–36.

Valentine, B.A., de Lahunta A, Divers T.J., Ducharme N.G., and Orcutt R.S.. "Clinical and Pathologic Findings in Two Draft Horses with Progressive Muscle Atrophy, Neuromuscular Weakness, and Abnormal Gait Characteristic of Shivers Syndrome." J Am Vet Med Assoc. 1999 Dec 1; 215 (11): 1661–5, 1621.

Valentine, B.A. "Equine Polysaccharide Storage Myopathy." *Equine Veterinary Education*, October 2003, pp. 326–334.

Valentine, B.A. "Role of Dietary Carbohydrate and Fat in Horses with Equine Polysaccharide Storage Myopathy." *Journal of American Veterinary Association* (December 1, 2001), Vol 219, No. 11, pp. 1537–1544.

Van Den Hoven, R. "Mind Over Muscle." *Equine Veterinary Journal*, Vol. 23, No. 2 (1991), pp. 73–74.

Van De Lest, C.H., Brama, P.A., and Van Weeren, P.R " The Influence of Exercise on the Composition of Developing Equine Joints." *Biorheology* 2002; 39 (1,2): 183–191.

Van Weeren P.R., Knaap J, and Firth E.C. "Influence of Liver Copper Status of Mare and Newborn Foal on the Development of Osteochondrotic Lesions." *Equine Vet J* 2003 Jan; 35 (1): 67–71.

Vanselow, B.A., 1. Abetz, and A.R.B. Jackson. "BCG Emulsion Immunotherapy of Equine Sarcoid." *Equine Veterinary Journal*, Vol. 20, No. 6 (1988), pp. 444–447.

Viitanen, M.J., Wilson, A.M., McGuigan, H.R., Rogers, K.D., and May, S.A. "Effect of Foot Balance on the Iintra-articular Pressure in the Distal Interphalangeal Joint In Vitro." *Equine Vet J* 2003 Mar; 35 (2) : 184–9.

Voges, F.E., Kienzle, and Meyer, H.. "Investigations on the Composition of Horse Bones." *Equine Veterinary Science*, Vol. 10, No. 3 (1990), pp. 208–213.

Wagoner, D.M., ed. *Feeding To Win II*. Equine Research Publications, 1992.

Wagoner, D.M., ed. *The Illustrated Veterinary Encyclopedia for Horsemen*. Equine Research Publications, 1977.

Wagoner, D.M., ed. *Veterinary Treatments and Medications for Horsemen*. Equine Research Publications, 1977.

Wagoner, D.M., ed. *Breeding Management and Foal Development*. Equine Research Publications, 1982.

Waldsmith, Jim. The Equine Center. San Luis Obispo, California, personal communication.

Wallace, F.J, and. Emery, J.D. Cripps A.N. "An Assessment of Mucosal Immunization in Protection Against *Streptococcus Equi* Infection in Horses." Vet Immunol Immunopathol 1995; 48: 139–154.

Wanless, M. *The Natural Rider*. Summit Books, New York, New York, 1987.

Webb, N.G., Penny, R.H., and Johnston, A.M. "Effect of a Dietary Supplement of Biotin on Pig Horn Strength and Hardness." Vet Record 1984, Feb 25: 114 (8): 185–9.

Webb, S.P., G.D. Potter, et al. "Physiological Responses of Cutting Horses to Exercise Testing and to Training." *Equine Veterinary Science*, Vol. 8, No. 3 (1988), pp. 261–265.

Webbon, P.M. "Preliminary Study of Tendon Biopsy in the Horse." *Equine Veterinary Journal*, Vol. 18, No. 5, pp. 383–387.

Weese, J.S. "A Review of Probiotics: Are they Really Functional Foods?" *Proceedings of the American Association of Equine Practitioners* (2001), pp. 27–31.

Weese, .JS., Anderson, M.E., Lowe, A., and Monteith, G.J.. "Preliminary Investigation of the Probiotic Potential of Lactobacillus Rhamnosus Strain GG in Horses: Fecal Recovery Following Oral Administration and Safety." Can Vet J 2003 Apr; 44 (4): 299–302.

White, G.W. "Adequan: A Review for the Practicing Veterinarian." *Equine Veterinary Science*, Vol. 8, No. 6 (1988), pp. 463–467.

White, N.A. "Thromboembolic Colic in Horses." *Compendium on Continuing Education*, Vol. 7, No. 3 (March 1985), pp. 156–162.

Wilson, G.L. and M. Mueller. *The Equine Athlete*. Veterinary Learning Systems Co., Inc., New Jersey, 1982.

Wilson, W.D. "Streptococcus Equi Infections (Strangles) in Horses." *Equine Practice*, Vol. 10, No. 7 (July/August 1988), pp. 12–25.

Wood, C.H., T.T. Ross, et al. "Variations in Muscle Fiber Composition Between Successfully and Unsuccessfully Raced Quarter Horses." *Equine Veterinary Science*, Vol. 8, No. 3 (1988), pp. 217–220.

Woolen, N., DeBowes, R.M., Leipold, H.W., and Schneider, L.A.. "A Comparison of Four Types of Therapy for the Treatment of Full-Thickness Skin Wounds of the Horse." *Proceedings of the American Association of Equine Practitioners* (1988), pp. 569–576.

Wright, I.M. "Oral Supplements in the Treatment and Prevention of Joint Diseases: A Review of Their Potential Application to the Horse." *Equine Veterinary Education*, June 2001, pp. 179–184.

Yelle, M.T. "Clinical Aspects of *Streptococcus Equi* Infection." *Equine Veterinary Journal*, Vol. 19, No. 2 (1987), pp. 158–162.

Young L.E., Marlin D.J., Deaton C., Brown-Feltner H., Roberts C.A., Wood J.L. "Heart size estimated by echocardiography correlates with maximal oxygen uptake." Equine Vet J Suppl 2002 Sep; (34): 467–71.

Yovich, J.V., G.W. Trotter, C.W. McIlwraith, and R.W. Norrdin. "Effects of Polysulfated Glycosaminoglycan on Chemical and Physical Defects in Equine Articular Cartilage." *American Journal of Veterinary Research*, Vol. 48, No. 9 (September 1987), pp. 1407–1413.

Index

Page numbers in *italic* indicate illustrations; those in **bold** indicate main discussions.

Abdominocentesis, 302, 303, *303*, 312
Abortion, 271, 272, 536, **556**
Abscesses
 hoof, 63, 64, **70–71**, *71*, 80
 injections, 438
 navicular syndrome, 86
Accommodation, 490
Acepromazine, 83
Acetazolamide, 177
Acetylcholine, 514, 526
Acoustical streaming for tendons, 198
Acquired angular limb deformity, 135
Acquired flexural contracture, *199*, 199–200
Action potential of muscle, 138
Acupressure for muscle, 178
Acupuncture for, 374
 back pain, 215, *215*
 mare, 542, *542*
 muscle, 178
 osteoarthritis, 129
Adenosine triphosphate (ATP), 138, 140, 141, 146, 164, 165, 169–170
Adipose tissue (fat reserves), 140, 325
Adrenaline (epinephrine), 439–440
Aerobic exercise
 bone response, 98, 99, 101
 cardiovascular system, 226
 metabolism, 140–141, 142, 143
 muscle endurance, 145–146, *146*, 151–152, 161
 spleen, 220
Agar-gel-immunodiffusion (AGID), 457
Age of horse impact on
 joints, 112
 strangles, 273–274
 vaccination, 265, 270, 272
Agglutinate, 425
Agonist muscles, 144, 145, *145*
AI (artificial insemination), 550, 551, *551*, **553–555**
Air quality impact on
 respiratory system, 254, 256–257
 trailering, *479–480*, 479–481
Airway, maintaining, 431, *431*
Airway inflammation disease, 260–261
Airways and airflow, 246–247
Alcohol as antiseptic, 407, 435
ALD (angular limb deformities), 22, 22–23, 23, 103, *134–135*, **134–136,** 535
Alkali disease (selenium poisoning), 57–58, **374–375**
Allergens, 252
Allergic reactions
 deworming, 471–472
 NSAIDs, 446
 skin, 377, *377–378*, 378, 389–391, *389–391*
Alopecia (hair loss), 374, 380, 385
Alpha-tocopheryl, 338
Altrenogest, 541, 551
Aluminum hydroxide buffer, 319–320
Alveolar-capillary interface, 249
Alveolar macrophages, 255
Alveoli, 221, *245*, 249
Amblyomma (tick), 387
American Quarter Horse Association (AQHA), 444. *See also* Quarter Horses
Ammonia, 257, 343
Amnionic sac, 560, 561, *561*
Amnion wound dressing, 415–416
Anabolic steroids and estrus, 543
Anaerobic bacteria, 422, *422*
Anaerobic exercises
 bone response, 98–99, 101
 cardiovascular system, 220, 228
 metabolism, 140, 141, 142, 143, 161
 skeletal muscle adaptations, 147–148, 150
Anaerobic threshold, 147–148, 149
Analgesia (pain relief), 178, 193–194, 198
Anamnestic antibody response, 265
Anaphylactic shock, 432, 434, **439–440,** 446
Anaphylaxis, 391
Anatomy and function, 7–11
 balance of horse, 10–11, *12*
 eye, *488–489*
 intestinal tract, *291*, 291–293
 joints, 9, *109*, 109–110
 legs, 8–9, *8–9*
 mare, 539
 muscle, 7–8, *8*, 10, *10*
 overview of, 8–9
 parts of horse, *9*
 skeletal system, 8, *8*
 spatial terminology, *11*
 stallion, 536
 symmetry, 8–9
 tendons and ligaments, *181*
 thirds of horse, balance, 10–11, *12*
 See also Conformation
Anchoring filaments, hoof, 42, 81
Anemia, 233, **241–243, 252–253,** 337, 457
Anesthesia injection test, 89, *89*, 90
Anestrus, 538, 539
Angioedema, 391
Angular limb deformities (ALD), 22, 22–23, 23, 103, *134–135*, **134–136,** 535
Anhidrosis, 361
Ankylosis of joint, 128
Antacids, 319–320, 336
Antagonist muscles, 144, 145, *145*
Anterior segment dysgenesis (ASD), 500
Anterior uveitis (ERU), 385–386, 445, *497–498*, **497–499,** 500
Antibiotics
 botulism, 527
 intestinal tract disease, 296
 muscle, 175
 ointments, absorption, 414–415
 skin, 375
 strangles, 275
 trailering, 482
Antibodies, 264–265, 266, 267
Antigenic drift, 266, 267
Antioxidants, 338
Antiseptic solutions, 405–406, 435–436
Antivenom, 432
Arabians
 cardiovascular system, 236
 conformation, 26, 29, 34, 35
 dental and oral cavity, 306, 310
 laminitis, 86
 muscle endurance, 143, 147, 167
 neurologic system, 518
 reproductive strategies, 535, 556
 respiratory system, 246, 250, 251
 skin as an organ, 360, 364, 372
Arachidonic acid prostaglandins, 444
Arched neck, 17, *17*, 18
Arrhythmias, 240, 279
Arteriovenous anastomoses (AVA), 357
Arthrodese, 128, *128*
Arthroscopic surgery, 123
Articular cartilage, joints, *109*, 110, 111, 116
Articular ringbone, 122, 128
Artificial insemination (AI), 550, 551, *551*, **553–555**
Arytenoid cartilages, 16

Arytenoid chondritis, 259
Ascarids (roundworms), 322, 460, *460*, 462, *462*, 467
Ascorbyl palmitate, 338
ASD (anterior segment dysgenesis), 500
Aspartate aminotransferase (AST), 170
Aspiration pneumonia, 295–296
Aspirin, 445
AST (aspartate aminotransferase), 170
Ataxia, 502, *502*, 504
Atlanto-axial "no" joint, 14
Atlanto-occipital "yes" joint, 14
Atlas vertebra, *8*, 14
Atrial fibrillation, 240
Ausculation, 293
AVA (arteriovenous anastomoses), 357
Avermectins, 466, *467*, 471
Avocado (*Persea americana*) toxicity, 283–284, 320
Avulsion, 187
Bacillus Calmette-Guerin (BCG) injections, 396, 396–397
Back at the knee (calf-kneed), 22, *22*, 24, 104
Backing a horse, restraint, 450
"Backing up the toe," 50, 60
Back pain, 203–217
  "cold-backed" horse and, 207
  conformation, *8–10*, *26–28*, *27*, *35*, *36*, *37*
  flexion tests for, 206
  hollow back vs. round back, 217, *217*
  identification of, *205*, 205–207
  manual stretch, 154–155, *155*
  misleading signs of, 207
  NSAIDs for, 215
  palpation of back, 205, *205*, 207
  signs of, 203–207, *204–205*
  therapy for, 214–217, *215–217*
  See also Back pain, causes of
Back pain, causes of, 207–214
  conformational faults, 212
  dental care (poor), 210
  dorsal spinous processes and, 212–213, *213–214*
  fistulous withers, 214, *214*
  fitness of horse and, 211
  fracture, *213*, 213–214
  hunter's bump and, *27*, 27, 30, *30*, **208**, *208*
  lameness, compensation, *211*, 211–212
  overriding ("kissing spines"), 30, **212–213**, *213*
  repetitive stress, 209
  rider and, *210*, 210–211
  roach back (kyphosis), 27, *27*, 30, *30*, **212**, *212*
  saddle fit and, *19*, *19*, *20*, 206–207, *209*, 209–210, *365*, 365–366
  scoliosis, 212
  shoeing issues, 211, *211*
  spinal infection, 214, *214*
  sway back (lordosis), 26, *27*, *27*,
212, **212**
  trauma, 207–211, *208–210*
  vertebral problems, 212–214, *212–214*
  See also Back pain
Bacteria infection
  identification of, 411
  lower respiratory, 273–279, *274*, 277
  neurologic system, 513–514, *514*
  stallion, culture, 537
  uterus, culture, 548, 548–549
Bacterial pneumonia, 259
Baking soda drench "milkshake," 336–337
Balance
  hoof, 53, *53*, 60, 62, *62*
  horse, 10–11, *12*
  neck and, *13*, 13–14, 15
  neurologic system, 501
Bandaging
  tendon injury from, 183
  tendons, **194**, *194*, 195, 196, 198, 202
  wounds, 416–419, *417*, *419*
Barefoot (unshod) foot, 58, 59
Barley, 330
Barn and cool-down, 160
Bars, hoof, *39*, 44, *44*
Basal cells, hoof, 40
Bascule, 14, *14*
Basement membrane, 42, 81
Base-narrow/wide chest, 20, *21*, *21*
Bastard strangles (metastatic strangles abscessation), 276–277
Baths, medicated for skin, 374
BCAAs (branched chain amino acids), 161
BCS (body condition scoring), 345–350, *347–350*. *See also* Nutritional management
"Beans" of smegma, 400, 401, *401*
Bedding dust, 256, 257, 261, 264, 481
Bee stings, 381, *381*
Beet pulp, 328–329
Belly lifts, 154
Belly tap (abdominocentesis), 302, 303, *303*, 312
Bench-kneed (offset cannon bones), 23, *23*, 24, 25, *25*, 104
Benign skin growths, 392
Benzimidazoles, 466, *467*, 471
Beveled (slippered) shoe, 60
Bicarbonate caution, 336
Big Head Disease (Nutritional Secondary Hyperparathyroidism), **107**, 329
Binocular vision, 488, 490–491
Biological control, external parasites, 383–384
Biorhythm and trailering, 484
Biotin, 67–68
Bit evasion, 248–249, 253
Biting midges (*Culicoides*), *378*, 378–379, 382, 383, 390
Bit seat, 286, *286*, 290
Bitting impact, respiratory system, 249–249, 253
Black flies (*Simulium*), 377, 377–378, 382
Black vs. white hoof, 47, *47*
Black walnut (*Juglans nigra*), 80
Black widow spider, 389
Bladder, ruptures, 563
Blanketing
  cool-down and, 159–160
  mare, 540
  respiratory system, 258
"Bleeders" (EIPH), *262*, 262–264
Bleeding, stopping, 426–427, *427*
Blindfold, 452
Blindness, 500
Blind spots, 490, 491, *491*
Blind staggers (moldy corn poisoning), 527
Blister beetle toxicity, 321
Block and tackle mechanics, muscle, 138
Blood boosters, 161–162
Blood lactate levels, 152
Bloodroot (*Sanguinaria canadensis*), 397
Blood tests, 457–458
Blood vessels
  cardiovascular system, 219, 221
  hoof, 42, *42*, 46
  skin, 357, *357*
Bloodworms (strongyles), 322, 460, *460–461*, 461–462, 467
Blunt trauma, 410–411, 423–424, **423–424**
Body clipping, 159, *159*
Body condition scoring (BCS), 345–350, *347–350*. *See also* Nutritional management
Body language of horse, 1, 6
Body trauma, neurologic system, 523, *523*
Body water balance, 333
Body weight and trailering, 483–484
Bog spavin, 31, **120**, *120*
Bone development, 95–107
  ample bone, 9, 24, 25, *25*
  bone mineral content, 99, 102, 105
  calcium reservoir, bone as, 96
  conformation impact, 95, *95*
  density of bone, 99
  extracorporeal shock wave therapy (ESWT), **106–107**, 130
  genetics impact, 98, 99
  ligaments interaction with, 99
  mineral within bone, 95–96
  muscle interaction with bone, 99–100
  Nutritional Secondary Hyperparathyroidism (Big Head Disease), **107**, 329
  parathyroid hormone and, 107, 164–165
  size of bone and performance, 98–99
  system, bone as a, 95–98
  tendons interaction with, 99
  therapy for, **106–107**, 130
  See also Bone response to conditioning;

Cannon bones; Pasterns; Remodeling process of bone
Bone response to conditioning, 100–105
   bone fractures, 103
   bucked shins, 101, 103, *103*
   "closed" growth plates, 102, 112, *112*
   fatigue state of bones, 103
   fractured splint, 104, 105, *105*
   high-speed training, 100–101
   interval training (IT), 100
   long, slow distance (LSD) training, 100
   nutritional management, 100, 105, 107
   overtraining, 102–105, *103–105*
   pastern joint and, 112, *112*
   peak strength, conditioning, 100–102
   performance and, 98–100
   remodeling process of bone and, 103
   splints, 24, **103–105**, *104–105*, 424, *424*
   strength, skeletal, 101
   See also Bone development; Remodeling process of bone
Bone spavin, 31, 33, **120**, *120*, 130, 211, *211*
Bone spurs (enthesiophytes), 90
Bony spine, 14, *14*
Booking to a stallion, 534
Boosters, 265, 266, 270, 456
Boots vs. shoes, 59, 59–60, 65
Borborygmi (waves of contractions), 301
Boredom relief, 477
Borium caulks, **62–63**, *63*, 97, 184, 211
Borrelia burgdorferi, 136
Bot flies (*Gasterophilus intestinalis*), 379, *460*, 462
Bot larvae and worms, 379, 460, *460*, 462–463, *462–463*, 467
Botulism, 505, **525–527**
Bowed tendon, 24, 26, 183, 184, **185**, *185*, 191, *191*
Bowel, *291*, 292
Bowker, Robert M., 87
Bow-legged (carpus varus), 22, 23, *23*, 24, 33, *33*
"Box" guidelines for balance, 10
Bradykinin and NSAIDs, 442
Braken fern (*Pterydium aquilinium*), 528
Branched chain amino acids (BCAAs), 161
Branching airways, 249
Brand inspection, 457
Bran for colic, 314–315
Breakover, hoof, 24, 49, **49–50**, 52, 60
Breathing, 249–251, *250*, 252
Breeding contract, 534
Breeding performance, stallion, 532–534, *533*
Breeding process, 550–553, *551–553*. *See also* Reproductive strategies

Broken-back hoof-pastern axis, **50–51**, *51*, 60, 183
Broken-forward hoof-pastern axis (club foot), 52, **52–53**, 87, *87*, 200, *200*
"Broken wind" (chronic obstructive pulmonary disease), **260**, 456
Bronchioles, *245*, 249, 261
Bronchoalveolar lavage, 262
Bronchoconstriction, 259, 260, 261
Bucked-kneed (over at the knee), 22, *22*, 24
Bucked shins, 101, 103, *103*
Buffalo gnats (*Simulium*), 377, 377–378, 382
Bursa injury, 114
Bursitis theory, navicular, 86
Bute. *See* Phenylbutazone
Calcium
   muscle, concentrations, 138, 169–170
   muscle performance and imbalance, 163–164, 165, 166
   reservoir, bone as, 96
Calcium bicarbonate caution, 336
Calcium-to-phosphorus (Ca:P) ratio, 327, 329, 337
Calf-kneed (back at the knee), 22, *22*, 24, 104
Calf roping, 141, 142
Calisthenics, 151
Calmness, creating, 447–448
Camped-out, 31, 32, *32*
Canker, 63, **73**
Cannon bones
   bone development, 98, *98*, 99, 100
   conformation, 8, 8–9, 23, *23*, 24–25, *25*, 35, 36, 37
   remodeling, 98, *98*
   tendons and ligaments, *181*, 185–187, *185–187*
Cantharidin toxicosis, 321
Capillary refill time (CRT), 231, *231*, 236
Capped elbow (shoe boil), 114, *114*
Capped hock, **114**, *114*, 475
Capsulitis, 111, 113, *113*
Carbohydrates
   laminitis and overload, 75, **76–77**, 82
   large intestine digestion, 292–293, 325
   muscle energy, 139, 142, 325
Carbon dioxide, 141, 249, 250
Carbon monoxide, 256
Cardiac recovery index (CRI), *230*, 230–231, 239
Cardiotachometer. *See* Heart rate monitor
Cardiovascular system, 219–243
   blood vessels, 219, 221
   combination exercise, 220
   electrocardiogram (ECG) studies, 221
   equipment, *222*, 222–224
   exercise and adaptions, 220–222
   heart efficiency, 220–221
   heart rate monitor (cardiotachometer), *222*, **222–224**, 229, *230*

   intestinal tract and, 221–222
   lactic acid, 220, 223
   long, slow distance (LSD) training, 223, **226–227**
   respiratory adaptations, 251–252
   respiratory rate, 221, 240, **250**, **251**, 300, 429
   spleen, 219–220
   vascular network, 219
   working heart rate, 223, 224
   See also Cardiovascular system response to conditioning; Exercise intolerance
Cardiovascular system response to conditioning, 224–233
   aerobic capacity, 226
   anaerobic workouts, 220, 228
   detraining, 233
   evaluating cardiovascular conditioning, 229–233, *230–231*
   intensity, increasing, 226–227
   interval training (IT), 227–228
   long, fast distance training, 229
   nutritional management, 231–232
   "progressive training" methods, 224
   repetition, value of, 225
   speed play (fartleks), 228
   strength training, 227
   swimming, value of, 225–226, *226*
   target heart rates, 226
   walking, value of, 225
   See also Cardiovascular system; Exercise intolerance
Carnitine, 161
Carotid artery, 441
Carpal hypoflexion, 135, *135*
Carpus valgus (knock-kneed), 22, 23, *23*, 24, 104, 134, *134*
Carrier horses, 241, 242, 272, 274–275, 455
Carrot stretches, 154–155, *155*
Caslick's surgery (episioplasty), 545–546, *546*
Cataplexy, muscle, 519
Cataract, 499, *499*, 500, 535
Catecholamines, 252
Catheter (IV), 441
Cattle implants for mare, 542
Cauda equina (PNE), **519**, 527
Caudal heel pain, 50
Caulks, shoes, **62–63**, *63*, 97, 184, 211
"Caved in," 36
Cavities (casies), 288
CBC (complete blood count), 457–458
Cecum, *291*, 292
C-ELISA (Competitive Enzyme-Linked Immunosorbent Assay), 457
Cell mediated immunity (CMI), 272
Cellular fluid, bone, 99
Cellulitis, 422, *422*, **438**, 475
Center of mass and balance, 10–11, *12*
Central sulcus, hoof, *39*, 44–45, 45
Cereal grain hay (oat hay), 327
Cerebrospinal fluid (CSF) tests, 512
Cervical joints, 8, *14*, 14–15

Cervical vertebral malformation (CVM), 132, **134**, 328, 511, **517**, 535
Cervix, 547
Chemicals
　fly control, 382–383
　fusion, joints, 116
　proud flesh, chemicals for, 416
　restraint with, 453–454
Chemistry panel, 458
Chemotherapeutic agents, 397
Chest conformation, 8–*10*, 20, 21, *21*, 36
Chewing, 282, *282*, 284, *284*
Chiggers (*trombiculiasis*), 385
Chiropractic for back pain, 215
Chlorhexidine, 406, 414, 428, 435, 561–562
Chloride imbalance, 163
Choke, 295–296, **295–297**, 328
Chondroids from strangles, 277
Chondroitin sulfate, 127
Chondroprotective drugs, 125–126
Chorioptic mange/mites, 369, 384
Chromium tripicolinate, 80
Chronic choke (esophageal obstruction), 284, **296**
Chronic obstructive pulmonary disease (COPD), **260**, 456
Ciliary muscles, *489*, 490
Cimetidine, 398–399
Circulating antibodies, 268
Circulatory compromise, laminitis, 75–76, *76*
Circumduction, 502
Circumflex artery, 75, 76, *76*
CK (creatine phosphokinase), 170
Claviceps spp., 558
Cleansing
　injection site, 435–436
　wounds, 403, 404, *405*, 405–406
Clenbuterol, 262, *262*
Climatic considerations, performance, 4
"Closed" growth plates, 102, 112, *112*
Clostridium
　intestinal tract, 294
　neurologic system, 513–514, 525, 526, 527
　wound management, 422, *422*, 430, 438
Clotrimazole, 374
Club foot (broken-forward hoof-pastern axis), 52, **52–53**, 87, *87*, 200, *200*
CMI (cell mediated immunity), 272
Coastal Bermuda grass (*Cynodon* spp.), 306
Coffin bone and joint
　arthritis, 90, 129
　conditioning response, 112, *112*
　hoof, *40*, 41, 42, 43, 45, 50, 52, 58
　laminitis, 81–82, 83, *83*, 84, *85*, 85
　navicular syndrome, 86, 87, *87*, 88
Coggins, LeRoy, 457
Coggins Test, 242–243, 455, **457**
"Cold-backed" horse, 207
Cold therapy
　joints, 131
　laminitis, 82
　muscle, 177–178
　tendons, 182–183, **192–194,** *193*, 198
Cold weather feeding, 341, 344–345
Colic, 297–323
　belly tap (abdominocentesis), 302, 303, *303*, 312
　blister beetle toxicity, 321
　bran for, 314–315
　cantharidin toxicosis, 321
　Coastal Bermuda grass (*Cynodon* spp.), 306
　cold water after exercise and, 317
　confinement effects, 305
　cool-down and, 157
　defined, 297
　dehydration effects, 300, *301*, 317–318, 333, *334*
　dental problems, 284, 285, 288
　displacement, 308, 309, *309*
　enteroliths, 306, *306*
　exercise and, 316–317
　feces and dehydration, 236, **237**, *237*, 302, 303, 317
　gaseous colic, **308–309**, 308–309, 327
　gastric ulcer syndrome (GUS), **318–320**, 326, 445–446
　heart rate and, 300, *301*
　hypermotile gut, 303
　ileum, *291*, 304, 308, 316
　impaction colic, 303–308, 316
　incarcerated piece of bowel, 308
　internal parasites and, 294, 321–322
　intussusception, 303, 309, 464
　life-style effects, 305
　lipomas (intestinal), 308–309, 309–310, *310*, 352
　mesentery (bowel lining) and, 297
　mesentery tear, 308
　mucous membranes and, 299–300, *299–300*
　necrosis (tissue death), 303
　nephrosplenic entrapment, 309
　non-strangulation infarction, 322
　NSAIDs and, 307, 320, 443
　nutritional management, 304–305, 305–306, 313, *313*, 315–316, 319, 322–323, 326, 328, 329
　obese horses and, 352
　organophosphate dewormers and, 303
　pain of horse, interpreting, 298–299
　peritonitis, 310, 429, 462, *463*
　plant toxicity, 320–321
　prevention of, 307, 313–315, 321, 322–323
　psyllium for, **313–314**, 332
　radiographs (X-rays), 312, *312*
　rectal examination, 301–302, 312
　reduced bowel function, effects of, 317
　respiratory rate and, 300
　risk factors (highest) for, 315–316
　roundworms (ascarids) and, 322, 460, 462, *462*
　sand colic, 302, 310–315, *311–313*
　shock, *299*, 299–300
　signs of, 297–298, *298*, 311, 318, 321
　spasmodic colic, 303
　stomach (nasogastric) tube, 296, *296*, **302**
　strangulation obstruction, 308
　strongyles (bloodworms) and, 322, 460, *460*, **461**
　surgery for, 298–299, 315
　torsion (twist), 30, 308, 309
　treatment for, 319–320
　trotting a horse for, 298
　tying-up syndrome, 171
　ulcerative colitis, 320
　ultrasound for, 302, 312
　undetermined diagnosis, 302
　vital signs, 299–301, *299–301*, 367
　volvulus, 308, *308–309*
　walking a horse for, 298, 299
　water drinking importance, 296, 304–305, 313
　See also Intestinal tract
Collagen, 97, 419
Collapsed heels, 60, 63, *63*
Collateral cartilage complex theory, navicular, 87–88
Collateral ligaments, 182
Colon, *291*, 292, 293
Color vision, 492
Colostrum, 557, 561
Combination exercise, 142–143, 220
Combined driving, 142, 162, 222
Companionship for trailering, 482
Competing excessively, avoiding, 6
Competition regulations, NSAIDs, **443–444**, 457
Competitive Enzyme-Linked Immunosorbent Assay (C-ELISA), 457
Complete blood count (CBC), 457–458
Complete feed pellets, 328, 332–333, 476
Compression and tension, bone, 97
Compressive strain, bone, 96
Concavity (dishing), 54, 55, *55*, 74, 84, *85*, 85
Concentrates, feed, 326, 328, 329–330, 332
Concentric contraction, 139
Concussion, hoof, 40–42, *42*, 45–46, 48, 52
Concussion injury, tendons, 184
Conditioning
　body condition scoring (BCS), 345–350, *347–350*
　levels of, 224, 225, *225*
　respiratory system, 251
　skin as an organ, 359–360, *360–361*, 362
　strategies, 4, 5–6
　See also Bone response to conditioning; Cardiovascular system response to conditioning; Muscle response to conditioning

Confinement impact on
    colic, 305
    dental problems, 281, 282, 285, 305
    muscle injury, 178
    stress, 473–474, 476
Conformation, 7–38
    back, 8–10, 26–28, 27, 35, 36, 37
    back pain, 212
    bone development, 95, 95
    cannon bone, 8, 8–9, 23, 23, 24–25, 25, 35, 36, 37
    chest, 8–10, 20, 21, 21, 36
    croup, 8–10, 28, 28–29, 29, 35–36
    dressage horses, 13, 13, 16, 17, 18, 23, 28, 31, 37
    eyes, 9, 12
    fetlocks, 8–9, 34
    forearm, 8–10, 24, 36, 37
    forelimb alignment, 22, 22–23
    head, 8–10, 11–12
    hind legs, lower portion of, 8–9, 34
    hindquarters, 8–10, 28–30, 28–31, 35, 36, 37
    hocks, 8–9, 9, 31–34, 33–34, 35, 37
    ideal conformation, 7
    jaws, 8–9, 12
    joints, 111
    jumpers, 14, 14, 16, 23, 25, 26, 28, 36–37
    knees (carpus), 8, 8–10, 9, 22, 22–23, 24, 35
    loins, 9–10, 27–28, 28, 35, 36
    lower portion of rear limb, 8–9, 34
    neck, 8–10, 11, 13–15, 13–18, 17–18, 35, 36–37
    nostrils, 9, 11
    osteoarthritis and, 22, 24, 33, 34
    pasterns, 8–9, 25–26, 25–26, 36
    pelvis and croup angle, 28–30, 29–30
    shoulder, 8–10, 20–22, 21, 35, 36, 37
    sports specific, 34–37
    stifle, 8–10, 9, 29, 30, 30, 31, 32, 32, 33, 33, 36, 37
    stretching through the topline (longitudinal flexion), 18–19
    stride length and, 15, 20–22, 21, 31
    tendons and ligaments, 183–184
    throatlatch, 9, 12, 15
    upper arm, 8–10, 21, 22–23
    Western pleasure horses, 34–36
    withers, 8–10, 18–20, 19, 35, 36
    See also Anatomy and function; Back pain
Congenital angular limb deformity, 134–135, 135
Congenital flexural contracture, 198–199
Conjunctivitis, 493, 493
Contaminated medication, 434
Continuous dewormers (Strongid-C), 466–467, 467, 469–470
Continuous wave ultrasound, 197
Contours (hoof), abnormal, 54–55, **54–56**, 74, 79
Contracted heels (narrow heels), 48, 49, 49, 86

Contracted tendons, 328, 564, **564**
Contraction, wounds, **407–410**, 408–410, 419
Contraction of muscle, 138–139
Convection, 257
Convective cooling, skin, 359
Cook, W. Robert, 258
Cool-down exercises, 156–160
    barn and, 160
    blanketing and, 159–160
    body clipping and, 159, 159
    bone response to conditioning, 105
    colic and, 157
    cool weather, 158–159, 158–160
    drying the hair coat, 159
    enclosed barn and, 160
    fat insulation, delaying cool-down, 158
    food after, 157
    insulation, delaying cool-downs, 158, 158, 159, 159
    joints, 131
    lactic acid, removal of, 156
    massage, 157, 157
    rump rug for, 158, 158
    sponging head, neck, chest, legs, 157, 157
    walking, 156, 156, 159
    warm weather cool-downs, 157, 157–158
    water after, 157
    wet horse, blanketing, 160
    See also Muscle response to conditioning; Warm-up exercises
Cooling a fever, 429–430, 430
Cooling methods, 357–359, 358
COPD (chronic obstructive pulmonary disease), **260**, 456
Copper deficiency and DOD, 337
Coprophagy (manure eating), 461
Coral snakes, 430
Corium, hoof, 41, 41–42, 42, 84
Corn, 329–330, 332, 342
Cornea, 488–489, 489–490
Corneal edema, 495, 495
Corneal ulcer or laceration, 376, **494–496**, 495
Corneocytes, hoof, 40
Corns, hoof, 63, 64, **71–72**, 72
Coronary band, 40, 41, 41, 56, 56, 67
Corpora nigra, 488, 489
Corrective shoeing, 62
Cortical walls, 97
Corticosteroids for
    back pain, 215
    bone response to conditioning, 105
    healing wounds, 416
    laminitis, 78, 79
    navicular syndrome, 92–93
    osteoarthritis, 127
Corticosteroids/hyaluronic acid ("white acid"), 127
Cortisol, 257–258, 481–482
Corynebacteria organisms, 174–175, 176, 377
Coughing, 255
Counterbalance, 13–14, 13–14
Coupling, 26

Cow-hocked, 32, 33, 33, 34, 35
"Cow" sense, 35
COX-1/2 (cyclooxygenase), 444, 445
CPK (creatine phosphokinase), 170
Cracked heels (scratches), 367–369, **367–371**, 384
Cracks, hoof, 55, 55, 57–58, 57–58, 60
Cramps, muscle, 168–169, 168–169
Cranial nerves, 501, 502
Creatine phosphokinase (CPK), 170
"Creeping" of cartilage, 110
Crepitation, 422, 438
Crevices (sulci), hoof, 39, 44–45, 45, 73
CRI (cardiac recovery index), 230, 230–231, 239
Cribbing, 285, 288, 288, 289, 475
Crookedness of limbs, 8–9
Cross-protective antibodies, 265
Cross-reactivity caution, 162
Cross-ties, 449–450
Cross-training, 150–151
Cross-ventilation, 256–257
Croup conformation, 8–10, 28, 28–29, 29, 35–36
CRT (capillary refill time), 231, 231, 236
Cryotherapy. See Cold therapy
CSF (cerebrospinal fluid) tests, 512
Cumulative overuse, tendons, 183
Cup of hoof, 36, 48, 48
Curb (inflammation of plantar tarsal ligament), 31, 34, **187**, 187
Custom-tailored training, 3–5
Cutaneous habronemiasis (summer sores), 383, **388–389**, 395, **463**, 467, 536
Cutting. See Reining and cutting
CVM (cervical vertebral malformation), 132, **134**, 328, 511, **517**, 535
Cyclooxygenase (COX-1/2), 444, 445
Cyproheptidine, 78
Cysts (demineralization) and navicular syndrome, 90
Cytology evaluation of uterus, 549
DDFT. See Deep digital flexor tendon
DDSP (dorsal displacement of the soft palate), **259**, 511
Dead-end hosts, 504
Debridement, 404, 405, 405, 408, 408
Debulking, wounds, 408, 408
Deep digital flexor tendon (DDFT)
    hoof and, 40, 45, 46, 49, 50, 181
    injury, 181, 187–188, 187–188
    laminitis, 81, 83, 181
    navicular syndrome, 85, 86, 87, 87, 88, 181
Deerflies (Chrysops), 241–242, 376, 382
Deer ticks, 388
Degenerative joint disease (DJD), 109. See also Osteoarthritis
Degenerative myocardial disease, 240
Degenerative suspensory desmitis, 188–189, 189
Dehydration impact on
    cardiovascular system, 234, 235, **235–239**, 237–238

colic, 300, *300,* 317–318, 333, *334*
cycle, 333, *334*
feces, 236, **237,** *237,* 302, 303, 317
muscle, 166
respiratory system, 253–254
trailering, 484
tying-up syndrome, 167
Delayed patella release (upward fixation of the patella), 31, 33, **118–119,** *119,* 518
Demodectic mange/mites, 384
Density of bone, 99
Dental and oral cavity, 281–323
    bit seat, 286, *286,* 290
    chewing and teeth wear, 282, *282, 284, 284*
    eruption process of teeth, 282, 285, *285*
    evolution of horse, 281
    molars, 282, 286
    nutritional demands and, 282, *282, 284, 284*
    temporomandibular joint (TMJ), 288, 289
    wear of teeth, 282
    See also Dental problems; Intestinal tract
Dental problems, 282–291
    avocado (*Persea americana*) toxicity, 283–284, 320
    back pain and, 210
    cavities (casies) 288
    colic from, 284, 285, 288
    confinement impact on, 281, 282, 285, 305
    cribbing, 285, 288, *288,* 289, 475
    equine dentistry, 289–291, *290*
    floating teeth, 286, 289–290, *290*
    health signs of, 284, *284*
    hooks on teeth, 285, 288, *288,* 290, *290*
    hypersalivation, 282–283
    incisor overgrowth, 286–287, *287*
    incisors, 285, 289, 289
    overbite, 287, *287*
    parrot mouth, 12, 287, 535
    performance signs of, 285–286
    prevention of, 282, 283, 290–291
    ramps on teeth, 285, 288
    retained caps, 286
    salivation, excessive, 282–283
    sharp points on teeth, 286
    vesicular stomatitis (VSV), 283, *283*
    wave mouth, 285, 287
    wear abnormalities, 286–288, *287–288*
    wolf teeth, 286, *286*
    See also Dental and oral cavity
Dermatitis, 367
Dermatophilus congolensis, 369, 371, *375*
Dermatophytosis, 372–374, *373*
Dermocenter (tick), 387, 387–388
Desmitis (injury to ligament), 183
Desmotomy of navicular suspensory ligaments, 93

Detomidine, 453
Detraining, 151–152, 233, 252
Developmental Orthopedic Disease (DOD), 131–136
    acquired angular limb deformity, 135
    angular limb deformities (ALD), 22, 22–23, *23,* 103, *134–135,* **134–136,** 535
    congenital angular limb deformity, 134–135, *135*
    epiphysitis (physeal dysplasia), *132,* **132–133,** 199, *199,* 328, 337, 353
    flexural contracture, 52, 132
    nutritional imbalance, 131–132, 133, 134, 135, 329, 337
    osteochondrosis (OCD), 120, 132, **133–134,** 328, 337, 353, 517, 535
    shoes and pads for, 136
    surgery for ALD, 136
    wobbler syndrome (cervical vertebral malformation), 132, **134,** 328, 511, **517,** 535
    See also Joint injury and disease
Deworming, 264, 459, 460, *460,* **466–472,** *467,* 540
Dew poisoning (rain scald), 369, 371, 375
Diaphragm, 247, 249, 250, 252
Diarrhea, 284, **293–295,** 311, 333, *334,* 336
Diastole (filling stage), 221
Dietary manipulation of muscle endurance, 160–165, *164. See also* Muscle endurance
Digestive system. *See* Dental and oral cavity; Intestinal tract
Digital cushion, hoof, 40, *40,* 42, *42,* 46, 52, 58
Digital pulse, hoof, 69
Dimethyl glycine (DMG), 161
Dimethyl sulfoxide (DMSO) for
    laminitis, 80
    osteoarthritis, 127–128
    tendon injury, 195
    West Nile Virus (WNV), 506
    wounds, 415
Discharge (exudate), 404
Dishing (concavity), 54, 55, *55,* 74, 84, 85, *85*
Displacement, colic, 308, 309, *309*
Distal intertarsal joint, 32
Distal sesamoid bone, 85, 86, 87, *87,* 182
Distal sesamoideon ligaments, *181,* 184
Distal suspensory impar ligament, 87–88
Distemper. *See* Strangles
DJD. *See* Degenerative joint disease
D-L methionine, 68
DMG (dimethyl glycine), 161
DMSO. *See* Dimethyl sulfoxide
DNA polymerase chain reaction (PCR) test, 512
DOD. *See* Developmental Orthopedic Disease
Domperidone, 559

Dorsal colon, *291,* 292
Dorsal displacement of the soft palate (DDSP), **259,** 511
Dorsal laminar arteries, 75, 76, *76*
Dorsal spinous processes, 212–213, *213–214*
"Downhill" frame, 35
Draft horses, 47, 172, 369, 518
Drainage, wounds, 411, *411*
Dressage horses
    back pain, 213
    bone development, 98
    cardiovascular system, 220
    conformation, 13, *13,* 16, 17, 18, 23, 28, 31, 37
    joints, 111
    muscle endurance, 142, 148, 152
    respiratory system, 247
Dressings, hoof, 67
Drift, virus, 266, 267
Droplet nuclei, 255
Drug names, uses, actions, 368–370
Drug testing profile, 458
Drying the hair coat, cool-down, 159
Dryland distemper (pigeon breast, pigeon fever), *174,* **174–176,** 273, 377
Dryland pasture, roughage, 281, *281*
Dummy foal (NMS), 563
Duran, Stephen, 340
Dynamic balance, hoof, 53, *53*
Dystocia, 559–560
Dystrophic calcification, 338
Ear gnats (*Simulium*), 377, 377–378, 382
Ear inflammation, 514–515, *515*
"Earring down," 451
Eastern equine encephalitis (EEE), **508,** 540
Eccentric contraction, muscle, 139
ECD (Equine Cushing's Disease), **77–78,** *77–78,* 500
ECF (extracellular fluid), 235
ECG (electrocardiogram) studies, 221
Echocardiography studies, 221
Effusion (filling of joint capsule), 118, *118*
Egg bar shoes, **91,** *91,* 124, 188
Ehrlichia equi (Anaplasma phagocytophila), 201, 388
Ehrlichia risticii, 294
EHV1/4 (equine herpesvirus), 268, **270–273,** *271,* 456, 497, **508–509,** 511, 516, 536, 540
EIA (equine infectious anemia), **241–243,** 376, 457, 536
EIPH (exercise-induced pulmonary hemorrhage), 262, 262–264
Electrical muscle stimulation (EMS), 138, 139, 179
Electrical therapies for muscle, 178–180
Electroanalgesia for muscle, 179
Electrocardiogram (ECG) studies, 221
Electrolyte supplementation, 333–337
    antacids with, 336

body water balance regulated by, 333
cautions, 336–337
commercial electrolyte products, 335–336
dehydration cycle, 333, 334
depletion, tying-up syndrome, 169, 171, 333, 334
diarrhea from excess, 336
dietary manipulation of muscle endurance, 152, 162–165, 164
dosages of, 335, 335, 336, 340
electrical impulses mediated by, 333
electrolyte depletion, 169, 171, 333, 334
hot climate feeding, 344
imbalance, exercise intolerance, 236, 240
loss, 296
muscle and, 152, 162–165, 164
reabsorption, intestinal tract, 292, 293
salt content in, 335–336
sodium bicarbonate drench ("milk shake"), 336–337
sweating and electrolytes, 162–163, 164, 165, 333, 334, 356
See also Nutritional management
Electromyography, 518
Electrostimulation for back pain, 214
Emaciated horse (BCS 1), 345, 346, 347, 347
Embryonic migration, 550
Embryo transfer (ET), 555
EMND (equine motor neuron disease), 511, **517–518**
Empyema from strangles, 277
EMS (electrical muscle stimulation), 138, 139, 179
Encephalomalacia (moldy corn poisoning), 527
Endopararites, 459. See also Internal parasites and control
Endophytic fungus (*Neotyphodium, Acremonium*), 558
Endorphins, 178, 451–452
Endoscope, 259, 262, 264
Endotoxin, 293, 294, 300, 300, 317
Endurance exercise. See Aerobic
Energy absorption, hoof, 40–42, 42, 45–46, 48, 52
Energy and nutritional management, 325–326
Energy production, muscle, 140–143
Enhanced cyclic loading, joints, 111
Enkephalins, 178, 451–452
Enteroliths, 306, 306
Enthesiophytes (bone spurs), 90
Environmental management
external parasites, 381
internal parasites, 459, 465–466
Environmental stress, trailering, 478–484, 479
Enzymatic damage, joints, 115, 115–116
Enzymes (degraded), removing from joint, 122–123
Enzymes and damage, tying-up syndrome, 170, 458
Eohippus, 104
Epaxial muscles, 208
Epidermal lamellae, hoof, 42
Epidermis, hoof, 66
Epiglottic entrapment, 259
Epinephrine (adrenaline), 439–440
Epiphora, 492
Epiphysitis (physeal dysplasia), 132, **132–133**, 199, 199, 328, 337, 353
Episioplasty (Caslick's surgery), 545–546, 546
Epithelial cells, 255, 261
Epithelialization, 407, 408, 408, 419
EPM (equine protozoal myelitis), 500, 505, **510–513**, 511, 516, 517, 520
EPO (erythropoietin), 161–162
Epsom salt soaks, 70, 70, 71, 195
EPSSM (equine polysaccharide storage myopathy), 165, 167, **172–173**, 518, 541
Equine Cushing's Disease (ECD), **77–78**, 77–78, 500
Equine dentistry, 289–291, 290. See also Dental and oral cavity
Equine distemper. See Strangles
Equine encephalitis (sleeping sickness), 381, 505, **508**, 540
Equine granutocytic ehrlichiosis (*Anaplasma phagocytophila*), 388
Equine herpesvirus (EHV1/4), 268, **270–273**, 271, 456, 497, **508–509**, 511, 516, 536, 540
Equine infectious anemia (EIA), **241–243**, 376, 457, 536
Equine influenza ("flu"), **267–270**, 268, 456, 497, 540
Equine metabolic syndrome (peripheral cushingold syndrome), 78, **78–80**, 353
Equine motor neuron disease (EMND), 511, **517–518**
Equine polysaccharide storage myopathy (EPSSM), 165, 167, **172–173**, 518, 541
Equine protozoal myelitis (EPM), 500, 505, **510–513**, 511, 516, 517, 520
Equine recurrent uveitis (ERU), 385–386, 445, 497–498, **497–499**, 500
Equine relapsing fever (EIA), **241–243**, 376, 457, 536
Ergogenic acids, 160–162
Ergot alkaloids, 558
ERU (equine recurrent uveitis), 385–386, 445, 497–498, **497–499**, 500
Eruption process, teeth, 282, 285, 285
ERV (rhinovirus), 268, **272–273**, 456
Erythema and NSAIDs, 442
Erythropoietin (EPO), 161–162
Eschar formation from burns, 425–426
Esophageal obstruction (chronic choke), 284, **296**
Esophagus, 292, 296
Estrus cycle, 534, 539, **540–543**, 542
detecting for breeding, 550–551, 551–552, 552
ESWT. See Extracorporeal shock wave therapy
ET (embryo transfer), 555
Evaporative cooling, skin, 357, 358, 358
Evolution of horse, 281
Ewe neck, 17–18, 17–18
Exercise-induced pulmonary hemorrhage (EIPH), 262, 262–264
Exercise intolerance, 233–243
anemia, 233, **241–243, 252–253**, 337, 457
dehydration, 234, 235, **235–239**, 237–238, 300, 300
electrolyte imbalance, 236, 240
equine infectious anemia (EIA), **241–243**, 376, 457, 536
fatigue, signs of, 239, 239–240
heart irregularities, 233, 240
overtraining, 234
stress indicators, 239, 239–240
See also Cardiovascular system; Cardiovascular system response to conditioning
Exercise physiology, insights, 1. See also Conditioning; Organ systems and performance
Exertional rhabdomyolysis, 166
Exhalation, 247, 250
Expiration date, drugs, 433
Extensor muscles, 139
External parasites and control, 376–389
avermectins, 466, 467, 471
bee stings, 381, 381
benzimidazoles, 466, 467, 471
biological control, 383–384
biting midges (*Culicoides*), 378, 378–379, 382, 383, 390
black flies (*Simulium*), 377, 377–378, 382
black widow spider, 389
bot flies (*Gasterophilus intestinalis*), 379, 460, 462
chemical fly control, 382–383
chiggers (*trombiculiasis*), 385
chorioptic mange/mites, 369, 384
deerflies (*Chrysops*), 241–242, 376, 382
demodectic mange/mites, 384
environmental management, 381
equine granutocytic ehrlichiosis (*Anaplasma phagocytophila*), 388
face flies (*Musca autumnalis*), 376, 382
facemasks for, 381–382, 382, 399
feed-through fly control (*tetrachlorv inphos*), 383
flies and gnats, 376–382, 377–382, 384
focal ventral midline dermatitis, 379–380
horn flies (*Haematobia*), 379–380, 382

horseflies (*Tabannus*), 241–242, 376, 382
houseflies (*Musca domestica*), 376, 382
ivermectin and, 383, 384, 385–386, 387, 389, 466, 467, 469
lice (pediculosis), 386, 386–387
microfilaria and, 385, *385*
mosquitoes, 380, *380–381*, **381**, 383, 390, **507–508**
nodular necrobiosis, *380*, **380–381**, 442
NSAIDs for, 389
Onchocerca worm, 383, *385*, **385–386**, 390, 467, 497
organophosphates, 303, 466, 467
pelodera strongyloides, 386
pinworms (*Oxyuris equi*), 379, *379*, *460*, *460*, *463–464*, **463–464**, 467
piperazine, 466, 467
praziquantel, 466, 467
psoroptic mange, 384
pyrethins, pyrethoids for, 383, 387
Queensland's itch (summer itch), *378*, 378–379
"rat" tail from, 378, *378*
rhabditic dermatitis, 386
sarcoptic mange/mites, 384
scabies (psoroptic mites), 384
spinous ear tick (*Otobius*), 171, 387, **387, 515,** 516
stable flies (*Stomoxys calcitrans*), 376–377, 382
stinging wasps (*parasitoids*) for, 383–384
straw-itch mites, 385
stress from, 376
summer sores (*Habronema, Draschia*), 383, **388–389**, 395, **463**, 467, 536
ticks, 171, 387, **387, 515,** 516
warbles (heel flies) (*Hypoderma*), **380,** 513
See also Internal parasites and control; Preventive health; Skin diseases
Extracellular fluid (ECF), 235
Extracorporeal shock wave therapy (ESWT)
bone development, **106–107**, 130
osteoarthritis, **106–107**, 130
tendon and ligament injury, 187, **198**
Exuberant granulation (proud flesh), 388, 394, 407, *407*, 408, 409, *409*, **416,** 418
Exudate (discharge), 404
Eye injury and disease, 492–500
anterior segment dysgenesis (ASD), 500
blindness, 500
cataract, 499, *499*, 500, 535
conjunctivitis, 493, *493*
corneal edema, 495, *495*
corneal ulcer or laceration, 376, **494–496**, *495*
epiphora, 492
equine recurrent uveitis (ERU), 385–386, 445, 497–498, **497–499,** 500
eyelid trauma, 494, *494*
facemasks for, 496–497, *497*
flourescein dye, 495, *495*
human ophthalmic lubricating ointments for, 496
irrigation for, 496
lipopigment deposition in retina, 518
managing a painful eye, 496–497, *497*
"menace response," 500, 502
NSAIDs for, 496
ocular discharge (abnormal), 492–493, *493*
phthisis bulbi, 498, *498*
synechia, 498
tumors of eye, 499, *499*
See also Eyes
Eyes, 487–500
accommodation, 490
anatomy of eye, 488–489
binocular vision, 488, 490–491
blind spots, 490, 491, *491*
ciliary muscles, *489*, 490
color vision, 492
conformation, 9, 12
cornea, 488–489, 489–490
corpora nigra, 488, *489*
focus and perception, 490–492, *491*
index of refraction, 489–490
lens, 489, 489–490
mental perception, 487–488
nasolacrimal duct, 492, *493*
panoramic field of vision, 490, *491*
pupil, 488–489
refraction, 489–490
retina, 489, *489*, 490
riding and, 487–488, 491–492
spooky behavior, 487–488, 491–492
third eyelid (nictitating membrane), 488, **490,** 516
See also Eye injury and disease
Eyeworms (*Thelazia*), 376, 383, 467
Face flies (*Musca autumnalis*), 376, 382
Facemasks, 381–382, *382*, 399, 496–497, *497*
Facial wounds, 411–412, *412, 413, 413*
Fainting spell (syncope), 240, 520
Fallen horse, 520–524, *522–523*
Farrier care, 4, 6. *See also* Hoof; Shoes and pads
Fartleks (speed play), 228
Fascia, muscle, 137, 144, 145, *145*
Faster gaits, muscle conditioning, 150
Fast twitch high oxidative muscle fibers (FTH, Type II A), 143–144, 145, 146, 147, 148, 225, 228
Fast twitch low oxidative (FT, Type II B), 143, 144, 145, 146, 147, 225
Fat, nutritional management, 326
Fat for energy, 330–331, 332, 342
Fat horse (BCS 8), 346, 347–349, *349*
Fatigue
bones, fatigue state of, 103
delaying, 148, 330
muscle, 165–166, 184, 343, 483
signs of, 239, 239–240
Fats, muscle fuel, 139, 140, 143, 160
Fatty acids, muscle fuel, 139–140, 141–142, 160
Fecal analysis, internal parasites, 465
Feces and dehydration, 236, **237,** 237, 302, 303, 317
Fédération Equestre Internationale (FEI), 102, 444, 542, 568
"Feed for a better horse," 68–69
Feed supplements, 328–329
Feed-through fly control (*tetrachlorvinphos*), 383
Fermentation process in intestinal tract, 292, 294
Fescue toxicosis, 558–559
Fetlocks
conformation, 8–9, 34
tendons and ligaments, *181*, 187–189, *187–189*
Fetlock valgus (splayfooted), 22, 23, *23*
Fetlock varus (pigeon-toed), 22, 23, *23*, 36, 134
Fever (febrile), 429–430, *430*
Fever impact on hoof, 55
Fiber, 139, 160, 326, 328, 340
Fiber-optic exam of uterus, 550
Fibrin and granulation tissue repair, 191, *191*
Fibroblastic sarcoids, 388, 394, *394*, 395
Fibroblasts, 407, 419
Fibrocartilage, hoof, 46
Fibromas, 395
Fibrosis (scarring), 200
Fibrotic myopathy, 172, *173*, **173–174,** 197, 438–439
Field fitness test, 232–233
First aid kit, 428–429
Fistulograms, 421–422
Fistulous withers, 214, *214*
Fitness indicators, 229–232, *230–231*
Flaccid paralysis, 526
Flares, hoof, 54, 55, *55*, 56
Flat sole, hoof, 48, *48*
Flehmen, 298, *298*
Fleshy horse (BCS 7), 346, 347–349, *349*
Flexibility exercises, 149
Flexion, poll and neck, 247–248, 253
Flexion tests
back pain, 206
joints, 115, *115*, 118
navicular syndrome, 88–89
Flexural contracture, 198–201, *199–200*. *See also* Tendons and ligaments injury and disease
Flexural limb deformity, 564, *564*
Flexural strain, bone, 96–97
Flies and gnats, 376–382, 377–382, 384
Flight instinct, 447, 448, 449, 450
Floating teeth, 286, 289–290, *290*
Flourescein dye, 495, *495*

"Flu" (equine influenza), **267–270**, *268*, 456, 497, 540
Fluids
  loss, 296, 333, *334*
  reabsorption of, intestinal tract, 292, 293
  replacement of, wounds, 428, *428*
Flunixin meglumine, 444, 445. *See also* Nonsteroidal anti-inflammatory drugs (NSAIDs)
Fly control strategies, 381–384, *382*
Flymasks for skin disease, 372
Fly sheets, 381, 382, *382*
Fly traps, 384
Foal by side and breeding, 554
Foaling and complications, 557–565
  amnionic sac, 560, 561, *561*
  bladder, ruptures, 563
  chlorhexidine for umbilical problems, 561–562
  colostrum, 557, 561
  contracted tendons, 328, *564*, **564**
  dystocia, 559–560
  fescue toxicosis, 558–559
  flexural limb deformity, 564, *564*
  immunoglobulin g (IgG), 561
  meconium impaction, 563
  neonatal isoerythrolysis (NI), 563–564
  neonatal maladjustment syndrome (NMS), 563
  newborn foal, 558, 559, *559*
  normal foal, 565, *565*
  passive transfer and antibody protection, 561
  placenta, 560–561, *560–561*
  placentitis, 563
  premature foal, 565
  prolactin and, 558
  retained fetal membranes, 560–561, *560–561*
  septicemia, 497, 562
  sick foal, signs of, 564–565
  udder edema, 557, 558, *558*
  umbilical problems ("navel ill"), 561–563, *562*
  waxing of nipples, 557, 558, *558*
  See also Mare; Reproductive disease and problems; Reproductive strategies
Foal restraint, 453
Focal ventral midline dermatitis, 379–380
Focus and perception, 490–492, *491*
Focused shock wave machine, 106
Follicles, mare, 538, 547, *547*, 552
Food allergies, 390
Foot. *See* Hoof
Forage poisoning (botulism), 505, **525–527**
Forearm, conformation, 8–*10*, 24, 36, 37
Forehand, traveling on the, 16, 17
Foreign particles, respiratory system, 254–255
Foreleg movement and neck, 15, 16

Forelegs, manual stretch, 154, *154*
Forelimb alignment, 22, *22–23*
Fracture and back pain, *213*, 213–214
Fractured splint, 104, 105, *105*
Free fatty acids, 140, 141, 146
Freeze-dried (lyophilized) form injectable medication, 434
Frictional forces between bones, 110
Frog
  hoof, 39, 40, 44–45, *44–45*
  laminitis and, 83, 84, *84*
  navicular syndrome and, 86
Frog wedge test, 89
Front-end stress impact, navicular syndrome, 86
Front symmetry, 8–9
Frost nails, 63
Fructan (oligofructose), 76–77, 80, 82
FT, Type II B (fast twitch low oxidative), 143, 144, 145, 146, 147, 225
FTH, Type II A (fast twitch high oxidative muscle fibers), 143–144, 145, 146, 147, 148, 225, 228
Fullered (full-swedge) shoes, 63
Fungal infection, skin, 369, 372–374, 373
Fungal spores, 256
Furosemide, 263
Fusarium moniliforus, 527
Fusion for
  joints, 116
  osteoarthritis, *128*, 128–129
GAGs (glycosaminoglycans), 125–126
Gait of horse
  breathing and, *250*, 250–251, 254
  joints and, 117–122, *118–121*
  navicular syndrome, 85, 88, 93
  neurologic system, 502, *502–503*, 503
Gaseous colic, **308–309**, *308–309*, 327
Gas expulsion, 292
Gastric ulcer syndrome (GUS), **318–320**, 326, 445–446
Gastrointestinal tract (GI). *See* Intestinal tract
"Gate theory" of pain relief, 178
GBF (germinated barley foodstuff), 320
Gelatinization, injectable medication, 434
Generic vs. name brand, 433
Gene therapy for osteoarthritis, 131
Genetics
  bone development and, 98, 99
  hoof and, 46, 69
  improvement, reproduction, 531, *531*
  navicular syndrome and, 86
  remodeling bone and, 96
Gene transfer vector (IL-1Ra), 131
Gentamycin, 506
Geometric balance, hoof, 53, *53*
Germinated barley foodstuff (GBF), 320
GI. *See* Intestinal tract
Girths, 20, 21, *21*, 366
Glandular mucosa, 318
Glucocorticoids, 78

Glucosamine, 126–127
Glucose, muscle fuel, 139, 140, 147, 325
Glucose intolerance (insulin resistance), **79–80**, 126, 353
Glycine, 161, 514
Glycogen
  depletion, muscle, 166, 169–170, 330
  muscle fuel, 139, 140, 141–142, 143, 146, 148, 160, 325, 326
Glycosaminoglycans (GAGs), 125–126
Glycosaminoglycans (proteoglycans), 110, 111, 125, 446
GnRH (gonadotropic-releasing hormone), 539, **541–542**, 552
Goiter, 337
Gonadotropic-releasing hormone (GnRH), 539, **541–542**, 552
Grain
  colic caution, 319
  digestion in small intestine, 292, 293
  hot climate feeding, 341–342
  overload, laminitis, 75, **76–77**, 82, 329
Gram-positive organisms, 77
Granulation tissue
  tendon and ligament repair, 191, *191*
  wound healing, 407, *407*, 408, 409, *409*
Grass hay, 327, 332
Gravel, 70
Grazing muzzle, 352, *352*
Grease heel (scratches), 367–369, **367–371**, 384
"Green" ("hot") splint, 104, *104*
Grooming and skin, 366
Ground abrasion and moisture, hoof, 66
Growth of hoof, 40–43, *40–43*
Growth plates and bone response to conditioning, 102, 103, 112, *112*
Growth rate differences, hoof, 54, *54*, 84, 85, 85
Guide to Plant Poisoning of Animals, A (Knight), 529
GUS (gastric ulcer syndrome), **318–320**, 326, 445–446
Gut sounds
  cardiovascular system, conditioning, 231–232
  intestinal tract, 291, 293, 301, *301*, 311–312, 317
Guttural pouch infection, 277
HA. *See* Hyaluronic acid
Habronema spp., 383, **388–389**, 395, **463**, 467
Hair loss (alopecia), 374, 380, 385
Halters, 450, *450*
Harvest mites (*trombiculiasis*), 385
HA (hemagglutinin) spikes, 264
Hay
  dust and respiratory system, 256, 257, 261, 264
  nutritional management, 326–328
HBOT (hyperbaric oxygen therapy), 420–421
HCG (human chorionic gonadotropin), 539, 552

Head
  carriage and neck, 16–18, *17–18*
  conformation, 8–*10*, 11–12
  position in trailer, *480*, 480–481
  trauma, 522–523, *523*
Head bumper, 485
Headshaking, 515–516
Healing wounds, 407–421
  amnion wound dressing, 415–416
  bacteria, identification of, 411
  bandaging, 416–419, *417, 419*
  chemicals for proud flesh, 416
  collagen and remodeling, 419
  contraction, **407–410,** *408–410,* 419
  debulking, 408, *408*
  dimethyl sulfoxide (DMSO) gel, 415
  drainage, 411, *411*
  epithelialization, 407, 408, *408,* 419
  facial wounds, 411–412, *412,* 413, *413*
  granulation tissue, 407, *407,* 408, 409, *409*
  hyperbaric oxygen therapy (HBOT), 420–421
  keloid formation, 420, *420*
  poultice, 418
  proud flesh (exuberant granulation), 388, 394, 407, *407,* 408, 409, *409,* **416,** 418
  remodeling of wound, 418–420, *429–420*
  rope burns, 426
  scar tissue, 183, 420, *420*
  second intention healing, 426
  sugar (granulated) dressing, 415
  sutures, 411–412, *412,* 413, *413*
  systemic antibiotics for, **410–411,** *411,* 428
  topical ointments, 412, **414–416,** 428
  See also Wound management
Health inspection, 455–456
Health management strategies, 4, 5. *See also* Preventive health
Heart efficiency, cardiovascular system, 219, 220–221
Heart irregularities, 233, 240
Heart rate
  cardiovascular system, 220
  colic and, 300, *301*
  elevation, persistent, 239–240
  trailering stress, 484
Heart rate monitor (cardiotachometer)
  cardiovascular system, 222, **222–224,** 229, 230
  muscle conditioning, **149–150,** 152, 224
Heart rate recovery, 223, **229,** 230
Heat and respiratory system, 253–254, 255, 256
Heat and tendon injury, *189,* 189–190
Heat dissipation, 146, 149, 252, 356–357, *357*
Heat exhaustion and obese horses, 352, 429
Heat from joint injury, 113, *113*
Heat from metabolism of fuel, 2

Heat increment (HI) of feed, 341, 342
Heat index, 361–362, *362*
Heat stress, **359–363,** *360–363,* 429
Heat therapy for tendon injury, 192–193, 194–195
Heave line, 260
Heaves (RAO), 256, **259–262,** *260,* 267, 456, 543–544
Heel flies (warbles), **380,** 513
Heels
  cracks, 57, *57*
  expansion and shoeing, 59
  hoof, *39,* 40
  navicular syndrome, 85–86, 88
  support and shoeing, 60, 62, *62–63, 63, 65,* 65
Helicobacter pylori, 318
Hemagglutinin (HA) spikes, 264
Hematoma, 423, 424, *424*
Hemicircumferential periosteal transection with periosteal stripping, 136
Hemidesmosomes, hoof, 42, 80
Hemoglobin, 249, 251, 337
Hemorrhage, 426–428, *427–428*
Herbs for estrus, 542
Herd health, 265, 455–459, 465
Herd instinct, 447, 448, 449, 472, 476, 482
Hereditary Equine Regional Dermal Asthenia (HERDA, *Hyperelastosis cutis*), 392
Heritable abnormalities, 535
HFEA (high frequency electroanalgesia), 179
High fiber feed supplements, 328–329
High frequency electroanalgesia (HFEA), 179
High intensity work, 141
High ringbone, 121, 122, 128
High-set neck, 17, *17*
High-speed training, 100–101
High withers, 19, *19*
Hill exercises, 148, 150, 151
Hind legs, lower portion of, 8–9, 34
Hind legs, manual stretch, 154, *154*
Hindquarters
  conformation, 8–*10,* 11, 28–30, 28–31, 35, 36, 37
  neck and, 13–14, *13–14,* 17–18
Hip (gluteal) muscles, 9–*10,* 27, 28, 436
Histamine, 398–399, 442
Hives (urticaria), 389–*391,* **389–392,** 440
Hoary alyssum (*Berteroa incana*), 80
Hobble, 452–453
Hocks
  conformation, 8–9, *9,* 31–34, *33–34,* 35, 37
  pain, 116, *116–117,* 117, 119–121, *120–121*
Hollow back vs. round back, 217, *217*
Hoof as visual record of stress, 54–58
  alkali disease (selenium poisoning), 57–58, **374–375**
  contours, abnormal, *54–55,* **54–56,** 74, 79

  coronary band response to uneven stresses, 56, *56*
  cracks, 55, *55,* 57–58, *57–58,* 60
  dishing (concavity), 54, 55, *55,* 74, 84, 85, *85*
  flares, 54, 55, *55,* 56
  growth rate differences, 54, *54,* 84, 85, *85*
  heel crack, 57, *57*
  quarter cracks, 57, *57*
  ridges/ ripples, 54, 74, 79
  sand cracks, 57, 58, *58,* 67
  selenium toxicity, **57–58,** *58,* 162, 173, 338
  sheared heels, 56–57, *57*
  shoeing and, 53, *53,* 55, 60–61, *60–61*
  toe crack, 57, *57*
  See also Hoof characteristics; Hoof lameness; Hoof structure and growth; Laminitis; Navicular syndrome; Shoes and pads
Hoof characteristics, 47–53
  angle of hoof, 48–49, *50*
  balance of hoof, 53, *53*
  breakover, 24, *49,* **49–50,** 52, 60
  broken-back hoof-pastern axis, **50–51,** *51,* 60, 183
  club foot (broken-forward hoof-pastern axis), 52, **52–53,** 87, *87,* 200, *200*
  color and strength of hoof, 47, *47*
  contracted heels (narrow heels), 48, 49, *49,* 86
  differences (large) in size of feet, 48, 49, *49*
  hoof-pastern axis, 48–49, 50–51, *50–51,* 60, 87, *87*
  integrity of hoof wall, 47
  isoxsuprine hydrochloride, 68
  size of hoof, 48, 48–49
  supplements, 67–68
  under-run heels, 60, 63, *63*
  See also Hoof as visual record of stress; Hoof lameness; Hoof structure and growth; Laminitis; Long-toe low-heel (LTLH); Navicular syndrome; Shoes and pads
Hoof extension test, 89
Hoof lameness, 69–73
  abscesses, 63, 64, **70–71,** *71,* 80
  canker, 63, **73**
  corns, 63, 64, **71–72,** *72*
  digital pulses for identifying, 69
  Epsom salt soaks for, 70, *70,* 71
  gravel, 70
  sole bruises, 64, 65, **70,** *70*
  subsolar abscess, 70
  thrush (pododermatitis), 63, **73**
  white line disease, 44, **73,** 74, *74*
  See also Hoof as visual record of stress; Hoof characteristics; Hoof structure and growth; Laminitis; Navicular syndrome; Shoes and pads

Hoof-pastern axis, 48–49, 50–51, *50–51*, 60, 87, *87*
Hoof strike, *49*, 49–50
Hoof structure and growth, 39–47
  bars, *39*, 44, *44*
  coffin bone, *40*, 41, 42, 43, 45, 50, 52, 58
  concussion, 40–42, *42*, 45–46, 48, 52
  coronary band, 40, 41, *41*
  digital cushion, 40, *40*, 42, *42*, 46, 52, 58
  dressings and supplements, 66–69
  "feed for a better horse," 68–69
  frog, *39*, 40, 44–45, *44–45*
  genetic predisposition, 46, 69
  growth of hoof, 40–43, *40–43*
  health of hoof, 42, *42*, 46–47, *47*
  heels, *39*, 40
  hoof wall, *39–43*, **40–43**, 47, 48, 49, *49*, 55, 60, *60–61*, 61, 66
  impact energy absorption, 40–42, *42*, 45–46, 48, 52
  interactive structures, *39*, 45, 45–46
  laminae, 40, 41, *41*, 42, 44, 74
  moisture loss in hoof, 66–67
  navicular structures, *40*, *45*, 45, 49
  parts of hoof, 39–40
  "quick" (corium), 41, *41–42*, 42, 84
  remodeling of hoof, 42–43, *43*
  weight-bearing structures, 40, 44–45, *44–45*
  white line, *39*, 44, *44*
  See also Hoof as visual record of stress; Hoof characteristics; Hoof lameness; Laminitis; Navicular syndrome; Shoes and pads
Hoof tester exam, 88, *89*, 89
Hooks on teeth, 285, 288, *288*, 290, *290*
Hormonal manipulation, mare, 539, 541–542
Horner's syndrome, 516–517
Horn flies (*Haematobia*), 379–380, 382
Horn tubules, hoof, 40, 59, 66–67, 84
Horse and rider team, 1, 5, 6
Horseflies (*Tabannus*), 241–242, 376, 382
Horsetail (*Equisetum* spp.), 528
Hot climate feeding, 341–344, *343*. *See also* Nutritional management
"Hot" nail, 72–73
"Hot" ("green") splint, 104, *104*
Houseflies (*Musca domestica*), 376, 382
Housing and lower respiratory problems, 261
Human chorionic gonadotropin (HCG), 539, 552
Human-horse bond (partnership), 1
Human ophthalmic lubricating ointments, 496
Humerus (arm bone), *8*, 20, *21*, 22, 23
Hunter's bump, 27, *27*, 30, *30*, **208**, *208*
Hyaluronic acid (HA)
  joints, 110
  navicular syndrome, 92
  osteoarthritis, 125
Hydration assessment, 235, 235–236
Hydrogen peroxide, 407
Hydrotherapy for tendon injury, 195–196
Hydroxyapatitie crystals, 96
Hygiene
  preventive health and, 459
  skin and, 367, 367–368, 371
Hygromas, **114,** *114,* 475
Hyoid apparatus, 247
Hyperbaric oxygen therapy (HBOT), 420–421
Hyperesthesia (touch sensitivity), 518
Hyperglycemia, 79–80
Hyperimmune plasma, 505–506
Hyperkalemic periodic paralysis (HYPP), **176–177,** 520
Hypermotile gut, 303
Hyperplasia, 144
Hypersalivation, 282–283
Hyperthermia for skin growths, 397
Hypothalamus, 538
Hypoxia, 238
HYPP (hyperkalemic periodic paralysis), **176–177,** 520
Hypsodont teeth, 282
IAD (inflammatory airway disease), 259, **261–262,** 267, 270
Ice-free water, 345
Ice nails, 63
ICF (intracellular fluid), 235
ID (intradermal injection), 442
Ideal condition (BCS 5), 346, 347, 348, *348*
Ideal conformation, 7
Idle horses and nutrition, 339
IFCL (inferior check ligament), *181*, 186, *186*
IgG (immunoglobulin g), 561
IL-1Ra (gene transfer vector), 131
Ileum, *291*, 304, 308, 316
Ilium, *8*, 30
IM (intramuscular injection), 119, 434, *436–437*, **436–440,** 454
Imagining a fit horse, 2–3
Imbalance and lameness, 53, *53*, 55, 59, 60, 88
Immune function and trailering, 481–482
Immune system and vaccination, 265
Immunizations. *See* Vaccinations
Immunoglobulin g (IgG), 561
Immunoglobulins and respiratory system, 257–258
Immunologically naïve horses, 267
Immunotherapy, 396
Impact energy absorption, hoof, 40–42, *42*, 45–46, 48, 52
Impaction colic, 303–308, 316
Inactivated ("killed") vaccines, 266
Inapparent carrier of EIA, 241
Incarcerated piece of bowel, 308
Incisor overgrowth, 286–287, *287*
Incisors, 285, 289, *289*
Index of refraction, 489–490
Inferior check ligament (IFCL), *181*, 186, *186*
Inferior digital check ligament surgery, 200
Inflammation
  burns, 425
  impact, hoof, 56
  joints, 115–116, *115–117*, 117
  osteoarthritis, 122–123, *123*
  tendon injury, 192–198, *193–194*
Inflammatory airway disease (IAD), 259, **261–262,** 267, 270
Influenza virus ("flu"), **267–270,** *268*, 456, 497, 540
Infrared thermography, 102, 113, 179
Ingesta (food material), 292
Inhalation, 246–247
Initial treatment, wounds, 403
Injectable medication, 432–442
  abscesses from injections, 438
  active ingredient, 433
  alcohol as antiseptic, 407, 435
  anaphylactic shock from, 432, 434, **439–440,** 446
  antiseptic solutions, 435–436
  carotid artery caution, 441
  cellulitis, 422, *422*, **438,** 475
  cleaning injection site, 435–436
  contaminated medication, 434
  environmental stress of, 434
  epinephrine (adrenaline) for anaphylactic shock, 439–440
  expiration date, 433
  flu-like symptoms from, 439
  freeze-dried (lyophilized) form, 434
  gelatinization, 434
  generic vs. name brand, 433
  injectable medication
    catheter (IV), 441
  intradermal injection (ID), 442
  intramuscular injection (IM), 119, 434, *436–437*, **436–440,** 454
  intravenous injections (IV), 434, *436*, **440–441,** *441*, 454
  label, 433–434, 435
  muscle soreness from, 439, *439*
  neck injections, 436, *436*
  needles and syringes, 435, 437–438
  NSAIDs for, 439
  oral preparations vs., 440
  pectoral injections, 437
  pre-injection procedure, 435–436
  refrigeration, 433
  rump injections, 436, 437, *437*
  sedimentation, 434
  storage, 434–435
  subcutaneous injection, 441–442
  thigh injections, 437, *437*
  thrombophlebitis from, 441
  vitamins (injectable), 435
  See also Wound management
Injectable polysulfated glycosaminoglycans, 125–126
Injectable vaccines, 266
Injections for navicular syndrome, 92–93

Insect transmission of EIA, 241–242, 376
Insensitive laminae, hoof, 40, 44
Insulation, delaying cool-downs, 158, *158*, 159, *159*
Insulin resistance (glucose intolerance), **79–80**, 126, 353
Intensity, cardiovascular system, 226–227
Interactive structures, hoof, *39, 45*, 45–46
Interferon, 506
Internal blistering for back pain, 215
Internal parasites and control, 459–472
    allergic reactions to deworming, 471–472
    bot larvae and worms, 379, 460, *460*, 462–463, *462–463*, 467
    colic and, 294, 321–322
    continuous dewormers, 466–467, *467*, 469–470
    deworming, 264, 459, 460, *460*, **466–472**, *467*, 540
    environmental management, 459, 465–466
    eyeworms (*Thelazia*), 376, 383, 467
    fecal analysis monitoring, 465
    Habronema spp., 383, **388–389**, 395, **463**, 467
    intestinal threadworms (*Strongyloides westeri*), 464, 467
    lungworms, 464, 467
    natural immunity to parasites, 465
    performance impacted by, 459, 461
    pinworms (*Oxyuris equi*), 379, *379*, 460, *460*, 463–464, **463–464**, 467
    pyrantel (Strongid-C), 466–467, *467*, 469–470
    roundworms (ascarids), 322, 460, *460*, 462, *462*, 467
    stomach worms, *460*, 462–462, *462–463*
    strongyles (large and small) (blood worms), 322, 460, *460–461*, 461–462, 467
    tapeworms, 460, *460*, 464, 467
    Trichostrongylus axei, 463
    See also External parasites and control; Preventive health
Interosseous ligament inflammation, 104
Interval training (IT), 100, 149–150, 227–228
Intestinal symptoms, NSAIDs, 296, **445–446**
Intestinal threadworms (*Strongyloides westeri*), 464, 467
Intestinal tract, 291–323
    anatomy and function, *291*, 291–293
    borborygmi (waves of contractions), 301
    carbohydrates, digestion in large intestine, 292–293, 325
    cardiovascular system and, 221–222, 231–232
    electrolytes, reabsorption of, 292, 293
    endotoxin, 293, 294, 300, *300*, 317
    esophageal obstruction (chronic choke), 284, **296**
    esophagus and stomach, 292, 296
    feeding and, 340–341
    fermentation process in, 292, 294
    fluids, reabsorption of, 292, 293
    grain, digestion in small intestine, 292, 293
    gut sounds, 291, 293, 301, *301*, 311–312, 317
    intestinal transit, 293, 304
    large colon, *291*, **293**, 310
    large intestine (LI), *291*, **292–293**, 294
    motility of, 293, 304
    nutritional management, 296–297, 340–341
    pelvic flexure, *291*, 292, 309
    peristalsis and, 293, 314–315
    small colon, *291*, 292, 293
    small intestine (SI), *291*, 292, 293
    stomach, *291*, 291–292, 293
    volatile fatty acids (VFAs) from vdigestion, 292–293, 325
    water drinking importance, 296, 304–305, 313
    See also Colic; Dental and oral cavity; Intestinal tract disease
Intestinal tract disease, 293–297
    aspiration pneumonia, 295–296
    choke, 295–296, **295–297**, 328
    diarrhea, 284, **293–295**, 311, 333, *334*, 336
    electrolyte loss, 296
    fluid loss, 296, 333, *334*
    internal parasites and, 294, 321–322
    Potomac Horse Fever, **294–295**, 388
    stomach (nasogastric) tube for, 296, 296, **302**
    treatment for, 296, **445–446**
    See also Colic; Dental and oral cavity; Intestinal tract
Intra-articular anti-inflammatory medication, 92–93
Intracellular fluid (ICF), 235
Intradermal injection (ID), 442
Intramuscular estrogen therapy, 119
Intramuscular injection (IM), 119, 434, 436–437, **436–440**, 454
Intranasal vaccines, 266, 270, 277–278
Intravenous drugs, 434
Intravenous (IV) fluids, 359
Intravenous injections (IV), 434, 436, **440–441**, *441*, 454
Intussusception, 303, 309, 464
Inversion, 240
Iodine, 337
Iontophoresis, 130
Iron, 337
Irrigation for eye injury, 496
Irritation, neurologic system, 514–520, *515*
Isolation and stress, 473–474, 476
Isolation of sick horse, 269, 275
Isometric contraction, 139
Isoxsuprine hydrochloride, 68, 83
IT (interval training), 100, 149–150, 227–228
IV (intravenous injections), 436, **440–441**, *441*, 454
Ivermectin, 383, 384, 385–386, 387, 389, 466, *467*, 469
IV (intravenous) fluids, 359
Ixodes ticks, 136
Jaws, conformation, 8–9, 12
Jaw width, respiratory system, 258–259, 264
Joint effusion (windpuffs), 26, 33, 113, *113*
Joint injury and disease, 112–122
    articular ringbone, 122, 128
    bog spavin, 31, **120**, *120*
    bone spavin, 31, 33, **120**, *120*, 130, 211, *211*
    bursa injury, 114
    capped elbow (shoe boil), 114, *114*
    capped hock, **114**, *114*, 475
    capsulitis, 111, 113, *113*
    chemical fusion for, 116
    cold (ice) therapy for, 131
    delayed patella release (upward fixation of the patella), 31, 33, **118–119**, *119*, 518
    effusion (filling of joint capsule), 118, *118*
    enzymatic damage, *115*, 115–116
    flexion tests for, 115, *115*, 118
    fusion for, 116
    high ringbone, 121, 122, 128
    hock pain, signs of, 116, *116–117*, 117, 119–121, *120–121*
    hygromas, **114**, *114*, 475
    inflammation, 115–116, *115–117*, 117
    infrared thermography for, 113
    intramuscular estrogen therapy, 119
    kneecap (patella), 118–119, *119*
    low ringbone, 121–122
    Lyme disease, **136**, 388, 497
    musculoskeletal stress, 112, *112*
    non-arthritic ringbone, 122, 128
    pain from, 112–113, *112–113*
    punctures, 421–422
    radiographic (X-ray) evaluation, 115, 120, 121, *121*, 122
    ringbone, 22, 25, 112, *121*, **121–122**, 128–129
    soft tissue injury, 114, *114*
    stifle pain, signs of, 117–118, *118*
    surgical fusion for, 116
    synovitis, 111, 113, *113*
    windpuffs (joint effusion), 26, 33, 113, *113*
    See also Developmental Orthopedic Disease (DOD); Joints; Osteoarthritis
Joints, 109–136
    anatomy and function, 9, *109*, 109–110
    articular cartilage, *109*, 110, 111, 116

back pain and therapy, 215
exercise effect, 110, 111–112, 131
joint capsule, *109*, 109–110, 116
ligaments and, *109*, *109*, 116
NSAIDs for, 446
proteoglycans (glycosaminoglycans) and, 110, 111, 125, 446
range of motion, 110–111
synovial joint, *109*, 109–110
"wear and tear," 111–112
See also Joint injury and disease
Jugular refill time, 231, *231*
Jumpers
  back of horse, 204, 213
  bone development, 100, 108
  cardiovascular system, 226
  conformation, 14, *14*, 16, 23, 25, 26, 28, 36–37
  joints, 111
  muscle endurance, 143, 148, 156
  navicular syndrome, 86
  respiratory system, 247, 258
Kaptchuk, Ted J., 1
Keloids, 395, 420, *420*
Kenney classification system, 549–550
Keratin, hoof, 40, 67, 73
Keratinocytes, hoof, 40
Kick chains, 476–477
Kick wounds, 423, *423*
"Killed" (inactivated) vaccines, 266
Killed virus vaccine, 506
Kissing spines (vertebral impingement), 30, **212–213**, *213*
Klebsiella, 549
Kneecap (patella), 118–119, *119*
Knees (carpus), conformation, 8, *8–10*, *9*, 22, *22–23*, 24, 35
Knight, Anthony P., 529
Knock-kneed (carpus valgus), 22, 23, *23*, 24, 104, 134, *134*
Kronfeld, D.S., 340
Kyphosis (roach back), 27, *27*, 30, *30*, **212**, *212*
Label, drugs, 433–434, 435
Labia, 544–545, *545*
Lactate dehydrogenase (LDH), 170
Lactate testing, 458
Lactic acid
  cardiovascular system, 220, 223
  muscle fuel, 141, 142, 147, 164
  removal, cool-down, 156
  tolerance, 147, 149, 150, 152, 161, 170
Lactobacillus, 77, 331
Lameness. *See* Back pain; Hoof lameness; Joint injury; Laminitis; Muscle injury and disease; Navicular syndrome; Tendons and ligaments injury and disease
Laminae, hoof, 40, 41, *41*, 42, 44, 74
Laminitis, 74–85
  acepromazine for, 83
  acute laminitis, 81, 84
  acute phase of, 81
  basement membrane and anchoring points failure, 42, 81

characteristics of, 74, *74*
chromium tripicolinate for, 80
chronic laminitis, 84
circumflex artery, 75, 76, *76*
coffin bone and, 81–82, 83, *83*, 84, 85, *85*
consequences of, 81–82
cryotherapy (ice therapy), 82
cyproheptidine for, 78
deep digital flexor tendon (DDFT) and, 81, 83, *181*
defined, 74, 75, 76, *76*
developmental phase, 75, 77, 81, 82
dimethyl sulfoxide (DMSO) for, 80
dorsal laminar arteries, 75, 76, *76*
exercise restriction for, 83
frog support for, 83, 84, *84*
grading of severity of, 74–75
growth rate differences in hooves, 54, *54*, 84, 85, *85*
hoof wall irregularities and, 55
isoxsuprine hydrochloride for, 68, 83
matrix metalloproteinases (MMPs) and, 75, 77, 81, 82, 337
nitroglycerine for, 83
NSAIDs for, 82
nutritional management, 78, 80, 82, 327, 329
Obel Grade 1-4 (pain response), 75
pain from, 74, *74*, 81
pentoxyfylline for, 83
pergolide for, 78
prevention of, 82
radiographic (X-ray) evaluation, 83
severity, grading of, 74–75
shoeing and, 64, 83
solar bruising and, 70
stomach tubing, grain overload, 82–83
Styrofoam for, 83, 84, *84*
therapy for, 82–83
vasoconstriction and, 75, 82
vasodilation and, 82, 83
veterinary attention for, 82
vitamin E for insulin resistance, 80
white line disease, 44, **73**, 74, *74*
See also Hoof lameness; Laminitis, causes of
Laminitis, causes of, 75–81
  abscesses and, 80
  carbohydrate overload, 75, **76–77**, 82
  circulatory compromise, 75–76, *76*
  corticosteroids and, 78, 79
  Equine Cushing's Disease (ECD), **77–78**, *77–78*, 500
  equine metabolic syndrome (peripheral cushingold syndrome), 78, **78–80**, 353
  fructan (oligofructose) and, 76–77, 80, 82
  glucocorticoids and, 78
  grain overload, 75, **76–77**, 82, 329
  Gram-positive organisms and, 77
  hemidesmosomes damage, 80
  hyperglycemia and, 79–80
  insulin resistance (glucose intolerance), **79–80**, 126, 353

mechanical causes, 80–81, *81*
metabolic causes, 75–80, *76–79*
momentum and, 79
obese horses, 353
oxidative stress, 80
pasture (rich) overload, 75, **76–77**, 82
pituitary pars intermedia dysfunction (PPID), 77–78, *77–78*
plant toxicity, 80
road founder, 80, 81, *81*
support founder, 80–81, *81*
Landeau, L.J., 47
Lanyon, 100
Large colon, *291*, *293*, 310
Large intestine (LI), *291*, **292–293**, 294
Laryngeal hemiplegia (RLN), 12, 16, 246, 247, **258–259**, 263, 511
Laryngo-palatal dislocation, 248
Larynx, 245, 246, 247, 258
Laser-facilitated joint fusion, 128, *128*
Lateral (ungual) cartilages, 42, *42*, 46, 58
Lathyrism (*Lathyrus hirsutus*), 529
Lavage, 405, *405*
Lawns (grazing areas), 459
LDH (lactate dehydrogenase), 170
Legs of horse, 8–9, *8–9*
Legume hay, 164–165, 327–328, 332
Lens, eyes, 489, *489–490*
Leptospirosis, 497
"Letdown" period, 543
Levers, muscle, 137–138
LFEA (low frequency electroanalgesia), 179
LFG (live foal guarantee), 534, 554
LI (large intestine), *291*, **292–293**, 294
Lice (pediculosis), 386, *386–387*
Ligaments
  bone interaction, 99
  joints and, 109, *109*, 116
  tendons vs., *181*, 181–182, 190
  See also Tendons and ligaments
Lighting and estrus cycle, 539–540
Limb crookedness, 8–9
Limb interference, 20, 21, *21*
Limb swelling from strangles, 201
Lip chain, 452, *452*
Lipids, muscle, 143, 160
Lipomas (intestinal), 308–309, *309*–310, *310*, 352
Lipopigment deposition in retina, 518
Live foal guarantee (LFG), 534, 554
Lockjaw, 514
Locomotor-respiration coupling, *250*, 250–251, 254
Locoweed (*Astragalus* spp., *Oxytropis* spp.), 199, **528**
Loins, conformation, *9–10*, 27–28, *28*, 35, 36
Loner horses, 476
Long, fast distance training, 229
Long, slow distance (LSD) training, 100, 148, 182, 223, **226–227**
Long back, 26, 27, *27*
Longing to check gaits, 69
Longitudinal flexion, 18–19
Long muscles, 137–138

Long neck, 15, 16
Long pastern, 25, 25–26, 26
Long-toe low-heel (LTLH)
  back pain, 211
  fallen horse, 524
  hoof and, 24, 50, 51–52, 51–52, 57, 60
  moisture and, 66–67
  navicular syndrome, 88
  tendons and ligaments, 183–184, 186
Lordosis (sway back), 26, 27, 27, 212, **212**
Low bow, 187–188, 187–188
Lower portion of rear limb, 8–9, 34
Lower respiratory problems, 259–279
  airway inflammation disease, 260–261
  bacterial infections, 273–279, 274, 277
  bacterial pneumonia, 259
  bronchoconstriction, 259, 260, 261
  chronic obstructive pulmonary disease (COPD), **260**, 456
  exercise-induced pulmonary hemorrhage (EIPH), 262, 262–264
  inflammatory airway disease (IAD), 259, **261–262**, 267, 270
  lung abscesses, 259
  nasal discharge, 268, 268, 271, 271, 273
  nutritional management, 261–262
  pleuropneumonia, 259, **273**, 480
  recurrent airway obstruction (RAO), 256, **259–262**, 260, 267, 456, 543–544
  therapy for, 262, 262–264
  vaccinations for, 262, 264
  viral infections, 259
  See also Respiratory illness; Respiratory system; Respiratory viruses
Lower respiratory tract, 245, 245, 249–251, 250
Low frequency electroanalgesia (LFEA), 179
Low ringbone, 121–122
Low-set hocks, 32
Low-set neck, 16, 17
Low withers, 19, 20
LSD (long, slow distance) training, 100, 148, 182, 223, **226–227**
L-S joint (lumbosacral joint), 8, 14, 28, 28–29
LTLH. See Long-toe low-heel
Lumbosacral joint (L-S joint), 8, 14, 28, 28–29
Lung abscesses, 259
Lungs, 245, 249
Lungworms, 464, 467
Lupine (Lupinus argenteus), 528
Lyme disease, **136**, 388, 497
Lymphangitis, 202, 202
Lymph nodes swelling, 273, 274, 274, 275
Lyophilized (freeze-dried) form injectable medication, 434
Macrophages, 255
Magnesium imbalance, 163–164
Magnets for osteoarthritis, 130
Magnetic resonance imaging (MRI), **90**

Maiden mare, 547
Malignant cancer, 392
Malignant edema, 422–423, 423
Mallow (Malva spp.), 529
Manipulative therapy for back pain, 215
Manual stretching, 153–155, 154–155
Manure eating (coprophagy), 461
Mare, 538–550
  abortion, 271, 272, 536, **556**
  acupuncture for, 374, 542, 542
  altrenogest for, 541, 551
  anabolic steroids and estrus, 543
  anestrus, 538, 539
  bacteria culture of uterus, 548, 548–549
  blanketing, 540
  Caslick's surgery (episioplasty), 545–546, 546
  cattle implants for, 542
  cervix, 547
  cytology evaluation of uterus, 549
  deworming, 540
  embryonic migration, 550
  estrus, 534, 539, **540–543**, 542
  fiber-optic exam of uterus, 550
  foal by side and breeding, 554
  follicles, 538, 547, 547, 552
  gonadotropic-releasing hormone (GnRH), 539, **541–542**, 552
  herbs for, 542
  hormonal manipulation, 539, 541–542
  human chorionic gonadotropin (HCG), 539, 552
  hypothalamus, 538
  Kenney classification system, 549–550
  labia, 544–545, 545
  "letdown" period, 543
  lighting and cycle, 539–540
  maiden mare, 547
  mastitis, 546
  maturity of mare and breeding, 544
  mechanical control, estrus, 542, 542
  melatonin, 538
  nutritional management, 540, 544
  ovariectomy, 542–543
  ovaries, 538, 539
  ovulation, 541, 542
  perineum, 544–545, 545
  physical exam, 543–544
  pineal gland, 538, 539
  pre-breeding program, 534, 543–550, 545–549
  pregnancy check, 552–553, 553
  preventive medicine, 540
  progesterone, 539
  prostaglandins, 539, 550, 551
  rectal examination, 546
  reproductive cycle, 538–540, 539
  seasonally polyestrus, 538
  "silent" heats, 534, 551
  surgical options, 542–543
  third degree perineal laceration, 546
  transitional period, 538

twins, 552, 553, 553
udder evaluation, 546
ultrasound exam, 546, 547, 547
uterine biopsy, 549, 549–550
uterine cysts, 546
uterus, 539, 548–549, 548–550
uterus, infected, 532
vaccinations, 540
vagina, 532, 539, 545, 545
vaginal exam, 547–548, 548
vestibular seal, 545
weight concerns, 544
  See also Conformation; Foaling and complications; Reproductive disease and problems; Reproductive strategies; Stallion
Massage for
  back pain, 214
  cool-down and, 157, 157
  coronary bands, 42, 67
  muscle, 178
  osteoarthritis, 129
  tendon injury, 195–196
  tying-up syndrome caution, 171
Mast cells, 261
Mastitis, 546
Matrix metalloproteinases (MMPs)
  hoof structure, **42–43**, 43, 337
  laminitis and, 75, 77, 81, 82, 337
Maximal exercise. See Anaerobic exercise
MCA (mucociliary apparatus), 255, 268, 273
McClure, Scott, 106–107
MDI (metered dose inhaler), 262, 262
Mechanical causes, laminitis, 80–81, 81
Mechanical concerns, skin, 364–367, 365–366
Mechanical control, estrus, 542, 542
Meconium impaction, 563
Medial to lateral hoof imbalance, 88
Meibomian glands, 492
Melanocytes and skin, 364–365, 365, 396
Melanomas, **397–399**, 398–399, 499, 499, 536, 545
Melatonin, 538
"Menace response," 500, 502
Mental perception and eyes, 487–488
Mentation, neurologic system, 501
Mesentery (bowel lining), 297
Mesentery tear, 308
Metabolic alkalosis, **152**, 163, **170**
Metabolic causes, laminitis, 75–80, 76–79
Metabolism, muscle, 140–143
Metastatic strangles abscessation, 276–277
Metered dose inhaler (MDI), 262, 262
Microfilaria and external parasites, 385, 385
Microminerals, 133–134, 337–338
Microstreaming, 198
"Milkshake" (sodium bicarbonate drench), 336–337
Milkweed (Asclepias spp.), 529

Millipore filter system, 434
Minerals and trace microminerals, 337–338
Mineral within bone, 95–96
Mitochondria, **140–141,** 143, 228, 249, 251
Mixed sarcoids, 394, *394*
MMPs. *See* Matrix metalloproteinases
Moderate conditioned horse (BCS 5), 346, 347, 348, *348*
Moderately fleshy horse (BCS 6), 346, 347, 348, *348,* 350, *350*
Modification by viruses, 266–267
Modified live vaccines, 266
Moisture content of hay, 327
Moisture loss in hoof, 66–67
Molars, 282, 286
Mold in hay, 327
Moldy corn poisoning (encephalomalacia), 527
Momentum and laminitis, 79
Moon blindness (ERU), 385–386, 445, *497–498,* **497–499,** 500
Mosquitoes, 380, *380–381,* **381,** 383, 390, **507–508**
Motility of intestinal tract, 293, 304
Motility of semen, 537
Motor endplates/neutrons, 138
Motor points, muscle, 178
Mounted suppling exercises, 155, *155–156,* 156
Movement (work of) in fit horse, 2
Moving horse and back pain, 205–206
MRI (magnetic resonance imaging), **90**
Mucociliary apparatus (MCA), 255, 268, 273
Mucociliary-apparatus-clearance, 261
Mucociliary escalator, 479–480
Mucocutaneous junctions, 372
Mucous membranes and colic, 299–300, *299–300*
Mud fever (scratches), 367–369, **367–371,** 384
Muscle endurance, 137–180
  action potential, 138
  anatomy and function, 7–8, *8,* 10, *10*
  bone interaction, 99–100
  calcium concentrations, 138, 169–170
  contraction of muscle, 138–139
  dietary manipulation of, 160–165, *164*
  electrical stimulation, 138, 139, 179
  ergogenic acids and, 160–162
  fascia, 137, 144, 145, *145*
  fast twitch high oxidative muscle fibers (FTH, Type II A), 143–144, 145, 146
  fast twitch low oxidative (FT, Type II B), 143, 144, 145, 146
  fatigue, 148, 165–166, 184, 330, 343, 483
  joints, stress, 112, *112*
  levers, 137–138
  myoglobin, 143, *167,* **167–168,** 337
  nerve impulses, 138, 139, 149
  pulleys, 137–138
  shoeing and, 58–59
  slow twitch high oxidative muscle fibers (ST, Type 1), 143, 144, 145, 146
  stretching, 149, 153–156, *154–156*
  tendinous attachment to bone, 137, 138, 144, 145, *145*
  See also Muscle fuels and energy; Muscle injury and disease; Muscle response to conditioning
Muscle fuels and energy, 139–143
  adenosine triphosphate (ATP), 138, 140, 141, 146, 164, 165, 169–170
  adipose tissue (fat reserves), 140, 325
  aerobic (endurance) metabolism, 140–141, 142, 143
  anaerobic (sprint) metabolism, 140, 141, 142, 143, 161
  by-products, 141, 142, 147
  carbohydrates, 139, 142, 325
  conserving glycogen, 141–142
  energy production, 140–143
  fats, 139, 140, 143, 160
  fatty acids, 139–140, 141–142, 160
  fiber, 139, 160
  free fatty acids, 140, 141, 146
  glucose, 139, 140, 147, 325
  glycogen, 139, 140, 141–142, 143, 146, 148, 160, 325, 326
  lactic acid, 141, 142, 147, 164
  metabolism, 140–143
  mitochondria and, **140–141,** 143, 228, 249, 251
  oxygen and, 140, 141, 142
  volatile fatty acids (VFAs), 139–140, 141, 325
  See also Muscle endurance; Muscle injury and disease; Muscle response to conditioning
Muscle injury and disease, 165–180
  causes of, 165
  dryland distemper (pigeon breast), *174,* **174–176,** 273, 377
  electrolyte depletion (cause), 169
  endorphins, pain relief, 178, 451–452
  equine polysaccharide storage myopathy (EPSSM), 165, 167, **172–173,** 518, 541
  fatigue, 148, 165–166, 184, 330, 343, 483
  fibrotic myopathy, 172, *173,* **173–174,** 197, 438–439
  "gate theory" of pain relief, 178
  glycogen depletion, 166, 169–170, 330
  hyperkalemic periodic paralysis (HYPP), **176–177,** 520
  metabolic alkalosis (cause), **152,** 163, **170**
  neuromuscular depression, 163
  neuromuscular hyperirritability, 163–165, *164,* 166
  NSAIDs for, 175
  pulled muscles, 165
  strained muscles, 165
  temperature (elevated), 166, 169–170
  therapy for, 177–180
  thumps (synchronous diaphragmatic flutter), *164,* **164–165,** 170, 239, 333, 334
  trigger points, 178, 179
  ulcerative lymphangitis, 175
  white muscle disease, 173, 338
  See also Muscle endurance; Muscle fuels and energy; Muscle response to conditioning; Tying-up syndrome
Muscle response to conditioning, 144–160
  aerobic skeletal muscle adaptations, 145–146, *146,* 151–152, 161
  agonist muscles, 144, 145, *145*
  anaerobic skeletal muscle adaptations, 147–148, 150
  anaerobic threshold, 147–148, 149
  antagonist muscles, 144, 145, *145*
  blood lactate levels, 152
  calisthenics, 151
  conditioning levels, 224, 225, *225*
  cross-training benefits, 150–151
  deep footing exercises, 150, 151
  detraining, 151–152
  electrolytes and, 152, 162–165, *164*
  evaluating muscular efficiency, 152
  faster gaits, 150
  fast twitch high oxidative muscle fibers (FTH, Type II A), 145, 146, 147, 148, 225, 228
  fast twitch low oxidative (FT, Type II B), 145, 146, 147, 225
  fatigue, delaying, 148, 330
  flexibility exercises, 149
  heart rate monitor, **149–150,** 152, 224
  heat dissipation, improving, 146, 149
  hill exercises, 148, 150, 151
  interval training (IT), 149–150
  lactic acid tolerance, 147, 149, 150, 152, 161, 170
  long, slow distance (LSD) training, 148
  metabolic alkalosis, **152,** 163, **170**
  neuromuscular reflexes, 144, 145, *145*
  oxidative capacity within muscle, 146, *146,* 152
  rehabilitation, 152
  slow twitch high oxidative muscle fibers (ST, Type 1), 145, 146, 225
  strength training, 148–149, 150, 151
  stretching exercises, 149
  sweating, improving, 146, 149
  training responses, 144–145, *145*
  See also Cool-down exercises; Muscle endurance; Muscle fuels and energy; Muscle injury and disease; Warm-up exercises
Muscle soreness from injectable medication, 439, *439*
Musculotendinous attachments, 24
Mutation of viruses, 266, 267
Myeloencephalopathy (viral neurologic disease), 271, 272
Myocardium and cardiovascular system, 220–221

Myofascial tightening, 93
Myofibrils, muscle, 138
Myofibroblast cells, 407–408
Myoglobin, muscle, 143, *167*, **167–168**, 337
Myositis (muscle inflammation), 277–278. *See also* Tying-up syndrome
Name brand vs. generic, 433
Narcolepsy, 519–520
Narrow (contracted) heels, 48, 49, *49*, 86
Nasal discharge, 268, *268*, 271, *271*, 273
Nasal passages, 246, *246*, 254–255
Nasal strips, 263–264
Nasogastric (stomach) tube, 296, *296*, **302**
Nasolacrimal duct, 492, *493*
Nasopharyngeal swabs, 276
Nasopharynx, 246, *248*
National Animal Health Monitoring System (NAHMS), 267
Natural cover, 550
Natural immunity to parasites, 465
"Navel ill" (umbilical problems), 561–563, *562*
Navicular structures, hoof, *40*, 45, *45*, 49
Navicular syndrome, 85–93
   abscesses and, 86
   anesthesia injection test, 89, *89*, 90
   breed types and, 86
   characteristics of, 85–86, *86*, 88
   coffin bone, 86, 87, *87*, 88
   coffin joint arthritis, 90, 129
   contracted heels and, 48, 49, *49*, 86
   corticosteroids for, 92–93
   cysts (demineralization) and, 90
   deep digital flexor tendon (DDFT) and, 85, 86, 87, *87*, 88, *181*
   defined, 85–86
   desmotomy of navicular suspensory ligaments for, 93
   diagnostic tests, 88–90, *89*, *91*
   egg bar shoes for, 91, *91*
   enthesiophytes (bone spurs) and, 90
   exercise for, 93
   flexion tests, 88–89
   foot size (small) and, 86, *86*
   frog and, 86
   frog wedge test, 89
   front-end stress impact, 86
   gait of horse, 85, 88, 93
   genetics, 86
   hard surfaces impact, 86
   heel soreness and, 85–86, 88
   hoof extension test, 89
   hoof tester exam, 88, 89, *89*
   hyaluronic acid for, 92
   injections for, 92–93
   intra-articular anti-inflammatory medication for, 92–93
   isoxsuprine hydrochloride for, 68, 92
   myofascial tightening, 93
   navicular bone (distal sesamoid bone), 85, 86, 87, *87*, *182*
   navicular bursa, 85
   nerve blocks, diagnostic, 89, 89–90
   neurectomy for, 93
   nonsteroidal anti-inflammatory drugs (NSAIDs) for, 93
   nuclear scintigraphy, 90
   padding the foot for, 64
   palmar digital nerve (PDN) block, 89, 89–90
   palmar digital neurectomy for, 93
   pasterns (upright), 25, 86, *86*, 87
   pentoxyfylline for, 92
   polysulfated glycosaminoglycans for, 92
   radiographic (X-ray) evaluation, 90, 91, *91*
   sclerosis (increased mineralization) and, 90
   shoeing, 90–92, *91–92*, 93
   surgical options, 93
   synovial invaginations and, 90
   synthetic shoes for, 91–92, *92*
   ultrasound test, 90
   See also Hoof lameness; Navicular syndrome, causes of
Navicular syndrome, causes of, 86–88
   bone remodeling theory, 86
   bursitis theory, 86
   collateral cartilage complex theory, 87–88
   distal suspensory impar ligament, changes to, 87–88
   long-toe low-heel (LTLH), 88
   medial to lateral hoof imbalance, 88
   sheared heels, 57, *57*
   thrombosis/ischemia theory, 86, 92
   See also Navicular syndrome
Neck
   conformation, 8–10, 11, *13–15*, 13–18, *17–18*, 35, 36–37
   injections, 436, *436*
   manual stretch, 154–155, *155*
Necrosis (tissue death), 71, 303
Needles and syringes, 435, 437–438
Neonatal isoerythrolysis (NI), 563–564
Neonatal maladjustment syndrome (NMS), 563
Neoprene equipment, 366–367
Neospora hughesi, 510
Nephrosplenic entrapment, 309
Nerve blocks, diagnostic, navicular syndrome, 89, 89–90
Nerve impulses, muscle, 138, 139, 149
Nervousness impact, intestinal tract, 294
Neurectomy, 93
Neurologic injury and disease, 504–529
   ataxia, 502, *502*, 504
   bacterial infection, 513–514, *514*
   body trauma, 523, *523*
   botulism, 505, **525–527**
   cerebrospinal fluid (CSF) tests, 512
   dimethyl sulfoxide (DMSO) for WNV, 506
   DNA polymerase chain reaction (PCR) test, 512
   ear inflammation, 514–515, *515*
   Eastern equine encephalitis (EEE), **508**, 540
   equine encephalitis (sleeping sickness), 381, 505, **508**, 540
   equine herpesvirus (EHV1/4), 268, **270–273**, *271*, 456, 497, **508–509**, 511, 516, 536, 540
   equine motor neuron disease (EMND), 511, **517–518**
   equine protozoal myelitis (EPM), 500, 505, **510–513**, *511*, 516, 517, 520
   fallen horse, 520–524, *522–523*
   headshaking, 515–516
   head trauma, 522–523, *523*
   Horner's syndrome, 516–517
   irritation, compression, 514–520, *515*
   lockjaw, 514
   moldy corn poisoning (encephaloma lacia), 527
   muscle fasciculations, 504
   narcolepsy, 519–520
   nigropallidal encephalomalacia, 528
   nonsteroidal anti-inflammatory drugs (NSAIDs) for WNV, 506
   nutrition-related, 525–529
   nystagmus, 515
   opisthotonus, 520
   otitis media-interna, 514–515, *515*, 516
   plant toxicity and, 525, 527–529
   polyneuritis equi (PNE), **519**, 527
   rabies, 505, **509**
   recumbency, 504, **521–522**, *522*
   scavengers and EPM, 510, 513
   seizures, 520
   shivers, 172, **518**
   spinal taps, 512
   spinal trauma, 522, *522–523*, 523
   stringhalt, 172, **524–525**
   sweeny, 524
   syncope (fainting spell), 240, 520
   tetanus, 404, **422**, 431, **513–514**, 540
   tick paralysis, 515
   toxicoinfectious infection, 525
   trauma, 520–525, *522–523*
   Venezuelan equine encephalitis (VEE), 508
   vertebral fracture, 522
   viral infection, 504–509, *505*
   vitamins for, 518
   Western blot assay test, 512
   Western equine encephalitis (WEE), **508**, 540
   West Nile virus (WNV), 381, **504–508**, *505*, 540
   wobbler syndrome (cervical vertebral malformation), 132, **134**, 328, 511, **517**, 535
   See also Neurologic system
Neurologic system, 501–529
   acetylcholine and, 514, 526
   balance, 501
   circumduction, 502
   cranial nerves, 501, 502
   electromyography, 518
   gait evaluation, 502, *502–503*, 503
   "menace response," 500, 502
   mentation, 501
   obstacle testing, 502–503
   obturator nerve, 525

proprioception, 501, 502, 503, *503*
rapid eye movement (REM) sleep, 519
slow-wave sleep (SWS), 519
strength and posture, 501, 503
suprascapular nerve, 524
sway test, 503
tail-pull test, 503
testing, 501–504
trigeminal nerve, 516
vestibular system, 501
See also Neurologic injury and disease
Neuromuscular hyperirritability, 163–165, *164,* 166
Neuromuscular reflexes, 144, 145, *145*
Neutrophil, 261
Newborn foal, 558, 559, *559*
New horses and nutritional management, 473
NI (neonatal isoerythrolysis), 563–564
Nictitating membrane (third eyelid), 488, **490**, 516
Nightshade (*Solanum eleagnifolium*), 529
Nigropallidal encephalomalacia, 528
Nitazoxanide, 513
Nitric oxide (NO), 264
Nitrofurazone, 416
Nitroglycerine, 83
Nitrovasodilators, 264
NMS (neonatal maladjustment syndrome), 563
NO (nitric oxide), 264
Nociceptors, 178
Nodular necrobiosis, *380,* **380–381**, 442
"No" joint (atlanto-axial joint), 14
Non-arthritic ringbone, 122, 128
Nonsteroidal anti-inflammatory drugs (NSAIDs), 442–446
  abuse of, 442, 443
  allergic reactions from, 446
  alternatives to, 446
  arachidonic acid prostaglandins, 444
  aspirin, 445
  back pain, 215
  benefits of, 442–443
  bradykinin and, 442
  cautionary situations, 443–444
  colic and, 307, 320, 443
  competition regulations, **443–444**, 457
  cyclooxygenase (COX-1/2), 444, 445
  double-dosing, 443
  erythema and, 442
  external parasites and control, 389
  eye injury and disease, 496
  flexural contracture, 200
  flunixin meglumine, 444, 445
  histamines and, 442
  injectable medication and, 439
  intestinal symptoms, 296, **445–446**
  intestinal tract, 296, **445–446**
  joint effects from, 446
  kidneys and, 446
  lameness and, 443
  laminitis, 82
  method of action, 442–443

muscle injury, 175
navicular syndrome, 93
osteoarthritis, 127, 130
phenylbutazone (bute), 442, 444–445
prepurchase exams and, 443
prostaglandins and, 442, 443, 444, 446
renal papillary necrosis, 446
skin disease and, 371, 390
strangles, 275
tendon and ligament injury, 196–197
toxicity, 445–446
vaccinations and, 456–457
West Nile Virus (WNV), 506
wounds, 428–429, 429–430, 431
See also Wound management
Non-strangulation infarction, 322
Normal foal, 565, *565*
"No-see-ums" (*Culicoides*), 378, 378–379, 382, 383, 390
Nostrils, 9, 11, 245, 246, 247
NSAIDs. *See* Nonsteroidal anti-inflammatory drugs
Nuchal ligament, 14, *14,* 19, 436
Nuclear scintigraphy, 90, 102
Nutritional management, 325–353
  antioxidants, 338
  body condition scoring (BCS) system, 345–350, *347–350*
  bone conditioning, 100, 105, 107
  calcium-to-phosphorus (Ca:P) ratio, 327, 329, 337
  cardiovascular system, 231–232
  cold weather feeding, 341, 344–345
  colic, 304–305, 305–306, 313, *313,* 315–316, 319, 322–323, 326, 328, 329
  critical temperature and feeding, 344
  dental and oral cavity, 282, *282,* 284, *284*
  Developmental Orthopedic Disease (DOD), 131–132, 133, 134, 135, 329, 337
  dietary manipulation of muscle endurance, 160–165, *164*
  energy, 325–326
  Equine Cushing's Disease (ECD), 78
  equine metabolic syndrome (peripheral cushingold syndrome), 78, **78–80**, 353
  equine polysaccharide storage myopathy (EPSSM), 165, 167, **172–173**, 518, 541
  fat, 326
  guidelines for, 326, 329
  hot climate feeding, 341–344, *343*
  hyperkalemic periodic paralysis (HYPP), 177
  intestinal tract, 296–297, 340–341
  laminitis, 78, 80, 82, 327, 329
  lower respiratory problems, 261–262
  mare, 540, 544
  microminerals, 133–134, 337–338
  minerals and trace microminerals, 337–338
  obese horses (BCS 9), 346, *349,* 349–353, *352, 353,* 474

  protein, 327, 328, 329, 330, 332
  replenishing energy, 339–340
  respiratory illness, 252, 269
  soy products, 332
  trailering and, 481
  tying-up syndrome, 327, 333, *334*
  vitamins, 80, 331, 332, **338**, 482
  weight vs. volume of feed, 326, 330
  See also Electrolyte supplementation; Roughage; Water
Nutritional Secondary Hyperparathyroidism (Big Head Disease), **107**, 329
Nutrition-related neurologic injury and disease, 525–529
Nystagmus, 515
Oats, 329–330, 332
Obel Grade 1-4 (pain response), 75
Obese horses (BCS 9), 346, *349,* 349–350, 349–353, *352, 353,* 474
Obstacle testing, neurologic system, 502–503
Obturator nerve, 525
Occiptus, 14
Occlusion (even contact) of molars, 286
Occult sarcoids, 394–395, *395–396,* 396, 397
OCD (osteochondrosis), 120, 132, **133–134**, 328, 337, 353, 517, 535
Ocular discharge (abnormal), 492–493, *493*
Offset cannon bones, 23, *23,* 24, 25, *25,* 104
Offset knees, 36
Oligofructose (fructan), 76–77, 80, 82
Omeprazole, 319
Onchocerca worm, 383, 385, **385–386**, 390, 467, 497
"On the bit," 15, 248, 249, 491
Open mind of rider for learning, 5
Opisthotonus, 520
Optimizing performance, 5–6
Oral cavity. *See* Dental and oral cavity
Oral glycosaminoglycans, 126–127
Oral vs. injectable medication, 440
Organophosphates, 303, 466, 467
Organ systems and performance, 1–6
  custom-tailored training, 3–5
  human-horse bond (partnership), 1
  imagining a fit horse, 2–3
  optimizing performance, 5–6
  talent of horse and, 1, 3, 7
  team effort for performance, 1, 5, 6
  whole, viewing body as a, 1, 3
  See also Anatomy and function; Back pain; Bone development; Cardiovascular system; Conformation; Dental and oral cavity; Eyes; Hoof; Intestinal tract; Joints; Muscle endurance; Neurologic system; Nutritional management; Preventive health; Reproductive strategies; Respiratory system; Skin as an organ; Tendons and ligaments; Wound management

Osteoarthritis, 122–131
  alternative therapies, 129–130
  back pain and, 214
  coffin joint arthritis, 90, 129
  conformation and, 22, 24, 33, 34
  egg bar shoes for, 91, *91*, 124
  hock joints, 116, *116–117*, 117, 121, *121*
  inflammation, controlling, 122–123, *123*
  nonsteroidal anti-inflammatory drugs (NSAIDs) for, 127, 130
  osteochondrosis fragments, 123, *123*
  radiographic (X-ray) evaluation, 116, 117, *117*, 121, *121*
  shoeing and, 116, 123–124, *124*
  surgery for, 123
  surgical options, 123, *128*, 128–129
  tendon dorsiflexion, **124**, *124*, 184, 196
  therapy for, 122–131, *123*, *128*
  villonodular synovitis, 123, *123*
  See also Joint injury and disease; Joints
Osteoblasts, remodeling bone, 96
Osteochondrosis (OCD), 120, 132, **133–134**, 328, 337, 353, 517, 535
Osteocytes, 96
Otitis media-interna, 514–515, *515*, 516
Outdoor stabling for stress, 477
Ovariectomy, 542–543
Ovaries, 538, 539
Over at the knee (bucked-kneed), 22, *22*, 24
Overbite, 287, *287*
Overriding ("kissing spines"), 30, **212–213**, *213*
Overtraining
  avoiding, 6
  bone response, 102–105, *103–105*
  exercise intolerance, 234
  remodeling bone, 103
Ovnicek, Gene, 48
Ovulation, 541, 542
Oxidative capacity within muscle, 146, *146*, 152
Oxidative stress, laminitis, 80
Oxygen
  cardiovascular system, 228
  muscle endurance, 140, 141, 142
  respiratory system, 249, 250, 251, 252
Oxytetracycline, 200
Packed cell volume (PCV), 241
Padding for stall kickers, 476
Padding the foot, 64–65, *64–65*
Paddling, 20, 111
Pain and estrus, 543
Pain of horse, interpreting, 298–299
Pain relief (analgesia), 178, 193–194, 198
Paired serology, 269
Palmar digital nerve (PDN) block, 89, 89–90
Palmar digital neurectomy, 93
Panoramic field of vision, 490, *491*
Panting, heat dissipation, 240, 252
Papillomas (warts), **392**, *392*, 393, 536
Papules, 385
Parasites. *See* External parasites and control; Internal parasites and control
Parasitoids (stinging wasps), 383–384
Parathyroid hormone, 107, 164–165
Parrot mouth, 12, 287, 535
Passive transfer and antibody protection, 561
Pasterns
  bone development, 99
  bone response to conditioning, 112, *112*
  conformation, 8–9, 25–26, *25–26*, 36
  navicular syndrome, 25, 86, *86*, 87
  tendon injury and, 183–184
Pasture, 282, *282*, **329**, 459
Pasture overload, laminitis, 75, **76–77**, 82
Patchy shedding, 374
PCR (polymerase chain reaction) test, 276
PCV (packed cell volume), 241
PDN (palmar digital nerve) block, 89, 89–90
Peak strength of bone, 100–102
Pectoral injections, 437
Pedunculated sarcoids, 394
Pelleted feeds, 328, 332–333, 476
Pelodera strongyloides, 386
Pelvic flexure, *291*, 292, 309
Pelvis and croup angle, 28–30, *29–30*
PEMF (pulsing electromagnetic fields), 179–180
Penis, 400, *400*, **536**, *536*
Pentoxyfylline, 83, 92
Perfusion of different organs, 221–222
Pergolide, 78
Perineum, 544–545, *545*
Periodic ophthalmia (ERU), 385–386, 445, 497–498, **497–499**, 500
Periople of hoof, 59, 66, 67
Periosteum, 103
Peripheral cushingold syndrome (equine metabolic syndrome), 78, **78–80**, 353
Peristalsis, 293, 314–315
Peritendinous, 191
Peritonitis, 310, 429, 462, *463*
Permeability features of hoof, 66
Personality conflicts between horses, 477
Petechiations, 271, 277, 388
Pharyngeal lymphoid hyperplasia, 259
Pharyngitis, 247
Phayrnx, 247
Phenylbutazone (bute), 442, 444–445. *See also* Nonsteroidal anti-inflammatory drugs (NSAIDs)
Pheromones in fly traps, 384
Phonophoresis, 198
Phosphate molecules, muscle, 140
Phosphocreatine, 141
Photoactivated vasculitis, 368, 371
Photon absorptiometry, 102
Photophobia, 385
Photosensitivity ("sunburn"), 368–369, *369*, *371*, 371–372, 385
Phthisis bulbi, 498, *498*
Physeal dysplasia (epiphysitis), 132, **132–133**, 199, *199*, 328, 337, 353
Physical exam mare, 543–544
Physical exam stallion, 535
Physical restraint, 450–453, *450–453*
PI (povidone iodine), 406, 414, 428, 435
Pigeon-breasted horse, 23
Pigeon breast/fever (dryland distemper), *174*, **174–176**, 273, 377
Pigeon-toed (fetlock varus), 22, 23, *23*, 36, 134
Pineal gland, 538, 539
Pinworms (*Oxyuris equi*), 379, *379*, 460, *460*, 463–464, **463–464**, 467
Piperazine, 466, 467
Piroplasmosis, 435
Pitcher plant (*Sarapin*), 215
Pitting edema, 389, 390, *390*
Pituitary pars intermedia dysfunction (PPID), 77–78, *77–78*
Pit vipers, 430
Placenta, 560–561, *560–561*
Placentitis, 563
Plaiting, 20, 206, 208
Plantar tarsal ligament, 31, 34, **187**, *187*
Plant toxicity, 571–573
  colic, 320–321
  flexural contracture, 199
  laminitis, 80
  neurologic injury and disease, 525, 527–529
  skin disease, 368, 369, 375
Pleuritis, 429
Pleuropneumonia, 259, **273**, 480
PNE (polyneuritis equi), **519**, 527
Pododermatitis (thrush), 63, **73**
Points of hocks, 8–9, *9*
Pollen and skin, 390
Pollitt, Chris, 76, 82, 317
Polymerase chain reaction (PCR) test, 276, 512
Polyneuritis equi (PNE), **519**, 527
Polysulfated glycosaminoglycans (PSGAGs), 92, 125–126
Ponazuril, 513
"Popped" splint, 104
Post-legged, 32, *32*, 33, *33*
Potassium in muscle, 138, 163
Potomac Horse Fever, **294–295**, 388
Poultices, 195, 418
Povidone iodine (PI), 406, 414, 428, 435
PPID (pituitary pars intermedia dysfunction), 77–78, *77–78*
Praziquantel, 466, 467
Prednisolone, 262
Pregnancy check, 552–553, *553*
Premature foal, 565
Prepuce (sheath), 79, **400**, *400*
Prepurchase exams and NSAIDs, 443
Preventive health, 455–485
  blood tests, value of, 457–458
  brand inspection, 457
  chemistry panel, 458
  Coggins Test, 242–243, 455, **457**
  Competitive Enzyme-Linked Immunosorbent Assay (C-ELISA), 457
  complete blood count (CBC), 457–458

drug testing profile, 458
health inspection, 455–456
herd health, 265, 455–459, 465
hygiene (good), 459
lactate testing, 458
quarantine, 260, 270, 276, **458–459**, 465
Synthetic Antigen ELISA (SA-ELISA), 457
vaccination protection, 456–457
See also External parasites and control; Internal parasites and control; Stress; Trailering stress
Primary immunization, 265
Probiotics, 331–332
Progesterone, 539
"Progressive training" methods, 224
Prolactin and foaling, 558
Proprioception, 501, 502, 503, *503*
Propulsive forces, bone, 97
Prostaglandins
inhibiting, 127
mare and, 539, 550, 551
NSAIDs and, 442, 443, 444, 446
Protective bandages/boots, 485, *485*
Protein
climate feeding, 342–343
muscle, 139
nutritional management, 327, 328, 329, 330, 332
Proteoglycans (glycosaminoglycans), 110, 111, 125, 446
Proud flesh (exuberant granulation), 388, 394, 407, *407*, 408, 409, *409*, **416**, 418
Proximal intertarsal joint, 32
Proximal suspensory ligament, *181*, *186*, 186–187
Pseudomonas, 549
PSGAGs (polysulfated glycosaminoglycans), 92, 125–126
Psoroptic mites (scabies), 384
Psychological stress, 472–478
Psyllium, **313–314**, 332
Pulled muscles, 165
Pulleys, muscle, 137–138
Pulsing electromagnetic fields (PEMF), 179–180
Pulsing wave ultrasound, 198
Puncture wounds, 403, 410, *421–422*, **421–423**
Pupil, eyes, *488–489*
Purina *Race of Champions*, 221
Purpura hemorrhagica, 201, 277, 277–278, **391**
Pyloric sphincter, 317
Pyrantel (Strongid-C), 466–467, *467*, 469–470
Pyrethins, pyrethoids, 383, 387
Pyrimethamine, 512
Quadriceps, *10*, 27
Quarantine, 260, 270, 276, **458–459**, 465
Quarter cracks, hoof, 57, *57*
Quarter Horses
cardiovascular system, 220
conformation, 31, 35
muscle, 142, 143, 147, 172, 176
navicular syndrome, 86, *86*
neurologic system, 518
nutritional management, 337
skin as an organ, 360, 392
Queensland's itch (summer itch), 378, 378–379
"Quick" (corium), hoof, 41, *41–42*, 42, 84
Quick turns, tendon injury, 184
Rabies, 505, **509**
Radial shock wave machine, 106
Radiographic (X-ray) evaluation
bone response to conditioning, 102
colic, 312, *312*
flexural contracture, 200–201
joints, 115, 120, 121, *121*, 122
laminitis, 83
navicular syndrome, 90, 91, *91*
osteoarthritis, 116, 117, *117*, 121, *121*
Radius, 8, 24
Rain scald (rain rot), 369, 371, 375
Ramps on teeth, 285, 288
Range of motion, joints, 110–111
RAO (recurrent airway obstruction), 256, **259–262**, *260*, 267, 456, 543–544
Rapid eye movement (REM) sleep, 519
"Rat" tail from parasites, 378, *378*
Rattlesnakes, 430
RBCs (red blood cells), 221, 241, 457
Rear symmetry, 9
Recombinant DNA vaccine, 506–507
Recovery period, respiratory viruses, 269–270
Rectal examination, 301–302, 312, 546
Rectal temperature
colic and, 301
cooling and, 359
exercise intolerance, 237–238, 239, 240
fever, 429
Rectum, *291*, 292
Recumbency, 504, **521–522**, *522*
Recurrent airway obstruction (RAO), 256, **259–262**, *260*, 267, 456, 543–544
Recurrent exertional rhabdomyolysis (RER), **166–167**, 541
Recurrent laryngeal nerves, 16
Recurrent laryngeal neuropathy (RLN), 12, 16, 246, 247, **258–259**, 263, 511
Red blood cells (RBCs), 221, 241, 457
Red maple toxicity and anemia, 241
Refraction, 489–490
Refrigeration, injectable medication, 433
Rehabilitation, muscle, 152
Reining and cutting
bone development, 86
conformation, 23, 25, 26, 28, 31, 34–36
exercises, 151
joints, 111
muscle endurance, 139, 143, 148
navicular syndrome, 86
Remodeling bone theory, navicular, 86
Remodeling of
hoof, 42–43, *43*
wound, 418–420, *429–420*
Remodeling process of bone, 96–98
cannon bone, 98, *98*
collagen, 97
compression and tension, 97
compressive strain, 96
flexural strain, 96–97
genetics and, 96
hydroxyapatite crystals, 96
multiple forces, 97
osteoblasts, 96
osteocytes, 96
osteoid, 96
overtraining and, 103
propulsive forces, 97
rotational strain, 97
shearing strain, 97
strain and deformation, 96–97, *97*
strength of bone, 97–98, *98*
stress, bone response to, 96–97, *97*
swing phase of limb strain, 97, 120
tensile strain, 96
torque strain, 97
torsion (twisting), 97
training response, 96–97, *97*, 98, 99
Wolff's Law, 97
See also Bone development; Bone response to conditioning
REM (rapid eye movement) sleep, 519
Renal papillary necrosis, 446
Repetition, cardiovascular system, 225
Repetitive stress and back pain, 209
Replenishing energy, 339–340
Replication of a virus, 264–265
Reproductive disease and problems, 555–565
cervicitis, 547
combined immunodeficiency disease (CID), 535
contagious equine metritis (CEM), 536–537
equine coital exanthma, 536
equine viral arteritis (EVA), 268, 536, **555–557**
granulosa cell tumor, 555, *555*
hernia, 535
mare reproductive loss syndrome (MRLS), 555
parrot mouth, 12, 287, 535
retained testicle (cryptorchidism), 535
shedding stallions, 556–557
tipped vagina, **545**, *545*, 548, *548*
urine pooling (*vesiculo-vaginal reflux*), 532, 545, **547**
uterine infection (metritis), 544
vaginitis, 547
"windsucking" vagina (pneumovagina), 544, 545
See also Foaling and complications; Reproductive strategies
Reproductive strategies, 531–565
artificial insemination (AI), 550, 551, *551*, **553–555**
breeding evaluation, 532
breeding process, 550–553, *551–553*
embryo transfer (ET), 555
estrus, detecting for breeding, 550–551, *551–552*, 552

genetic improvement, 531, *531*
natural cover, 550
pregnancy check, 552–553, *553*
scientific interference, 531–532
See also Conformation; Foaling and complications; Mare; Reproductive disease and problems; Stallion
RER (recurrent exertional rhabdomyolysis), **166–167**, 541
Resistance exercises, 150
Respiratory adaptations, 251–252
Respiratory cooling, 357–358, *358*
Respiratory illness, 252–279
   air quality impact, 254, 256–257
   anemia, 233, **241–243**, 252–253, 337, 457
   arytenoid chondritis, 259
   coughing, 255
   dorsal displacement of the soft palate (DDSP), **259**, 511
   epiglottic entrapment, 259
   foreign particles, defense, 254–255
   mucociliary apparatus (MCA), 255, 268, 273
   nutritional management, 252, 269
   pharyngeal lymphoid hyperplasia, 259
   recurrent laryngeal neuropathy (RLN), 12, 16, 246, 247, **258–259**, 263, 511
   stress factors, 257–258
   trailering and, 253, 479–480, 481–482
   upper respiratory problems, 254–255, 258–259
   ventilation benefits, 256–257, 264, 480
   See also Lower respiratory problems; Respiratory system; Respiratory viruses; Strangles
Respiratory rate, 221, 240, **250, 251**, 300, 429
Respiratory system, 245–252
   airways and airflow, 246–247
   alveoli, *245*, 249
   bit evasion, 248–249, 253
   breathing, muscles, 249–251, *250*, 252
   bronchioles, *245*, 249, 261
   carbon dioxide, 249, 250
   cardiovascular adaptations, 251–252
   diaphragm, 247, 249, 250
   exhalation, 247, 250
   flexion, poll and neck, 247–248, 253
   functional adaptation, 251–252
   hemoglobin, 249, 251, 337
   inhalation, 246–247
   laryngo-palatal dislocation, 248
   larynx, *245, 246*, 247, 258
   locomotor-respiration coupling, *250*, 250–251, 254
   lower respiratory tract, *245*, *245*, 249–251, *250*
   lungs, *245*, 249
   nostrils, *245, 246*, 247
   oxygen, 249, 250, 251, 252
   respiratory rate, 221, 240, **250, 251**, 300, 429
   "second wind," 252

soft palate, 247, 248, *248*, 259
sternothyrohyoideus, 247
thoracic cavity, *245*, 249
trachea, 246, 247, *248*
upper respiratory tract, *245–246*, 245–249, *248*
   See also Cardiovascular system; Lower respiratory problems; Respiratory illness; Respiratory viruses; Strangles
Respiratory viruses, 264–273
   age of horse and vaccination, 265, 270, 272
   antibodies, 264–265, 266, 267
   antigenic drift, 266, 267
   boosters, 265, 266, 270, 456
   cell mediated immunity (CMI) and, 272
   diagnosis, 268–269
   drift, 266, 267
   equine herpesvirus (EHV1/4), 268, **270–273**, *271*, 456, 497, **508–509**, 511, 516, 536, 540
   equine influenza ("flu"), **267–270**, *268*, 456, 497, 540
   hemagglutinin (HA) spikes and, 264
   herd health, 265, 455–459, 465
   influenza virus ("flu"), **267–270**, *268*, 456, 497, 540
   isolation of sick horse, 269
   modification by viruses, 266–267
   nasal discharge, 268, *268*, 271, *271*, 273
   petechiations, 271, 277, 388
   prevention of, 265, 270, 279
   quarantine of new horse, 269, 270, **458–459**
   recovery period, 269–270
   replication of a virus, 264–265
   rhinovirus (ERV), 268, **272–273**, 456
   spread of, 264, 267–268, 271–272, 274, 275
   tracheobronchitis, 272–273
   vaccinations (immunizations), 265–266, 270, 272, 279, 456
   viral duplication, 266–267
   viral neurologic disease (myeloencephalopathy), 271, 272
   See also Lower respiratory problems; Respiratory illness; Respiratory system; Strangles
Rest for
   back pain, 205, 214
   cardiovascular system, 233, 234
   fit horse, 2
   hoof lameness, 69
   muscle, 152
   osteoarthritis, 122
Resting heart rate, 229, 230, 252
Restraint, safe and effective, 446–454
   backing a horse, 450
   behavior of horses and, 447, 448, 449
   blindfold, 452
   calmness, creating, 447–448
   chemical restraint, 453–454
   cross-ties, 449–450

"earring down," 451
endorphins, 178, 451–452
equipment, safe, 448
flight instinct, 447, 448, 449, 450
foal restraint, 453
halters, 450, *450*
handlers, 449
herd instinct, 447, 448, 449, 472, 476, 482
hobble, 452–453
letting go, avoiding, 449
lip chain, 452, *452*
physical restraint, 450–453, *450–453*
standing positions, 449
stocks, 453, *453*
stud chain, 452
tranquilizers, 453–454
twitch, *451*, 451–452
war bridle, 452
work areas, safe, 448
See also Wound management
Retained caps, 286
Retained fetal membranes, 560–561, *560–561*
Retina, 489, *489*, 490
Retropharyngeal lymph nodes, 273, 274, *274*
Rhabditic dermatitis, 386
Rhinopneumonitis (equine herpesvirus), 268, **270–273**, *271*, 456, 497, **508–509**, 511, 516, 536, 540
Rhinovirus (ERV), 268, **272–273**, 456
Rhizoctonia leguminicola, 282
Rice bran, 331
Rider and horse back pain, *210*, 210–211
Ridges, hoof, 54, 74, 79
Riding and vision of horse, 487–488, 491–492
Riding instruction, 6
Rim pads/shoes, 63, 65
Ringbone, 22, 25, 112, *121*, **121–122**, 128–129
Ringworm, 372–374, *373*
Ripples, hoof, 54, 74
RLN (recurrent laryngeal neuropathy), 12, 16, 246, 247, **258–259**, 263, 511
Roach back (kyphosis), 27, *27*, 30, *30*, **212**, *212*
Road founder, 80, 81, *81*
Roaring (RLN), 12, 16, 246, 247, **258–259**, 263, 511
"Rockered" (rolled) toe, 50, 60
Rodier, A.V., 484
Rope burns, 424–426, *425*
Rotational strain, bone, 97
Roughage, 326–332
   alternatives, 328–329
   barley, 330
   beet pulp, 328–329
   cereal grain hay (oat hay), 327
   cold weather feeding and, 344
   complete feed pellets, 328, 332–333, 476
   concentrates, 326, 328, 329–330, 332
   corn, 329–330, 332, 342

fat for energy, 330–331, 332, 342
feed supplements, 328–329
fiber, 326, 340
grass hay, 327, 332
guidelines for, 326, 329
hay, 326–328
high fiber feed supplements, 328–329
legume hay, 164–165, 327–328, 332
moisture content of hay, 327
mold in hay, 327
nutritional value of hay, 327
oats, 329–330, 332
pasture, 282, *282*, **329**, 459
pelleted feeds, 328, 332–333, 476
probiotics, 331–332
psyllium, **313–314**, 332
rice bran, 331
rye, 330
sweet feed, 330
vegetable oil, 330–331
water and, 333
wheat bran, 329
See also Nutritional management
Roughs (ungrazed grass around feces), 459
Round back vs. hollow back, 217, *217*
Roundworms (ascarids), 322, 460, *460*, 462, *462*, 467
Rubin, S.T., 100
Rump injections, 436, *437*, 437
Rump rug for cool-down, 158, *158*
Russian knapweed (*Acroptilon repens*), 528
Rye, 330
Sacroiliac area and back pain, 207, 208
Sacroiliac ligaments, 30
Sacrum, 8, 30
Saddle fit, 19, *19*, 20, 206–207, *209*, 209–210, 365, 365–366
Saddle sores, 364–367, *365–366*
Saddling issues, 4–5, 6
SA-ELISA (Synthetic Antigen ELISA), 457
Saline solution irrigation, 496
Salivation, excessive, 282–283
Salmonella spp., 294
Salt block, 333
Salt content in electrolytes, 335–336
Sand colic, 302, 310–315, *311–313*
Sand cracks, hoof, 57, 58, *58*, 67
Sarcocystis falcatula, 510
Sarcoids, 393–396, **393–397**, 536
Sarcoplasmic reticulum, muscle, 138
Sarcoptic mange/mites, 384
Scabies (psoroptic mites), 384
Scaffold for healing, 425
Scalenus muscles, 19
Scapula (shoulder blade), 8, 20, *21*, 23
Scarring (fibrosis), 200
Scar tissue, 183, 420, *420*
Scavengers and EPM, 510, 513
SCC (squamous cell carcinomas), 372, 388, 395, **399**, 400, *400*, 490, 499, *499*, 536, 545
Scientific interference, reproduction, 531–532

Sclerosis, 90
Scoliosis, 212
Scope, 26, 36
Scratches (grease heel), 367–369, **367–371**, 384
Scrubbing wound, 405
SDF (synchronous diaphragmatic flutter), *164*, **164–165**, 170, 239, 333, *334*
SDFT (superficial digital flexor tendon), *181*, 181–182, 183, *185*, **185–186**
Seasonally polyestrus, 538
Secondary bacterial infection, 273
Second intention healing, 426
"Second wind," 252
Secretory antibodies, 268
Sedatives, 453–454
Sedimentation, injectable medication, 434
Seizures, neurologic, 520
Selenium, 162, 173, **337–338**
Selenium poisoning (alkali disease), 57–58, **374–375**
Selenium toxicity, **57–58**, *58*, 162, 173, 338
Self-exercise and stress, 477
Semen
  evaluation, 534, 537–538
  extenders, 538
  frozen, 550, 551, *551*, 554
Sense of humor, 5
Sensitive laminae, hoof, 42, 44, 74
Septicemia, 497, 562
Sequestrum, 424, *424*
Seroma, 423, *423*
Serotonin, 178
Serum antibodies, 505
Serum hepatitis, 422
Sesamoiditis, 26
Sessile sarcoids, 394
SET (standard exercise test), 232–233
Shaker foal syndrome (botulism), 505, **525–527**
Sharp points on teeth, 286
"Shave job," 361, *361*
Sheared heels, 56–57, *57*
Shearing strain, bone, 97
Sheath cleaning, 399–401, *400–401*
Shin splints, 103
Shipping boots, 485, *485*
Shipping fever, 273, 480
Shivers, 172, **518**
Shock and colic, *299*, 299–300
Shock wave therapy. See Extracorporeal shock wave therapy (ESWT)
Shoe boil (capped elbow), 114, *114*
Shoes and pads, 58–65
  "backing up the toe," 50, 60
  back pain and, 211, *211*
  balance of hoof, 60, 62, *62*
  boot alternatives, 59, 59–60, 65
  breakover and, 50, 60
  broken-back hoof-pastern axis, **50–51**, *51*, 60, 183
  caulks, **62–63**, *63*, 97, 184, 211
  collapsed heels, 60, 63, *63*
  corns from, 63, 64, **71–72**, *72*
  corrective shoeing, 62

daily care importance, 63
Developmental Orthopedic Disease (DOD), 136
egg bar shoes, **91**, *91*, 124, 188
flexural contracture, 200
fullered (full-swedge) shoes, 63
heel expansion, 59
heel support, 60, 62, *62–63*, *63*, 65, *65*
hoof as visual record of stress, 53, *53*, 55, 60–61, *60–61*
hoof-pastern axis, 48–49, 50–51, *50–51*, 60
hoof wall flexibility, 60, *60–61*, 61
"hot" nail, 72–73
imbalance and lameness, 53, *53*, 55, 59, 60, 88
injury vs. protection, 58–63, *59–63*
joints and, 111
laminitis and, 64, 83
musculoskeletal structures and, 58–59
navicular syndrome, 90–92, *91–92*, 93
osteoarthritis, 116, 123–124, *124*
padding the foot, 64–65, *64–65*
protection, shoeing for, 59
rim pads/shoes, 63, *65*
"rockered" (rolled) toe, 50, 60
"short shod," 61, *61*
size of shoe, 60, *60–61*, 61
slippered (beveled) shoe, 60
synthetic shoes, 91–92, *92*
tendon injury, 183, 188
tincture of iodine, 65, 406
toe grabs, **63**, *63*, 97, 211
traction devices, 62–63, *63*
unshod (barefoot) foot, 58, 59
wedge pads, 60, 65, *65*
widest part of frog, 60, 61, *61*
wide-web shoes, 65, *66*, 66
See also Hoof; Long-toe low-heel (LTLH)
Short back, 26, 27, *27*
Short muscles, 137–138
Short neck, 15, *15*
Short pastern, 25, *25*
"Short shod," 61, *61*
Shoulder, conformation, 8–10, 20–22, *21*, 35, 36, 37
Show classes, 142
SI (small intestine), *291*, 292, 293
Sick foal, signs of, 564–565
Sickle-hocked, 31, 32, *32*, 33–34, *34*, 35
Sidebone, hoof, 46–47, *47*
Side symmetry, 9
"Silent" heats, 534, 551
Silver sulfadiazine, 367, 414, 428
Siring records, stallion, 538
Skeletal system, 8, *8*
Skin as an organ, 355–401
  anhidrosis, 361
  arteriovenous anastomoses (AVA), 357
  blood vessels, 357, *357*
  conditioning, 359–360, *360–361*, 362
  convective cooling, 359
  cooling methods, 357–359, *358*
  evaporative cooling, 357, *358*, 358
  heat dissipation, 356–357, *357*
  heat index, 361–362, *362*

heat stress, **359–363,** *360–363,* 429
rectal temperature and cooling, 359
respiratory cooling, 357–358, *358*
selenium toxicity, **57–58,** *58,* 162, 173, 338
sheath cleaning, 399–401, *400–401*
smegma, 400, 401, *401*
sweating excessively, 361
thermistor, 362–363, *363*
thermoregulation role, 355–363
trailering and heat, 360–361, *362*
water application, 358–359, *362*
See also Dehydration; Skin diseases; Skin growths
Skin diseases, 363–399
allergic reactions, 377, *377–378,* 378, 389–391, *389–391*
alopecia (hair loss), 374–375, 380, 385
anaphylaxis, 391
angiodema, 391
anti-inflammatory treatment, 370–371
chorioptic mange/mites, 369, 384
dermatitis, 367
Dermatophilus congolensis, 369, 371, 375
dermatophytosis, 372–374, *373*
diagnosis of, 363–364
drug allergies and, 390
food allergies and, 390
fungal infection, 369, 372–374, *373*
girths and, 366
hair loss associated with, 374–375, 385
Hereditary Equine Regional Dermal Asthenia (HERDA, *Hyperelastosis- cutis),* 392
hives (urticaria), *389–391,* **389–392,** 440
hygiene and, 367, *367–368,* 371
mechanical concerns, 364–367, *365–366*
melanocytes and, 364–365, *365,* 396
NSAIDs for, 371, 390
patchy shedding, 374
photoactivated vasculitis, 368, 371
photosensitivity ("sunburn"), 368–369, *369, 371,* 371–372, 385
pitting edema, 389, 390, *390*
plant toxicity and, 368, 369, 375
purpura hemorrhagica, 201, 277, 277–278, *391*
rain scald (dew poisoning), 369, 371, 375
ringworm, 372–374, *373*
saddle sores, 364–367, *365–366*
scratches (grease heel), 367–369, **367–371,** 384
selenium poisoning (alkali disease), 57–58, **374–375**
skin scald, 374
treatment for, 371–372, 374
white pastern disease (scratches), 367–369, **367–371,** 384
See also External parasites and control; Skin as an organ; Skin growths
Skin growths, 392–399
Bacillus Calmette-Guerin (BCG)

injections, *396,* 396–397
benign, 392
bloodroot *(Sanguinaria canadensis)* extract for, 397
fibroblastic sarcoids, 388, 394, *394,* 395
fibromas, 395
keloids, 395, 420, *420*
malignant cancer, 392
melanomas, **397–399,** *398–399,* 499, *499,* 536, 545
occult sarcoids, 394–395, *395–396,* 396, 397
sarcoids, 393–396, **393–397,** 536
squamous cell carcinomas (SCC), 388, 395, **399,** 400, *400,* 490, 499, *499,* 536, 545
surgery for, 395–396
treatment for, 396, 397, 398–399
warts (papillomas), **392,** *392,* 393, 536
See also Skin as an organ; Skin diseases
Skin pinch test, 235, *235–236*
Skin scald, 374
Skin tension and contraction, 408–409, *409*
Slaframine toxin, 282–283
Sleeping sickness (equine encephalitis), 381, 505, **508,** 540
Slippered (beveled) shoe, 60
Sloping shoulder, 20–22, *21*
Slow healing, 418
Slow twitch high oxidative muscle fibers (ST, Type 1), 143, 144, 145, 146, 225
Slow-wave sleep (SWS), 519
Small colon, *291,* 292, 293
Small intestine (SI), *291,* 292, 293
Smegma, 400, 401, *401*
Snakebite, 430–432, *431*
Social acclimation and stress, 472–473, *473*
Sodium bicarbonate drench ("milkshake"), 336–337
Sodium hyaluronate. *See* Hyaluronic acid
Sodium imbalance, muscle endurance, 163
Soft laser for osteoarthritis, 129
Soft palate, 247, 248, *248,* 259
Soft tissue injury, joints, 114, *114*
Solar bruising and laminitis, 70
Sole bruises, hoof, 64, 65, **70,** *70*
Sole callus, hoof, 39, 44, *44*
Sorghum-sudan grass, 527–528
Soy products, 332
Spasmodic colic, 303
Spatial terminology, *11*
Speed play (fartleks), 228
Sphincter, 292
Spinal infection, 214, *214*
Spinal taps, 512
Spinal trauma, 522, *522–523,* 523
Spinous ear tick *(Otobius),* 171, 387, **387, 515,** 516
Spinous processes, 212–213, *213–214,* 345
Splayfooted (fetlock valgus), 22, 23, *23*

Spleen, cardiovascular system, 219–220
Splint boots, 104, 105, *105*
Splints, 24, **103–105,** *104–105,* 424, *424*
Splints for flexural contracture, 200
Sponging, cool-down, 157, *157*
Spooky behavior, 487–488, 491–492
Sports specific conformation, 34–37
Spread of respiratory viruses, 264, 267–268, 271–272, 274, 275
Sprint exercise. *See* Anaerobic
Squamous cell carcinomas (SCC), 372, 388, 395, **399,** 400, *400,* 490, 499, *499,* 536, 545
Squamous mucosa, 318
ST, Type 1 (slow twitch high oxidative muscle fibers), 143, 144, 145, 146, 225
Stable flies *(Stomoxys calcitrans),* 376–377, 382
Stallion, 532–538
bacterial culture, 537
bad-tempered, 532, 533, *533*
booking to a stallion, 534
breeding contract, 534
breeding performance, 532–534, *533*
health, maintaining, 535
heritable abnormalities, 535
live foal guarantee (LFG), 534, 554
penis, 400, *400,* **536,** *536*
physical exam, 535
questionable breeder, 538
reproductive exam, 535–538, *536*
satisfactory breeder, 538
season for breeding, 538
semen, frozen, 550, 551, *551,* 554
semen evaluation, 534, 537–538
semen extenders, 538
siring records, 538
stress and fertility, 537–538
teasing programs, 534–535
testicles, 535–536, *536*
unsatisfactory breeder, 538
venereal disease, 536–537
See also Conformation; Mare; Reproductive disease and problems; Reproductive strategies
Stall-kicking, 475–477
Stamina, improving, 148
Stance phase of limb loading, 99, 120
Standard exercise test (SET), 232–233
Staphylococcal sp., 369, 371
Stereotypic behaviors, stress, 474–477
Sternothyrohyoideus, 247
Stethoscope, 222, *222*
Stifle
conformation, 8–10, 9, 29, 30, *30,* 31, 32, *32,* 33, *33,* 36, 37
pain, signs of, 117–118, *118*
Stinging wasps *(parasitoids),* 383–384
"Stocked-up" legs, 68, 196
Stocks, restraint, 453, *453*
Stomach, *291,* 291–292, 293
Stomach (nasogastric) tube, 296, *296,* **302**
Stomach tubing, grain overload, 82–83
Stomach worms, *460,* 462–462, *462–463*
Storage, injectable medication, 434–435

Strain and deformation, bone, 96–97, 97
Strained muscles, 165
Strangles (*Streptococcus equi*, equine distemper), 273–279
  age of horse and, 273–274
  antibiotics for, 275
  bastard strangles (metastatic strangles abscessation), 276–277
  boosters, 276
  carrier horses, 274–275
  chondroids from, 277
  complications from, 276–278, *277*
  diagnosis of, 268, 273, 276
  empyema from, 277
  guttural pouch infection, 277
  hot packs for, 275
  intranasal vaccine, 277–278
  isolation of sick horse, 275
  limb swelling from, 201
  lymph nodes swelling, 273, 274, *274*, 275
  nasal discharge, 268, *268*, 271, *271*, 273
  nasopharyngeal swabs, 276
  NSAIDs for, 275
  polymerase chain reaction (PCR) test, 276
  prevention of, 275–276, 279
  purpura hemorrhagica from, 277, 277–278
  quarantine of new horse, 276, **458–459**
  retropharyngeal lymph nodes and, 273, 274, *274*
  risk of, 273–275
  sanitation for controlling, 275
  spread of, 274, 275
  submandibular lymph nodes and, 273, 274, *274*
  surgical lancing for, 275
  vaccination (immunization) strategies, 275–276, 278–279
  See also Lower respiratory problems; Respiratory illness; Respiratory system; Respiratory viruses
Strangulation obstruction, 308
Straw-itch mites, 385
Strength
  bone, 97–98, *98*
  hoof, 47, *47*, 66
  neurologic system, 501, 503
  skeletal, 101
Strength training
  back pain and, *216*, 216–217
  cardiovascular system, 227
  muscle endurance, 148–149, 150, 151
Streptococcus
  cardiovascular system, 240
  eyes, 497
  laminitis, 77
  preventive health, 480
  reproductive strategies, 549
  respiratory system, 268, 273
  skin as an organ, 371, 391
Stress, 472–484
  boredom relief, 477
  confinement impact, 473–474, 476
  cribbing, 285, 288, *288*, 289, 475
  defined, 472
  environment, changing for, 477–478
  exercise intolerance, 239, *239*, 239–240
  external parasites and, 376
  fertility, stallion, 537–538
  handlers, changing, 477–478
  herd instinct, 447, 448, 449, 472, 476, 482
  isolation impact, 473–474, 476
  loner horses, 476
  movement (abnormal) and, 475
  mucociliary escalator and, 479–480
  outdoor stabling for, 477
  performance exercise and, 477
  personality conflicts between horses, 477
  psychological stress, 472–478
  respiratory system, 257–258
  self-exercise and, 477
  social acclimation and, 472–473, *473*
  stall-kicking and, 475–477
  stereotypic behaviors, 474–477
  toys for boredom relief, 477
  wood chewing and, 474–475
  See also Preventive health; Trailering stress
Stress-related failure, tendons, 183
Stretching
  back pain and, 216
  muscle endurance, 149, 153–156, *154–156*
  osteoarthritis and, 129
Stretching through the topline, 18–19
Stride length and conformation, 15, 20–22, *21*, 31
Stringhalt, 172, **524–525**
Strongyles (large and small) (bloodworms), 322, 460, *460–461*, 461–462, *467*
Strongylus, 321–322, 461
Stud chain, 452
Studs on shoes, 62–63, *63*
Stull, C.L., 484
Subchondral bone, joints, *109*, 110, 116
Subclinical infection, 267
Subcutaneous injection, 441–442
Submandibular lymph nodes, 273, 274, *274*
Submaximal exercise. *See* Aerobic exercise
Subsolar abscess, hoof, 70
Sugar (granulated) dressing, 415
Sulci (crevices), hoof, *39*, 44–45, *45*, 73
Sulfadiazine, 512
Summer itch (Queensland's itch), 378, 378–379
Summer sores (*Habronema, Draschia*), 383, **388–389**, 395, *463*, *467*, 536
Sunburn (photosensitivity), 368–369, *369*, *371*, 371–372, 385
Superficial digital flexor tendon (SDFT), *181*, 181–182, 183, *185*, **185–186**
Superior check desmotomy, 197, 200
Superior check ligament surgery, 200
Supplements, hoof, 67–68
Support bandages for tendons, **196**, 202
Support founder, 80–81, *81*
Suppressor T-cells, 398–399
Suprascapular nerve, 524
Surgery for
  angular limb deformities (ALD), 136
  colic, 298–299, 315
  joint fusion, 116
  mare, 542–543
  navicular syndrome, 93
  osteoarthritis, 123, *128*, 128–129
  proud flesh, 416
  recurrent laryngeal neuropathy (RLN), 259
  skin growths, 395–396
  strangles, lancing, 275
  tendons, 197
Suspensory desmitis, 26
Suspensory ligament injury, 33, 34
Suspensory ligaments, *181*, 182
Sutures, 411–412, *412*, 413, *413*
Swamp fever (EIA), **241–243**, 376, 457, 536
Sway back (lordosis), 26, 27, *27*, 212, **212**
Sway test, 503
Sweat bandages, **195**, 198, 418
Sweat glands, 356
Sweating
  calcium lost in, 96
  electrolytes and, 162–163, 164, 165, 333, 334, 356
  excessively, 361
  muscle endurance, 146, 149
  protein role in, 343, *343*
Sweeny, 524
Sweet feed, 330
Swelling
  joint injury, 113, *113*
  tendon injury, *189*, 189–190, **192–198**, *193–194*
Swimming, 225–226, *226*
Swing phase of limb strain, 97, 120
SWS (slow-wave sleep), 519
Symmetry of horse, 8–9
Synchronous diaphragmatic flutter (SDF), *164*, **164–165**, 170, 239, 333, 334
Syncope (fainting spell), 240, 520
Synechia, 498
Synovial invaginations, 90
Synovial joint, *109*, 109–110
Synovitis, 111, 113, *113*
Synthetic Antigen ELISA (SA-ELISA), 457
Synthetic shoes, 91–92, *92*
Systemic antibiotics, **410–411**, *411*, 428
Systemic illness, tendon injury, 201–202, *201–202*
Systems. *See* Organ systems and performance
Tack equipment, 4–5, *6*, 448
Tailhead, 345
Tail-pull test, 503
Tail wrap, 485

Talent of horse, 1, 3, 7
Tapetum, 489
Tapeworms, 460, *460,* 464, *467*
Target heart rate, 226
Tarsometatarsal joint, 32, 121, *121,* 130
Tarsus valgus, 134
Tattooing, skin, 372
Taylorella equigenitalis, 536–537
Team effort for performance, 1, 5, 6
Teasing programs, 534–535
Temperature (elevated), muscle injury, 166, 169–170
Temperature changes (rapid), respiratory system, 258
Temporomandibular joint (TMJ), 288, 289
Tendinitis (injury to tendon), 183
Tendinous attachment, 137, 138, 144, 145, *145*
Tendon dorsiflexion, **124,** *124,* 184, 196
Tendons and ligaments, 181–202
  anatomy of, *181*
  conditioning levels, 224, 225, *225*
  exercise, response to, 182–183
  ligaments vs. tendons, *181,* 181–182, 190
  long, slow distance (LSD) training, 182
  shoes and pads for, 183
  superficial digital flexor tendon (SDFT), *181,* 181–182, 183
  suspensory ligaments, *181,* 182
  See also Cool-down exercises; Tendons and ligaments injury, causes of; Tendons and ligaments injury and disease; Warm-up exercises
Tendons and ligaments injury, causes of, 183–189
  areas, injury-prone, 184–189, *185–189*
  bandage, incorrectly applied, 183
  cannon bones, *181,* 185–187, *185–187*
  concussion injury, 184
  conformation, 183–184
  contracted tendons, 328, *564,* **564**
  curb (inflammation of plantar tarsal ligament), 31, 34, **187,** *187*
  deep digital flexor tendon (DDFT), *181,* 187–188, *187–188*
  degenerative suspensory desmitis, 188–189, *189*
  distal sesamoidean ligaments, *181,* 184
  fetlocks, *181,* 187–189, *187–189*
  inferior check ligament (IFCL), *181,* 186, *186*
  long-toe low-heel (LTLH), 183–184, *186*
  low bow, 187–188, *187–188*
  muscle fatigue, 148, 165–166, 184, 330, 343
  plantar tarsal ligament, 31, 34, **187,** *187*
  predisposing factors to, 183–184
  proximal suspensory ligament, *181,* 186, 186–187

  shoes and pads for, 188
  stress-related failure, 183
  superficial digital flexor tendon (SDFT), *185,* **185–186**
  terrain (difficult), 4, 184
  turns, quick, 184
  volar anular ligament (VAL), 188, *188*
  See also Tendons and ligaments; Tendons and ligaments injury and disease
Tendons and ligaments injury and disease, 189–202
  bandaging, **194,** *194,* 195, 196, 198, 202
  bowed tendon, 24, 26, 183, 184, **185,** *185,* 191, *191*
  fibrin and granulation tissue repair, 191, *191*
  flexural contracture, 198–201, *199–200*
  granulation tissue repair, 191, *191*
  heat and, *189,* 189–190
  inflammation, controlling, 192–198, *193–194*
  lymphangitis, 202, *202*
  NSAIDs for, 196–197
  pain and, *189,* 189–190
  pain relief (analgesia), 193–194, 198
  peritendinous, 191
  punctures, 421–422
  repair, 190–192, *191*
  signs of injury, 189–190, *189–190*
  "stocked-up" legs, 68, 196
  success vs. recurrence, 192
  superior check desmotomy, 197, 200
  surgery for, 197, 200
  sweat bandages, **195,** 198, 418
  swelling and, *189,* 189–190, **192–198,** *193–194*
  systemic illness, 201–202, *201–202*
  therapy for, 192–198, *193–194,* 200–201
  See also Tendons and ligaments; Tendons and ligaments injury, causes of
TENS (transcutaneous electrical nerve stimulation), 178
Tensile strain, bone, 96
"Tented" skin, 235, *235*
Teratogens ingestion, 199
Terrain considerations, 4, 184
Testicles, 535–536, *536*
Tetanus, 404, **422,** 431, **513–514,** 540
Tetany, 164
Theiler's disease, **422**
Thermal therapy, 129, 192
Thermistor, 152, 224, 362–363, *363*
Thermoregulation role, skin, 355–363
Thiabendazole, 374
Thigh injections, 437, *437*
Thin horse (BCS 3), 345, 346, 348, *348,* 350, *350*
Third degree perineal laceration, 546
Third eyelid (nictitating membrane), 488, **490,** 516

Thirds of horse, balance, 10–11, *12*
Thirst reflex, 236
Thoracic cavity, *245,* 249
Thoracolumbar area, 207
Thorax, 246, 247
Thoroughbreds
  bone development, 100, 103
  cardiovascular system, 222, 236
  conformation, 7, 35
  muscle endurance, 143, 167
  navicular syndrome, 86
  neurologic system, 518
  nutritional management, 337
  reproductive strategies, 550, 556
  respiratory system, 252, 258
  skin as an organ, 360, 364
Thoroughpin, 31, 33–34
Throatlatch, conformation, 9, 12, 15
Thrombophlebitis, 441
Thrombosis/ischemia theory, navicular, 86, 92
Thrush (pododermatitis), 63, **73**
Thumps (synchronous diaphragmatic flutter), **164,** **164–165,** 170, 239, 333, *334*
Tibiotarsal joint, 32
Ticks, 171, *387,* **387, 515,** 516
Tidal volume, 251
Tie-back surgery for RLN, 259
Tied-in behind the knees, 22, *22,* 24
Timber racing, 152, 162, 220, 252
Time constraints, 3–4
Tincture of iodine, 65, 406–407
Tissue death (necrosis), 71, 303
TMJ (temporomandibular joint), 288, 289
Toe crack, hoof, 57, *57*
Toed-in (varus), 25, *25,* 53
Toed-out (valgus), 34, 36, 53
Toe grabs on shoes, **63,** *63,* 97, 211
Toe length, hoof, 48
Toes, hoof, 40
Tongue, 248, *248*
Topical ointments, 412, **414–416,** 428
Topographical/directional terms, *11*
Torque strain, bone, 97
Torsion (twisting), bone, 97
Torsion (twist), colic, 30, 308, 309
Touch sensitivity (hyperesthesia), 518
Tourniquet, 427
Toxicoinfectious infection, 525
Toys for boredom relief, 477
Trachea, 246, 247, *248*
Tracheobronchitis, 272–273
Tracheotomy, 431, *431*
Traction devices on shoes, 62–63, *63*
Trailering stress, 478–485
  air quality and, *479–480,* 479–481
  ambient temperature and, 478–479
  antibiotics (unnecessary), 482
  behavioral adaptations, 482–483
  biorhythm, 484
  body orientation and, 483
  body weight and, 483–484
  companionship for, 482
  cortisol and, 257–258, 481–482

dehydration effects of, 484
environmental stress of, 478–484, 479
head bumper for, 485
head position in trailer, 480, 480–481
heart rate as indicator of, 484
heat and, 360–361, 362
humidity, decreased, 480
immune function and, 481–482
muscular fatigue from, 483
nutritional management, 481
performance and, 6
protective bandages/boots, 485, 485
respiratory illness, 253, 479–480, 481–482
shipping boots for, 485, 485
vehicle vibration impact, 482–483
ventilation in trailer, 480
white blood cell count and, 484
See also Stress
Training, custom-tailored, 3–5
Tranquilizers, 453–454
Transcutaneous electrical nerve stimulation (TENS), 178
Transitional period, mare, 538
Transition zones, tendon injury, 192
Trauma
back pain, 207–211, 208–210
neurologic system, 520–525, 522–523
Traumatic arthritis. *See* Degenerative joint disease (DJD)
Trichostrongylus axei, 463
Trigeminal nerve, 516
Trigger points, muscle, 178, 179
Triglycerides, 140
Trotting a horse, 153, 298
Tryptophan, reducing, 161
Tuber sacrale of the pelvis, 27, 27, 30, 30
Tubules, hoof, 40, 41, 41, 51, 51
Tumors of eye, 499, 499
Turns, quick, tendon injury, 184
Twins, 552, 553, 553
Twitch, 451, 451–452
Tying-up syndrome, 166–171
calcium-phosphorus (Ca:P) ratio, 337
cramps in muscles, 168–169, 168–169
dehydration (cause), 167
dietary manipulation of muscle endurance, 164, 165, 338
electrolyte depletion (cause), 169, 171, 333, 334
enzymes and damage, 170, 458
metabolic alkalosis (cause), **152, 163, 170**
muscle tone, 168–169, 168–169
nutritional management, 327, 333, 334
recurrent exertional rhabdomyolysis (RER), **166–167,** 541
signs of, **166,** 166, 207, 511
temperature of muscles, 169–170
urine (discolored), 167–168, 167–168, 171
See also Muscle injury and disease
Type 1 (slow twitch high oxidative muscle fibers), 143, 144, 145, 146, 225
Type II A (fast twitch high oxidative muscle fibers), 143–144, 145, 146, 147, 148, 225, 228
Type II B (fast twitch low oxidative), 143, 144, 145, 146, 147, 225
Udder edema, 557, 558, 558
Udder evaluation, 546
Ulcerative colitis, 320
Ulcerative lymphangitis, 175
Ultrasound for
back pain, 214
colic, 302, 312
mare, 546, 547, 547
muscle, 178
navicular syndrome, 90
osteoarthritis, 129
tendons, 190, 190, 197–198
Umbilical problems ("navel ill"), 561–563, 562
Under-run heels, 60, 63, 63
Ungual (lateral) cartilages, 42, 42, 46, 58
United States Department of Agriculture (USDA), 242, 557
United States Equestrian Federation (USEF), 443–444, 542
Unshod (barefoot) foot, 58, 59
Upper arm, conformation, 8–10, 21, 22–23
Upper respiratory problems, 254–255, 258–259
Upper respiratory tract, 245–246, 245–249, 248
Upward fixation of the patella (delayed patella release), 31, 33, **118–119,** 119, 518
Urine
dehydration and, 236
protein and, 343
tying-up syndrome, 167–168, 167–168, 171
Urticaria (hives), 389–391, **389–392,** 440
Uterine biopsy, 549, 549–550
Uterine cysts, 546
Uterus, 539, 548–549, 548–550
Uterus, infected, 532
Vaccinations (immunizations)
lower respiratory problems, 262, 264
mare, 540
NSAIDs and, 456–457
preventive health, 456–457
respiratory viruses, 265–266, 270, 272, 279, 456
strangles, 275–276, 278–279
West Nile Virus (WNV), 506–507
Vagina, 532, 539, 545, 545
Vaginal exam, 547–548, 548
Vagus nerve, 16
VAL (volar anular ligament), 188, 188
Valgus (toed-out), 34, 36, 53
Varus (toed-in), 25, 25, 53
Vascular network, 219
Vasculitis, 201
Vasoconstriction, 75, 82
Vasodilation, 82, 83
Vegetable oil, 330–331
Vehicle vibration, trailering, 482–483
Venereal disease, 536–537
Venezuelan equine encephalitis (VEE), 508
Ventilation, 256–257, 264, 480
Ventral colon, 291, 292
Verrucous sarcoids, 394, 394
Vertebral fracture, 522
Vertebral impingement (kissing spines), 30, **212–213,** 213
Vertebral problems, 212–214, 212–214
Vertical shoulder, 22
Vesicular stomatitis (VSV), 283, 283
Vestibular seal, 545
Vestibular system, 501
VFAs. *See* Volatile fatty acids
Videotaping hoof lameness, 69
Villonodular synovitis, 123, 123
Viral duplication, 266–267
Viral infection
lower respiratory problems, 259
neurologic system, 504–509, 505
See also Respiratory viruses
Viral neurologic disease (myeloencephalopathy), 271, 272
Viral shift, 266
Viruses, respiratory illness, 252
Visual streak of retina, 490
Vital signs, 367
colic and, 299–301, 299–301
wound management and, 427–428
Vitamins
injectable, 435
insulin resistance, 80
neurologic injury and disease, 518
nutritional management, 80, 331, 332, **338,** 482
Vitiligo, 372
Vocal folds, 246
Volar anular ligament (VAL), 188, 188
Volatile fatty acids (VFAs)
digestion, 292–293, 325
muscle fuels, 139–140, 141, 325
Volvulus, 308, 308–309
VSV (vesicular stomatitis), 283, 283
Walking a horse
cardiovascular system, 225
colic, 298, 299
cool-down, 156, 156, 159
warm-up, 153
Warbles (heel flies) (*Hypoderma*), **380,** 513
War bridle, 452
Warmth and contraction, 410, 410, 418
Warm-up exercises, 153–156
back, manual stretch, 154–155, 155
belly lifts, 154
bone response to conditioning, 105
carrot stretches, 154–155, 155
forelegs, manual stretch, 154, 154
hind legs, manual stretch, 154, 154
joints, 131
manual stretching, 153–155, 154–155
mounted suppling exercises, 155, 155–156, 156
neck, manual stretch, 154–155, 155
sport-specific warm-up exercises, 156
stretching, 153–156, 154–156
trotting, 153

walking, 153
    See also Cool-down exercises;
        Muscle response to conditioning
Warm weather cool-downs, 157, 157–158
Warts (papillomas), **392,** 392, 393, 536
Water
    cool-down and, 157
    dietary manipulation of muscle
        endurance, 165
    doctoring, 236
    hot climate feeding, 341, 343
    intestinal tract and, 296, 304–305, 313
    muscle by-product, 141
    normal intake, 236
    nutritional management, 326, 328,
        332–333, 340, 341, 343, 345
    roughage and, 333
    skin application, 358–359, 362
Water hemlock (Cicuta maculata), 529
Water-soluble ointments, 412, 414
Wave mouth, 285, 287
Waxing of nipples, 557, 558, 558
Weak flexor tendons, 201
"Wear and tear," joints, 111–112
Web That Has No Weaver, The
    (Kaptchuk), 1
Wedge pads, 60, 65, 65
Weight-bearing structures, hoof, 40,
    44–45, 44–45
Weight concerns, mare, 544
Weight of horse from muscle, 137
Weight vs. volume of feed, 326, 330
Western blot assay test, 512
Western equine encephalitis (WEE),
    508, 540
Western pleasure horses conformation,
    34–36
West Nile virus (WNV), 381, **504–508,**
    505, 540
Wet horse, blanketing, 160
Wheat bran, 329
White, Nat, 315

"White acid" (corticosteroids/hyaluronic
    acid), 127
White blood cell count, 484
White line, hoof, 39, 44, 44
White line disease, 44, **73,** 74, 74
White muscle disease, 173, 338
White pastern disease (scratches),
    367–369, **367–371,** 384
White vs. black hoof, 47, 47
Whole, viewing body as a, 1, 3
Widest part of frog, shoeing to, 60, 61, 61
Wide-web shoes, 65, 66, 66
Windpuffs (joint effusion), 26, 33, 113,
    113
Windswept rear legs, 134, 135, 135
Winging, 20, 111
Withers, conformation, 8–10, 18–20,
    19, 35, 36
WNV (West Nile virus), 381,
    504–508, 505, 540
Wobbler syndrome (CVM), 132, **134,**
    328, 511, **517,** 535
Wolff's Law, 97
Wolf teeth, 286, 286
Wood chewing, 474–475
Work areas, safe, 448
Working heart rate, 223, 224
Wound management, 403–454
    airway, maintaining, 431, 431
    anaerobic bacteria and, 422, 422
    antiseptic solutions, 405–406
    antivenom, 432
    bleeding, stopping, 426–427, 427
    chlorhexidine for, 406, 414, 428, 435
    cleansing, 403, 404, 405, 405–406
    compounds that slow healing,
        406–407, 412
    cooling a fever, 429–430, 430
    damage, assessing, 403–404, 404
    debridement, 404, 405, 405, 408, 408
    first aid kit, 428–429
    fluids, replacement of, 428, 428

    hemorrhage control, 426–428, 427–428
    inflammation from burns, 425
    initial treatment, 403
    lavage, 405, 405
    NSAIDs for, 428–429, 429–430, 431
    povidone iodine (PI) for, 406, 414,
        428, 435
    scrubbing wound, 405
    shaving hair around area, 404–405
    tetanus, 404, **422,** 431, **513–514,** 540
    tincture of iodine, 406–407
    tourniquet, 427
    tracheotomy, 431, 431
    vital signs, monitoring, 367, 427–428
    See also Healing wounds; Injectable
        medication; Nonsteroidal anti-
        inflammatory drugs (NSAIDs);
        Restraint, safe and effective;
        Wounds, types of
Wounds, types of, 403–454
    blunt trauma, 410–411, 423–424,
        423–424
    fever (febrile), 429–430, 430
    fistulograms, 421–422
    hematoma, 423, 424, 424
    joint punctures, 421–422
    kick wounds, 423, 423
    malignant edema, 422–423, 423
    partial thickness burns, 425
    puncture wounds, 403, 410, 421–422,
        421–423
    rope burns, 424–426, 425
    sequestrum, 424, 424
    seroma, 423, 423
    snakebite, 430–432, 431
    tendon punctures, 421–422
X rays. See Radiographic (X-ray)
Xylazine, 453
Yellow star thistle (Centaurea solsti-
    tialis), 528
"Yes" joint (atlanto-occipital joint), 14
Zinc, 337